Paleopathology of Children

To Charlotte and Keith, for showing the way.

Paleopathology of Children
Identification of Pathological Conditions in the Human Skeletal Remains of Non-Adults

Mary Lewis

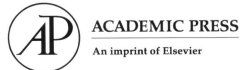

Academic Press is an imprint of Elsevier
125 London Wall, London EC2Y 5AS, United Kingdom
525 B Street, Suite 1800, San Diego, CA 92101-4495, United States
50 Hampshire Street, 5th Floor, Cambridge, MA 02139, United States
The Boulevard, Langford Lane, Kidlington, Oxford OX5 1GB, United Kingdom

Copyright © 2018 Elsevier Inc. All rights reserved.

No part of this publication may be reproduced or transmitted in any form or by any means, electronic or mechanical, including photocopying, recording, or any information storage and retrieval system, without permission in writing from the publisher. Details on how to seek permission, further information about the Publisher's permissions policies and our arrangements with organizations such as the Copyright Clearance Center and the Copyright Licensing Agency, can be found at our website: www.elsevier.com/permissions.

This book and the individual contributions contained in it are protected under copyright by the Publisher (other than as may be noted herein).

Notices
Knowledge and best practice in this field are constantly changing. As new research and experience broaden our understanding, changes in research methods, professional practices, or medical treatment may become necessary.

Practitioners and researchers must always rely on their own experience and knowledge in evaluating and using any information, methods, compounds, or experiments described herein. In using such information or methods they should be mindful of their own safety and the safety of others, including parties for whom they have a professional responsibility.

To the fullest extent of the law, neither the Publisher nor the authors, contributors, or editors, assume any liability for any injury and/or damage to persons or property as a matter of products liability, negligence or otherwise, or from any use or operation of any methods, products, instructions, or ideas contained in the material herein.

Library of Congress Cataloging-in-Publication Data
A catalog record for this book is available from the Library of Congress

British Library Cataloguing-in-Publication Data
A catalogue record for this book is available from the British Library

ISBN: 978-0-12-410402-0

For information on all Academic Press publications visit our website at
https://www.elsevier.com/books-and-journals

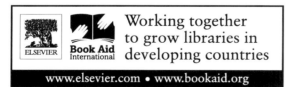

Publisher: Sara Tenney
Acquisition Editor: Elizabeth Brown
Editorial Project Manager: Joslyn Chaiprasert-Paguio
Production Project Manager: Lisa Jones
Designer: Mark Rogers

Typeset by TNQ Books and Journals

Contents

Acknowledgments	xi

1. Biology and Significance of the Nonadult Skeleton

Introduction	1
Skeletal Development and Ossification	3
Intramembranous Ossification	3
Endochondral Ossification	3
Bone Formation and Remodeling	4
Pattern and Timing of Ossification	5
Immune System Development	5
Immunity in the Newborn	5
Immunity in the Child	6
Immunity in the Adolescent	6
Exploring Immunodeficiency in Bioarchaeology	7
Factors in Pediatric Paleopathology	8
Themes in Child Paleopathology	8
Hidden Heterogeneity of Frailty and Selective Mortality	8
Measuring Specificity	9
A "Slew" of Possibles: Methodological Rigor, Transparency, and Objectivity	10
Differential Diagnosis	10
Comorbidity and Cooccurrence	11
References	12

2. Congenital Conditions I: Anomalies

Introduction	17
Terminology	18
Timing	18
Cranium	19
Premature Cranial Suture Closure	20
Microcephaly	26
Hydrocephaly	26
Congenital Deafness (Aural Stenosis and Aural Atresia)	28
Spine	29
Congenital Lordosis, Kyphosis, and Scoliosis	29
Occipitalization (Atlantooccipital Fusion)	29
Lumbarization and Sacralization	30
Spondylolysis	30
Sagittal Clefting	30
Cleft Neural Arches	31

Thorax	32
Supernumerary Ribs	32
Bifid Ribs, Costal Fusion	33
Extremities	33
Talipes Equinovarus (Clubfoot)	33
Radioulnar Synostosis	33
Polydactyly and Syndactyly	34
Neural Tube Defects	34
Congenital Herniation (Dystrophism)	34
Anencephaly	35
Cleft Palate	37
Spina Bifida	39
References	40

3. Congenital Conditions II: Skeletal Dysplasias and Other Syndromes

Introduction	45
Skeletal Dysplasias	46
Achondroplasia	46
Acromesomelia	48
Mesomelia	48
Thanatophoric Dwarfism	48
Developmental Dysplasia of the Hip and Congenital Hip Dislocation	49
Metaphyseal Dysplasia (Pyle's Disease)	52
Fibrous Dysplasia	53
Congenital Syndromes	53
Binder Syndrome (Maxillonasal Dysplasia)	53
Klippel–Feil Syndrome	55
Down Syndrome (Trisomy 21) and Other Aneuploid Conditions	57
Osteogenesis Imperfecta	60
Osteopetrosis (Osteosclerosis Fragilis)	61
Cerebral Palsy	63
References	64

4. Dental Disease, Defects, and Variations in Dental Morphology

Introduction	67
Teething	67
Dental Caries	68
Paleopathology	70
Dental Calculus	76
Periapical Cavitation	77
Periodontal Disease (Periodontitis)	77
Antemortem Tooth Loss	78
Dental Anomalies	79
Hypodontia	79
Hyperdontia (Supernumerary Teeth)	80
Natal and Neonatal Teeth	80
Dental Fusion	81
Macrodontia and Microdontia	83
Talon Cusps	83
Dental Trauma	83
Dental Modification	84

Disruption in Dental Development	84
Dental Enamel Hypoplasia	84
Turner's and Skinner's Teeth	85
References	86

5. Trauma and Treatment

Introduction	91
Principles of Pediatric Trauma	92
Greenstick Fractures	92
Plastic Deformation	93
Buckle Fractures	94
Physeal Fractures	94
Long Bone Fractures	96
Complications Specific to Child Trauma	96
Premature Fusion	96
Fragment Overlap	97
Overgrowth	97
Healing	98
Identifying Postcranial Injuries	100
Callus	101
Cortical Striations	102
Angulation	102
Cranial Fractures	102
Facial Fractures	103
Spinal Injuries	104
Tetanus	106
Spondylolysis and Spondylolisthesis	106
Clay-Shoveler's Fractures	107
Rib Fractures	108
Age-Related Injuries	108
Birth Trauma	108
Erb's and Klumph's Palsy (Congenital Brachial Palsy)	109
Toddler's Fractures	110
Juvenile Osteochondritis Dissecans	110
Slipped Femoral Epiphysis	111
Other Forms of Trauma	112
Dislocations	112
Myositis Ossificans Traumatica (Heterotrophic Ossification)	114
Treatment: Autopsies and Surgical Intervention	115
Trepanation	115
Themes in the Study of Child Trauma	117
Violence Associated With Extreme Cultural Conflict	117
Culturally Sanctioned Ritual Violence	118
Caregiver-Induced Violence and Neglect	119
Activity-Induced Injuries	121
Structural Violence	122
References	123

6. Infectious Diseases I: Infections of Nonspecific Origin

Introduction	131
Subperiosteal New Bone Formation	131

	Infective Osteitis	133
	Osteomyelitis	134
	Infantile Osteomyelitis	136
	Brodie's Abscess	136
	Spinal Osteomyelitis	137
	Chronic Sinusitis	137
	Otitis Media and Mastoiditis	140
	Endocranial Lesions	141
	Infantile Cortical Hyperostosis	145
	References	147

7. Infectious Diseases II: Infections of Specific Origin

	Smallpox (Osteomyelitis Variolosa)	151
	Rubella	152
	Poliomyelitis	153
	Tuberculosis	155
	Cranium	156
	Mandible	158
	Scapula	158
	Spine	158
	Ribs	160
	Joints	160
	Long Bones	161
	Hands and Feet	162
	Paleopathology	162
	Leprosy	164
	Infantile Leprosy	164
	Pathogenesis in Children	166
	Nerve Damage	167
	Skeletal Manifestations	167
	Paleopathology	171
	Treponemal Diseases	172
	Yaws	175
	Endemic Syphilis (Bejel, Treponarid)	176
	Congenital Syphilis	176
	Paleopathology	182
	References	185

8. Hemopoietic and Metabolic Disorders

	Hemopoietic Disorders	193
	Cribra Orbitalia, Porotic Hyperostosis, and the "Cribrous Syndrome"	194
	Thalassemia	200
	Sickle Cell Anemia	203
	Leukemia	206
	Hemophilia A and B	207
	Metabolic Disorders	209
	Rickets and Osteomalacia (Vitamin D Deficiency)	209
	Infantile Scurvy (Vitamin C Deficiency)	213
	Comorbidity and Cooccurrence in Rickets and Scurvy	218
	References	218

9. Neoplastic Disease, Tumors, and Tumor-Like Lesions

Introduction	225
Classification of Lesions and Terminology	226
Recognition of Tumors	226
Benign Primary Tumors	230
Osteoid Osteoma	230
Osteoblastoma (Codman's Tumor)	230
Giant-Cell Tumor (Osteoclastoma)	231
Osteochondroma	231
Hereditary Multiple Osteochondromas	232
Chondromas and Ollier's Disease	232
Chondroblastoma	234
Chondromyxoid Fibroma	234
Desmoid Fibroma (Desmoplastic Fibroma)	234
Fibrous Cortical Defects	234
Nonossifying Fibroma	235
Osteofibrous Dysplasia	235
Bone Cysts	236
Unicameral (Solitary) Bone Cyst	236
Aneurismal Bone Cyst	236
Langerhans Cell Histiocytosis	236
Eosinophilic Granuloma	238
Hand–Schüller–Christian Disease	238
Letterer–Siwe Disease	239
Malignant Primary Tumors	240
Osteosarcoma (Osteogenic Sarcoma)	240
Ewing's Sarcoma	240
Chordoma	241
Non-Hodgkin's Lymphoma	242
References	242

10. Juvenile Arthropathies, Circulatory, and Endocrine Disorders

Juvenile Idiopathic Arthritis	245
Systemic Arthritis	247
Seronegative Idiopathic Arthritis	248
Juvenile-Onset Adult-Type Rheumatoid Arthritis	249
Juvenile-Onset Ankylosing Spondylitis	250
Juvenile Psoriatic Arthritis	250
Hemophilic Arthritis	252
Schmorl's Nodes	252
Circulatory Disorders	252
Osteochondroses	252
Osgood–Schlatter Disease	254
Blount's Disease (Tibia Vara)	255
Legg–Calvé–Perthes' Disease	255
Scheuermann's Disease (Juvenile kyphosis, Spinal Osteochondrosis)	256
Endocrine Disturbances	258
Hypopituitarism (Pituitary Dwarfism)	259
Hyperpituitarism (Pituitary Gigantism, Acromegaly)	259
Hypothyroidism (Myxedema)	260
Hyperthyroidism (Thyrotoxicosis)	261
Cushing's Disease	261

Hypogonadism	261
Hypergonadism	262
Hypoparathyroidism	262
Hyperparathyroidism	262
References	263

11. Miscellaneous Conditions

Infantile Cranial Lacunae	267
Cranial Modification	267
Anteroposterior Deformation	268
Circumferential or Circular Deformation	268
Juvenile Paget's Disease (Infantile Hereditary Hyperphosphasia, Hyperostosis Corticalis Deformans)	269
Phossy Jaw	269
Bladder Stone Disease	270
Lead Poisoning	271
Transverse Lines in Bone	271
Harris Lines	271
Lead Lines	272
Bismuth Lines	273
Metaphyseal Bands of Leukemia	273
Scurvy Line	273
Healing and Healed Rickets	273
Osteopathia Striata	274
Bone Length Discrepancy	274
Fluctuating and Directional Asymmetry	274
Pathological Asymmetry	275
References	278

Index	283

Acknowledgments

I am indebted to my friends and colleagues from around the world for their unwaveringly generosity in providing their expertise, photographs, publications, unpublished data, assistance, access to collections, and permission to include images of their wonderful cases. I have been sent many examples of child skeletal pathology over the years, and while not every remarkable child made it into this book, they remain in the archive and are not forgotten.

I thank Jelena Beklavac and Richard Dabb (Museum of London Archaeology), Robert Kruszynski (The Natural History Museum, London), Daniel Antoine (The British Museum), Jason L. King (CAA Archeology, Kampville), and Simon Roffey (University of Winchester) for granting permission to include images of the individuals that they curate. I thank Sarah Lucas (University of Reading) for creating Fig. 2.1, and Louise Loe (Oxford Archaeology), Rebecca Gowland (Durham University), Maria Liston (University of Waterloo), and Petra Verlinden (University of Sheffield) who all generously took the time to rephotograph their skeletons for inclusion in the book. Petra also contributed her great expertise by coauthoring the trauma chapter. I had a very enjoyable day at the British Museum photographing the child with osteogenesis imperfecta, and I am grateful to Daniel Antoine for all his help and expertise. So many other colleagues have provided tremendous support in responding to my (sometimes endless) queries and sharing their cases and images: Anne Rohnbogner, Ceri Falys, Elsa Tomasto-Cagigao, Fiona Shapland, Judith Arnett, Sharon Clough, Caroline Arcini, Nancy Tayles, Corinne Duhig, Charlotte Roberts, Jane Buikstra, Katie Tucker, Joël Blondiaux, Simon Hillson, Alan Ogden, Malin Holst, Handan Üstündag, Gaynor Western, Jelena Beklavac, and Rebecca Redfern. Every effort has been made to acknowledge copyright holders, but in the few cases where this has not been possible, any omissions brought to my attention will be remedied in any future editions. Thanks also go to Joslyn Paguio and all the team at Elsevier for their good natured, but firm nudging and help pulling everything together.

As always I am thankful for my friends and colleagues in the Department of Archaeology at the University of Reading. They provide such a stimulating place to work and have allowed me the time and moral support needed to finish this book. It was sorely needed when I broke my right wrist 2 months before the deadline! Finally, I am grateful to my friends and family for their continued interest, encouragement, and endless glasses of wine! And to Jack, for the walks.

Chapter 1

Biology and Significance of the Nonadult Skeleton

Chapter Outline

Introduction	1
Skeletal Development and Ossification	3
Intramembranous Ossification	3
Endochondral Ossification	3
Bone Formation and Remodeling	4
Pattern and Timing of Ossification	5
Immune System Development	5
Immunity in the Newborn	5
Immunity in the Child	6
Immunity in the Adolescent	6
Exploring Immunodeficiency in Bioarchaeology	7
The Developmental Origins of Health and Disease Hypothesis	7
Factors in Pediatric Paleopathology	8
Themes in Child Paleopathology	8
Hidden Heterogeneity of Frailty and Selective Mortality	8
Measuring Specificity	9
A "Slew" of Possibles: Methodological Rigor, Transparency, and Objectivity	10
Differential Diagnosis	10
Comorbidity and Cooccurrence	11
References	12

INTRODUCTION

A child's skeleton carries a wealth of information about their physical and social life; from their birth, growth and development, diet and age at death, to the social and economic factors that exposed them to trauma and disease at different stages of their brief lives. Cultural attitudes dictated where and how infants and children were buried, when they assumed their gender identity, if they were sacrificed or exposed to physical abuse, and at what age they were set to work or considered adults. As vulnerable members of a society who are wholly dependent on the care of others, understanding the survival of infants has the potential to provide an accurate measure of a population's ability to adapt to their particular environmental circumstances (Mensforth et al., 1978). Children have emerged as important social actors in the past, contributing to material culture and influencing the archeological record (Baxter, 2006, 2008), and we are increasingly aware of their importance to our understanding of past society, culture, and the life lived (Halcrow and Tayles, 2011). A child's genetic inheritance may determine their level of frailty and susceptibility to disease and death, but their health is profoundly influenced by overlapping and interconnected socioeconomic layers, comprising their family, immediate social environment, and cultural norms that dictate their lives (World Health Organisation, 1993) (Fig. 1.1). As children age and begin to interact with their peers and their wider surroundings they are exposed to new physical hazards and pathogens (Halcrow and Tayles, 2011; Kamp, 2006), and these risks increase as they enter adolescence (Lewis et al., 2015). Hence, our understanding of disease and trauma in a child in the past must also be informed by their physical age and transforming social identity that influenced their freedoms and experience of risk.

Early reports of pathological lesions in children's skeletal remains are rare, perhaps due to a previous misconception that these individuals would have died too soon for lesions of chronic disease to be expressed on their skeleton. Child paleopathology had a few early pioneers. The earliest report of pathology in a child from an archeological context was by Shattock (1905) who identified bladder stones in a 16-year-old and an "adolescent male" from Egypt. In 1915, Bolk examined premature cranial suture closure in nonadult skulls from a cemetery in Amsterdam, while Derry (1938) described tuberculosis in a 9-year-old. Williams et al. (1941) suggested multiple myeloma for the lytic lesions present in a 10-year-old from 13th-century Rochester, New York, and 10 years later, Stewart and Spoehr (1951) argued for the presence of yaws in a 14-year-old from Malaysia. This case still remains as one of the few examples of yaws in the paleopathological literature. In England, Brothwell (1958) identified leprosy in an isolated child skull from medieval Scarborough Castle, and Wells (1961) described the first case of Scheuermann's disease in paleopathology in

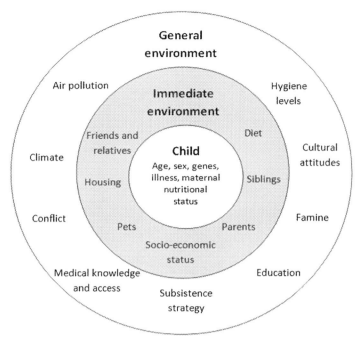

FIGURE 1.1 Overlapping and interconnected socioeconomic factors that influence children's health and their lived experience. *After the World Health Organisation, 1993. The Health of Young People. A Challenge and a Promise. WHO, Geneva, p. 3.*

the spine of a 16-year-old female from Bronze Age Dorset. Brothwell (1960) continued to highlight the importance of examining nonadult skeletons adding a potential case of Down syndrome to his body of research. In the 1970s, studies that focused on dental disease (Lunt, 1972; Moore and Corbett, 1973, 1975, 1976) and physiological stress indicators demonstrated the potential of population analysis over individual case studies for understanding child health (Cook and Buikstra, 1979; Mensforth et al., 1978; Mulinski, 1976). A series of articles by Ortner et al. (Ortner and Utermohle, 1981; Ortner, 1984; Ortner and Hunter, 1981) highlighted juvenile arthritis, osteomyelitis, and scurvy, while Hinkes (1983), Hummert (1983), and Storey (1986) carried out the first large-scale studies that concentrated on the health of children from the Grasshopper Pueblo, Sudan, and Mexico, respectively. At the same time, Schultz (1984) began extensive research into the histological evidence for disease in prehistoric child samples from numerous sites across Europe. By the late 1990s studies of nonadult paleopathology had become more commonplace, and today the discipline has fully matured. Our analysis has gone beyond simple identification to a more nuanced approach to the investigation of comorbidity and cooccurrence of disease in childhood (Crandall and Klaus, 2014; Schattmann et al., 2016; Snoddy et al., 2016) and the role children play in our understanding of sacrifice, caregiving, and violence in the past (Crandall et al., 2012; Kato et al., 2007; Klaus, 2014a; Mays, 2014). Advances have been made in the identification of accidental and nonaccidental trauma (Verlinden and Lewis, 2015; Wheeler et al., 2013), tuberculosis (Lewis, 2011; Santos and Roberts, 2001), mercury treatment in syphilis (Ioannou et al., 2015), anemia, rickets, scurvy (Brickley and Ives, 2008; Stark, 2014; Zuckerman et al., 2014), and upper respiratory tract infections (Krenz-Niedbała and Łukasik, 2016a,b), while dental disease is now receiving much more detailed attention (Halcrow et al., 2013). Scurvy is perhaps the most commonly reported child disease in the paleopathological literature. Initially, only reported as isolated cases, it has become recognized as a powerful tool in understanding issues surrounding food shortages, weaning practices, subsistence transitions, social control and marginalization, genetic susceptibility, and the coexistence of cancer and gastrointestinal diseases (Bourbou, 2014; Buckley, 2014; Crandall, 2014; Halcrow et al., 2014; Lewis, 2010). Reflecting advances in adult paleopathology, the identification of diseases in a child's remains through the use of ancient deoxyribonucleic acid (aDNA) analysis is also on the increase (Dabernat and Crubézy, 2010; Montiel et al., 2012; Pálfi et al., 2000; Rubini et al., 2014).

Despite the rising popularity of nonadult paleopathology, there are still challenges. Many pertain to the nature of growing bone. For example, rickets appears readily as large quantities of structurally inferior new bone are rapidly deposited at the growth plate, while in mature bone a slower rate of turnover means lesions take much longer to appear and are more subtle (Brickley et al., 2005). Conversely, accelerated growth then allows the inferior bone to be quickly replaced by normal tissue as the minerals needed for normal bone formation are once again received, causing both the macroscopic and radiographic signs of the disease to disappear from the skeleton within months (Harris, 1933). The highly plastic nature of children's bones means that they are less prone to complete fracture, but instead suffer partial breaks (greenstick fractures), buckling or bowing deformities that are hard to identify in dry bone (Lewis, 2000, 2007, 2014). We are still unable to effectively distinguish between new bone formation as the result of infection or trauma, from that which forms as part of the normal growth process in young children, often hindering our ability to explore such pathology in children younger than 4 years of age. In addition, the utility of subperiosteal new bone as an indicator of general physiological stress has been called into question (Weston, 2012; but see Klaus, 2014b). To accurately diagnose pathological conditions on a child's remains, it is crucial to have a comprehensive understanding of growth and development; the differences between adult and pediatric bones, or child and adolescent skeletons; and the different responses each age group has to disease and trauma.

SKELETAL DEVELOPMENT AND OSSIFICATION

During early embryonic development there are three primary germ layers from which all of the structures of the body develop: the ectoderm, mesoderm, and endoderm. The outer layer (or ectoderm) gives rise to the hair, nails, and skin; the inner layer (endoderm) is responsible for the development of the digestive tract and respiratory systems. The mesoderm condenses to form the mesenchyme or embryonic connective tissue from which the bones, cartilage, muscles, and circulatory system arise around the 12th week of gestation (Humphries, 2011). Cells arising from the mesenchyme migrate to specific locations from where ossification (osteogenesis) of bones of the skeleton will begin. Osteogenesis occurs through both intramembranous (within membrane) and endochondral (from cartilage) ossification.

Intramembranous Ossification

The flat bones of the skull (frontal, parietal), clavicle, and maxilla form within a thickened connective membrane in a process referred to as intramembranous ossification. Cells arising from the mesenchyme differentiate into osteoblasts producing a network of spicules (trabecule) around which collagen fibers are deposited on condensed vascular connective tissue (Humphries, 2011; Steiniche and Hauge, 2003). The membrane is directly ossified by osteoblasts without the need for a cartilage precursor, allowing for the accelerated bone formation necessary to accommodate the rapidly growing brain, which achieves 50% of its weight by the end of the first year. Growth gradually slows until around 7 years when the skull reaches its adult dimensions (Feik and Glover,

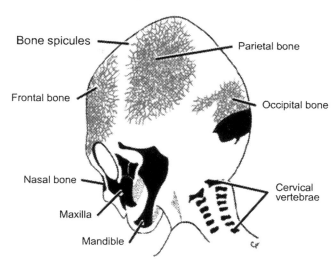

FIGURE 1.2 Development of the skull with solid black areas at the base of the skull forming endochondrally and hatched areas showing the spread of spicules from a center of ossification within connective tissue. *From Sadler, T., 2012. Langman's Medical Embryology. Lippincott: Williams & Wilkins, London, p. 134.*

1998). Bone is deposited in irregular concentric layers composed of woven bone. At birth the cranial vault has one layer, with the inner and outer lamina (tables) and inner diploë not clearly defined until the 4th year (Steiniche and Hauge, 2003). Dimensional growth of the cranial vault is achieved at the sutures. By the 2nd year of life, the bones of the sutures have interlocked and growth continues by bone absorption and deposition at the skull tables (Feik and Glover, 1998). The development of the rest of the skull occurs through both endochondral ossification (mandible, cranial base) and a combination of endochondral and intramembranous ossification (temporal, sphenoid, occipital) (Humphries, 2011). Understanding the pattern and timing of cranial vault development is crucial for the interpretation of the appearance of dry bone when considering the presence of possible endocranial lesions in infants and young children (Fig. 1.2).

Endochondral Ossification

The cartilage template on which endochondral ossification occurs is produced by the chondrification of other mesenchyme cells, which separate into fibroblasts and chondroblasts. The cartilage template develops through both interstitial and appositional growth. Appositional growth occurs where layer after layer of cartilage is deposited on the perichondrium (the precursor to the periosteum) that lines the outer surface of the model (Humphries, 2011). Multifocal or interstitial growth occurs as the template's central cells swell and blood vessels form to produce the primary center of ossification contained within a collar of bone. Osteoblasts are released and begin to deposit osteoid (the precursor to mineralized bone) to form the bone shaft or diaphysis (Steiniche

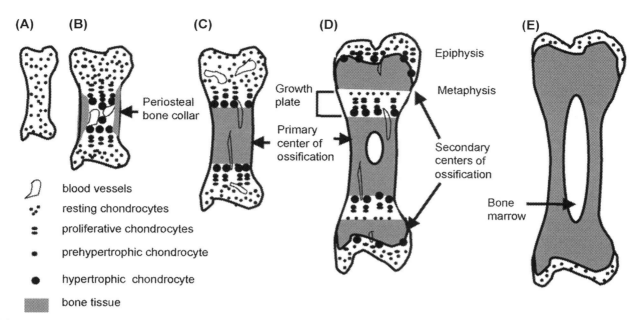

FIGURE 1.3 Endochondral development of a long bone. (A) Embryonic cartilage model. (B) Initiation of formation of the primary center of ossification at the center of the cartilage model, with chondrocyte hypertrophy and vascular invasion. (C) Primary center of ossification is established. (D) Secondary centers of ossification (epiphyses) appear and are separated from the primary center of ossification by the growth plate. (E) In the adult, the growth plate has been consumed and the epiphyses have fused to the diaphysis ending longitudinal growth. *After Mackie, E., Ahmed, Y., Tatarczuch, L., Chen, K., Mirams, M., 2008. Endochondral ossification: how cartilage is converted into bone in the developing skeleton. The International Journal of Biochemistry & Cell Biology 40, 46–62, p. 48.*

and Hauge, 2003). This process continues along the template, while blood vessels form at the end of the model to produce a secondary center of ossification, or epiphysis (Fig. 1.3). The growing end of the shaft (or metaphysis) and epiphyses are separated by a zone of cartilage known as the growth plate (or physis) allowing the bone to increase in length. This plate varies in thickness throughout the growth period, until it is eventually consumed by bone and the epiphyses fuse marking the end of bone growth (Humphries, 2011).

Endochondral growth at the growth plate is achieved by the construction of an extracellular matrix through a proliferation of chondrocytes organized in zones. The zone furthest away from ossification is occupied by resting chondrocytes, adjacent to which are hypertrophied chondrocytes, which deposit the matrix and eventually become flattened and die. The matrix is then invaded by blood vessels, bone marrow cells, osteoclasts, and osteoblasts, with the latter depositing osteoid onto the matrix. Endochondral growth is regulated by the growth hormone and thyroid hormone (Mackie et al., 2008). In the child, vitamin D deficiency disrupts the quality of new bone deposition at both the endochondral and intramembranous sites, resulting in a combination of rickets and osteomalacia, respectively (Pettifor and Daniels, 1997).

Bone Formation and Remodeling

Osteoblasts (bone formers) are the main cells responsible for bone development and remodeling (Marks, 1979). They are single nucleated cells that synthesize alkaline phosphate and regulate the deposition of the bone matrix molecules, including type 1 collagen and a variety of proteins (Walsh et al., 2003). Once surrounded by a mineralized bone matrix they are considered osteocytes (bone maintainers). Despite their isolated location within fluid spaces or lacunae, osteocytes continue to communicate with each other via canaliculi that connect the lacunae. Osteoclasts (bone absorbers) are hematopoietic in origin and are multinucleated cells around 10 times larger and less numerous than osteoblasts. They secrete protons and hydrolyses that degrade the organic and inorganic constituents of the bone tissue (Walsh et al., 2003). Bone can be divided into two distinct types: woven and lamellar bone. Woven or immature bone (also known as fiber bone) is arranged randomly in a meshwork pattern, whereas lamellar or mature bone is organized in parallel sheets or lamellae. Woven bone is formed during rapid bone formation such as during the growth and development of perinates and infants (Ortner, 2003). After 4 years of age the main bone deposited is lamellar bone (Steiniche and Hauge, 2003), and any additional woven bone may be seen as part of a pathological process (Ortner, 2003). Throughout the growth process an increase in the diameter of the bone, or "bone modeling," occurs as new bone is deposited on the external (periosteal) surface of the shaft by osteoblasts, which line the inner layer of the periosteum. Funnelization, or the process by which the diaphysis remains tapered and the metaphysis flared, occurs with resorption under the periosteum producing a porous or "cutback zone." At the same time, bone is removed on the internal (endosteal) surface of the shaft to maintain the proportions of the medullary cavity (Schönau and Rauch, 2003).

Skeletal growth is accelerated up to 37 weeks of gestation and then after birth, with bone turnover rates higher in premature babies than full-term infants (Mora et al., 2003). Bone tissue continues to be removed and replaced throughout life in a process known as "bone remodeling" (Frost, 1964), producing more numerous and intercutting Haversian systems (or osteons) as the bone ages. In healthy children, the amount of bone added and removed is perfectly balanced, but when this equilibrium is disrupted, the features indicative of bone pathology (e.g., hypertrophic or atrophic bone) become evident. Normal bone development is not only dependent on a normal nutritional and endocrine environment, but on normal muscular activity. In the child, muscles are attached to the periosteum rather than the bone itself, and loss of muscle pull causes the normally relaxed periosteum to become tightly bound to the cortex with a loss of osteogenic activity, eventually causing hypotrophy (atrophy) of the bone. Epiphyseal activity due to effects on the cartilage in disuse may also cause a loss in bone length during paralysis (Ring, 1961).

Pattern and Timing of Ossification

The number of bones in the nonadult range from 156 to 450, as ossification centers appear and fuse (e.g., 156 at birth and 332 at age of 6 years) compared to 206 in the adult (Lewis, 2007:26). Almost all of the primary ossification centers are present between 7 and 12 weeks in utero, with the secondary ossification centers appearing over a much longer period from birth to puberty. The skeletal elements ossify from "head to tail" in the axial skeleton and from proximal to distal in the appendicular skeleton. The clavicle is the first bone to ossify followed by the mandible and maxilla, which stimulate the development of the dental follicles (Long, 2012; Retrouvey et al., 2012). Humphrey (1998) demonstrated that in the growing skeleton, the cranium is the earliest to reach adult proportions and starts with an increase in frontal breadth, ending in the mandible and mastoid process. Long bone diameters reach adult proportions last, with long bone length being followed by the completion of growth in the pelvis, scapula, and clavicle. Later growing bones are more sexually dimorphic than the earlier growing elements, with males growing faster and for longer during puberty. This allows for males, who previously lag behind the females, not only to catch up in size but to overtake the females at the end of the adolescent growth spurt (Humphrey, 1998). Careful attention to the timing and fusion of the epiphyses is essential, and in younger skeletons an unfused neural arch, sacral laminae, or dens "epiphysis" (ossiculum terminale) may hinder diagnosis of congenital or traumatic conditions such as spina bifida, Klippel–Feil syndrome, or aplasia of the odontoid process, before 12 or 15 years of age.

IMMUNE SYSTEM DEVELOPMENT

The main organs involved in the production of cells responsible for the human immune system are the bone marrow, thymus, spleen, and lymph nodes (Abbas et al., 2014). The cells of the immune system are derived from stem cells that originate from the fetal liver and bone marrow. Immune cells signal each other through cell surface molecules and soluble messengers (cytokines, chemokines, and interleukins). When pathogens breach the body's barrier defenses (i.e., skin and mucosa), it reacts in two ways, through innate and then adaptive immunity. Both mechanisms have a humoral and cellular response to a pathogen. Innate immunity describes mechanisms that exist before infection. It comprises physical barriers such as the skin, and antimicrobial substances produced by the epithelial surfaces; phagocytic cells (neutrophils, macrophages) and natural killer cells, blood proteins, and cytokines that regulate and coordinate the other cells of innate immunity (Abbas et al., 2014). Innate immunity is mainly concerned with containing microbes on first contact, while adaptive immunity is involved in the final clearance of the invader from the body (Goenka and Kollmann, 2015). The adaptive immune response is characterized by its ability to build an immunological memory for a particular microbe that, while causing an initial delay in the immune response, leads to more rapid and enhanced responses to the microbe on each reinfection (Cant et al., 2008). For this reason it is also known as acquired or specific immunity (Abbas et al., 2014). The adaptive immune response is controlled by T and B lymphocytes producing T-receptor cells and microbe targets or antigens (Abbas et al., 2014; Cant et al., 2008). Humoral immunity is mediated by molecules in the blood or antibodies, which are immunoglobins produced by B lymphocytes in the bone marrow. Antibodies recognize the microbial antigens and neutralize the infectivity of the microbe. They are highly specialized and in turn activate other immune mechanisms, with some activating phagocytic cells and other inflammatory mediators (or mast cells) from leukocytes. The most dominant types of antibody are IgM, IgA, and IgG, followed by IgD and IgE (Abbas et al., 2014).

Immunity in the Newborn

While the form of immunity induced by exposure to foreign antigens is known as active immunity, passive immunity describes the transfer of lymphocytes from an immunized individual to another unexposed individual, such as from a mother to her child. During the critical few months of a newborns' life they move from a sterile uterine environment to one teeming with new pathogens for which they have no acquired immunity, meaning they are at unprecedented risk of infection and death (Goenka and Kollmann, 2015). Mothers provide protection in the form of transplacental antibodies, antiinfective factors in amniotic fluid, and through colostrum (the thicker and yellowish 'first milk') and breast milk enabling newborns to fight infections before he/she has the ability to create their own antibodies (Palmeira and Carneiro-Sampaio, 2016). It is the IgG molecules that cross the placenta in large numbers and provide a high degree of passive immunity to the newborn (Abbas et al., 2014; Janeway et al., 1997). Depending on the mother's previous exposure, IgG can protect the newborn against infections such as tetanus, diphtheria, rubella, mumps, and measles (Hoshower, 1994). Antibodies have a half life of 21 days and maternal antibodies transferred to the child during the last month of pregnancy may still be present 3 months after birth. Secretory IgA antibodies are present in large amounts in colostrum (released for 2–5 days postpartum) and breast milk, which along with other bioactive factors provide protection against infections without causing inflammation, while also supporting the child's developing mucosal system in the digestive and respiratory tract (Palmeira and Carneiro-Sampaio, 2016). IgA antibodies are absorbed through the mucosa of the urinary tract, rather than the gut (Newman, 1995), and compensate for the minimal production of secretory antibodies by the newborn in the first 6 months of life (Palmeira and Carneiro-Sampaio, 2016). Breast milk has been demonstrated to provide protection against acute diarrhea, respiratory tract infections, otitis media, neonatal septicemia, *Escherichia coli*, streptococci, *Salmonella*, and viral infections such as poliomyelitis (Hoshower, 1994). Studies have also shown that the milk of mothers with preterm babies contains higher concentrations on immune proteins than full-term milk (Trend et al., 2016). Long term, breast feeding lowers the risk of childhood tumors and in later life, diabetes, rheumatoid arthritis, Crohn's disease, and obesity (Palmeira and Carneiro-Sampaio, 2016).

In the face of bacterial invasion, the innate neonatal immune system will respond by releasing phagocytes and antigen presenting cells, with additional protection provided by maternal antigens. This is normally an effective response to infection, but in the neonate an immature regulatory response can cause a fatal buildup of proinflammatory cytokines causing septic shock and multiple organ failure. A gradual maturation of the antigen response to produce specific antigens is only seen after 2 years (McKintosh and Stenson, 2008). While these complicating factors associated with an immature immune system will be increased in preterm children, there is evidence that they will develop more robust immune systems earlier than their full-term counterparts (McKintosh and Stenson, 2008). Fetuses and newborns also have a limited ability to mount a cellular immune response compared to adults. Granulocytes do not form in large numbers until after birth, while macrophages are the first and neutrophils are the last cells to appear in the blood during fetal life (Holt and Jones, 2000). Neutrophils are short-lived cells that die soon after phagocytosis becoming a major component of pus. Macrophages by contrast are more robust and form an important front line of defense against infection (Janeway et al., 1997).

Immunity in the Child

Childhood immunity is defined as the period from 2 years to the start of gonadal steroid production that precedes the onset of puberty (McDade, 2003). From two years, breast milk cannot supply the immunological resistance needed and passive immunity is no longer effective, meaning children now need to rely on their own immunological defenses (McDade, 2003). This may explain why mortality rates between the ages of 1 and 5 years, while lower than for the infant, are five times higher than in an adult, and by 5–15 years mortality rates are twice as high as they are in adulthood. T and B lymphocytes steadily decline in comparison to their number at infancy, while lymphocytes bearing memory cell markers increase as children are exposed to an ever increasing number of pathogens in their environment. Studies have shown that high-pathogen loads put a strain on the body's resources as the activation of the immune system is compromised in favor of optimal growth. However, in those with better nutritional resources, this trade-off is less apparent (McDade, 2003).

Immunity in the Adolescent

With an increase in demands for resources during the pubertal growth spurt, the trade-off between the immune system and physiological development becomes more apparent with mortality from infection increasing to 2.5 times that of late childhood (McDade, 2003). The influence of the sex hormones on the immune system is demonstrated by the types of diseases that reveal themselves, with females more prone to autoimmune diseases and males more likely to experience chronic inflammatory disease and infections (Bupp, 2015). Stini (1985, p. 213) argued that the difference in immune system capability between males and females arises during adolescence as female bodies prepare for pregnancy. Androgens and estrogens have different moderating effects on the immune system, with testosterone being more immunosuppressive, and estrogen causing suppressed cell-mediated immunity coupled with advanced B lymphocyte activity and antibody production (McDade, 2003). As a result, adolescents are increasingly susceptible to chronic infections such as tuberculosis and leprosy, with other infections appearing due to their tendency of exposure to a riskier lifestyle through experimentation with sex and drugs (Lewis et al., 2015). The influence of the sex hormones on cellular and hormonal immune response may explain why at puberty, adolescents develop adult-type tuberculosis, which is no longer contained, but attacked increasing the risk of the mycobacteria being released into the bloodstream (Marais et al., 2005). The health of a pregnant adolescent female has a direct influence on the fetus and hence the next generation. For example, fetal growth impairment which is more common in pregnant women under the age of 18 years, has been shown to predispose the child to diabetes in later life (Sawyer et al., 2012).

Exploring Immunodeficiency in Bioarchaeology

A normally functioning cortex is essential to the immune system, as it is essential for the production of sufficient helper, effector, and killer cells by the T cells that pass through the cortex (Clark et al., 1986). As bone and neurological growth follow a similar growth trajectory, limitations in early bone development are likely to reflect damage to the neurological and immune systems that would leave individuals vulnerable throughout their life. The relationship between immunity and growth in childhood has been explored in bioarchaeology through tooth and vertebral neural canal (VNC) dimensions, and head circumference where reduced size has been consistently shown to affect adult health (Clark et al., 1986). Dimensions of the VNC, unlike stature and are not affected by catch-up growth. Tracking reduced dimensions along the anterior–posterior (AP) and transverse (TR) axis has allowed for a more detailed understanding of stress events at ages 6 and 17 years, respectively (Watts, 2013). Several studies have shown individuals with reduced TR and AP neural arch size have a reduced life span (Clark et al., 1986; Watts, 2013). Head circumference is also vulnerable to stunting due to its relationship with the thalamus gland that also influences the function of immature T cells, which migrate from the bone marrow to the thalamus early in life where they become functionally mature (Clark et al., 1986).

The Developmental Origins of Health and Disease Hypothesis

More recently bioarchaeologists have begun to engage with the Developmental Origins of Health and Disease (DOHaD) hypothesis. This stems from Barker's (2012) assertion that good nutritional health of the mother is crucial to the prevention of chronic disease in their offspring in later life (e.g., coronary heart disease, diabetes, and breast cancer). For example, individuals with type 2 diabetes have been shown to be small for gestational age and grow slowly for the first 2 years after birth. Malnutrition and other stressors during fetal development permanently alter gene expression. Humans are plastic during their development and an adverse environment can affect the body structure and the function of different systems at critical periods of growth in utero (Barker, 2012). As the developing fetus thrives on maternal stores of protein and fat in tissue laid down before pregnancy, the nutritional health of the mother at conception is vital. This nutritional status at the time of conception and throughout pregnancy affects the growth trajectory of the fetus. Dietary improvements result in faster fetal growth, particularly in males, suggesting they are more sensitive to environmental stressors than females (Barker, 2012). As females are born with all the ovum they will ever release, the quality of these eggs is a reflection of their mother's maternal nutritional state (Barker, 2012), and hence the damaging effect of poor nutrition is transferred from generation to generation. The impact of poor maternal nutrition may also be felt during breastfeeding, leading to stunted growth in the young child (Gowland, 2015). Gowland (2015) has criticized our lack of engagement with key concepts of phenotypic plasticity that have long held the attention of medical and social sciences. In particular, we have ignored the concept that the health of a given population cannot be understood simply in terms of their immediate environment, but that "individual biographies should be viewed as nested or 'imbedded' within the lives of others" (Gowland, 2015, p. 530). Epigenetic processes (or gene expression) form the basis of phenotypic flexibility that allows the organism to respond to adverse environmental circumstances. While epigenetics may help us to understand generational responses to stress in the past, there are two major hurdles identified by Klaus (2014b). First, that we cannot see the changes of gene expression at the skeletal level or recognize changes on dry bone and second, that we have yet to understand how genetic flexibility impacts specific skeletal phenotypes leading to common stress indicators such as enamel hypoplasia. Temple's (2014) study of enamel hypoplasia and longevity in late Jomon foragers from Japan may provide one way for us to explore this. He demonstrated that those with earlier forming dental defects had a significantly greater risk of forming later enamel defects and dying younger indicating a trade-off between growth and immune competence in later life. Gowland (2015) suggests that evidence for growth retardation in those under 3 years of age may provide a context for our understanding of adult health in any given sample, with children acting as proxies for their "invisible" mothers (Barker, 2012; Gowland, 2015; Waterland and Michels, 2007). In addition, perinates may have the potential to reveal information about maternal nutritional status through examination of δ^{15} nitrogen levels, which are now considered to also reflect an ill or malnourished mother, rather than simply providing a breastfeeding signal (Beaumont et al., 2015).

FACTORS IN PEDIATRIC PALEOPATHOLOGY

The juvenile skeleton differs from the adult in its biomechanics, morphology, anatomy, and physiology and is characterized by nutritionally dependent rapid growth (Humphries, 2011). There are several key factors that need to be considered when assessing skeletal pathology in children. These make the frequency and nature of disease expression different to that of adults:

1. Rapid bone remodeling
2. Bone plasticity
3. The presence of a cartilaginous growth plate
4. A looser, thicker, and more active periosteum
5. Large amounts of red bone marrow

The implications of rapid bone remodeling on the expression and repair of pathological conditions have already been discussed in regard to rickets, with the presence of the cartilaginous growth plate increasing the distribution of rickets lesions in the child (Chapter 8). Young bone is more porous and flexible than mature bone, as sparse Haversian systems mean that the canals occupy a greater portion of the cortex. Coupled with greater amounts of collagen and a fluid growth plate, this means nonadult bone can withstand greater pressure before breaking (Humphries, 2011). Fractures are often incomplete (i.e., greenstick, bowed) and heal rapidly as fracture lines, calluses, and deformities are quickly incorporated into the normal dimensions of the growing bone (Chapter 5). However, the presence of the vulnerable growth plate (or physis) means that in the child, the complications of trauma can include premature epiphyseal fusion, shortening, overgrowth, or joint angulation if one area of the growth plate is "tethered" (Verlinden and Lewis, 2015). Whereas after 18 months and before fusion, the growth plate can provide protection against the spread of infection between the epiphysis and metaphysis (Resnick and Kransdorf, 2005, p. 715). The pediatric periosteum is thicker, stronger, and more biologically active than an adult's due to the need for constant remodeling during growth (Wilber and Thompson, 1998). Although more firmly attached to the metaphyses through a dense network of fibers (zone of Ranvier), the periosteum is more loosely attached to the diaphyses. When inflamed through trauma or infection, a child's periosteum is more likely to be ripped away from large portions of shaft, resulting in widespread hematomas. More numerous and active osteoblasts are then more likely to cause bone hypertrophy (Humphries, 2011). Conversely, due to this loose connection the periosteum is less likely to be torn during a traumatic event allowing for tissue continuity and stability for healing (Johnston and Foster, 2001, p. 29). In the skull, however, the more loosely adhered dura mater in a child is more susceptible to rupture (Mack et al., 2009).

The distribution and expression of lesions is further complicated by a transforming immune system and the gradual replacement of red with yellow bone marrow as the child ages (Kricun, 1985). This has implications for the expression of hemopoietic disorders such as iron deficiency anemia, the formation of cribra orbitalia, and the hematogenous spread of infections that often accumulate in the joints (Chapter 6). The ready supply of iron not only provides the perfect environment for bacteria replication, but also means that hyperemia caused by hypervascularity at the infected site can result in overgrowth (Trueta, 1959). The recognition of overgrowth or shortening is, however, dependent on the age at which the child is affected. Any difference in one bone compared to the opposite side will only be evident if there is enough normal longitudinal growth left for these discrepancies to emerge (Chapter 11).

THEMES IN CHILD PALEOPATHOLOGY

Hidden Heterogeneity of Frailty and Selective Mortality

Hidden heterogeneity describes the various degrees of susceptibility to disease and death of individuals in any given population. Frailty, where the individual has a decreased resistance to stressors, is highly individualistic and unrelated to age or the presence of chronic disease (Fried et al., 2009). An individual's likelihood to succumb is the result of hidden factors such as genetic predisposition, socioeconomic status, and microenvironment. As frail individuals die more readily, they may be overrepresented within the mortuary sample, dying with higher rates of pathology, or short stature that attests to their lower immune competence (Wood et al., 1992). Given that bioarchaeologists can only normally recognize lesions after an individual has suffered for some time (i.e., they were strong enough to mount some resistance or overcome the infection), the idea that lesions equate to poor health and that no lesions equate to good health is far too simplistic (Siek, 2013). Those interested in children wrestle with the fact that biologically they have failed to reach reproductive age, represent the nonsurvivors in that community, and hence, are potentially all frail. That said, Dewitte and Stojanowski (2015) emphasize the importance of a child's remains in understanding hidden frailty. They represent a group where ages can be more precisely determined, and coupled with the use of multiple stress indicators they allow the infant, child, and adolescent to be used to explore the details of frailty and longevity in the early part of the life course.

Several scholars have cautioned against the belief that we are measuring "health" in past populations as opposed to the prevalence of indicators of physiological stress (Temple and Goodman, 2014). Health, in the modern sense, refers to the complete physical, mental, and social well-being of an individual, not just the absence of disease or infirmity (Reitsema and McIlvaine, 2014). Health may be culturally embedded and this is not easily identified through the analysis of human skeletal remains. While it may be beyond our reach to measure such a holistic concept as "health," we may be able to explore different levels of frailty within a population and between groups. A measure of frailty that can be used to assess an individual's current functionality and susceptibility to future assaults requires the examination of multiple stress indicators, rather than a single biomarker (Temple and Goodman, 2014). In 2016, Marklein et al. suggested the use of the "Frailty Index" by which an individual's vulnerability to disability, decreased mobility, reduced activity levels, need for long-term care, and mortality could be measured and compared to others. In modern clinical medicine the index utilizes up to 70 biomarkers including hormonal markers that are currently impossible to apply to skeletal material (Marklein et al., 2016). Physiological stress markers have dual meaning, as they represent both a survival of past stress events and indicate ongoing and cumulative stress at the time of death. The use of biomarkers such as osteoporosis or periodontal disease are heavily weighted toward an adult's remains but many of the markers proposed in the index are applicable to children, in addition to several others (i.e., disuse atrophy, see Table 1.1). The use of femoral length per quartile as a measure of stunted growth is problematic when scoring children's remains as they are still growing, but large nonadult samples where dental ages will allow comparisons of growth may prove useful.

We have the potential to score healing and active rickets and scurvy in nonadult remains, and while degenerative joint disease is rare in younger individuals, it has been shown to be present in an adolescent's skeletal remains (Lewis, 2016). In children, these lesions may be truncated, but they are no less useful, and improvements in aDNA sequencing are enabling us to identify pathogens in individuals where skeletal lesions have not had time to develop (Wright and Yoder, 2003). Dewitte and Stojanowski (2015) highlight the importance of using short-term cemeteries with precise chronologies to explore issues of frailty and selectivity, taking a multidisciplinary bioarcheological approach that emphasizes the cultural context and seeks to address, rather than to avoid, issues of heterogeneity of frailty.

Measuring Specificity

Wright and Chew (1999) explored issues of selective mortality in rural Guatemala. High levels of porotic hyperostosis indicative of childhood anemia had been noted in the adult skulls of ancient Mayans and interpreted as suggesting poor levels of nutrition in the past. Similar high levels of anemia in modern children from the region, however, were not reflected in the prevalence of porotic hyperostosis in modern adult crania from forensic contexts. This suggested that circumstances in the past were more conducive to survival with childhood anemia than they were in the modern population. This example highlights the fact that the presence of a lesion does not always infer illness and that the absence of a lesion does not always infer health. Nor is

TABLE 1.1 Frailty Index Measured Through Multiple Indicators of Stress, Revised for Use in a Nonadult's Remains

Stress Category	Frailty Variable	Scores and Measurements	Frailty Score "1"
Growth	Femoral length	Length in quadrants	Shortest lengths
	Enamel hypoplasia	Present/absent	Present
Nutrition and infection	Osteomyelitis	Active, healing, absent	Active
	Subperiosteal new bone	Active, healing, absent	Active
	Periodontal disease	Present/absent	Present
	Cribra orbitalia	Active, healing, absent	Active
	Rickets and osteomalacia	Active, healing, absent	Active
	Scurvy	Active, healing, absent	Active
	Neoplasms	Present/absent	Present
Activity	Osteoarthritis	Present/absent	Present
	Disuse atrophy	Present/absent	Present
Trauma	Fracture	Present/absent	Present

Adapted from Marklein, K.E., Leahy, R.E., Crews, D.E., 2016. In sickness and in death: assessing frailty in human skeletal remains. American Journal of Physical Anthropology 161 (2), 208–225, p. 5.

there a one-to-one relationship between diseases and their corresponding lesions. Individuals vary in their expression of a disease, and as our skeletal samples only represent a small cohort of the original living population we cannot take lesion frequency in a mortality sample and simply extrapolate that into disease frequency in the living population from which they were derived (Boldsen, 2001). To explore this fully, we need to embrace current concepts of lesion specificity and host sensitivity; using clinically diagnosed individuals and healthy controls from a suitable preantibiotic reference population to build a suite of diagnostic criteria for the conditions we wish to study (Weston, 2008). Boldsen (2001) argues that we should be applying modern basic epidemiological concepts to study disease frequency which involves including negative cases, and standardized descriptive terminology, to predict the number of cases we may expect to manifest certain lesions within a specific disease complex.

Boldsen and Milner (2012) divide their mortality samples by (1) sensitivity: individuals who have a particular disease and show lesions that can be recognized as diagnostic of that disease (true positive) and (2) specificity: a group of individuals without the disease who are recognized as being disease free (true negative). As not all people with the same disease show the same distribution of lesions, not all lesions are distinctive enough to be diagnostic of a disease, and not all individuals with a disease will show lesions, any mortuary sample will include people who:

1. lack lesions because they are disease free (true negative);
2. lack lesions despite suffering from the disease being examined (false negative);
3. show diagnostic lesions for the disease being examined and suffer from that disease (true positive);
4. show lesions similar to the disease being examined, but suffer from another disease (false positive).

To tackle issues of sensitivity, this approach takes the bold step in suggesting the presence of disease without the empirical skeletal evidence. For nonadult paleopathologists Boldsen's model is complicated by the different susceptibility to disease in children of different ages, and because of this, Boldsen's study of leprosy in Tirup, Denmark only included individuals over the age of 14 years (Boldsen, 2001). As children often reflect the endemic nature of a disease within a population, more detailed research using reference child populations is desirable.

A "Slew" of Possibles: Methodological Rigor, Transparency, and Objectivity

In 2016, Zuckerman et al. provided an unblinking critique of current paleopathological practice. They accuse many researchers of failing to adhere to scientific rigor, engage in hypothesis testing, or to adopt methodological advances relevant to the discipline, resulting in "an obfuscating slew of 'possible' cases" (2016: 381). Following Boldsen and Milner (2012), they highlighted the need for us to advance the discipline by considering the specificity of each lesion to the disease in question, ensuring that such lesions do not occur in other conditions. Evidence-based criteria should be developed by testing the expression of the lesions in a variety of museum-based pathological skeletons with known conditions and in healthy individuals (i.e., negative cases) (Zuckerman et al., 2016).

Bone has a limited ability to respond to a particular stress insult, and in the absence of soft tissue we are left with a defined sequence of changes (Ortner, 2012):

a. abnormal bone formation
b. abnormal absence of bone
c. abnormal bone size
d. abnormal bone shape

Our current classification system is complex and riddled with pitfalls, as a disease may be classed according to the cause (e.g., pathogen) or pathogenesis of the disease (Ortner, 2012). For example, joint disease may be inflammatory in origin and circulatory diseases often develop after a traumatic event. Assignment may also be arbitrary, reflecting evolving clinical practice or historical patterns as in the case of Langerhans cell histiocytosis and leukemia. Both are blood-born disorders once classified as neoplastic. We also rely on good preservation to map the pattern of diseases throughout the skeleton and help us classify and perhaps diagnose a condition. However, when it comes to diagnosing a condition in a child, we also need to be conscious of the changes in skeletal response due to age that dictates which areas of the skeleton are most vulnerable and when, and incorporates transitions within the immune system. Many conditions will produce the same type of lesion, such as porosity seen in the initial stages of inflammation due to an infection, or that as the result of rickets, scurvy, and anemia. We have yet to fully understand the impact of one disease process or treatment on the visibility and expression of another (e.g., rickets and scurvy; mercury and congenital syphilis) (Chapters 7 and 8).

Differential Diagnosis

Klepinger (1983) considers that some diseases paleopathologists encounter may no longer exist, disappearing before they were ever recorded in the clinical literature, while others may have evolved through time. We may encounter diseases at the early or terminal phases of expression or during the healing process, stages that are rarely documented clinically. We need to merge our processual, biocultural, and evolutionary analysis of disease with data or method-driven approaches using clinically diagnosed comparatives to enable us to view the entirety of each particular disease expression on the skeleton (Zuckerman et al., 2016). When considering a diagnosis it is important to consider many possible conditions (a list of differential diagnoses), casting the net widely and then narrowing down the likely causes using specific diagnostic criteria, within the context of the geographic location, culture, and the age and sex of the individual. Some conditions will be more common in adults or the elderly, while others commonly affect infants or children. While these considerations may not immediately eliminate a specific condition from the list, it makes it less likely. An excellent example of this type of approach is demonstrated by Bauduer et al. (2014) who examined destructive lesions on the skull of a 20-year-old female. They began by describing the macroscopic, radiographic, and CT scan appearance of the lesions, their distribution on the skull (e.g., that they spared the facial bones), their size, involvement of the cranial tables, appearance of the edges, and whether the lesions converged. The list of classifications that caused abnormal removal of bone was created (i.e., traumatic, metabolic, neoplastic, congenital, infectious) and eliminated one by one, exploring infections and neoplasia in more detail. Once a neoplastic condition was determined the nature of the lesion and the age, sex, and geographical origin of the individual was used to isolate a specific diagnosis, noting that the lack of postcranial bones made a definitive diagnosis impossible. The examination should, wherever possible, include radiographs. Anterioposterior and mediolateral views, and an X-ray of the unaffected bone from the other side is desirable, but not always practical in large-scale studies taking place in local museums where the facilities are limited and permission is rarely given to remove the skeleton. However, a detailed description and photographs are essential. De Boer et al. (2013) reviewed the significance of histology in the diagnosis of specific conditions in skeletonized remains, and while advocating its use in the differential diagnosis process, they argued that histology could currently only provide a specific diagnosis for a few conditions: osteoporosis, Paget's disease, hyperparathyroidism, and, potentially, osteomalacia.

An accurate description of lesions underpins a thorough examination and allows for any diagnosis to be challenged at a later date even in the absence of the bone itself, which may have been lost or reburied. With this in mind, Appleby et al. (2015, p. 20) proposed the adoption of descriptive terminology ratified by the United Nations and used by forensic practitioners to describe the lesions of torture. They provided standard terms that reflect the strength of the lesion in the determination of a specific diagnosis. Matthias et al. (2016) later removed the fourth criterion, arguing that the difference between 'highly consistent' and 'typical' was too vague. Four options are provided here:

1. "Not consistent": the lesion could not have been caused by the condition described.
2. "Consistent with": the lesion could have been caused by the condition described but is nonspecific, and there are many other possible causes.
3. "Highly consistent": the lesion could have been caused by the condition described, but there are a few other possible causes.
4. "Diagnostic of": this lesion could not have been caused in any way other than the condition describes (i.e., it is pathognomonic).

The overall evaluation of lesions and their distribution throughout the skeleton (i.e., the bones affected) is crucial, as is consideration of the age of the individual when trying to determine a definitive diagnosis. There should also be recognition that individuals may be suffering from more than one related condition at their time of death (comorbidity) or may exhibit lesions characteristic of another earlier unrelated disease, or secondary condition (cooccurrence). The healed and active appearance of lesions is crucial in determining possible comorbidity from cooccurence.

Comorbidity and Cooccurrence

As it is unlikely a malnourished child will be deficient in just one nutrient, the presence of lesions in the skeleton relating to more than one nutritional condition is likely high (Armelagos et al., 2014; Crandall and Klaus, 2014). We also know that in the past conditions such as rickets left children susceptible to potentially fatal diseases such as whooping cough (Hardy, 1992), and that malnutrition and infection are inextricably linked (Jones and Berkley, 2014). But our identification of comorbidity, where several conditions are active at once, or cooccurrence where one disease may manifest after another, is still in its early stages, and the issues are highly complex. For example, if a child is suffering from rickets and marasmus (severe protein–calorie deficiency) and has retarded growth, the signs and symptoms of rickets will not appear unless the marasmus is cured (Griffith, 1919). Hence, children suffering from a suite of nutritional diseases may not show any visible signs of disease on the skeleton. While the relationship between rickets, scurvy, and anemia is acknowledged, we are only now developing detailed descriptions that may enable us to identify their comorbidity in the past (e.g., Schattmann et al., 2016; Zuckerman et al., 2014). For example, Klaus (2013) suggested that new bone formation in the cranium caused by rickets is much finer than that produced in scurvy. It is also not clear which of the conditions, rickets or scurvy, will dominate in cases of comorbidity, with some studies showing vitamin C deficiency can inhibit or eliminate traces of rickets

(Bromer and Harvey, 1948) and others that rickets will be the dominant manifestation (Follis et al., 1940).

This book attempts to provide a comprehensive guide to the recognition and diagnosis of pathological conditions in a child's skeletal remains, taking into account the differences in the biomechanics, morphology, anatomy, and physiology of pediatric bone. Disease classifications may overlap, but wherever possible the underlying cause of the condition, differential diagnoses, and modern frequency in different sexes and age groups are highlighted. Understanding and documenting the occurrence and frequency of these pathological conditions has the potential to provide an in-depth appreciation of living conditions and socioeconomic factors in the past. A child's importance lies in the fact that they represent the most vulnerable members of any given society, from babies that rely entirely on the help of others, to toddlers exploring their environment, and adolescents whose psychological and physiological transitions render them exposed to stress, trauma, and disease.

REFERENCES

Abbas, A.K., Lichtman, A.H., Pillai, S., 2014. Cellular and Molecular Immunology. Elsevier Health Sciences.

Appleby, J., Thomas, R., Buikstra, J., 2015. Increasing confidence in paleopathological diagnosis – application of the Istanbul terminology framework. International Journal of Paleopathology 8, 19–21.

Armelagos, G.J., Sirak, K., Werkema, T., Turner, B.L., 2014. Analysis of nutritional disease in prehistory: the search for scurvy in antiquity and today. International Journal of Paleopathology 5, 9–17.

Barker, D., 2012. Developmental origins of chronic disease. Public Health 126 (3), 185–189.

Bauduer, F., Bessou, M., Guyomarc'h, P., Mercier, C., Castex, D., 2014. Multiple calvarial lytic lesions: a differential diagnosis from Early Medieval France (5th to 7th c. AD). International Journal of Osteoarchaeology 24 (5), 665–674.

Baxter, J., 2006. Making space for children in archaeological interpretations. Archaeological Papers of the American Anthropological Association 15, 77–88.

Baxter, J., 2008. The archaeology of childhood. Annual Review of Anthropology 37, 159–175.

Beaumont, J., Montgomery, J., Buckberry, J., Jay, M., 2015. Infant mortality and isotopic complexity: new approaches to stress, maternal health, and weaning. American Journal of Physical Anthropology 157 (3), 441–457.

Boldsen, J., Milner, G., 2012. An epidemiological approach to paleopathology. In: Grauer, A. (Ed.), A Companion to Paleopathology. Wiley Blackwell, Chichester, pp. 114–132.

Boldsen, J.L., 2001. Epidemiological approach to the paleopathological diagnosis of leprosy. American Journal of Physical Anthropology 115 (4), 380–387.

Bolk, L., 1915. On the premature obliteration of sutures in the human skull. American Journal of Anatomy 17 (4), 495–523.

Bourbou, C., 2014. Evidence of childhood scurvy in a middle Byzantine Greek population from Crete, Greece (11th–12th centuries A.D.). International Journal of Paleopathology 5, 86–94.

Brickley, M., Ives, R., 2008. The Bioarchaeology of Metabolic Bone Disease. Academic Press, Oxford.

Brickley, M., Mays, S., Ives, R., 2005. Skeletal manifestations of vitamin D deficiency osteomalacia in documented historical collections. International Journal of Osteoarchaeology 15, 389–403.

Bromer, R.S., Harvey, R.M., 1948. The roentgen diagnosis of rickets associated with other skeletal diseases of infants and children. Radiology 51 (1), 1–10.

Brothwell, D., 1958. Evidence of leprosy in British archaeological material. Medical History 2, 287–291.

Brothwell, D., 1960. A possible case of mongolism in a Saxon population. Annals of Human Genetics 24 (2), 141–150.

Buckley, H., 2014. Scurvy in a tropical paradise? Evaluating the possibility of infant and adult vitamin C deficiency in the Lapita skeletal sample of Teouma, Vanuatu, Pacific Islands. International Journal of Paleopathology 5, 72–85.

Bupp, M.R.G., 2015. Sex, the aging immune system, and chronic disease. Cellular Immunology 294 (2), 102–110.

Cant, A., Davies, E., Cale, C., Gennery, A., 2008. Immunodeficiency. In: McIntosh, N., Helms, P., Smyth, R., Logan, S. (Eds.), Forfar and Arneil's Textbook of Pediatrics. Churchill Livingstone, London, pp. 1139–1176.

Clark, G., Hall, N., Armelagos, G.A., Panjabi, M.M., Wetzel, F., 1986. Poor growth prior to early childhood: decreased health and life-span in the adult. American Journal of Physical Anthropology 70, 145–160.

Cook, D.C., Buikstra, J.E., 1979. Health and differential survival in prehistoric populations: prenatal dental defects. American Journal of Physical Anthropology 51, 649–664.

Crandall, J., Martin, D., Thompson, J., 2012. Evidence of child sacrifice at La Cueva de los Muertos Chiquitos (660–1430 AD). Landscapes of Violence 2 (2).

Crandall, J.J., 2014. Scurvy in the greater American southwest: modeling micronutrition and biosocial processes in contexts of resource stress. International Journal of Paleopathology 5, 46–54.

Crandall, J.J., Klaus, H.D., 2014. Advancements, challenges, and prospects in the paleopathology of scurvy: current perspectives on vitamin C deficiency in human skeletal remains. International Journal of Paleopathology 5, 1–8.

Dabernat, H., Crubézy, E., 2010. Multiple bone tuberculosis in a child from Predynastic upper Egypt (3200 BC). International Journal of Osteoarchaeology 20 (6), 719–730.

De Boer, H., Van der Merwe, A., Maat, G., 2013. The diagnostic value of microscopy in dry bone palaeopathology: a review. International Journal of Paleopathology 3 (2), 113–121.

Derry, D., 1938. Pott's disease in ancient Egypt. The Medical Press and Circular 197, 196–199.

DeWitte, S., Stojanowski, C., 2015. The osteological paradox 20 years later: past perspectives, future directions. Journal of Archaeological Research 23 (4), 397–450.

Feik, S., Glover, J.E., 1998. Growth of children's faces. In: Clement, J., Ranson, D. (Eds.), Craniofacial Identification in Forensic Medicine. Arnold, London, pp. 204–224.

Follis, R.H., Jackson, D.A., Park, E.A., 1940. The problem of the association of rickets and scurvy. American Journal of Diseases of Children 60, 745–747.

Fried, L.P., Xue, Q.-L., Cappola, A.R., Ferrucci, L., Chaves, P., Varadhan, R., Guralnik, J.M., Leng, S.X., Semba, R.D., Walston, J.D., 2009. Nonlinear multisystem physiological dysregulation associated with frailty in older women: implications for etiology and treatment. The Journals of Gerontology Series A: Biological Sciences and Medical Sciences 64A (10), 1049–1057.

Frost, H.M., 1964. Dynamics of bone remodelling. In: Frost, H.M. (Ed.), Bone Biodynamics. J & A Churchill, London, pp. 315–333.

Goenka, A., Kollmann, T.R., 2015. Development of immunity in early life. Journal of Infection 71, S112–S120.

Gowland, R.L., 2015. Entangled lives: implications of the developmental origins of health and disease hypothesis for bioarchaeology and the life course. American Journal of Physical Anthropology 158 (4), 530–540.

Griffith, J., 1919. The Diseases of Infants and Children. W.B. Saunders and Company, London.

Halcrow, S., Harris, N., NBeavan, N., Buckley, H., 2014. First bioarchaeological evidence of probable scurvy in southeast Asia: multifactorial etiologies of vitamin C deficiency in a tropical environment. International Journal of Paleopathology 5, 63–71.

Halcrow, S., Harris, N., Tayles, N., Ikehara-Quebral, R., Pietrusewsky, M., 2013. From the mouths of babes: dental caries in infants and children and the intensification of agriculture in mainland southeast Asia. American Journal of Physical Anthropology 150, 409–420.

Halcrow, S., Tayles, N., 2011. The bioarchaeological investigation of children and childhood. In: Agarwal, S., Glencross, S. (Eds.), Social Bioarchaeology. Wiley-Blackwell, Chichester, pp. 333–360.

Hardy, A., 1992. Rickets and the rest: child-care, diet and the infectious children's diseases, 1850–1914. Social History of Medicine 5 (3), 389–412.

Harris, H.A., 1933. Bone Growth in Health and Disease. Oxford University Press, London.

Hinkes, M., 1983. Skeletal Evidence of Stress in Subadults: Trying to Come of Age at Grasshopper Pueblo. University of Arizona, Arizona.

Holt, P., Jones, C., 2000. The development of the immune system during pregnancy and early life. Allergy 55 (8), 688–697.

Hoshower, L.M., 1994. Brief communication: immunologic aspects of human colostrum and milk – a misinterpretation. American Journal of Physical Anthropology 94, 421–425.

Hummert, J., 1983. Cortical bone growth and dietary stress among subadults from Nubia's Batn El Hajar. American Journal of Physical Anthropology 62, 167–176.

Humphrey, L.T., 1998. Growth patterns in the modern human skeleton. American Journal of Physical Anthropology 105 (1), 57–72.

Humphries, A., 2011. Basic juvenile skeletal anatomy and growth and development. In: Ross, A., Abel, S. (Eds.), The Juvenile Skeleton in Forensic Abuse Investigations. Humana Press, New York, pp. 19–31.

Ioannou, S., Sassani, S., Henneberg, M., Henneberg, R.J., 2015. Diagnosing congenital syphilis using Hutchinson's method: differentiating between syphilitic, mercurial, and syphilitic-mercurial dental defects. American Journal of Physical Anthropology 159, 617–629.

Janeway, C.A., Travers, P., Walport, M., Shlomchik, M.J., 1997. Immunobiology: The Immune System in Health and Disease. Current Biology, Singapore.

Johnston, E., Foster, B., 2001. The biologic aspects of children's fractures. In: Beaty, J., Kasser, J. (Eds.), Rockwood and Wilkins' Fractures in Children Fifth Edition. Lipencott Williams and Wilkins, Philadelphia, pp. 21–48.

Jones, K.D., Berkley, J.A., 2014. Severe acute malnutrition and infection. Paediatrics and International Child Health 34 (Suppl. 1), S1–S29.

Kamp, K., 2006. Dominant discourses: lived experiences: studying the archaeology of children and childhood. Archaeological Papers of the American Anthropological Association 15, 115–122.

Kato, K., Shinoda, K., Kitagawa, Y., Manabe, Y., Oyamada, J., Igawa, K., Vidal, H., Rokutanda, A., 2007. A possible case of prophylactic suprainion trepanation in a child cranium with an auditory deformity (pre-Columbian Ancon site, Peru). Anthropological Science 115, 227–232.

Klaus, H., 2013. Subadult scurvy in Andean South America: evidence for vitamin C deficiency in the late pre-hispanic and colonial Lambayeque valley, Peru. International Journal of Paleopathology 5, 34–45.

Klaus, H., 2014a. A history of violence in the Lambayeque valley: conflict and death from the late pre-hispanic apogee to European colonization of Peru (AD 900–1750). In: Knusel, C., Smith, M. (Eds.), The Routledge Handbook of the Bioarchaeology of Human Conflict. Routledge, London, pp. 389–414.

Klaus, H.D., 2014b. Frontiers in the bioarchaeology of stress and disease: cross-disciplinary perspectives from pathophysiology, human biology, and epidemiology. American Journal of Physical Anthropology 155 (2), 294–308.

Klepinger, L.L., 1983. Differential diagnosis in paleopathology and the concept of disease evolution. Medical Anthropology 7 (1), 73–77.

Krenz-Niedbała, M., Łukasik, S., 2016a. Prevalence of chronic maxillary sinusitis in children from rural and urban skeletal populations in Poland. International Journal of Paleopathology 15.

Krenz-Niedbała, M., Lukasik, S., 2016b. Skeletal evidence for otitis media in medieval and post-medieval children from Poland, Central Europe. International Journal of Osteoarchaeology. http://dx.doi.org/10.1002/oa.2545.

Kricun, M., 1985. Red-yellow marrow conversion: its effect on the location of some solitary bone lesions. Skeletal Radiology 14, 10–19.

Lewis, M., 2000. Non-adult palaeopathology: current status and future potential. In: Cox, M., Mays, S. (Eds.), Human Osteology in Archaeology and Forensic Science. Greenwich Medical Media Ltd, London, pp. 39–57.

Lewis, M., 2010. Life and death in a Civitas capital: metabolic disease and trauma in the children from late Roman Dorchester. Dorset. American Journal of Physical Anthropology 142, 405–416.

Lewis, M., 2011. Tuberculosis in the non-adults from Romano-British Poundbury Camp, Dorset, England. International Journal of Paleopathology 1 (1), 12–23.

Lewis, M., 2014. Sticks and stones: exploring the nature and significance of child trauma in the past. In: Knusel, C., Smith, M. (Eds.), The Routledge Handbook of the Bioarchaeology of Human Conflict. Routledge, London, pp. 39–63.

Lewis, M., 2016. Work and the adolescent in medieval England (AD 900–1550). The osteological evidence. Medieval Archaeology 60 (1), 138–171.

Lewis, M.E., 2007. The Bioarchaeology of Children: Perspectives from Biological and Forensic Anthropology. Cambridge University Press, Cambridge.

Lewis, M.E., Shapland, F., Watts, R., 2015. The influence of chronic conditions and the environment on pubertal development. An example from medieval England. International Journal of Paleopathology 12, 1–10.

Long, F., 2012. Prenatal bone development. In: Glorieux, F., Pettifor, J., Jüppner, M. (Eds.), Pediatric Bone: Biology and Diseases. Academic Press, New York, pp. 39–53.

Lunt, D.A., 1972. The dentition in a group of mediaeval Scottish children. British Dental Journal 132, 443–446.

Mack, J., Squier, W., Eastman, J.T., 2009. Anatomy and development of the meninges: implications for subdural collections and CSF circulation. Pediatric Radiology 39 (3), 200–210.

Mackie, E., Ahmed, Y., Tatarczuch, L., Chen, K., Mirams, M., 2008. Endochondral ossification: how cartilage is converted into bone in the developing skeleton. International Journal of Biochemistry & Cell Biology 40, 46–62.

Marais, B., Donald, P., Gie, R., Schaaf, H., Beyers, N., 2005. Diversity of disease in childhood pulmonary tuberculosis. Annals of Tropical Paediatrics: International Child Health 25 (2), 79–86.

Marklein, K.E., Leahy, R.E., Crews, D.E., 2016. In sickness and in death: assessing frailty in human skeletal remains. American Journal of Physical Anthropology 161 (2), 208–225.

Marks, S., 1979. The cellular basis for extremity bone loss in leprosy. International Journal of Leprosy 47 (1), 26–32.

Matthias, A.E., McWhinney, L.A., Carpenter, K., 2016. Pathological pitting in ankylosaur (Dinosauria) osteoderms. International Journal of Paleopathology 13, 82–90.

Mays, S., 2014. The bioarchaeology of the homicide of infants and children. In: Thompson, J., Alfonso-Durruty, M., Crandall, J. (Eds.), Tracing Childhood Bioarchaeological Investigations of Early Lives in Antiquity. University of Florida Press, Gainesville, pp. 99–122.

McDade, T.W., 2003. Life history theory and the immune system: steps toward a human ecological immunology. American Journal of Physical Anthropology 122 (S37), 100–125.

McKintosh, N., Stenson, B., 2008. The newborn. In: McIntosh, N., Helms, P., Smyth, R., Logan, S. (Eds.), Forfar and Arneil's Textbook of Pediatrics. Churchill Livingstone, London, pp. 191–366.

Mensforth, R.P., Lovejoy, O.C., Lallo, J.W., Armelagos, G.J., 1978. The role of constitutional factors, diet and infectious disease in the etiology of porotic hyperostosis and periosteal reactions in prehistoric infants and children. Medical Anthropology 2 (1), 1–59.

Montiel, R., Solórzano, E., Díaz, N., Álvarez-Sandoval, B., González-Ruiz, M., Cañadas, M., Simões, N., Isidro, A., Malgosa, A., 2012. Neonate human remains: a window of opportunity to the molecular study of ancient syphilis. PLoS One 7 (5).

Moore, W.J., Corbett, E., 1973. The distribution of dental caries in ancient British populations II. Iron Age, Romano-British and mediaeval periods. Caries Research 7, 139–153.

Moore, W.J., Corbett, E., 1975. Distribution of dental caries in ancient British populations III. The 17th century. Caries Research 9, 163–175.

Moore, W.J., Corbett, E., 1976. Distribution of dental caries in ancient British populations IV. The 19th century. Caries Research 10, 401–414.

Mora, S., Bachrach, L., Gilsanz, V., 2003. Biochemical markers of bone metabolism. In: Glorieux, F., Pettifor, J., Jüppner, M. (Eds.), Pediatric Bone: Biology and Diseases. Academic Press, New York, pp. 303–327.

Mulinski, T.M.J., 1976. The Use of Fetal Material as a Measure of Stress at Grasshopper Pueblo. Society for Amercan Archaeology, St. Louis, U.S.A.

Newman, J., 1995. How breast milk protects newborns. Scientific American 273 (6), 76–79.

Ortner, D., 2003. Identification of Pathological Conditions in Human Skeletal Remains. Academic Press, New York.

Ortner, D., 2012. Differential diagnosis and issues in disease classification. In: Grauer, A. (Ed.), A Companion to Paleopathology. Wiley Blackwell, Chichester, pp. 250–267.

Ortner, D., Utermohle, C., 1981. Polyarticular inflammatory arthritis in a pre-Columbian skeleton from Kodiak Island, Alaska, USA. American Journal of Physical Anthropology 56 (1), 23–31.

Ortner, D.J., 1984. Bone lesions in a probable case of scurvy from Metlatavik, Alaska. MASCA Journal 3, 79–81.

Ortner, D.J., Hunter, S., 1981. Hematogenous osteomyelitis in a Precolumbian child's skeleton from Maryland. MASCA Journal 1 (8), 236–238.

Pálfi, G., Ardagna, Y., Maczel, Y., Berato, J., Aycard, P., Panuel, M., Zink, A., Nerlich, A., Dutour, O., 2000. Traces des infections osseuses dans la série anthropologique de la Celle (var, France): Résultats preliminaries. In: Paper presented at the Colloque 2000 du Groupe des Palaeopathologistes des Langue Francaise, February 11–13. Toulon.

Palmeira, P., Carneiro-Sampaio, M., 2016. Immunology of breast milk. Revista da Associação Médica Brasileira 62 (6), 584–593.

Pettifor, J., Daniels, E., 1997. Vitamin D deficiency and nutritional rickets in children. In: Feldman, D., Glorieux, F., Pike, J. (Eds.), Vitamin D. Academic Press, New York, pp. 663–678.

Reitsema, L.J., McIlvaine, B.K., 2014. Reconciling "stress" and "health" in physical anthropology: what can bioarchaeologists learn from the other subdisciplines? American Journal of Physical Anthropology 155 (2), 181–185.

Resnick, D., Kransdorf, M., 2005. Bone and Joint Imaging, Elsevier Saunders, Philadelphia.

Retrouvey, J.-M., Goldberg, M., Schwartz, S., 2012. Dental development and maturation, from the dental crypt to the final occlusion. In: Glorieux, F., Pettifor, J., Jüppner, H. (Eds.), Pediatric Bone. Academic Press, London, pp. 83–108.

Ring, P., 1961. The influence of the nervous system upon the growth of bones. Journal of Bone and Joint Surgery 43B (1), 121–140.

Rubini, M., Erdal, Y., Spigalman, M., Zaio, P., Donogue, H., 2014. Paleopathological and molecular study on two cases of ancient childhood leprosy from the Roman and Byzantine empires. International Journal of Osteoarchaeology 24 (5), 570–582.

Sadler, T., 2012. Langman's Medical Embryology. Lippincott: Williams & Wilkins, London.

Santos, A.L., Roberts, C.A., 2001. A picture of tuberculosis in young Portuguese people in the early 20th century: a multidisciplinary study of the skeletal and historical evidence. American Journal of Physical Anthropology 115 (1), 38–49.

Sawyer, S.M., Afifi, R.A., Bearinger, L.H., Blakemore, S.-J., Dick, B., Ezeh, A.C., Patton, G.C., 2012. Adolescence: a foundation for future health. Lancet 379 (9826), 1630–1640.

Schattmann, A., Bertrand, B., Vatteoni, S., Brickley, M., 2016. Approaches to co-occurrence: scurvy and rickets in infants and young children of 16–18th century Douai, France. International Journal of Paleopathology 12, 63–75.

Schönau, E., Rauch, F., 2003. Biochemical markers of bone metabolism. In: Glorieux, F., Pettifor, J., Jüppner, M. (Eds.), Pediatric Bone: Biology and Diseases. Academic Press, New York, pp. 339–357.

Schultz, M., 1984. The diseases in a series of children's skeletons from Ikiz Tepe, Turkey. In: Capecchi, V., Rabino Massa, E. (Eds.), Proceedings of the Fifth European Meeting of the Paleopathology Association, Siena, Italy. Siena: Tipografia Senese, pp. 321–325.

Shattock, S., 1905. A prehistoric or predynastic Egyptian calculus. Transactions of the Pathological Society, London 56, 275–291.

Siek, T., 2013. The Osteological paradox and issues of interpretation in palaeopathology. Explorations in Anthropology 13 (1), 92–101.

Snoddy, A., Buckley, H., Halcrow, S., 2016. More than metabolic: considering the broader paleoepidemiological impact of vitamin D deficiency in bioarchaeology. American Journal of Physical Anthropology 160 (2), 183–196.

Stark, R.J., 2014. A proposed framework for the study of paleopathological cases of subadult scurvy. International Journal of Paleopathology 5, 18–26.

Steiniche, T., Hauge, E., 2003. Normal structure and function of bone. In: Yuehuei, H., Martin, K. (Eds.), Handbook of Histology Methods for Bone and Cartilage. Humana Press, New Jersey, pp. 59–72.

Stewart, T.D., Spoehr, A., 1951. Evidence on the paleopathology of yaws. Bulletin of the History of Medicine 26 (6), 538–553.

Stini, W.A., 1985. Growth rates and sexual dimorphism in evolutionary perspective. In: Gilbert, R.I., Mielke, J.H. (Eds.), The Analysis of Prehistoric Diets. Academic Press, Inc.: Harcourt Brace Jovanovich, New York, pp. 191–226.

Storey, R., 1986. Perinatal mortality at pre-Columbian Teotihuacan. American Journal of Physical Anthropology 69, 541–548.

Temple, D.H., 2014. Plasticity and constraint in response to early-life stressors among late/final Jomon Period foragers from Japan: evidence for life history trade-offs from incremental microstructures of enamel. American Journal of Physical Anthropology 155 (4), 537–545.

Temple, D.H., Goodman, A.H., 2014. Bioarcheology has a "health" problem: conceptualizing "stress" and "health" in bioarcheological research. American Journal of Physical Anthropology 155 (2), 186–191.

Trend, S., Strunk, T., Lloyd, M.L., Kok, C.H., Metcalfe, J., Geddes, D.T., Lai, C.T., Richmond, P., Doherty, D.A., Simmer, K., 2016. Levels of innate immune factors in preterm and term mothers' breast milk during the 1st month postpartum. British Journal of Nutrition 115 (07), 1178–1193.

Trueta, J., 1959. The three types of haematogenous osteomyelitis. Journal of Bone and Joint Surgery 41B, 671–680.

Verlinden, P., Lewis, M., 2015. Childhood trauma: methods for the identification of physeal fractures in nonadult skeletal remains. American Journal of Physical Anthropology 157 (3), 411–420.

Walsh, W., Walton, M., Bruce, W., Yu, Y., Gillies, R., Svehla, M., 2003. Cell structure and biology of bone and cartilage. In: Yuehuei, H., Martin, K. (Eds.), Handbook of Histology Methods for Bone and Cartilage. Humana Press, New Jersey, pp. 35–58.

Waterland, R.A., Michels, K.B., 2007. Epigenetic epidemiology of the developmental origins hypothesis. Annual Review of Nutrition 27, 363–388.

Watts, R., 2013. Childhood development and adult longevity in an archaeological population from Barton-upon-Humber, Lincolnshire, England. International Journal of Paleopathology 3, 95–104.

Wells, C., 1961. A case of lumbar osteochondritis from the Bronze Age. Journal of Bone and Joint Surgery 43 (3), 575.

Weston, D., 2008. Investigating the specificity of periosteal reactions in pathology museum specimens. American Journal of Physical Anthropology 137 (1), 48–59.

Weston, D., 2012. Nonspecific infection in paleopathology. In: Grauer, A. (Ed.), A Companion to Paleopathology. Wiley Blackwell, Chichester, pp. 492–512.

Wheeler, S., Williams, L., Beauchesne, P., Dupras, T., 2013. Shattered lives and broken childhoods: evidence of physical child abuse in ancient Egypt. International Journal of Paleopathology 3, 71–82.

Wilber, J., Thompson, G., 1998. The multiply injured child. In: Green, N., Swiontkowski, M. (Eds.), Skeletal Trauma in Children, W.B. Saunders Company, Philadelphia, pp. 71–102.

Williams, G., Ritchie, W., Titterington, P., 1941. Multiple bony lesions suggesting myeloma in a Pre-Columbian Indian aged ten years. American Journal of Roentgenology 46, 351–355.

Wood, J.W., Milner, G.R., Harpending, H.C., Weiss, K.M., 1992. The osteological paradox. Problems of inferring prehistoric health from skeletal samples. Current Anthropology 33 (4), 343–370.

World Health Organisation, 1993. The Health of Young People. A Challenge and a Promise. WHO, Geneva.

Wright, L., Chew, F., 1999. Porotic hyperostosis and paleoepidemiology: a forensic perspective on anaemia among the ancient Maya. American Anthropologist 100 (4), 924–939.

Wright, L.E., Yoder, C.J., 2003. Recent progress in bioarchaeology: approaches to the osteological paradox. Journal of Archaeological Research 11 (1), 43–70.

Zuckerman, M., Garofalo, E., Frolich, B., Ortner, D., 2014. Anemia or scurvy: a pilot study on differential diagnosis of porous and hyperostotic lesions using differential cranial vault thickness in subadult humans. International Journal of Paleopathology 5, 27–33.

Zuckerman, M., Harper, K., Armelagos, G., 2016. Adapt or Die: three case studies in which the failure to adopt advances from other fields has compromised paleopathology. International Journal of Osteoarchaeology 3 (26), 375–383.

Chapter 2

Congenital Conditions I: Anomalies

Chapter Outline

Introduction	**17**	Lumbarization and Sacralization	30
Terminology	18	Spondylolysis	30
Timing	18	Sagittal Clefting	30
Cranium	**19**	Cleft Neural Arches	31
Premature Cranial Suture Closure	20	**Thorax**	**32**
Scaphocephaly	22	Supernumerary Ribs	32
Brachycephaly	22	Bifid Ribs, Costal Fusion	33
Plagiocephaly	23	**Extremities**	**33**
Trigonocephaly	23	Talipes Equinovarus (Clubfoot)	33
Oxycephaly	23	Radioulnar Synostosis	33
Cloverleaf Deformity	25	Polydactyly and Syndactyly	34
Crouzon's Syndrome (Craniofacial Dysotosis Type 1)	25	**Neural Tube Defects**	**34**
Microcephaly	26	Congenital Herniation (Dystrophism)	34
Hydrocephaly	26	Anencephaly	35
Congenital Deafness (Aural Stenosis and Aural Atresia)	28	Cleft Palate	37
Spine	**29**	Other Facial Clefts	39
Congenital Lordosis, Kyphosis, and Scoliosis	29	Spina Bifida	39
Occipitalization (Atlantooccipital Fusion)	29	**References**	**40**

INTRODUCTION

Congenital anomalies encompass a wide range of anatomical variations and defects that occur during embryonic and fetal development and that are present at or shortly after birth (Moore and Persaud, 2008). Defects in nerves, muscles and bones are a major cause of infant mortality and are classified as anatomical, functional (e.g., mental retardation, deafness, blindness), metabolic, behavioral, or hereditary (Castilla et al., 2001; Moore and Persaud, 2008). Many congenital abnormalities are genetic in origin resulting from a single gene mutation or a chromosomal disorder (Waldron, 2009), but up to 60% are of unknown etiology and occur through a complex mixture of intrinsic (genetic) and extrinsic (environmental) factors (Aufderheide and Rodriguez-Martín, 1998; Moore and Persaud, 2008). Developmental anomalies of the skeleton are a popular topic in paleopathology, and there are many case studies in the literature. While spontaneous defects are of limited use when trying to understand the impact of the environment on a child's health in the past, understanding the causative factors of other congenital conditions may prove more lucrative.

Teratology is a branch of science that studies the causes, mechanisms, and patterns of abnormal development and its environmental agents, or teratogens (Moore and Persaud, 2008). The most common teratogens resulting in congenital defects are drugs (e.g., thalidomide), chemicals (e.g., nicotine, alcohol), infections (e.g., rubella, syphilis), and radiation (Moore and Persaud, 2008). Teratogens that may have had an influence on fetal development in the past include maternal alcohol abuse, resulting in mental retardation, microcephaly, maxillary hypoplasia, and joint anomalies; the herpes complex virus that causes microcephaly, growth retardation, and hearing loss; the rubella virus (or German measles) that can result in deafness, microcephaly, and blindness; chicken pox (varicella zoster virus) causing muscle atrophy, hand deformation and mental retardation, and iodine deficiency that again might be identified through microcephaly as well as other skeletal malformations (Moore, 1988; Walker, 1991).

Estimating the modern frequency of congenital diseases is problematic as not all countries have the same level or detail of recording, but around 40% of people with major and minor congenital malformations die in infancy (Moore, 1988). Hence, perinates and infants provide a crucial source of information about congenital anomalies in the past, but their remains present particular challenges. Babies with visible abnormalities may have been the victims of infanticide and disposed of away from the community meaning they are lost to the archeological record. But even those that do make it into the cemeteries may go unnoticed. Perinatal skeletal remains are often not recovered and are rarely examined for congenital defects. How might skeletal underdevelopment of a particular bone due to premature birth be distinguished from malformation as the result of a congenital condition? How can we identify cleft palate before the palatine suture has fused? Some conditions are guaranteed to end in the death of the child after a few hours or days; anencephaly and spina bifida cystica are not compatible with life, but how can we recognize the unfused elements of an open sacrum or cranial vault when many of the deformations will only be evident on a cartilage template? The tiny size of these perinatal skeletal remains also means that many abnormalities will go unrecognized. Newly prematurely fused sutures may not have had time to develop the complex array of morphological changes that make craniosynostosis recognizable in older children or adults. Equally, fusion of sutures in later childhood, once the skull has finished growing, may mean that prematurely fused sutures in a normally shaped skull will be overlooked. While such challenges exist, several cases of congenital defects have been identified in nonadult remains, and careful examination of anatomical specimens to map the morphology of certain conditions is now beginning to emerge. Many defects will appear in isolation, but teratogens can produce a complex pattern of related abnormalities (Castilla et al., 2001) that may aid in their identification and interpretation. Many defects often occur together such as clubfoot and cleft palate; anencephaly and spina bifida cystic; and Down syndrome and heart defects (Freeman et al., 1998). We may also be able to identify "microsigns" of birth defects in infant remains. For example, Chemke and Robinson (1969) noted the presence of the third fontenelle, located 2 cm in front of the posterior fontenelle on the sagittal suture in infants born with Down syndrome, in those with rubella, or with congenitally dislocated hips. Overall, the identification of congenital defects relies on familiarity with the normal morphology of the bones of the nonadult skull and postcranium. Better recording of these anomalies will enable us to gather information on what types of congenital conditions were present in the past, what environmental conditions may have led to their occurrence, maternal health, and different attitudes to the physically impaired (Aufderheide and Rodriguez-Martín, 1998).

Terminology

The terminology used to describe congenital anomalies is complex and beset with controversy over which term best describes any one set of changes seen at birth. Despite this, there are four significant types of congenital anomaly:

1. Malformation: a morphological defect of an organ or a part of an organ, present during initial tissue development.
2. Disruption: a breakdown of previously normal tissue, an organ or a part of an organ as the result of an extrinsic factor (pollutant, trauma, infection).
3. Deformation: a change in form, shape, or position of a part of the body as a result of abnormal mechanical pressure on otherwise normal tissue. Deformations tend to occur in the third trimester when most normal development of tissues has occurred (Walker, 1991).
4. Dysplasia: the morphological results of abnormal cell and tissue organization. These conditions will be discussed in Chapter 3.

Defects may be further subdivided into those that are aplastic (total failure to develop) or hyperplastic (overdevelopment) (Walker, 1991). Dysostoses are malformations of individual bones, either singly or in combination (Moore and Persaud, 2008). Congenital anomalies will be discussed according to their location on the skeleton. Not all skeletal variations mentioned here would have been symptomatic, while others would have had fatal consequences. These more serious anomalies resulting from defects in the neural tube development are discussed at the end of this chapter.

Timing

The developing child is most vulnerable to environmental disruption during periods of rapid differentiation. Any teratogens present in the first 2 weeks of fetal development usually result in spontaneous abortion at 6–8 weeks (Moore, 1988). As this is before any centers of ossification have developed, these cases will be invisible in the archeological record. The timing of major events in prenatal development is divided into 23 stages based on external and internal morphological criteria being reached. The critical periods for the development of the limbs, organs, and central nervous system are provided in Fig. 2.1.

The embryonic period (2–8 weeks) is when major development of all systems occurs through cellular differentiation and signaling that determines the precise role of each cell. Major morphological abnormalities normally occur during this period. The homeobox or Hox genes (Hox a-5 and Hox c-8 genes) regulate the differentiation process of the axial and appendicular skeleton, and it is mutations in these genes that are responsible for malformations (Scheuer and Black, 2000, p. 172).

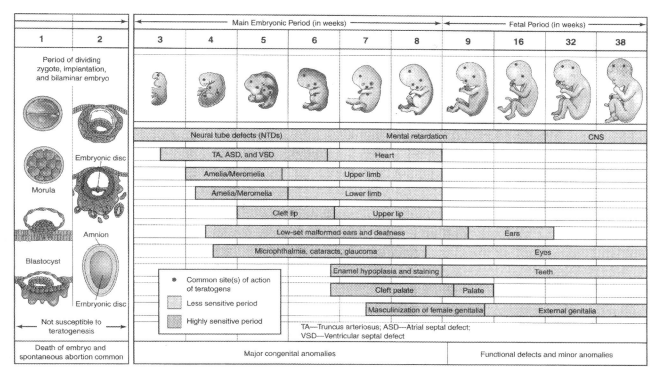

FIGURE 2.1 Critical periods in prenatal development. The embryo is not susceptible to teratogens during the first 2 weeks of development. After 2 weeks a teratogen may damage all or most of the developing cells causing death, or damage only a few cells allowing the embryo to recover without defects. Areas to the left of each bar denote a highly sensitive period when major defects may be produced, while those to the right denote a less sensitive period when more minor defects may appear. *From Moore, K., Persaud, T., 2008. The Developing Human, Saunders, Philadelphia, p. 473.*

The fetal period begins in the eighth week and is characterized by cell differentiation and growth, an increasing complexity of structures, and fetal weight gain during the third trimester (Walker, 1991). Skeletal development begins as bone mineral is deposited directly in mesenchyme (or membrane) for the clavicle, mandible, and bones of the skull vault (Krakow et al., 2009). Endosteal (within a cartilage template) mineralization forms the rest of the skeletal structure with limb abnormalities occurring in the early fetal period. The ilium and scapula begin ossification by 12 weeks, and the metacarpals and tarsals by 12–16 weeks (Krakow et al., 2009). Throughout, successful cell differentiation and ossification relies on a good maternal oxygen supply through the bloodstream (Waldron, 2009).

CRANIUM

In comparison to an adult, the immature cranium has a larger neural portion, smaller face and cranial base, more prominent frontal and parietal eminences, larger orbits, broader nasal aperture, and underdeveloped mastoid processes (Caffey, 1945). Five major sutures are present on the cranium. The coronal, lambdoid, and squamosal sutures are bilateral, while there is a single sagittal and metopic suture at the midline (Cohen, 2005). There are six constant fontanelles; four at each corner of the parietals and two at the midline where the frontal and occipital bone meet. In addition, four accessory fontanelles are present at birth along the sagittal suture (Fig. 2.2).

Development of the cranium occurs in the second to third fetal months, with foci of ossification appearing within membrane and spreading rapidly, fusing with others. At birth, there are around 45 separate bones of the cranium. The most rapid growth of the cranium occurs between 1 and 2 years of the child's life, with growth slowest from the age of 7 years until the pubertal growth spurt. Full adult size and proportions are reached at around 20 years. Although there is a variation in the timing of the closure of the fontanelles, the posterior fontanelle usually closes between birth and 2 months, and the anterior fontanelle by the second year. The metopic suture normally begins its closure at 2 years, but in 10% of cases it remains open into adulthood (Cohen, 2005). Caffey (1945) warns against overdiagnosis of cranial anomalies due to the great variety in the appearance of the normal skull. He points out that most skulls are asymmetrical with the left side usually larger than the right at the frontal regions, and that a flattened occipital may occur if the child is habitually laid on their back. Exaggerated endocranial vascular markings are also an unreliable indication of cranial pressure as they vary widely and may be entirely absent (Caffey, 1945).

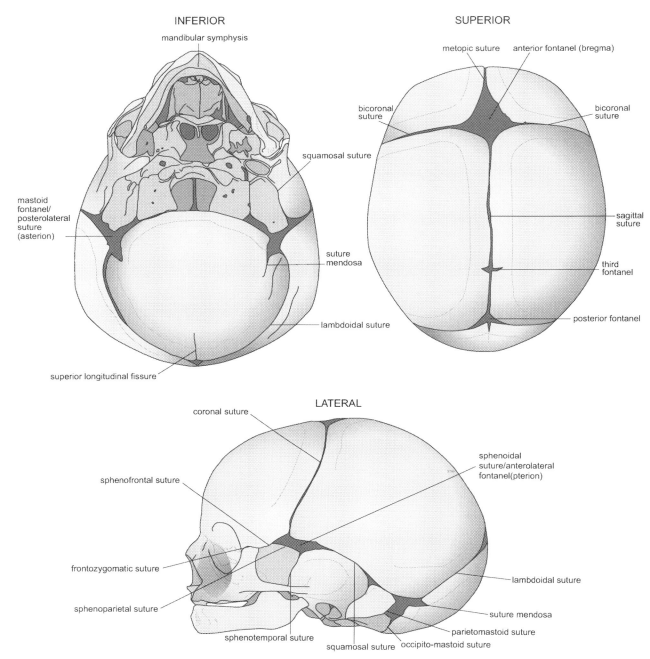

FIGURE 2.2 Location of the main fontanels and sutures of the infant skull.

Premature Cranial Suture Closure

Cranial sutures function to (1) allow the newborn passage through a narrow birth canal, (2) act as shock absorbers, (3) permit brain growth, and (4) prevent the skull plates from separating (Cohen, 2005). The occurrence of premature fusion of these sutures was first recognized by Virchow in 1851. Craniosynostosis refers to the process of premature suture fusion causing craniostenosis or an abnormal cranial shape (Cohen, 2005). Congenital cranial fusion, where the bones fail to differentiate and the suture is absent, is known as "sutural agenesis" (Barnes, 1994). The closure and gradual obliteration of the cranial sutures normally occurs between 22 and 72 years of age (Cohen, 2005), although this process is highly variable (Hershkovitz et al., 1997). Craniosynostosis may occur in isolation (primary) or as part of a syndrome (secondary) and can be simple (one suture) or compound (several sutures) (Jabs, 1998). Factors leading to craniosynostosis are very complex and little understood. Over 169 monogenetic disorders and 90 syndromes have been associated with premature suture fusion, and only one-third of craniosynostosis cases have a clear etiology (Jabs, 1998; Oostra et al., 2005). These include hyperthyroidism, vitamin D deficiency, Hurler's syndrome, genetic anemia (Khanna et al., 2011), head binding, and birth trauma (Aufderheide and Rodriguez-Martín, 1998). This wide variety of causes means that, in isolation, premature cranial suture closure may contribute little to our understanding of the past.

On radiograph, craniosynostosis is recognized as a straight rather than serrated line, with bony bridging along the suture (Benson et al., 1995). Craniostenosis is caused by a cessation of growth on the affected site with compensatory growth at the remaining open sutures (Duncan and Stojanowski, 2008). This compensatory growth is particularly evident at sutures that are parallel to the affected side (Jane et al., 2000). Morphological changes to the skull are varied, and the terminology is complex and often applied differently, making the comparative research difficult. For example, oxycephaly refers to either all of the cranial sutures being closed or the closure of the coronal plus one other suture, and there is no term for the premature fusion of the squamosal sutures where the temporal bone meets the parietal bone (Cohen, 2005). Many researchers have called for the abandonment of these terms altogether and instead, for the focus to be on listing the sutures affected (Barnes, 1994). The most common terms and their alternatives are provided in Table 2.1. The sagittal suture is the most frequently affected by premature fusion (around 50% modern cases), followed by the coronal, metopic, and lambdoidal sutures or a combination of them all (Benson et al., 1995; Cohen, 2005). Fusion of the squamosal sutures is rarely reported in the clinical literature, and this may be because it is less important for the development of the shape of the skull and goes unnoticed (Duncan and Stojanowski, 2008).

Bolk (1915) was the first to examine premature cranial suture closure in 1820 nonadult skulls from a cemetery in Amsterdam. The sagittal suture was affected in 47 (2.5%) skulls with total obliteration in 19 individuals (40%). Twenty-four (51%) of the cases occurred in those between the ages of 3 and 7 years leading Bolk to mistakenly conclude that fusion of the sagittal suture after 7 years was a part of the normal growth process. Importantly, Bolk (1915) noted that premature sagittal suture closure after the age of 6 years did not cause a change in normal cranial

TABLE 2.1 Terminology, Sutures Affected, and Morphological Features of Craniostenosis

Type	Sutures Involved		Other Terms
Simple Craniosynostosis			
Scaphocephaly	Sagittal	Narrow and elongated cranium with occipital and frontal bossing, and bilateral temporoparietal narrowing.	Dolichocephaly, clinocephaly
Brachycephaly	Bicoronal and/or lambdoidal	Rounded skull with prominent frontal bones and a flattened occipital bone.	Brachiocephaly
Plagiocephaly (frontal)	Unilateral lambdoidal	Flattening of forehead on affected side with frontal bossing of opposing side.	
Plagiocephaly (occipital)	Unilateral coronal	Occipital and parietal flattening of affected side with parietal and frontal bossing of opposing side.	
Trigonocephaly	Metopic	Triangular-shaped skull. Elongated pointed forehead with central ridge, parietal, and occipital bossing.	
Compound Craniosynostosis			
Oxycephaly	All sutures, or coronals plus one other	Abnormally broad skull and tower-like forehead, wide set eyes (hypertelorism) and a cephalic index of over 85, internal digital impressions from intracranial pressure.	Acrocephaly, turricephaly, hypsicephaly
Cloverleaf deformity	Multiple or all	Skull has a three-lobed appearance of a cloverleaf from the front. There is bulging of the frontal eminences and a constricted upright parietal bone.	Kleeblattschädel

Adapted from Benson, M., Oliverio, P., Yue, N., Zinreich, S., 1995. Primary craniosynostosis: imaging features. American Journal of Radiology 166, 697.

morphology and that fusion of this suture always began at the obelion. Of the 725 children who died between the ages of 3–6 years, 68 (9.3%) demonstrated suture fusion of the mastooccipital suture, again leading Bolk to the conclusion that this was normal. In contrast, Bolk reported that premature coronal suture closure was rare (n = 6 or 0.3%) and could commence at any point along the suture. Four skulls (0.2%) displayed sphenofrontal suture closure, and three (0.1%) had premature fusion of the squamosal sutures. Bennett (1967) found 12 (1.2%) nonadult cases of premature suture closure in 1000 skulls from the Arizona State Museum, the majority derived from archeological excavations. Of the 12, 11 (92%) involved the sagittal suture, with 5 (45%) showing evidence for head binding. For this reason, Bennett (1967, p. 7) considered premature fusion to be a "symptom" of artificial cranial modification. Goode-Nell et al. (2004) reported craniosynostosis in 31% of nonadults (>25 years) from the African Burial Ground in New York. Of these, 80% were over the age of 6 years and the sagittal suture was again the most commonly affected. Oostra et al. (2005) examined craniosynostosis in an anatomical collection from Amsterdam. They recorded premature suture closure in 14.3% (n = 23/160) child skulls. Of these, 15 (9.3%) involved the sagittal suture, 5 (3.1%) the metopic suture, 2 (1.2%) the unicoronal suture, and 1 (0.6%) the bicoronal suture. The higher frequency of sagittal suture closure in children between 3 and 6 years was notable, and Oostra et al. (2005) suggest that many are missed archeologically as they rarely produce cranial deformity.

Scaphocephaly

Scaphocephaly (Greek: *scaphe* = boat) is caused by craniosynostosis of the sagittal suture and occurs in between 50% and 80% of all cases (Aufderheide and Rodriguez-Martín, 1998; McAlister and Herman, 2005). Fusion of the sagittal suture means biparietal or transverse expansion is no longer possible and so compensatory growth in the frontal and occipital directions occurs at the metopic, coronal, and lambdoidal sutures, causing a narrow elongated (boat-shaped) skull and prominent frontal and occipital bosses (Benson et al., 1995; Oostra et al., 2005). The extent of cranial deformity depends on the portion of the sagittal suture that is fused; whether the anterior, posterior, or the entire suture. The cephalic index is usually below 70 and the skull base and maxilla are narrowed, with underdevelopment of the wings of the sphenoid (Sheldon, 1943). Scaphocephaly is characterized by obvious ridging of the fused sagittal suture and forms a distinct subset of dolichocephaly, a term used by surgeons to describe cranial elongation without synostosis (Cohen, 2005). If the coronal suture is also closed, it may indicate Crouzon's syndrome (craniofacial dysostosis) or Carpenter's syndrome (Aufderheide and Rodriguez-Martín, 1998). Ortner (2003) presents a case of scaphocephaly in a 9-week-old infant with a clear sagittal ridge. The additional partial fusion of the frontal suture resulted in a pointed frontal bone (See Trigonocephaly section) and poorly developed sutures on the lateral aspect of the skull as the result of intracranial pressure (Ortner, 2003, p. 455). The fragile nature of this example suggests that many cases may not survive in the archeological record. Scaphocephaly in older children may be easier to identify, and there are many examples from archeological contexts (Barnes, 1994; Clough and Boyle, 2010; Hegyi et al., 2004; McKinley, 2008; Meyer et al., 2006; Goode-Nell et al., 2004; Zink et al., 2006; Wolff et al., 2014). One of the first to be identified was of a 4- to 6-year-old from Grasshopper Pueblo, Arizona (AD 1275–1400) by Bennett (1967) (Fig. 2.3). Wolff et al. (2014) reported on two cases of sagittal suture fusion in children aged 4–5 and 13–14 years from a 7th- to 8th-century cemetery in central Hungary. The youngest child had evidence for cranial modification, while the older child appeared to be suffering from rickets, with both conditions potentially providing an underlying etiology for the suture fusion.

Brachycephaly

Brachycephaly (Greek: *brakhu* = short) describes a decrease in the anterioposterior dimension of the skull, often as the result of bilateral premature fusion of the coronal sutures and compensatory growth at the parietal sutures. Anterior fusion causes pronounced frontal bossing, whereas the less

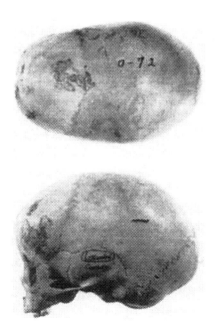

FIGURE 2.3 Sagittal suture fusion in a child (skull no. 72) from Grasshopper Pueblo, Arizona, with elongation of the cranial vault (scaphocephaly). *From Bennett, K., 1967. Craniostenosis: a review of the etiology and a report of new cases. American Journal of Physical Anthropology 27, 4.*

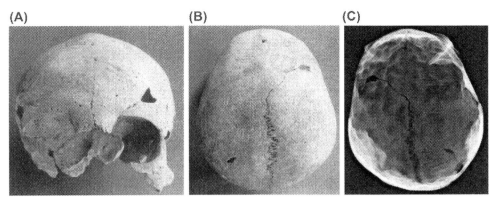

FIGURE 2.4 Child skull (skull b) from Lo Quarter, Sardinia, Italy, with bilateral fusion of the coronal sutures and mildly accentuated parietal growth. (A) The frontal view shows a prominent sagittal ridge on the superior aspect of the skull. (B) The coronal sutures are obliterated bilaterally (note the line on the left aspect is a postmortem break). (C) The radiograph demonstrates prominent convolutions indicative of increased cranial pressure (Giuffra et al., 2013, p. 135).

common posterior fusion results in a short broad or round skull and an occipital bone that juts out to form a shelf adjacent to the parietal bones (Jane et al., 2000). The cephalic index normally lies within 81–85. This round morphology can also be caused by bilateral lambdoidal synostosis, but this is rare (Oostra et al., 2005). Cases of brachycephaly are rarely reported, although Giuffra et al. (2013) presented a 9- to 10-year-old from the 16th-century Sardinian plague cemetery with bilateral fusion of the coronal sutures and a prominent ridge along the sagittal suture (Fig. 2.4).

Plagiocephaly

This is caused by closure of the coronal or lambdoidal sutures on one side, resulting in a lopsided skull with orbits of different heights (Aufderheide and Rodriguez-Martín, 1998). Fusion of the coronal suture causes the orbital portion of the skull to be displaced superiorly giving the orbits an upswept appearance ("harlequin eye") (Fig. 2.5). A bulging forehead, flattened orbital plate, and depression of the petrous bone are also characteristic (Benson et al., 1995; Pedersen and Anton, 1998). Plagiocephaly may also be caused by congenital muscular torticollis resulting from contraction of the sternocleidomastoid muscle. Torticollis has an unknown etiology and may cause problems during childbirth, resulting in facial asymmetry and a permanent sideways contraction of the head (Davidson et al., 2008). Plagiocephaly caused by craniosynostosis needs to be differentiated from positional plagiocephaly caused by a baby spending a prolonged amount of time lying on its back (Davidson et al., 2008). Bennett (1967) provides a case of occipital plagiocephaly in a child from Turkey Creek Arizona, and unilamboidal synostosis has been identified in an 8- to 12-year-old from Atapuerca, Spain, dating to the Middle Pleistocene (Gracia et al., 2009). Masnicová and Beňuš (2003) reported a more subtle case of left-sided coronal fusion and right-sided squamosal fusion in a medieval child from Devín in Slovakia.

Trigonocephaly

This form of craniostenosis results from fusion of the metopic suture, usually around birth. Symmetrical bone growth continues at the sagittal suture, with compensatory growth at the posterior aspect. There is asymmetrical growth at the coronal sutures resulting in a pear-shaped skull with flattened frontal eminences (Benson et al., 1995). The cranium is narrow anteriorly and broad posteriorly, and triangular in shape when viewed from the top (Oostra et al., 2005) (Fig. 2.6). The orbits are close-set (hypotelorism) with the intercanthal distance normally less than 15mm in an infant. A bony ridge will be evident at the glabella, and there may be anterior bowing of the coronal sutures. The cephalic index is normal (Aufderheide and Rodriguez-Martín, 1998). Richards (1985) reported trigonocephaly and microcephaly in a 6- to 10-year-old child from Santa Rosa Island, California.

Oxycephaly

Oxycephaly (or turricephaly) is one of the most severe cranial deformities and occurs when the lambdoid and coronal sutures fuse bilaterally resulting in a tall, cone-shaped head. Sheldon (1943) mentions overgrowth of the wings of the sphenoid causing the skull to bulge laterally above the ears. Where only the lambdoid sutures are involved, there may also be wide-set eyes (hypertelorism) and endocranial digital impressions from intracranial pressure (Aufderheide and Rodriguez-Martín, 1998). The eventual shape of an oxycephalic skull depends on the sutures involved and the extent of their involvement (i.e., partial or complete fusion). The age of the individual at onset influences the severity of the malformation as it dictates the amount of growth left to be achieved when fusion occurs (Oostra et al., 2005). The condition often results in microcephaly (Khanna et al., 2011) and may be related to Crouzon's syndrome (Aufderheide and Rodriguez-Martín, 1998; Oostra et al., 2005). Webb

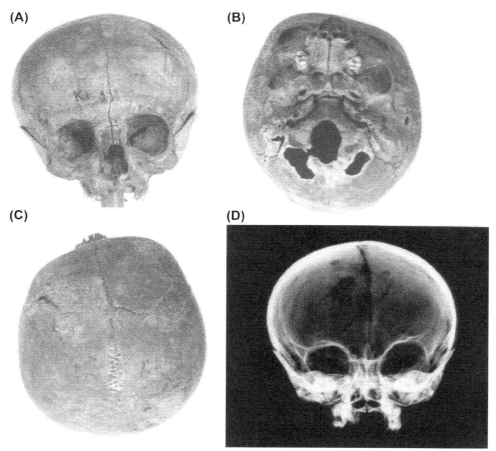

FIGURE 2.5 Plagiocephaly as the result of premature fusion of the left coronal suture (unicoronal synostosis) seen from the top (A) and base (B) with compensatory growth of the right frontal bone (C). The superior margin of the right orbit is flattened in comparison to the left, which appears larger, but Harlequin eye is not evident (D). *From Oostra, R.-J., van der Wolk, S., Maas, M., Hennekam, R., 2005. Malformations of the axial skeleton in the Museum Vrolik II: craniostenosis and suture related conditions. American Journal of Medical Genetics 136A, 331.*

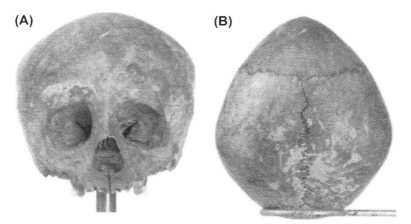

FIGURE 2.6 Trigonocephaly as the result of premature metopic suture fusion, resulting in hypotelorism (A), and a triangular-shaped vault when viewed from the top (B). *From Oostra, R.-J., van der Wolk, S., Maas, M., Hennekam, R., 2005. Malformations of the axial skeleton in the Museum Vrolik II: craniostenosis and suture related conditions. American Journal of Medical Genetics 136A, 332.*

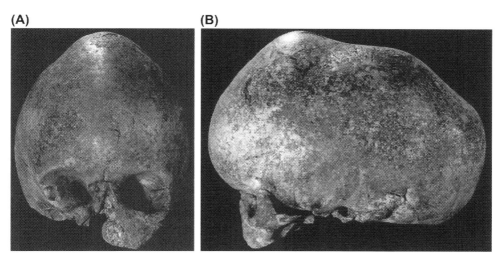

FIGURE 2.7 A possible case of oxycephaly in a 3- to 4-year-old child from prehistoric Moulamein, Australia. Premature fusion of the sagittal suture is also evident resulting in a tall (A) and elongated (B) cranial vault. Note the protrusion at the anterior fontanel or clown's cap deformity. *From Webb, S., 1995. Paleopathology of Aboriginal Australians, Cambridge University Press, Cambridge, p. 78, 80.*

(1995) describes oxycephaly in a 3- to 4-year-old from prehistoric Moulamein in Australia. The child displays a clown's cap deformity (protrusion at the anterior fontanelle) and has hypertrophy of the cranial and facial bones (Fig. 2.7). A case of bicoronal suture fusion with mild hydrocephaly was described by Pedersen and Anton (1998) in the tiny remains of an infant from an historic cemetery in Omaha. The infant was treated no differently to any of the other children at the site, whose bodies were all covered with red mercury lead pigment. When compared to the other infant skulls and a modern database, the affected skull demonstrated an enlarged anterior fontanel and shallow superior orbital margins resulting from a depressed frontal bone. The sphenoid suture was also fused bilaterally, and the authors suggested this may have been a case of Apert's syndrome (Pedersen and Anton, 1998). The poor preservation of the remains meant that cloverleaf deformity (see the following section) could not be ruled out.

Cloverleaf Deformity

Cloverleaf deformity describes a trilobed skull resulting from congenital hydrocephalus. It is caused by agenesis of the coronal and lambdoid sutures. Increased intracranial pressure causes bulging of the frontal eminences and at the parietosquamosal sutures, giving the skull a cloverleaf appearance when viewed from the front (Fig. 2.8). There is a downward displacement of the ears and exophthalmos (Angle et al., 1967). This form of deformation results in the brain being housed within a "rigid box" and subsequent mental retardation (Cohen, 2005, p. 319). The condition is related to thanatophoric dwarfism and usually causes in death in the perinatal period. However, it has been recorded in children as old as 8 years (Partington et al., 1971). Bennett (1967) describes a case of possible suture agenesis

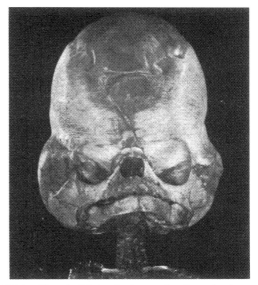

FIGURE 2.8 Cloverleaf deformity in a modern fetus showing a trilobed contour of the vault, shallow orbits, particularly of the superior margins, and reduced size of the mandible and maxilla in comparison to the nasal bones. The child was a thanatophoric dwarf. Curated at the Pathology Museum, St Bartholomew's Hospital (TE256). *From Partington, M., Gonzales-Crussi, F., Khakee, S., Wollin, D., 1971. Cloverleaf skull and thanatophoric dwarfism. Report of four cases, two in the same sibship. Archives of Disease in Childhood 46, 657.*

in a perinate from Utah that would likely have led to a cloverleaf deformity had the child lived.

Crouzon's Syndrome (Craniofacial Dysotosis Type 1)

Crouzon's syndrome is the most common syndrome leading to craniofacial anomalies. As it also features craniosynostosis, it is included here. Premature fusion of cranial base and lambdoid sutures results in individuals with protruding eyes (exophthalmos) and a brachyocephalic skull (Cohen and Krelborg, 1992). Hydrocephalus is usually present (Khanna et al., 2011), and coronal and sagittal suture fusion is also evident in 80% of cases (McAlister and Herman, 2005). Ossification of the stylohyoid ligament, deviation of the basal septum, and a hypoplastic maxilla give the mandible a prognathic appearance. A third of all cases also have spinal defects such as fusion of C2 and C3 (McAlister and Herman, 2005). Prokopec et al. (1984) presented a case of craniosynostosis in an aboriginal child that Barnes (1994, p. 154) later considered to be Crouzon's syndrome due to the formation of a clown's cap deformity. Campillo (2005) describes a second potential case in a 12-year-old from later medieval Spain, with ridging of the frontal bone and a beak-like appearance to the skull. Absence of the base of the skull meant that a diagnosis could not be confirmed.

Microcephaly

An abnormally small cranium can occur from an underlying condition that causes retarded brain growth (microencephaly) or affects normal growth at the sutures (e.g., hyperthyroidism or rickets) (Barnes, 1994; Oostra et al., 2005). The condition can occur both pre- and postnatally and results in mild-to-severe mental retardation and short stature (nanosomia). Microcephaly is not primarily caused by craniosynostosis, nor does craniosynostosis result in microcephaly; however, both conditions can occur together (Waldron, 2009). Microcephaly has been related to an autosomal recessive gene in siblings, but environmental factors such as fetal alcohol syndrome (Sampson et al., 1997), pre- and postnatal iodine deficiency (Hollowell and Hannon, 1997), radiation exposure during pregnancy, encephalitis and meningitis, birth trauma, and asphyxia have all been linked to the condition (Sheldon, 1943). A microcephalic skull displays recession of the frontal and parietal bones, a flattened occipital bone, a prominent nose, and a head circumference below 46 cm. Cranial capacity is usually less than 1000 cc (where 1000–1900 cc is considered normal), with the most extreme cases having a cranial capacity of only 600 cc (Waldron, 2009). Premature fusion of most of the sutures and the fontanel at bregma may result in a cone-shaped skull (Aufderheide and Rodriguez-Martín, 1998), and cranial lacunae may appear due to irregularity in the thickness of the cranial vault. Individuals may suffer epileptic seizures and limb paralysis, and many die in childhood (Aufderheide and Rodriguez-Martín, 1998).

Microcephaly needs to be diagnosed in comparison to measurements of skulls from children of similar ages and from the same sample. Richards (1985, p. 344) provides the following criteria for diagnosis:

1. small cranial vault with marked recession of the frontal bone and a vertical occipital bone
2. lack of premature suture closure
3. reduction in the volume of the brain (especially cerebral hemispheres)
4. reduced facial skeleton that is large in relation to the skull vault
5. micrognathia
6. smaller than average stature

One of the first cases of microcephaly to be reported in the archeological record was by Hrdlička (1918) in a 16-year-old female from Lima, Peru, with a cranial capacity of 490 cc compared to population norm of 1239 cc. The skull demonstrated restricted growth of the cranial vault relative to the development of the mandible and maxilla. Richards (1985) reported the youngest case of microcephaly in a 3-year-old from central California with a cranial capacity comparative to a 6-month-old from the same population (630 cc). The skull demonstrated severe malformation of the orbital surface and restricted growth of the frontal bone. In particular, the wings of the sphenoid were thickened with the orbital aspect of the greater wing being concave rather than flat. The postcranium developed normally, which enabled this case to be differentiated from pituitary dwarfism (Ortner, 2003).

Hydrocephaly

An abnormally enlarged skull results from an accumulation of cerebrospinal fluid in the subarachnoid space (Johanson et al., 2008). Cerebrospinal fluid is produced by the choroid plexus epithelial cells in the cerebral ventricular system (Johanson et al., 2008) and is essential for protecting the brain. The fluid contains proteins and chemicals similar to blood that keep the brain moist and remove waste material. Hydrocephalus may be caused by abnormal production of cerebrospinal fluid, defective absorption of the fluid at the sylvian aqueduct, or more commonly, blockage to the circulation of the cerebral ventricular system (Johanson et al., 2008; Murphy, 1996). A buildup of fluid or "water on the brain" causes increasing pressure on the brain resulting in headaches and a loss of balance. If left untreated hydrocephalus may cause blindness, deafness, and paralysis, and 50% of sufferers will die before the age of 5 years (Murphy, 1996). Today, hydrocephalus is congenital in 25% of all cases, but it is also related to prenatal trauma or anoxia, tumors, and infections such as mumps and measles (Laurence and Coates, 1962). Laurence and Coates (1962) presented a natural history of the disease without intervention. They followed 182 London children under 13 years of age who did not receive an operation for their condition. The majority of cases were caused by trauma or meningitis, and 34 had associated spina bifida cystic. Laurence and Coates (1962) observed that birth trauma resulted in hydrocephalus and cranial deformation around 2 months after delivery. After 5 years of age, 81 (44.5%) experienced spontaneous arrest of hydrocephalus, 9 (4.9%) still had a progressive disease, and 89 (48.9%) had died; 57% fell within the normal mental range, but 65% showed some form of physical handicap. Disabilities ranged from minor to blindness and quadriplegia with various degrees of brain damage or mental impairment (Laurence and Coates, 1962).

The features of a hydrocephalic skull include an enlarged cranium with frontal bossing, thinned cranial bones, bulging fontanels, interdigitalization of widened sutures, numerous wormian bones, and a flattened cranial base (Aufderheide and Rodriguez-Martín, 1998). Hydrocephalus is most likely to be identified in a child's remains or in adults who survived the condition in childhood. This is because the buildup of cerebrospinal fluid needs to occur around 6 months before the metopic suture and fontanels fuse for skull enlargement to occur (Murphy, 1996). In older children, hydrocephalus can result in increased intracranial pressure and an exaggerated depth to the sulcal and gyral impressions (known as copper or silver beaten skull). Children who develop the condition between 10 and 15 years of age suffer sutural separation of varying degrees. Between 9 months and 2 years, around 46% of cases will arrest when equilibrium is reached as pathological and compensatory processes no longer increase the size of the cranial vault, but a reduction of the deformity will not occur (Richards and Anton, 1991). Pretorius et al. (1985) reported that two-thirds of the fetal hydrocephalus cases in his study also had neural tube defects and that hydrocephalus had developed by 24-weeks gestation. The enlarged head of a fetus affected by this condition may cause trouble during childbirth (Roberts and Manchester, 2007), but cases of fetal remains with hydrocephalus have yet to be reported in the literature of archeological obstetric deaths.

As with microcephaly, hydrocephalus is best diagnosed using the mean cranial index of the skeletal sample from which the skull was derived (Waldron, 2009). To aid diagnosis, Richards and Anton (1991, p. 188) recommended several cranial measurements in addition to cranial capacity and established a set of criteria for the condition:

1. enlarged cranial vault based on maximum cranial dimensions with normal facial dimensions;
2. asymmetry of vault, thinning of cranial bones, cerebral imprinting;
3. interdigitation of sutures;
4. extra wormian bones.

At least 30 potential cases of hydrocephalus have been reported in the archeological record, dating from 10,000 BC to AD 1670 (Murphy, 1996) and around 11 of these cases are in children (Aufderheide, 2003; Tillier et al., 2001; Manchester, 1980; Murphy, 1996; Walker, 2012; Campillo, 2005; Kreutz et al., 1995; Held et al., 2010; Richards and Anton, 1991; Brothwell, 1967). Five have been identified in children who died around 3 years of age, while two cases have been identified in adolescents. Richards and Anton (1991) reported a case of hydrocephalus in a 10-year-old from California who exhibited the "setting-sun" sign of the orbits, where the eyes are pushed downward due to the posterioinferior inclination of the orbital plates and shallow orbital frontal junction (Fig. 2.9). The skeleton also displayed femoral atrophy indicating the presence of right-sided paraplegia. Manchester (1980) admits that his case from early medieval Eccles is problematic as sagittal

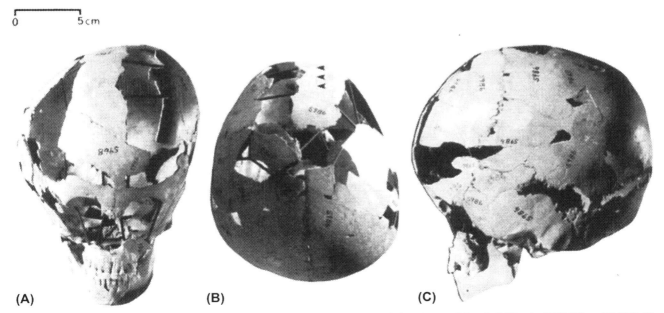

FIGURE 2.9 Hydrocephalus in the reconstructed skull of a 4-year-old (LMA 12-5986) from Protero Mound, California (2500 BC to AD 500). The cranial vault shows asymmetrical expansion (A) and has a triangular profile when viewed from above (B). Note the exaggerated proportions of the vault in comparison to the maxilla and mandible (C). *From Richards, G., Anton, S., 1991. Craniofacial configuration and postcranial development of a hydrocephalic child (ca. 2500 BC-500 AD): with a review of cases and comment on diagnostic criteria. American Journal of Physical Anthropology 85, 190.*

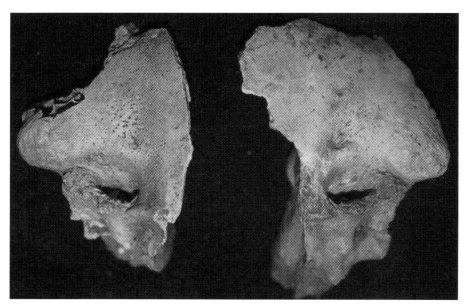

FIGURE 2.10 Bilateral aural stenosis (narrowing) of the external auditory meati in a 6- to 12-year-old from St Oswald's Priory in Gloucester, England (skeleton 74).

craniosynostosis may account for the hyperbrachycephalic skull, and the older age of the child (14–16 years) does not fit with the pathogenesis of the disease. The cranial capacity of the Eccles child was 1500 compared to 1650 cc in the Irish case presented by Murphy (1996) and 3200 cc in the example presented by Held et al. (2010). Manchester (1980) noted cranial asymmetry and had suggested the presence of an intracranial tumor as an underlying cause of hydrocephalus. Galdames et al. (2009) also reported cranial base asymmetry in all seven hydrocephalic skulls from an anatomical collection, with left-side asymmetry dominating. In their study, the greatest degree of asymmetry was seen in a newborn leading Galdames et al. (2009) to argue that asymmetry in hydrocephalus is caused by conditions within the uterus that limit bilateral cranial growth, rather than indicating the presence of an expanding cranial tumor.

Congenital Deafness (Aural Stenosis and Aural Atresia)

This congenital disorder is caused by hypoplasia or aplasia of the external auditory canal due to abnormal development of the first and second branchial arches. Congenital deafness can be the result of genetic mutations after exposure to teratogenic agents (Keenleyside, 2011), or associated with congenital conditions such as Goldenhar syndrome and Down syndrome (Balkany et al., 1979). The modern incidence is 1 in 10,000–20,000 births, and males are more commonly affected than females. Thirty percent of cases are bilateral, and the right side is more frequently affected than the left (Barnes, 1994). The defect can range from a narrowing of the external auditory meatus (stenosis) to its complete obliteration (atresia), and from normal formation of the middle and inner ear, to deformed and fused ossicles and rudimentary formation of the internal structures (Barnes, 1994). Depending on the severity of the deformation, the individual may have partial to complete hearing loss from birth, a small and underdeveloped ear (microtia) and in complete deafness, will be mute.

Reports of aural stenosis (Fig. 2.10) or atresia of the external auditory meatus are frequent in the paleopathological literature, and six reported cases are of children aged from 2 to 13 years of age (Farwell and Molleson, 1993; Hrdlička, 1938; Kato et al., 2007; Panzer et al., 2008, p. 188). Deaf-mute children may have received variable treatment from their society. For example, in ancient Rome a wealthy child who was expected to pursue an education would have been considered of inferior intellect by their society, whereas a similarly affected child of the lower classes may not have been so discriminated against (Laes, 2011). A 5-year-old found with auditory atresia at Romano-British Poundbury Camp was provided with an extraordinary elaborate burial in a stone-lined cyst grave (Farwell and Molleson, 1993, p. 188), and although the child was buried prone, which may suggest burial as an "other," this was by no means a unique burial position at the site (Fig. 2.11). Interestingly, Kato et al. (2007) reported on a case of 4- to 5-year-old deaf-mute from Ancon, Peru, with a subsequent healed trepanation on the occipital bone thought to have been related to an external ear deformity. The child also displayed perimortem drill holes on the frontal. One of the youngest reported cases of congenital atresia is a 1- to 2-year-old from medieval Barton-on-Humber in Lincolnshire with an affected right ear (Waldron, 2007, p. 115). Panzer et al. (2008) described a case of Goldenhar syndrome in a nonadult skull from Rain Chapel in Germany.

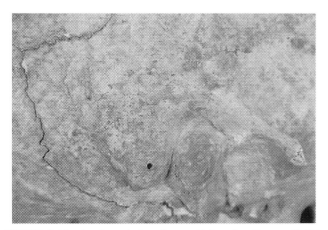

FIGURE 2.11 Aural atresia in a 5-year-old from late Romano-British Poundbury Camp, Dorset, England (skeleton 1114). *Photograph taken with kind permission from the Natural History Museum, London.*

The left temporal bone demonstrated bony atresia of the left external auditory canal, absent ear ossicles, and hypoplasia of the inner ear structures. The skull was also markedly asymmetrical. It is likely the child had evident soft tissue anomalies such as ear and eye deformities.

SPINE

The embryonic spine is made up of a series of bilaterally paired blocks or somites that give rise to the vertebrae and ribs during development. The vertebral bodies ossify from the central aspect outward, with each vertebra resulting from fusion of the caudal (bottom) half of one somite to the cranial (top) half of the adjacent one. Ossification commences in the lower thoracic region around the eighth fetal week, then proceeds caudally and cranially (Scheuer and Black, 2000). Ossification of the arches commences in the upper cervical vertebrae and proceeds through the thoracic, lumbar, and sacral segments. Fusion of the arches and pedicle boutons to the vertebral bodies starts around 3 years of age for the cervical vertebrae, finishing at 6 years for the lumbar (Walker, 1991). Changes in the morphology of the vertebrae are caused by "border shifting" in vertebral development, with the affected vertebra taking on the features of the adjacent vertebra above (cranial shifting) or below (caudal shifting) (Roberts and Manchester, 2007). Although spinal anomalies are commonly reported, anomalies of the upper and lower cervical spine are rare. When they do occur, congenital fusion of the cervical spine is most common in the first three vertebrae (75% cases) with the axis (C2) and third cervical vertebra (C3) most commonly affected (Guille and Sherk, 2002). Fifty percent of cases involve three or more elements. Congenital anomalies of the cervical spine may indicate malformations of other organs, especially the kidney and heart. They may be asymptomatic or associated with various syndromes including fetal alcohol syndrome (Guille and Sherk, 2002).

Congenital Lordosis, Kyphosis, and Scoliosis

Congenital lordosis is a rare congenital condition that results from a lack of segmentation or abnormal fusion of the posterior neural arches in combination with normal anterior development. The condition is generally mild and normally affects the thoracic vertebrae. Continued growth of the vertebral bodies anteriorly results in an increased and abnormal inward curve of the back (Kaplan et al., 2005). Congenital kyphosis is more common than lordosis and is related to agenesis or underdevelopment of the anterior vertebral bodies resulting in hemivertebrae. In kyphosis there is exaggerated forward (k-shaped) curvature of the thoracic spine resulting in a hunchback. It may also result from failure of the vertebral bodies to segment with an anterior bony bar forming between the vertebral bodies and restricting normal growth (Ozonoff, 2005). Congenital scoliosis may occur due to a complex array of spinal anomalies including wedge or hemivertebrae, supernumerary hemivertebrae, unilateral block vertebrae, or neural arch fusion. These anomalies may occur in isolation or in combination to produce an abnormal s-shaped curvature of the spine (Ozonoff, 2005, p. 1330). Ortner (2003, p. 464) provides a modern anatomical example of kyphoscoliosis with associated spina bifida cystic in an 8-year-old, illustrating the great extent of fragmentation that may occur in the spine. Another case of scoliosis was identified in the mummy of a 6-year-old from northern Chile, dating to 1000 BC (Gerszten et al., 2001).

Occipitalization (Atlantooccipital Fusion)

Partial or total fusion of atlas to the occipital facets results from segmental failure at the occipital–cervical border. It is the most common segmentation abnormality and seen in 1% of the general population (Aufderheide and Rodriguez-Martín, 1998). Occipitalization may also be associated with Down syndrome, achondroplasia, diastrophic dwarfism, spondyloepiphyseal dysplasia, Klippel–Feil syndrome, hyperparathyroidism, and C2–C3 fusion (Guille and Sherk, 2002; Senator and Gronkiewicz, 2012). Cervical–thoracic, thoracic–lumbar, and sacral–coccygeal transitions can also occur, but are less common (Aufderheide and Rodriguez-Martín, 1998).

Occipitalization develops during the third week of fetal life when the sclerotomes of the occipital and cervical vertebrae are forming and fail to divide (Senator and Gronkiewicz, 2012). Partial fusion of the anterior elements is the most common expression, but it may also include hypoplasia of the posterior elements. Occipitalization can result in premature deterioration of the atlantoaxial joint due to added mechanical stress, or spina bifida may occur on the posterior arch of the atlas. In a clinical study, 72% of those with occipitalization reported weakness, numbness or pain in the upper extremities, and dull headaches

(McRae and Barum, 1953). The defect can limit nodding or lateral rotation of the head, and neck ache may result from basilar compression of the odontoid process (Black and Scheuer, 1996). Symptoms appear gradually, usually after trauma to the neck, and may subsequently lead to death as the joint becomes less stable and the central nervous system becomes less tolerant to repeated knocks of the dens against the second cervical vertebra (Senator and Gronkiewicz, 2012). While occipitalization is usually asymptomatic in children and before the fourth decade of life, Gholve et al. (2007) reported spinal impingement in 45% of their child clinical cases leading to upper muscle weakness. A sagittal diameter under 13 mm may be associated with neural problems due to impingement of spinal cord in the cervical vertebrae (Guille and Sherk, 2002; Senator and Gronkiewicz, 2012). In unaffected individuals, this diameter normally measures over 30 mm and is often under 25 mm in those with occipitalization (Tun et al., 2004). Other deformities in the craniovertebral junction include congenital axis dysmorphism, where the dens of the axis is asymmetrical, misshapen, or deviated. This may occur in torticollis, where the odontoid process becomes tilted to one side, and is generally associated with deformities of the atlas (Travan et al., 2013). Travan et al. (2013) reported a case of axis asymmetry in an 8- to 10-year-old from Italy. The cause of death of the child was unknown, but the authors highlighted the risk of cranial–cervical dislocation and sudden death in such cases. A possible case of occipitalization with basilar compression and disuse atrophy of the humerus was noted in a 5- to 6-year-old from St Oswald's Priory in Gloucester (Fig. 2.12).

Lumbarization and Sacralization

Changes in the morphology of the fifth lumbar or first sacral vertebrae are caused by "border shifting" and are the most commonly reported spinal defects. Sacralization refers to partial or complete fusion of L5 to the sacrum, with the lumbar vertebra often developing rudimentary sacral alae (or enlarged transverse processes), resulting in a sacrum with six segments (Fig. 2.13). Lumbarization of S1 is less common and results from a failure of the sacral vertebra to fuse to the sacrum, leaving it with only four sacral segments (Ortner, 2003). In some cases the changes may be unilateral causing scoliosis of the spine. Determining which form of transitional vertebra has occurred is often difficult in paleopathology if the whole sacrum is not preserved (Roberts and Manchester, 2007), or if the sacrum is still unfused (i.e., before around 12 years of age). Despite this, at least six cases of lumbarization and sacralization in children have been identified in skeletal reports, with the youngest aged 6–8 years from Horncastle, England (Holst pers. comm.).

Spondylolysis

Detachment of the neural arch from the vertebral body crosses the boundary between a congenital and traumatic classification, as it is thought to be related to an underlying defect in the formation of the pedicles (Aufderheide and Rodriguez-Martín, 1998). The condition is uncommon in children before 5 years of age, but is present in 4%–8% of the general population today. Lesions may be unilateral, bilateral, complete, or partial. This condition is discussed more fully in Chapter 5.

Sagittal Clefting

Sagittal clefting is an anatomical defect in the vertebral body that occurs due to the irregular regression of the notochord from the centrum during fetal development (Merbs, 2004). The notochord represents the fetal spinal cord that

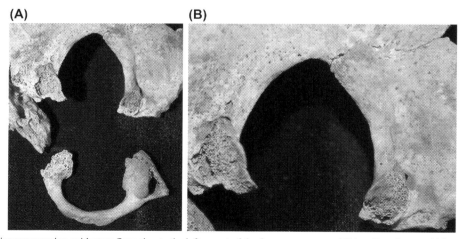

FIGURE 2.12 Basiliar compression evident as flattening to the left aspect of the foramen magnum (A) in a 5- to 6-year-old from St Oswald's Priory in Gloucester, England (AD 1540–1700, skeleton 368). Postmortem damage to the occipital facets suggests possible occipitalization due to fusion of the left facet during life (B). The compression led to disuse atrophy of the left arm.

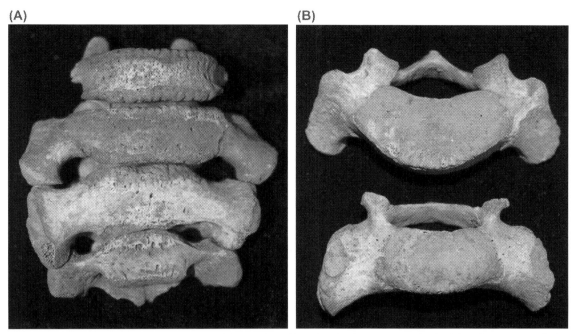

FIGURE 2.13 (A) Sacralization in a 6- to 7-year-old child from St Oswald's Priory in Gloucester, England, with rudimentary sacral alae of L5 (the second bone from the top in the image) and accessory facets on S1. (B) The rounded (top vertebra) as opposed to flattened profile (bottom vertebra) of the anterior aspect of the body indicates that it is a lumbar vertebra (AD 1120–1230, skeleton 129).

degenerates as it is gradually replaced by cells that will become the nucleus pulposus in the adult spine. In normal development, the notochord has disappeared by the 12th fetal week, and the midline cleft has been closed. Failure of the notochord to regress limits ossification at the midline resulting in a cleft, circular hole or complete separation of the two halves of the vertebra (butterfly vertebra) (Aufderheide and Rodriguez-Martín, 1998; Merbs, 2004). The vertebral bodies above and below the defect may alter their shape to compensate for the unusual morphology, and this may result in scoliosis, or later leave the spine vulnerable to compression fractures (Merbs, 2004). The defect occurs more commonly in males than females. It may occur in isolation, or in relation to another syndrome or defects, including block vertebrae, spina bifida, supernumerary vertebrae, lumbarization, and rib anomalies (Müller et al., 1986). The etiology behind sagittal clefting is unknown, but a genetic link is suspected (Merbs, 2004) as it has been identified in twins (van den Bos et al., 1984). While the atlas may also exhibit an unfused anterior arch, this clefting is not related to the notochord (Scheuer and Black, 2000). Peabody (1927) described a case of notochord regression failure in an infant who also exhibited sacralization of L5, fused vertebral centra, and rib fusion. The birth of the child was normal and he was able to walk, but the spinal deformity was progressive.

Merbs (2004) carried out a comprehensive review of vertebral anomalies in Inuit samples from Native Point and Silumuit, Canada. He identified sagittal clefts in four nonadults aged between 6- and 7-years. Vertebral clefts occurred most commonly in T8, followed by T6, while unfused posterior arches were more common in T11. Two children had identical forms of the defect, with both showing sagittal clefting of T8, severe clefting of T10, and a cleft posterior arch of T11, but evidence of kinship could not be determined. Merbs (2004) argued that, although the sample was limited, it was striking that those with the defects were less likely to make it to adulthood. Lewis (2008) reported a sagittal cleft of T8 in an 8- to 9-year-old from Chichester, Sussex. The child also had hypoplasia of the left neural arch of the axis. One of the most complex cases of vertebral clefting comes from medieval London, where Connell et al. (2012, p. 134) reported on a 12- to 17-year-old with a sagittal cleft of T5, aplastic arches of T6–9, and advanced kyphosis of the spine at a 180-degree angle. These lesions would have been evident from birth and are likely to have resulted in severe physical impairment of the adolescent. A perinate from St Oswald's Priory in Gloucester, England demonstrates sagittal clefting of the upper thoracic sternebra and bilateral costal fusion of the ribs at the vertebral ends. These defects suggest a disruption in somite differentiation and lack of notochord regression. The early death of this child may indicate that defects in the heart and lungs were also present at birth (Fig. 2.14).

Cleft Neural Arches

Unfused neural arches are commonly reported in the paleopathological literature, but caution should be used when

32 Paleopathology of Children

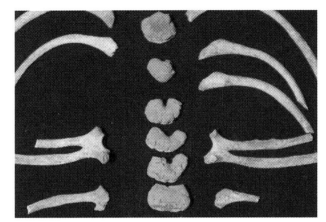

FIGURE 2.14 Multiple sagittal clefts and costal fusion in the thorax of a perinate from St Oswald's Priory in Gloucester, England (AD 1540–1700, skeleton 418) suggesting a disruption in somite differentiation and lack of notochord regression. More severe soft tissue deformities are likely to have been present resulting in the early death of the child.

identifying them in nonadult skeletal remains where the spine is still developing. The posterior synchondrosis of the lumbar vertebrae and sacrum are the last to fuse. Any defects will not be evident until the age at which normal fusion occurs has passed, or the posterior arch is clearly delayed in comparison to children of a similar age (Fig. 2.15). The posterior axis and atlas fuse between the ages of 3–4 and 4–5 years respectively, fusion of the posterior synchondrosis of the lumbar vertebrae occurs around 5–6 years of age, but fusion of the sacrum is not normally complete until around 15 years of age (Scheuer and Black, 2000). A brief survey of cleft neural arches reported in the gray and published literature revealed that of 24 nonadult cases, 15 (62.5%) were of L5, followed by the axis (n = 4) and T1 (n = 2), with reports of open neural arches for the atlas, L4 and S1 occurring only once.

THORAX

Supernumerary Ribs

These are common anatomical variations that result from elongation of the transverse process in a cervical or lumbar vertebra. In the cervical spine, ribs may occur in C5 to C7 but no higher (Black and Scheuer, 1997), and lumbar ribs are less common. Cervical and lumbar ribs may be bilateral or unilateral and comprise a vertebral head and short body. Although they are usually asymptomatic, well-developed cervical ribs tend to cause vascular problems with compression of the subclavian artery (Black and Scheuer, 1997). The etiology behind the development of these accessory ribs is unknown (Aufderheide and Rodriguez-Martín, 1998), but cervical ribs occur more frequently in females (Black and Scheuer, 1997). Black and Scheuer (1997) argued that true cervical ribs cannot

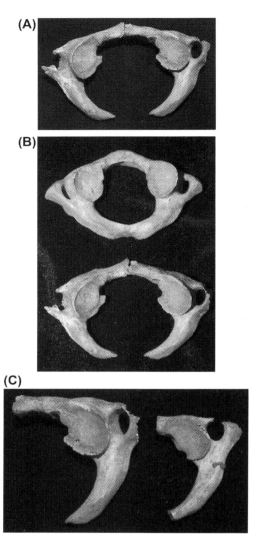

FIGURE 2.15 (A) Cleft neural arch of the atlas in an 8-year-old from St Oswald's Priory in Gloucester, England (AD 900–1348, skeleton 42), compared to a (B) complete atlas in a child of a similar age from the same site. (C) The margins of the posterior arch are tapered (left) in comparison to the more blunt profile of an unfused arch in a 5-year-old (right). Note also associated clefting of the anterior arch, which should fuse around 6 years of age (A).

be diagnosed in nonadults under the age of 10 years, as they do not fully develop until fusion of the transverse processes. This is disappointing as their occurrence in perinates may enable us to identify stillborn babies in the past. In a clinical study of 318 perinates born in Utah from 2006 to 2009, Furtado et al. (2011) reported a significantly higher prevalence of cervical ribs in stillborns (43%) compared to live-born children who died within the first year (12%). They conclude that cervical ribs signal a disadvantageous fetal environment that leads to a greater likelihood of stillbirth. Similarly, Bots et al. (2011) studied 199 stillborns and noted 40% had cervical ribs, and that extra ribs were likely to occur without any other skeletal defects.

Bifid Ribs, Costal Fusion

Fused ribs are usually associated with anomalies in the thoracic vertebrae. Irregular segmentation can cause a variety of morphological changes including bifurcation, flaring, and abnormal wideness, merging, and bridging (Barnes, 1994; Brues, 1946). Bifucation occurs primarily at the anterior ends and usually occurs on the right side, affecting the third and fifth ribs. Hinkes (1983) reported flared sternal ends in ribs 1–8 of a perinate from the Grasshopper Pueblo, Arizona, and Brothwell and Powers (2000) recorded merged ribs in a perinate and an infant from medieval Cannington, England. The infant was buried next to an adult female who also had a bifid rib.

EXTREMITIES

Talipes Equinovarus (Clubfoot)

Congenital talipes equinovarus is a common foot abnormality with a modern incidence of 1 in 800–1000 births. It is more common in boys than in girls (ratio 3.1:2), but the most severe cases are reported in females (Aufderheide and Rodriguez-Martín, 1998). Clubfoot can be bilateral or unilateral, and although there is a known family inheritance affecting male siblings (Davidson et al., 2008), the exact etiology is unclear (Aufderheide and Rodriguez-Martín, 1998). Clinically, deviation of the talus is evident in 24- to 26-week-old fetuses on ossification of the tarsus (Waisbrod, 1973). In fetal autopsies the navicular is found to cover the entire head of the talus, and the talus may be smaller and thinner than normal, with a long neck and pointed head. In the infant foot the talus shows medial and inferior deviation of the neck in relation to the head, and there may be talonavicular subluxation (Wright, 2011). The cuboid can become medially displaced and triangular in shape before 12 months of age, but may not show deformity until after 4 years when it becomes fully formed (Wright, 2011). Modern studies have shown that walking is possible, even on bilaterally affected feet, with the weight carried on the lateral margin of the foot. Equinovarus deformity may be a symptom of other congenital conditions such as Edward's syndrome (trisomy 18) or arthrogryposis multiplex congenital, a nonprogressive condition characterized by muscle weakness and joint deformities (Lloyd-Roberts and Lettin, 1970; Wright, 2011).

Such a common modern condition must have occurred in the past, but identification relies on good preservation, careful reconstruction of the foot and ankle, and comparison with the unaffected side (Roberts et al., 2004). Clubfoot is a progressive deformity, and as such may be difficult to identify in young children with more subtle changes. This might explain why the only cases that have been identified in the archeological record are of adults (Brothwell, 1967; Garlie et al., 2002; Johnson and Kerley, 1974; Mann and Owsley, 1989; Roberts et al., 2004). In archeological remains, disuse atrophy of the leg bones may be the most obvious sign, accompanied by medial displacement of the navicular and cuboid in relation to the talus and calcaneus, or inward rotation of the calcaneus under the talus, with regional hypoplasia of the carpals and metatarsals (Caffey, 1945). Brothwell (1967) and Morse (1978) have listed a number of indicators for the condition, and detailed examples of many of these changes are provided by Mann and Owsley (1989) and Wright (2011):

1. changes to the distal tibia articular process
2. cuboid with a pseudoheel, lacking the cuboid tuberosity
3. flattened areas on the superior aspects of the metatarsals, which have a medial deviation
4. small talus with a shortened or absent neck; it will always be abnormal
5. shortened and widened calcaneus
6. subluxation of the navicular with accessory articulations
7. posterior displacement of the fibula and flattened distal tibia

The youngest reported case of clubfoot in the archeological record is a 15- to 20-year-old male from Roman Gloucester (Roberts et al., 2004). This individual had marked atrophy of the left femur and tibia, and a severely bowed fibula likely due to mechanical loading and abnormal weight bearing on the lateral aspect of the foot. In the foot, the calcaneus had a pseudofacet for the talus, and the talus has reduced facets with a narrower head when compared to the right. When articulated, medial deviation of the talus was evident. There was buttressing on the lateral aspect of the left femur, and the pelvis demonstrated a shortening of the left os coxae perhaps due to abnormal weight transition through the sacroiliac joint. An additional atrophied left arm led Roberts et al. (2004) to conclude that clubfoot developed secondarily to paralysis in poliomyelitis.

Radioulnar Synostosis

Fusion of the radius and ulna results in an inability to pronate or supinate the forearm. The etiology is not understood and it may be inherited or related to fetal alcohol syndrome (Sampson et al., 1997). The condition has been divided into three distinct types (Aufderheide and Rodriguez-Martín, 1998):

1. True synostosis: where the proximal radius is underdeveloped and fused to the ulna. The radial shaft is longer and more robust than that of the ulna.
2. Congenital dislocation: due to underdevelopment of the radial head, with dislocation and subsequent fusion to the ulna at the proximal end.
3. Malformed radial head: later becomes fused to the proximal ulna.

Although considered rare in the clinical literature, several cases have been identified in the paleopathological literature including in fetal remains (Aufderheide and Rodriguez-Martín, 1998). Ortner (2003, p. 478) provides an example from the collection at the National Museum of Natural History in Washington with an underdeveloped radial head. A tiny example has been reported by Lorrio (2010) in a perinate from a double burial at El Molon in Spain. The normal appearance of the radial head suggests this may be a case of congenital dislocation.

Polydactyly and Syndactyly

Abnormalities of digits are common congenital malformations and can result in a series of changes in the hands and feet (Fig. 2.16). Polydactyly refers to the development of more than five digits on the hands and/or feet, which occur on the radial or tibial side (preaxial); on the ulnar or fibular side (postaxial) or more rarely, centrally (5% of cases). This is generally not an inherited anomaly (Caffey, 1945). In contrast, syndactyly is an inherited condition that causes a lack of differentiation, or fusion, of two or more digits (Waldron, 2009) and may occur in isolation or with lethal congenital syndromes (Aufderheide and Rodriguez-Martín, 1998). Syndactyly is especially common in native Africans (Davidson et al., 2008). Anomalies of the digits also include "symphalangism" where one phalanx is fused to another in the same digit, or "hyperphalangism" where there is an increase in the number of phalanges, usually in the thumb. Case et al. (2006) provide a comprehensive discussion of polydactyly and include several subclassifications: Type A describes a well-formed digit that either articulates with the fifth metatarsal, metacarpal, or phalanges or appears as a completely separate digit. This is more common in the foot, where there may also be a bifurcated "Y"-shaped metatarsal or phalanx, a metatarsal with a branch projection, or a block metatarsal with double phalanges. Type B describes a poorly formed digit made up of soft issue with no osseous defects. This type would be invisible archeologically, which may account for a general abundance of artistic and historic evidence compared to archeological findings.

Case et al. (2006) identified polydactyly in three nonadults from the prehistoric American Southwest. Each had a sixth digit on the fifth metatarsal (postaxial). The first, an infant from Tapia del Cerrito, had bilateral Y-shaped fifth metatarsals (Fig. 2.17). As these are usually associated with congenital heart disease, this was considered to be the cause of death.

NEURAL TUBE DEFECTS

Congenital Herniation (Dystrophism)

During embryonic development the central nervous system begins as a flat plate that becomes the neural tube by

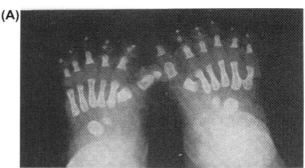
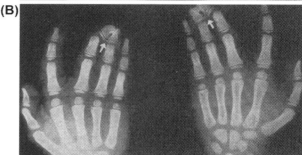
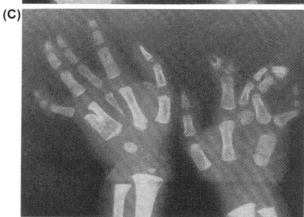

FIGURE 2.16 Clinical cases of abnormal digit formation in children showing the wide variety of skeletal malformations that may exist. (A) Polydactyly with oversegmentation of the digits and metatarsals in a 6-month-old; (B) symphalangism due to failure of segmentation of the distal phalanges in an 8-year-old; and (C) syndactyly due to irregular segmentation and hypoplasia of the phalanges and metacarpals. *From Caffey, J., 1945. Pediatric X-Ray Diagnosis, Year Book Medical Publishers, Inc., Chicago, p. 612.*

fusing along the median line, first in the cervical region, then progressing simultaneously caudally and cranially (Charon, 2004). The extremities of the neural tube (neuropores) then close. Disturbances to this fusion along the neural tube result in defects such as spina bifida cystica and anencephaly (Kalter, 2003). In congenital herniation of the cranium, failure of the anterior neuropore to fuse allows the meninges (meningocele) or the meninges and cephalic mass (meningoencephalocele) to protrude in a sac (or encephalocele) through a skull aperture. This aperture may be located on the sagittal plane of the occipital (75%), frontal (15%), or parietal bones (10%); however, lesions

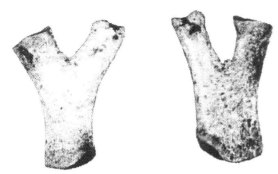

FIGURE 2.17 Bilateral Y-shaped metatarsals in an infant from prehistoric Tapia del Cerrito, Arizona (burial 4, feature 2). From Case, D., Hill, R., Merbs, C., Fong, M., 2006. Polydactyly in the prehistoric American Southwest. International Journal of Osteoarchaeology 16, 229.

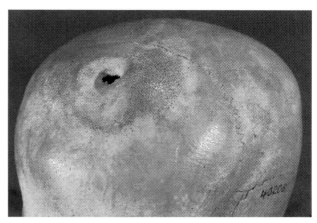

FIGURE 2.18 Congenital skull herniation in a 6- to 8-year-old from Ancon, Peru (FM 40208), viewed from the top. The lesion is located at the midline of the frontal bone and exhibits sloping, smooth, and well-circumscribed margins. The porous new bone surrounding the lesion is suggestive of an infection. From Ortner, D., 2003. Identification of Pathological Conditions in Human Skeletal Remains, Academic Press, New York, p. 460.

may also be evident on the roof of the orbit, nasal bones, or sella turcica (Aufderheide and Rodriguez-Martín, 1998; Barnes, 1994). The borders of the depression are sharply defined and surrounded by a buildup of bone due to pustulation of the soft tissue lesion (Barnes, 1994). In meningoencephalocele, the opening is larger giving the cranium a bifid appearance. Infants born with this defect will die, but individuals can survive with meningocele until adulthood. There may also be an aperture without any protrusion (cranium bifidumoccultum) (Caffey, 1945). Lesions may be mistaken for trepanations, but have a sharp anterior border and gradually sloping margins. It is not possible to determine which tissues are involved in dry bone defects (Ortner, 2003). Ortner (2003, p. 260) presents a likely case of a cranial herniation from Ancon, Lima in Peru, in a 6- to 8-year-old with depressed margins and associated inflammatory pitting (Fig. 2.18). An anatomical example of an anterior midline encephalocele in a 5-year-old is also presented (Ortner, 2003, p. 455). Diagnosis in archeological remains can be problematic, as demonstrated in a possible case from western central Asia (Blau, 2005). Postmortem surface erosion and a lack of a bony ridge made it difficult to confirm whether the aperture located on the frontal bone was the result of surgery, or a midline congenital malformation.

Anencephaly

Anencephaly is a lethal condition caused by severe malformation of the embryonic neural tube. It is the most common form of cranial malformation today (25% of all cases) occurring in 1 in 1000 births (Aufderheide and Rodriguez-Martín, 1998). Failure of the anterior neuropore to close results in cranial vault aplasia allowing the cerebral parenchyma to float in amniotic fluid and deteriorate, resulting in a mass of amorphous brain tissue, absence of a cranial vault, and rudimentary orbits at birth (Charon, 2004). The condition may be accompanied by cleft palate (Ortner, 2003) and craniorachischisis, where there is a failure of the vertebral lamina of the cervical and thoracic vertebrae to fuse exposing the neural canal. A deficiency in folic acid is strongly linked to its etiology today (Kalter, 2003), but anencephaly is also associated with mothers of low socioeconomic status and is more common in white populations (Aufderheide and Rodriguez-Martín, 1998).

Anencephaly has a long history, with the first account of a "headless infant" recorded in 426 BC and references to "monkey" and "elephant" infants thought to pertain to the condition (Charon, 2004). Ambrose Paré (AD 1585) writes about a female headless monster born in 1562. The oldest archeological case of anencephaly comes from an Egyptian catacomb in Hermopolis, built to house the mummies of sacred monkeys and ibises. The unusual shape and size of this "monkey" mummy called for greater investigation, and when unwrapped revealed a "fetal monstrosity" (Saint-Hillaire, 1826). This child was thought to have been given a sacred burial because it was interpreted as an animal born of a woman, and an omen of vengeance (Charon, 2004). An image of this mummy appears frequently in paleopathological textbooks, and an illustration of the skull elements is a useful aid to diagnosis. Charon (2004) provides a valuable account of eight anencephalic skulls in the Musee d'Homme in Paris and outlines several types of anencephaly including iniencephaly, amyelencephaly, and major meningoencephalocele. Charon's cases are of intact anatomical skulls, and many of the features identified may be difficult to identify in the more fragmented and tiny archeological material, or mistaken for nonhuman remains. In addition, the great variety of anencephalic forms makes it difficult to provide a single set of diagnostic criteria for archeological remains. Nevertheless, Dudar (2010) provides a quantitative diagnostic model using regression formulae for the

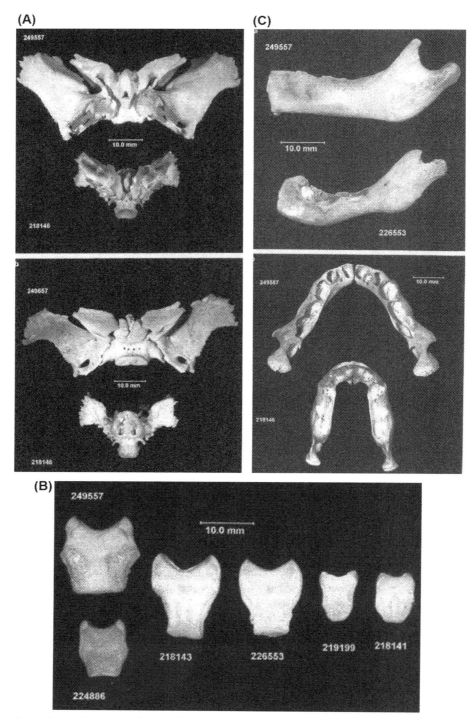

FIGURE 2.19 Comparisons of normal and anencephalic skull elements in perinates showing (A) the normal (top) and anencephalic (bottom) sphenoid; (B) varied morphology of the pars basiliaris; and (C) changes to the mandibular ramus (bottom) in comparison to normal (top). *From Dudar, J., 2010. Qualitative and quantitative diagnosis of lethal cranial neural tube defects from the fetal and neonatal human skeleton, with a case study involving taphonomically altered remains. Journal of Forensic Science 55 (4), 880, 881.*

diagnosis of anencephaly, prompted by the discovery of a 9.5-month fetus from Elmbank Pioneer cemetery, Toronto, Canada. The fetus had no cranial bones, but the surviving temporal bones, mandible, and sphenoid bones displayed morphological abnormalities (Fig. 2.19). Dudar (2010) suggests that flattened frontal bones, a normal skull base, and an unusual morphological appearance of the sphenoid body and wings may signal the presence of anencephaly.

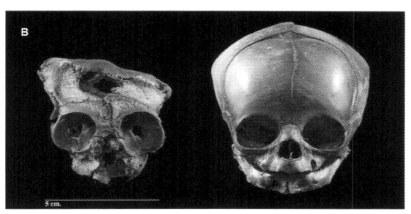

FIGURE 2.20 Comparison of an anencephalic skull of a modern 38-week-old (skeleton G294) with a normal infant. *From Irurita, J., Alemán, I., Viciano, J., López-Lázaro, S., Botella, M.C., 2015. Alterations of skull bones found in anencephalic skeletons from an identified osteological collection. Two case reports. International Journal of Legal Medicine 129 (4), 906.*

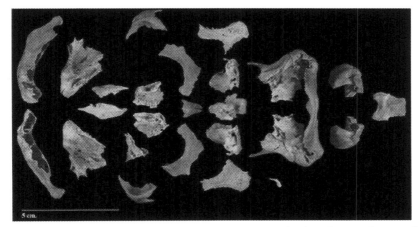

FIGURE 2.21 Individual elements of an anencephalic skull from a modern 40-week-old (G291) from the Granada Anatomical Collection. *From Irurita, J., Alemán, I., Viciano, J., López-Lázaro, S., Botella, M.C., 2015. Alterations of skull bones found in anencephalic skeletons from an identified osteological collection. Two case reports. International Journal of Legal Medicine 129 (4), 905.*

The absence of the cranial vault alone is more problematic, as it is often lost postmortem. Irurita et al. (2015) also provide a detailed analysis and illustrations of two anencephalic perinates from the San José cemetery in Granada, Spain (Figs. 2.20 and 2.21). They emphasize that while cranial deformities are evident, the difficulty in identifying individual cranial elements in such cases makes the application of regression formulae proposed by Dudar (2010) challenging and unnecessary for making a diagnosis.

An unusual case of holoprosencephaly was identified in a perinate from the Nasca culture in Peru (Tomasto-Cagigao, 2011). This abnormality is caused by the failure of the prosencephalon (the embryonic forebrain) to divide into the double lobes of the cerebral hemispheres, resulting in a single-lobed brain and severe skull and facial defects. The baby was buried with another perinate in the usual way within an urn (Fig. 2.22).

Cleft Palate

Cleft palate is caused by arrested development of the maxilla during embryogenesis, resulting in a midline defect that allows for communication between the oral and nasal cavities. Clefts may be partial, where the maxilla only is affected, or complete with clefting of both the maxilla and lip. Partial cleft palate is a relatively common developmental malformation. It is reported to be present in 1 in 1000 live births in white populations, 2 in 1000 in Asians, and 1 in 2000 live births in black individuals (Kalter, 2003), and it is more common in females than males (Aufderheide and Rodriguez-Martín, 1998; Sheldon, 1943, p. 51). There is great a variety in the severity of the condition which can be unilateral or bilateral, and range in severity from a minor cleft, to a "U"-shaped deformity of the whole hard palate that prohibits sucking (Roberts and Manchester, 2007). The

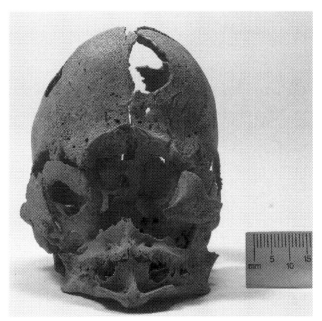

FIGURE 2.22 Holoprosencephaly in perinatal remains from Palpa, Peru (AD 335–440). *From Tomasto-Cagigao, E., 2011. A holoprosencephaly (cyclopia) case from the Nasca culture, Peru. In: Palaeopathology Association Meeting in South America IV. Lima, Peru, p. 117.*

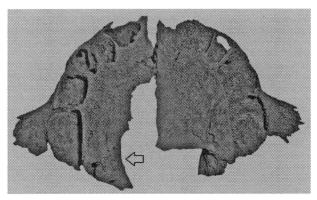

FIGURE 2.23 Infant from the Athenian Agora with cleft palate (left) and postmortem damage immediately above the defect. A normal left maxilla is shown for comparison on the right. *From Liston, M., Rotroff, S., 2013. Babies in the well: archaeological evidence for newborn disposal in Hellenistic Greece. In: Evans Grubbs, J., Parkin, T., Bell, R. (Eds.), The Oxford Handbook of Childhood and Education in the Classical World. Oxford University Press, Oxford, p. 75.*

left side of the palate is more commonly affected than the right (Orkar et al., 2002; Waldron, 2009). Although there is a strong familial link, cleft lip may be more influenced by environmental factors such as fetal exposure to tobacco smoke, rubella, and maternal folic acid deficiency. The association of cleft lip and/or palate with other congenital anomalies varies between countries, but can be as high as 90% for complete clefts, or as low as 8% for cleft lip alone (Orkar et al., 2002). Cleft lip has been associated with up to 400 different syndromes (Phillips and Sivilich, 2006) including Down syndrome, Apert's syndrome, and Klippel–Feil syndrome (Orkar et al., 2002). Those with bilateral cleft palate are more likely to suffer additional malformations (IPDTOC, 2011). In 50% of cases, cleft palate occurs in isolation (Wyszynski, 2002). Those affected may suffer respiratory and speech impairments, with hypodontia and dental agenesis also common due to the interruption of the dental lamina between the maxilla and nasal process. The lateral incisor on the side of the cleft is the most commonly affected tooth, but agenesis may also occur away from the cleft (Retrouvey et al., 2012). Lopes et al. (1991) reported an incidence of supernumerary teeth in 16% of individuals with cleft palate.

Whether the presence of adults with cleft palate in the past can provide evidence for social or parental investment in the individual's care depends on the severity of the condition, any additional skeletal defects, and the extent to which the hard palate is affected. Medical studies have shown children with either a cleft lip or a cleft palate can suckle successfully, whereas those with a combined cleft lip and palate need support to feed (Clarren et al., 1987). A differential diagnosis for cleft palate is a midline cyst, which will have an oval central shape, rather than on an opening one side or the other (Ortner, 2003). Attempts to repair a cleft lip ("harelip") or palate are known from China in AD 340, when soft tissue was stitched together. In the Leech Book of Bald (AD 920), the edges were excised and sewn together with silk, and covered with a red ointment. Paré introduced the use of thin silver or gold plates to bridge a cleft palate, with the first successful surgery of a hard palate carried out by Dieffenbach in 1828 (Kim, 2000). The surgical examples include children, but in most cases the operation involved repairing the surrounding soft tissue and would not be visible in skeletal remains. However, occasionally a surgeon is described as cutting away bone when the maxilla was deformed and projecting (Kim, 2000).

Several cases of cleft lip and/or palate have been identified in children from archeological contexts (Brothwell, 1967; Connell et al., 2012; Hegyi et al., 2002, 2003, 2004, p.133; Lewis, 2013; Liston and Rotroff, 2013). None of these cases are of the severest form, although the unilateral cleft palate with associated cleft atlas from later medieval St Mary Spital in London is one of the most well preserved (Connell et al., 2012, p. 133). In many cases, the palate is affected at the anterior margin (facial cleft resulting in a cleft lip), and in the case of the child from St Oswald's Priory in Gloucester, the dental changes (i.e., overcrowding, maleruption, supernumerary macrodont) were the first indication that a mild anterior cleft palate/lip may be present (Lewis, 2013). Liston and Rotroff (2013) present remarkable evidence for cleft palate in a series of infants from a well in an Athenian Agora. Of the 164 infants recovered, 9 (5.4%) of the full-term babies had evidence for malformed maxillae (Fig. 2.23), and it was suggested that their poor prospect of survival singled them out for disposal. Liston and Rotroff's (2013) case study shows how careful observation can reveal congenital defects in the tiniest of remains.

Other Facial Clefts

Cleft mandibles are rare malformations caused by developmental delay in mesenchymal growth at the ventral aspect of the mandible (Barnes, 1994). Hegyi et al. (2004) reported a partial cleft mandible in a child from 10th- to 12th-century Hungary (Fig. 2.24). Previously, Hegyi et al. (2002) had reported a case of nasal bone aplasia associated with cleft lip and palate in a medieval child from Csengele-Bogárhát, Hungary. Normally, each nasal bone is ossified in the third fetal month from one center in the membrane overlying the cartilaginous nasal capsule (Fig. 2.25).

Spina Bifida

There are two basic forms of this condition: spina bifida cystic and spina bifida occulta ("hidden"). Spina bifida cystica comes in a variety of forms, including protrusion of the nerve roots and meninges within a fluid sac (meningocele). This sac is covered by a layer of skin in 5% of cases, but in 60% of cases the spinal cord is left exposed (meningomyelocele) leading to infection (Sheldon, 1943). Most infants born with meningomyelocele will die shortly after birth. In contrast, individuals with spina bifida cystica with a minor meningocele can survive without symptoms into adulthood. The occulta form describes incomplete fusion of the posterior neural arches, mainly but not exclusively in the sacral and/or lumbar segments (Barnes, 1994). This form is usually asymptomatic, and in life the only evidence of the defect may be a dimple or a tuft of hair overlying the site. First described by von Recklinghausen in 1882, spina bifida occulta is one of the most common forms of neural tube defect and is thought to be present in around 5%–10% of the population. Males are more often affected than females, and many genetic and environmental factors have been associated with the condition, including maternal deficiencies in folic acid, vitamin B12, zinc, or selenium (Barnes, 1994).

In archeological remains, several adjacent neural arches need to be open before a diagnosis of spina bifida occulta

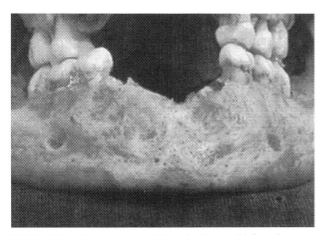

FIGURE 2.24 Cleft in the mandible of a 6-year-old from Szatymaz-Vasútállomás, Hungary (10th to 12th century AD, skeleton 146). *From Hegyi, A., Marcsik, A., Kocsis, G., 2004. Frequency of developmental anomalies on the skull and the axial skeleton from the archaeological periods (Hungary). Journal of Paleopathology 16 (1), 20.*

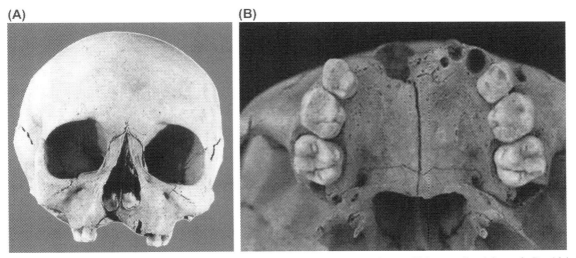

FIGURE 2.25 Aplasia of the (A) nasal bone and (B) associated cleft lip and palate in a 5- to 10-year-old from medieval Csengele-Bogárhát, Szegred, Hungary (skeleton 114). *From Hegyi, A., Marcsik, A., Kocsis, G., 2004. Frequency of developmental anomalies on the skull and the axial skeleton from the archaeological periods (Hungary). Journal of Paleopathology 16 (1), 20; and Hegyi, A., Marcsik, A., Kocsis, G., 2002. Developmental disorders of nasal bones in human osteoarchaeological samples. Journal of Paleopathology 14 (3), 117.*

is made, this is because the first, fourth, and/or fifth sacral neural arches often remain open in normal development (Roberts and Manchester, 2007). In addition, diagnosis can only been made in individuals over 15 years of age, when the sacrum would normally be completely fused. Cases of spina bifida cystica with meningomyelocele would likely only be identified in perinatal and infant material through careful examination of the unfused neural arches that may be altered in shape in response to pressure from the fluid-filled sac (Barnes, 1994, p. 49). In older children, there may be limb atrophy due to paralysis, an underdeveloped pelvis, hydrocephalus, or hemivertebrae and scoliosis (Ortner, 2003). To date, only two cases of possible spina bifida cystica have been described in nonadult skeletal remains. Dickel and Doran (1989) describe spina bifida of the neural arch from L3 to S2 and scoliosis in a 14- to 16-year-old from the Windover Site in Florida. The slight lateral spread of the marginal neural arches suggests the presence of a soft tissue cyst. The child also had a severe infection of the right tibia and fibula, and disuse atrophy of the long bones. Cone-shaped epiphyses were also evident and may indicate the child suffered from liver or kidney problems. The meningocele form of cystica would account for the individual's survival into adolescence (Fig. 2.26). The second case, described by Castro de la Mata and Bonavia (1980), is of a 6-year-old from the Peruvian coast with an open L5 and L6 and S1 to S5, as well as sacralization of a sixth lumbar vertebra. Three other nonadult cases of spina bifida also describe associated sacralization of a sixth lumbar vertebra (Bennett, 1972) or L5 (Papageorgopoulou and Xirotiris, 2009), and at Litten cemetery in Berkshire, England, a 15- to 16-year-old was recovered with an extra lumbar vertebra and spina bifida of L1 to L6 and the entire sacrum (Clough and Hardy, 2006).

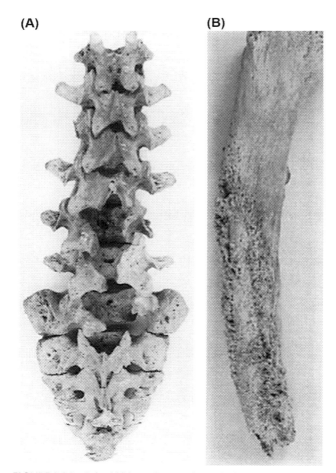

FIGURE 2.26 Spina bifida cystica (meningocele) in a 15- to 16-year-old from Windover Pond, Florida (7500 BP). (A) The neural arches have failed to form from L3 to S2. The splayed nature of the surviving neural elements suggests pressure from a cyst in life. (B) The right tibia shows active new bone formation and disuse atrophy. *From Dickel, D., Doran, G., 1989. Severe neural tube defect syndrome from the early archaic of Florida. American Journal of Physical Anthropology 80, 327–328.*

REFERENCES

Angle, C., McIntire, M., Moore, R., 1967. Cloverleaf skull: Kleeblattschädel-deformity. Archives of Pediatric and Adolescent Medicine 114 (2), 198–202.

Aufderheide, A.C., 2003. The Scientific Study of Mummies. Cambridge University Press, Cambridge.

Aufderheide, A.C., Rodriguez-Martín, C., 1998. The Cambridge Encyclopedia of Human Paleopathology. Cambridge University Press, Cambridge.

Balkany, T., Mischke, R., Downs, M., Jafek, B., 1979. Ossicular abnormalities in Down's syndrome. Otolaryngology Head Neck Surgery 87, 372–384.

Barnes, E., 1994. Developmental Defects of the Axial Skeleton in Palaeopathology. University of Colorado Press, Colorado.

Bennett, K., 1967. Craniostenosis: a review of the etiology and a report of new cases. American Journal of Physical Anthropology 27, 1–10.

Bennett, K., 1972. Lumbo-sacral malformations and spina bifida occulta in a group of proto-historic Modoc Indians. American Journal of Physical Anthropology 36, 435–440.

Benson, M., Oliverio, P., Yue, N., Zinreich, S., 1995. Primary craniosynostosis: imaging features. American Journal of Radiology 166, 697–703.

Black, S., Scheuer, L., 1996. Occipitalization of the atlas with reference to its embryological development. International Journal of Osteoarchaeology 6, 189–194.

Black, S., Scheuer, L., 1997. The ontogenetic development of the cervical rib. International Journal of Osteoarchaeology 7, 2–10.

Blau, S., 2005. An unusual aperture in a child's calvaria from western central Asia: differential diagnosis. International Journal of Osteoarchaeology 15, 291–297.

Bolk, L., 1915. On the premature obliteration of sutures in the human skull. American Journal of Anatomy 17 (4), 495–523.

Bots, J., Wijnaendts, L., Delen, S., Van Dongen, S., Heikinheimo, K., Galis, F., 2011. Analysis of cervical ribs in a series of human fetuses. Journal of Anatomy 219, 403–409.

Brothwell, D., 1967. Major congenital anomalies of the skeleton: evidence from earlier populations. In: Brothwell, D., Sandison, A. (Eds.), Diseases in Antiquity: A Survey of Diseases, Injuries and Surgery of Early Populations. Charles C. Thomas, Springfield, pp. 423–443.

Brothwell, D., Powers, R., 2000. The human biology. In: Rathtz, P., Hirst, S., Wright, S. (Eds.), Cannington Cemetery. English Heritage, London.

Brues, A., 1946. Alkali Ridge skeletons, pathology and anomaly. In: Brew, J. (Ed.), Archaeology of Alkali Ridge, Southeastern Utah. Harvard Press, Cambridge.

Caffey, J., 1945. Pediatric X-Ray Diagnosis. Year Book Medical Publishers, Inc., Chicago.

Campillo, D., 2005. Paleoradiology II. Congenital and hereditary malformations of the skeleton. Journal of Paleopathology 17 (2), 45–64.

Case, D., Hill, R., Merbs, C., Fong, M., 2006. Polydactyly in the prehistoric American Southwest. International Journal of Osteoarchaeology 16, 221–235.

Castilla, E., López-Camelo, J.S., Campaña, H., Rittler, M., 2001. Epidemiological methods to assess the correlation between industrial contaminants and rates of congenital anomalies. Mutation Research 489, 123–145.

Castro de la Mata, R., Bonavia, D., 1980. Lumbosacral malformations and spina bifida in a Peruvian preceramic child. Current Anthropology 21 (4), 515–516.

Charon, P., 2004. Contribution to osteo-archaeological knowledge of anencephaly. Journal of Paleopathology 16 (1), 5–13.

Chemke, J., Robinson, A., 1969. The third fontanelle. The Journal of Pediatrics 75 (4), 617–622.

Clarren, S., Anderson, B., Wolf, L., 1987. Feeding infants with cleft lip, cleft palate, or cleft lip and palate. Cleft Palate Journal 24 (3), 244–249.

Clough, S., Boyle, A., 2010. Inhumations and disarticulated human bone. In: Booth, P., Simmonds, S., Boyle, A., Clough, S., Cool, H., Poore, D. (Eds.), The Late Roman Cemetery at Lankhills, Winchester Excavations 2000-2005. Oxford Archaeology Ltd., Oxford, pp. 339–403.

Clough, S., Hardy, A., 2006. The Litten Cemetery, Newbury, Berkshire. Archaeological Excavation Report for West Berkshire Council. Oxford Archaeology, Oxford.

Cohen, M., 2005. Perspectives on craniosynostosis. American Journal of Medical Genetics 136A, 313–326.

Cohen, M., Krelborg, s, 1992. Birth prevalence studies of the Crouzon syndrome: comparison of direct and indirect methods. Clinical Genetics 41 (1), 12–15.

Connell, B., Gray Jones, A., Redfern, R., Walker, D., 2012. A Bioarchaeological Study of Medieval Burials on the Site of St Mary Spital. Museum of London Archaeology, London.

Davidson, J., Cleary, A., Bruce, C., 2008. Disorders of bones, joints and connective tissues. In: McIntosh, N., Helms, P., Smyth, R., Logan, S. (Eds.), Forfar & Arneil's Textbook of Pediatrics. Elsevier, Edinburgh, pp. 1385–1447.

Dickel, D., Doran, G., 1989. Severe neural tube defect syndrome from the early archaic of Florida. American Journal of Physical Anthropology 80, 325–334.

Dudar, J., 2010. Qualitative and quantitative diagnosis of lethal cranial neural tube defects from the fetal and neonatal human skeleton, with a case study involving taphonomically altered remains. Journal of Forensic Science 55 (4), 877–883.

Duncan, W., Stojanowski, C., 2008. A case of squamosal craniosynostosis from 16th century Southeastern United States. International Journal of Osteoarchaeology 18, 407–420.

Farwell, D.E., Molleson, T.I., 1993. Excavations at Poundbury 1966-80 Volume II: The Cemeteries. Dorset Natural History and Archaeological Society, Dorset.

Freeman, S., Taft, L., Dooley, K., Allran, K., Sherman, S., Hassold, T., Khoury, M., Saker, D., 1998. Population-based study of congenital heart defects in Down Syndrome. American Journal of Medical Genetics 80, 213–217.

Furtado, L., Thaker, H., Erickson, L., Shirts, B., Opitz, J., 2011. Cervical ribs are more prevalent in stillborn fetuses than in live-born infants and are strongly associated with fetal aneuploidy. Pediatric and Developmental Pathology 14 (6), 431–437.

Galdames, I., Zavando, M., Russo, P., 2009. Craniofacial asymmetries in subadults with hydrocephalus. International Journal of Odontostomat 3 (2), 163–166.

Garlie, T., Merrett, D., Meiklejohn, C., Finch, D., Waddell, B., 2002. Analysis of a foot deformity from a Laurel period (ca. 2000 BP) site in southeastern Manitoba: evidence for clubfoot. American Journal of Physical Anthropology (Suppl. 34), 75.

Gerszten, P.C., Gerszten, E., Allison, M.J., 2001. Diseases of the spine in South American mummies. Neurosurgery 48 (1), 208–213.

Gholve, P.A., Hosalkar, H.S., Ricchetti, E.T., Pollock, A.N., Dormans, J.P., Drummond, D.S., 2007. Occipitalization of the atlas in children. The Journal of Bone and Joint Surgery 89 (3), 571–578.

Giuffra, V., Bianucci, R., Milanese, M., Fornaciari, G., 2013. A probable case of non-syndromic brachycephaly from 16th century Sardinia (Italy). International Journal of Paleopathology 3, 134–137.

Goode-Nell, S., Shujja, K., Rankin-Hill, L., 2004. Subadult growth and development. In: Blakey, M.L., Rankin-Hill, L. (Eds.). Blakey, M.L., Rankin-Hill, L. (Eds), The New York African Burial Ground Skeletal Biology Final Report, vol. 1. Howard University for the United States General: Services Administration Northeast and Caribbean Region, Washington, DC, pp. 461–513.

Gracia, A., Arsuaga, J., Martinez, I., Lorenzo, C., Carretero, J., Bermúdez de Castro, J., Carbonell, E., 2009. Craniosynostosis in the Middle Pleistocene human cranium 14 from the Sima de los Huesos, Atapuerca, Spain. Proceedings of the National Academy of Sciences 106 (16), 6573–6578.

Guille, J., Sherk, H., 2002. Congenital osseous anomalies of the upper and lower cervical spine in children. Journal of Bone and Joint Surgery 84-A (2), 277–288.

Hegyi, A., Marcsik, A., Kocsis, G., 2002. Developmental disorders of nasal bones in human osteoarchaeological samples. Journal of Paleopathology 14 (3), 113–119.

Hegyi, A., Marcsik, A., Kocsis, G., 2003. Developmental disorders of nasal bones in human osteoarchaeological samples. Journal of Paleopathology 15 (2), 91–96.

Hegyi, A., Marcsik, A., Kocsis, G., 2004. Frequency of developmental anomalies on the skull and the axial skeleton from the archaeological periods (Hungary). Journal of Paleopathology 16 (1), 15–25.

Held, P., Schultz, M., Alt, K.W., 2010. Hydrocephalus in an 18th century subadult from Volklingen, Germany. In: Proceedings of the XVII European Meeting of the Paleopathology Association, p. 65.

Hershkovitz, I., Latimer, B., Dutour, O., Jellema, L., Wish-Baratz, S., Rothschild, C., Rothschild, B., 1997. Why do we fail in aging the skull from the sagittal suture? American Journal of Physical Anthropology 103 (3), 393–399.

Hinkes, M., 1983. Skeletal Evidence of Stress in Subadults: Trying to Come of Age at Grasshopper Pueblo. University of Arizona, Arizona.

Hollowell, J., Hannon, W., 1997. Teraogen update: iodine deficiency, a community teratogen. Teratology 55, 389–405.

Hrdlička, A., 1918. Skull of a midget from Peru. American Journal of Physical Anthropology 30, 77–81.

Hrdlička, A., 1938. Seven prehistoric American skulls with complete absence of external auditory meatus. American Journal of Physical Anthropology 92 (3), 355–377.

IPDTOC Working Group, 2011. Prevalence at birth of cleft lip with or without cleft palate: data from the international perinatal database of typical oral clefts (IPDTOC). Cleft Palate-Craniofacial Journal 48 (1), 66–81.

Irurita, J., Alemán, I., Viciano, J., López-Lázaro, S., Botella, M.C., 2015. Alterations of skull bones found in anencephalic skeletons from an identified osteological collection. Two case reports. International Journal of Legal Medicine 129 (4), 903–912.

Jabs, E., 1998. Towards understanding the pathogenesis of craniosynostosis through clinical and molecular correlates. Clinical Genetics 53, 79–86.

Jane, J., Lin, K., Jane, J.S., 2000. Saggital synostosis. Neurosurgery Focus 9 (3), 1–6.

Johanson, C., Duncan III, J., Klinge, P., Brinker, T., Stopa, E., Silverberg, G., 2008. Multiplicity of cerebrospinal fluid functions: new challenges in health and disease. Cerebrospinal Fluid Research 5 (10), 1–32.

Johnson, L., Kerley, E., 1974. Appendix B: report on pathological specimens from Mokapu. In: Snow, C. (Ed.), Early Hawaiians: An Initial Study of Skeletal Remains from Makapu, Oahu. The University of Kentucky Press, Lexington, pp. 149–158.

Kalter, H., 2003. Teratology in the 20th century. Environmental causes of congenital malformations in humans and how they were established. Neurotoxicology and Teratology 5546, 131–283.

Kaplan, K.M., Spivak, J.M., Bendo, J.A., 2005. Embryology of the spine and associated congenital abnormalities. The Spine Journal 5 (5), 564–576.

Kato, K., Shinoda, K., Kitagawa, Y., Manabe, Y., Oyamada, J., Igawa, K., Vidal, H., Rokutanda, A., 2007. A possible case of prophylactic supra-inion trepanation in a child cranium with an auditory deformity (pre-Columbian Ancon site, Peru). Anthropological Science 115, 227–232.

Keenleyside, A., 2011. Congenital aural atresia in an adult female from Apolloiona Pontica, Bulgaria. International Journal of Paleopathology 1 (1), 63–67.

Khanna, P., Thapa, M., Prasad, S., 2011. Pictorial essay: the many faces of craniosynostosis. Indian Journal of Radiology and Imaging 21 (1), 49–56.

Kim, S., 2000. A rosebud by any other name: the history of cleft lip and palate repair. In: Whitelaw, W. (Ed.), Proceedings of the 9th Annual History of Medicine Days. University of Calgary, Calgary, pp. 42–58.

Krakow, D., Lachman, R., Rimoin, D., 2009. Guidelines for the prenatal diagnosis of fetal dysplasias. Genetic Medicine 11 (2), 127–133.

Kreutz, K., Teichmann, G., Schultz, M., 1995. Palaeoepidemiology of inflammatory processes of the skull: a comparative study of two early medieval infant populations. Journal of Paleopathology 7 (2), 108.

Laes, C., 2011. Silent witnesses: deaf-mutes in Greco-Roman antiquity. Classical World 104 (4), 451–473.

Laurence, K., Coates, S., 1962. The natural history of hydrocephalus. Detailed analysis of 182 unoperated cases. Archives of Diseases in Childhood 37, 345–362.

Lewis, M., 2008. The children. In: Magilton, J., Lee, F., Boylston, A. (Eds.). Magilton, J., Lee, F., Boylston, A. (Eds.), Chichester Excavations 'Lepers Outside the Gate' Excavations at the Cemetery of the Hospital of St James and St Mary Magdalene, Chichester, 1986-87 and 1993, vol. 10. Council for British Archaeology Research Report, 158, York, pp. 174–186.

Lewis, M., 2013. Children of the Golden Minster: St Oswald's Priory and the impact of industrialisation on child health. Journal of Anthropology:959472. http://dx.doi.org/10.1155/2013/959472.

Liston, M., Rotroff, S., 2013. Babies in the well: archaeological evidence for newborn disposal in Hellenistic Greece. In: Evans Grubbs, J., Parkin, T., Bell, R. (Eds.), The Oxford Handbook of Childhood and Education in the Classical World. Oxford University Press, Oxford, pp. 62–83.

Lloyd-Roberts, G., Lettin, A., 1970. Arthrogryposis multiplex congenita. The Journal of Bone and Joint Surgery 52B (3), 494–508.

Lopes, L., Mattos, B., Andre, M., 1991. Anomalies in number of teeth in patients with lip and/or palate clefts. Brazilian Dental Journal 2 (1), 9–17.

Lorrio, A.J., 2010. Enterramientos infantiles en el oppidum en El Mólon (Camporrobles, Valencia). Cuadernos de Arqueología de la Universidad de Navarra 18, 201–262.

Manchester, K., 1980. Hydrocephalus in an Anglo-Saxon child from Eccles. Archaeologia Cantiana 96, 77–82.

Mann, R., Owsley, D., 1989. Anatomy of an uncorrected talipes equinovarus in a fifteenth-century American Inasian. Journal of the American Podiatric Medical Association 79 (9), 436–440.

Masnicová, S., Beňuš, R., 2003. Developmental anomalies in skeletal remains from the great Moravia and middle ages cemeteries at Delvín (Slovakia). International Journal of Osteoarchaeology 13, 266–274.

McAlister, W., Herman, T., 2005. Osteochondroplasias, dysostoses, chromosomal aberrations, mucopolysaccharidoses, and mucolipidoses. In: Resnick, D., Kransdorf, M. (Eds.), Bone and Joint Imaging. Elsevier Saunders, Philidelphia, pp. 1225–1298.

McKinley, J., 2008. Human remains. In: Mercer, R., Healy, F. (Eds.). Mercer, R., Healy, F. (Eds.), Hambledon Hill, Dorset, England Excavations and Survey of a Neolithic Monument Complex and Its Surrounding Landscape, vol. II. English Heritage, London, pp. 477–521.

McRae, D., Barum, A., 1953. Occipitalization of the atlas. American Journal of Roentgenology 70, 23–46.

Merbs, C., 2004. Sagittal clefting of the body and other vertebral developmental errors in Canadian Inuit skeletons. American Journal of Physical Anthropology 123, 236–249.

Meyer, C., Ruhli, F., Nicklisch, N., Weber, J., Alt, K., 2006. Beaten copper cranium-hyperostosis frontalis interna-craniosynostosis. Endocranial changes in a 17th century AD population from Hanau, Germany. In: Proceedings of the 16th Paleopathology Association European Meeting. Santorini, p. 90.

Moore, K.L., 1988. Essentials of Human Embryology. B.C. Decker Inc, Totonto.

Moore, K., Persaud, T., 2008. The Developing Human. Saunders, Philadelphia.

Morse, D., 1978. Ancient Disease in the Midwest. Ilinois State Museum, Springfield.

Müller, F., O'Rahilly, R., Benson, D., 1986. The early origins of vertebral anomalies, as illustrated by a 'butterfly vertebra'. Journal of Anatomy 149, 157–169.

Murphy, E.M., 1996. A possible case of hydrocephalus in a medieval child from Doonbought Fort, Co. Antrim, Northern Ireland. International Journal of Osteoarchaeology 6, 435–442.

Oostra, R.-J., van der Wolk, S., Maas, M., Hennekam, R., 2005. Malformations of the axial skeleton in the Museum Vrolik II: craniostenosis and suture related conditions. American Journal of Medical Genetics 136A, 327–342.

Orkar, K., Ugwu, B., Momoh, J., 2002. Cleft lip and palate: the Jos experience. East African Medical Journal 79 (10), 510–513.

Ortner, D., 2003. Identification of Pathological Conditions in Human Skeletal Remains. Academic Press, New York.

Ozonoff, M., 2005. Spinal deformities and curvatures. In: Resnick, D., Kransdorf, M. (Eds.), Bone and Joint Imaging, third ed. Elsevier Saunders, Philadelphia, pp. 1326–1334.

Panzer, S., Cohen, M.N., Esch, U., Nerlich, A., Zink, A., 2008. Radiological evidence of Goldenhar syndrome in a paleopathological case from a South German ossuary. HOMO-Journal of Comparative Human Biology 59, 453–461.

Papageorgopoulou, C., Xirotiris, N.I., 2009. Anthropological research on a Byzantine population from Korytiani, west Greece. Hesperia Supplements 43, 193–221.

Partington, M., Gonzales-Crussi, F., Khakee, S., Wollin, D., 1971. Cloverleaf skull and thanatophoric dwarfism. Report of four cases, two in the same sibship. Archives of Disease in Childhood 46, 656–664.

Peabody, C., 1927. Congenital malformation of spine. Journal of Bone and Joint Surgery 9, 79–83.

Pedersen, S., Anton, S., 1998. Bicoronal synostosis in a child from historic Omaha cemetery 25DK10. American Journal of Physical Anthropology 105, 369–376.

Phillips, S., Sivilich, M., 2006. Cleft palate: a case of disability and survival in prehistoric North America. International Journal of Osteoarchaeology 16, 528–535.

Pretorius, D., Davis, K., Manco-Johnson, M., Manchester, D., Meier, P., Clewell, W., 1985. Clinical course of fetal hydrocephalus: 40 cases. American Journal of Radiology 144, 827–831.

Prokopec, M., Simpson, D., Morris, L., Pretty, G., 1984. Craniostenosis in a prehistoric aboriginal skull: a case report. OSSA-International Journal of Skeletal Research 9 (11), 111–118.

Retrouvey, J.-M., Goldberg, M., Schwartz, S., 2012. Dental development and maturation, from the dental crypt to the final occlusion. In: Glorieux, F., Pettifor, J., Jüppner, H. (Eds.), Pediatric Bone. Academic Press, London, pp. 83–108.

Richards, G., 1985. Analysis of a microcephalic child from the late period (ca. 1100-17 AD) of central California. American Journal of Physical Anthropology 68, 343–357.

Richards, G., Anton, S., 1991. Craniofacial configuration and postcranial development of a hydrocephalic child (ca. 2500 BC-500 AD): with a review of cases and comment on diagnostic criteria. American Journal of Physical Anthropology 85, 185–200.

Roberts, C.A., Manchester, K., 2007. The Archaeology of Disease, Cornell University Press, Cornell.

Roberts, C., Knusel, C., Race, L., 2004. A foot deformity from a Romano-British cemetery at Gloucester, England, and the current evidence for Talipes in palaeopathology. International Journal of Osteoarchaeology 14, 389–403.

Saint-Hillaire, G., 1826. Note about an Egyptian monster found in the ruins of Thebes, in Egypt, by M. Passalascqua. Bulletin des Sciences Medicales 7, 105–108.

Sampson, P., Streissguth, A., Bookstein, F., Little, R., Clarren, S., Dehaene, P., Hanson, J., Graham, J., 1997. Incidence of fetal alcohol syndrome and prevalence of alcohol related neurodevelopment disorders. Teratology 56, 317–326.

Scheuer, L., Black, S., 2000. Developmental Juvenile Osteology. Academic Press, London.

Senator, M., Gronkiewicz, S., 2012. Anthropological analysis of the phenomenon of atlas occipitalisation exemplified by a skull from Twardogora (17th c.) – Southern Poland. International Journal of Osteoarchaeology 22, 749–754.

Sheldon, W., 1943. Diseases of Infancy and Childhood. J. & A. Churchill Ltd., London.

Tillier, A.-M., Arensburg, B., Duday, H., Vandermeersch, B., 2001. Brief communication: an early case of hydrocephalus: the middle Paleolithic Qafzeh 12 child. American Journal of Physical Anthropology 114, 166–170.

Tomasto-Cagigao, E., 2011. A holoprosencephaly (cyclopia) case from the Nasca culture, Peru. In: Palaeopathology Association Meeting in South America IV. Lima, Peru, p. 52.

Travan, L., Saccheri, P., Toso, F., Crivellato, E., 2013. Congenital axis dysmorphism in a medieval skeleton. Child's Nervous System 29, 707–712.

Tun, K., Okutan, O., Kaptanoglu, E., Gok, B., Solaroglu, I., Beskonakli, E., 2004. Inverted hypertrophy of occipital condyles associated with atlantooccipital fusion and basilar invagination: a case report. Neuroanatomy 3, 43–45.

van den Bos, R., Vielvoye, G., Blickman, J., 1984. Vertebral anomalies in monozygotic twins. Diagnostic Imaging in Clinical Medicine 53, 259–261.

von Recklinghausen, R., 1882. Ueber die Multiplen Fibrome der Haut und ihre Beziehung zu den Multiplen Neuromen. Hirschwald, Berlin.

Waisbrod, H., 1973. Congenital club foot. The Journal of Bone and Joint Surgery 55B (4), 796–801.

Waldron, T., 2007. St Peter's, Barton-upon-Humber, Lincolnshire. The Human Remains, vol. 2. Oxbow Books, Oxford.

Waldron, T., 2009. Palaeopathology. Cambridge University Press, Cambridge.

Walker, J., 1991. Musculoskeletal development: a review. Physical Therapy 71 (12), 878–889.

Walker, D., 2012. Disease in London, 1st-19th Centuries. Museum of London Archaeology, London.

Webb, S., 1995. Paleopathology of Aboriginal Australians. Cambridge University Press, Cambridge.

Wolff, K., Bernert, Z., Balassa, T., Szeniczey, T., Kiss, C., Hajdu, T., 2014. Two suture craniosynostoses: a presentation that needs to be noted. Journal of Craniofacial Surgery 25 (2), 714–715.

Wright, L., 2011. Bilateral talipes equinovarus from Tikal, Guatemala. International Journal of Paleopathology 1 (1), 55–62.

Wyszynski, D. (Ed.), 2002. Cleft Lip and Palate: From Origin to Treatment. Oxford University Press, New York.

Zink, A., Freisinger, P., Nerlich, A., 2006. Craniosynostosis in an Egyptian skeleton from the early dynastic period. In: Proceedings of the 16th Paleopathology Association European Meeting. Santorini, p. 132.

Chapter 3

Congenital Conditions II: Skeletal Dysplasias and Other Syndromes

Chapter Outline

Introduction	45
Skeletal Dysplasias	46
Achondroplasia	46
Acromesomelia	48
Mesomelia	48
Thanatophoric Dwarfism	48
Developmental Dysplasia of the Hip and Congenital Hip Dislocation	49
Metaphyseal Dysplasia (Pyle's Disease)	52
Fibrous Dysplasia	53
Congenital Syndromes	53
Binder Syndrome (Maxillonasal Dysplasia)	53
Klippel–Feil Syndrome	55
Down Syndrome (Trisomy 21) and Other Aneuploid Conditions	57
Osteogenesis Imperfecta	60
Osteopetrosis (Osteosclerosis Fragilis)	61
Cerebral Palsy	63
References	64

INTRODUCTION

The complex nature of congenital conditions means that in many cases they have little to tell us about environmental conditions of the past. The survival and burial of these unusual individuals may have more to contribute to our understanding of the treatment and care they experienced. Unfortunately, many case studies presented in the paleopathological literature are based on single crania or museum collections discovered out of their burial context. Where we do have burial records, the treatment of physically impaired children is rarely out of the ordinary, or their burial appears to have been prepared with greater attention to detail. For example, the deaf–mute child from Poundbury Camp, Dorset (Chapter 2), was among several individuals buried prone, none of the other skeletons had any pathologies to suggest this was the usual mode of burial for physically distinctive individuals. On the contrary, the child was given a cist burial, and slabs across the top of the grave suggest extra investment in their interment. The mummified child with osteogenesis imperfecta described by Gray (1969) was buried in a decorated coffin in the shape of Osiris, and Panzer et al.'s (2008) Goldenhar child was an isolated skull selected for secondary burial in an ossuary, deposited along with many others during clearance of a community cemetery. The severely disabled child with spina bifida cystic and subsequent paralysis described by Dickel and Doran (1989) was not afforded any special treatment. By contrast a less severely affected child with spina bifida recovered by Castro De la Mata (1980) was found within a specially dug pit, and covered with refuse material. While this may have the appearance of a derogatory grave, a necklace of seashells, cloth wrapping, and offerings between the child's feet suggest the view of the child may not have been a negative one. The two possible cases of Down syndrome in the United Kingdom, both from the early medieval period, were found in what are considered to be early hospital sites. While the reason for this is unlikely to have been to provide medical treatment, they seemed to have been singled out for charitable care. These examples suggest that societies in the past reacted differently toward individuals with physical impairments, and understanding the norms and values of human reaction at different times and in different places needs to be carried out with regard to additional iconographic, historical, and ethnographic information (Roberts, 2000).

Tilley (2012) presents a four-stage analytical approach to inferring the level of care an individual with a physical impairment may have received in the past which requires: (1) a detailed description of all lesions and possible diagnosis; (2) interpretation of the clinical and functional impact of the condition; (3) an assessment of the level of support required (e.g., resource demands, number of individuals involved); and (4) drawing together stages 1–3 to suggest the attitudes to caregiving in the community. Tilley (2012) describes care as being direct support for the impairment and/or accommodation for the individual's physical disability as they recover. Of course in cases of congenital deformities, while the individual may adapt, they will never recover, and their symptoms may become progressively worse as they age. The study of children with congenital conditions in particular may elucidate such attitudes in the past. A child with congenital hip dysplasia will be born without any outward signs of disease, but will gradually become more disabled as they grow. How society or a parent reacts to such young vulnerable individuals may be particularly telling. A survey of 260 cases of congenital disease in children from all periods across the world recorded in the published and unpublished literature revealed 49 individuals who would have been "physically distinctive" (e.g., polydactyly, short neck, cleft palate, deafness, club foot, and restricted movement). Of these, 18% (n=9) died before they were 3 years old, while a large number (n=23) of individuals survived into adolescence with a variety of physical impairments including club foot, Down syndrome, long-term paralysis, hip dislocations, cleft palate, and cranial malformations (Lewis, 2016). Looked at one way, this would imply social acceptance, but the fact that so many of the individuals died on the threshold of adulthood raises an interesting question. Were these individuals no longer cared for when they lost their protective "child" status? Of course, this may simply be a reflection of the dataset, which only includes individuals up to 17 years of age, and there are multiple cases of adults with limb paralysis in the archeological literature (Hawkey, 1998; Oxenham et al., 2009; Walker, 2012, p. 22). The following sections outline the diagnostic criteria for skeletal dysplasias and syndromes that have the potential to be recognized in a child's remains from archeological contexts and touches on some of the issues above.

SKELETAL DYSPLASIAS

There are several hundred forms of skeletal dysplasias which result from genetic mutations (Waldron, 2009). Today, skeletal dysplasia is rare with an incidence of 3.22 per 10,000 births (Stoll et al., 1989). A quarter of these are stillborn and another third die in infancy (Waldron, 2009), meaning that many of these conditions may only be recognized in perinatal and infant skeletal remains. Dysplasias are identified by an abnormal shape or size of the skeleton, an increase or decrease in the number of skeletal elements, and/or an abnormal bone texture due to disrupted bone mineralization and deposition (Waldron, 2009). Shortening of the extremities is a common feature, with a normal spine but shortened ribs resulting in a narrow thorax (Waldron, 2009, p. 198). Limb dysplasias are classified as follows:

1. Micromelic—shortening of whole limb
2. Rhizomelic—shortening of proximal segment (humerus, femur)
3. Mesomelic—shortening of middle limb segments (radius–ulna, tibia–fibula)
4. Acromelic—shortening of distal segment (hands, feet)

Today, the two most common types of skeletal dysplasia are achondroplasia and osteogenesis imperfecta (Stoll et al., 1989), with achondroplasia also the most common form of dwarfism identified in the archeological record.

"Dwarfism" is a term used to describe an individual with abnormally short stature (normally below 4 foot 10 inches or 147 cm in an adult). There are over 350 distinct forms, with achondroplasia and pituitary dwarfism (Chapter 10) being the most common (Krakow et al., 2009). The social treatment of dwarfs in past society has received much attention, and there is evidence to suggest they were often treated with veneration. For example, dwarfs appear in the art of Velasquez and Van Dyke and in the Royal courts of Spain. In England, the dwarfed figure of Turold, a Royal accountant is included on the Bayeux Tapestry, and the Egyptian gods Ptah and Bes were depicted as dwarfs (Kozma, 2008). Dawson (1938) also identified numerous images of achondroplasia in an elite tomb in Egypt. However, caution is advised when interpreting all diminutive figures as dwarfs, as in some artistic styles short stature is used to depict individuals of lower status, or children (Dasen, 1990; Dawson, 1938).

Achondroplasia

Achondroplasia is the most common of the nonlethal skeletal dysplasia. It is an autosomal dominant condition that results from a defect in the fibroblast growth factor receptor 3 gene located on chromosome 4p (Waldron, 2009). The modern incidence is 1 per 10,000 births (Roberts and Manchester, 2007). The term "achondroplasia" was first introduced by Parrot in 1876 to describe dwarflike features evident in fetuses with normal skulls but distinctive changes to their long bones (Harris, 1933, p. 153). As the name suggests, the condition is characterized by defective endochondral ossification affecting the limbs and cranial base, with normal intramembranous ossification of the skull vault, face, and clavicle. The short skull base results in a depressed nasal bridge and shortened facial area, while the long bones are shortened resulting in a disproportionate skeleton. Being the fastest growing, the femur is most severely affected, followed by the humerus, lower legs, and forearms (Ortner, 2003). Although the diaphyses form normally, the epiphyses can become "cone-shaped" and the metaphyses flared, while the fibula is generally longer than the tibia, and all the long bones appear thicker and shorter than normal (Harris, 1933; Nehme et al., 1975). Individuals usually only attain a height of around 130 cm. As the bodies of the spine form intramembranously, but the pedicles rely on endochondral expansion, the interpedicular spaces of the lumbar vertebrae fail to increase distally resulting in flattened, "bullet-shaped" vertebrae. As the child gets older, the vertebral bodies display posterior concavity and anterior edging, restricting the neural canal (Resnick and Kransdorf, 2005). The physical appearance of an achondroplastic is of prominent rhizomelia, with short hands, a brachycephalic skull, frontal bossing, a narrow foramen magnum, depressed nasal bridge, short vertebrae, squared iliac bones with a flat acetabular angle and a narrow sciatic notch, restricted neural canals (stenosis), and lumbar lordosis (Nehme et al., 1975; Wynne-Davis et al., 1981; Hecht et al., 1989; Hecht and Butler, 1990). The disproportions identified in adults are also evident in newborns (Harris, 1933). Neurological disorders are common, but life expectancy and mental capacity is normal (Waldron, 2009). Achondroplasia is linked to another form of dwarfism, hypochondroplasia, which in its mildest form is indistinguishable from the latter, although it tends not to involve the skull and face (Scott, 1976). Although the skeletal features of achondroplasia are quite distinctive, some features also occur in other dysplasias, such as multiple epiphyseal dysplasia, and should be among the differential diagnoses (Kozieradzka-Ogunmakin, 2011).

In a nonadult material, three possible cases of achondroplastic dwarfism have been identified. Ortner (2003) described a possible case of an older child from prehistoric Belle Glade in Florida with disproportionate widening and angulation of the distal femoral metaphyses, but preservation was poor and there was no skull. Sables (2010) presented suspected skeletal dysplasia in an 18- to 24-month-old from early medieval (AD 540–1020) Wales, UK. The child was found in a cist grave similar to others in the cemetery. The skeletal changes included shortened and broad long bones, flared metaphyseal distal ends, shortened humeral and femoral necks, reduction of the femoral trochanters, the beginnings of coxa vara, and extreme lateral bowing of the distal tibiae (Fig. 3.1). Again, there was no skull but unlike the case presented by Ortner (2003), the condition of the bone at the metaphyseal ends was normal suggesting a lack of chondral disruption. There was a lack of any spinal anomalies seen in other conditions such as chondrodysplasia punctate and camptomelic dysplasia, but diastrophic dysplasia characterized by club foot and cleft palate is a possible differential diagnosis.

A remarkable case study of the skeletal remains of a Dutch family from 19th-century Middenbeemster presents probable hypochondrodysplasia in an adult female. She was buried with three perinates, a 10-year-old girl and 21-year-old male, all identified through the documentary records as her offspring. While none of the perinates showed any signs of dysplasia, it was acknowledged that skeletal signs can be difficult to identify at such a young age. The 10-year-old daughter, however, showed some subtle signs that might be attributed to achondroplasia (Waters-Rist and Hoogland, 2013). There was minor dental developmental delay, with shorter diaphyses, and smaller scapulae and ilia than would be expected for a normal 10-year-old. While none of the bones were malformed, there was an extra (13th) thoracic vertebra and reduced sagittal diameters of the lumbar neural arches. The skull was also macrocephalic. It was acknowledged that these features could be explained by other conditions, such

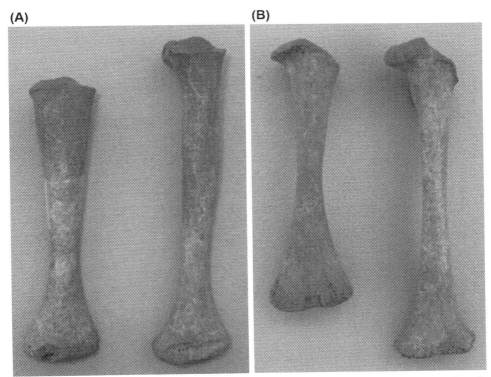

FIGURE 3.1 A child from Brownslade, Wales (AD 540–1020, skeleton PE315), showing shortening of the diaphyseal lengths and widened metaphyseal ends of the (A) humerus (left) and (B) femur (left). The bones are considerably shorter than those of a similarly aged child from the same site (on the right in A and B). The skull and feet were not preserved. *From Sables, A., 2010. Rare example of an early medieval dwarf infant from Brownslade, Wales. International Journal of Osteoarchaeology 20 (1), 50.*

as developmental stress, but the context of the case adds weight to the potential diagnosis of skeletal dysplasia. East and Buikstra (2001) presented a case of an achondroplastic female from Elizabeth Mounds, Tennessee with a fetus in utero that they suggested also had achondroplasia based on cranial and long bone measurements, but this case has yet to be fully published. Keith (1913) provides very useful comparative diagrams of the individual bones of an achondroplastic child against a normal child of the same age. The affected child displayed a reduced foramen magnum, absent suture mendosa, premature synostosis of the basioccipital suture, and short and broad wing of the pars lateralis. Frontal bossing was also evident as the brain grew and sought compensatory space.

Acromesomelia

Acromesomelic dysplasia is a rare autosomal recessive disorder causing disproportionate dwarfism characterized as the name suggests, by particularly short hands and feet (acromelia) and more pronounced shortening of the upper arms in comparison to the affected lower limbs (rhizomelia). The face retains its normal proportions. These changes become more pronounced as the child ages. For example, neonates will display short but normally proportioned upper limbs with foreshortened fingers. After 2 months the middle and proximal phalanges become broad and cone-shaped (Fig. 3.2). Shortening of the hands and feet is related to premature fusion of the epiphyses by about 2.5 years (Borrelli et al., 1983). The radius becomes markedly bowed with varying degrees of severity and is susceptible to subluxation and dislocation limiting pronation and supination of the elbow (Langer et al., 1977). The legs remain straight, but frontal and parietal bossing and thoracic kyphosis may be present, and there may also be flaring of the coastal margins of the ribs. The clavicles will appear normal. While intelligence of the individual with the condition is normal (Langer et al., 1977), adults are usually only 106–120 cm in height (Borrelli et al., 1983).

Frayer et al. (1988) have argued that Romito 2, a 17-year-old from an Upper Palaeolithic cave in Italy, displayed acromesomelic dwarfism. The skeleton was found in a shallow pit with an adult female (Romito 1) who is suggested to be cradling the adolescent in her arms. The skeleton is considered to be male based on mandibular and cranial robustness. The skull is brachycephalic with a cranial index of 82.5 and pronounced frontal and parietal bossing, a high and flat forehead, a tear drop–shaped foramen magnum, retarded growth of the sphenoid and basilar suture, a flattened face, and minor nasal projection. Similar to the Swiss case above, the ulnae are severely bowed, but only one radius survives. Given the absence of hand and foot bones, the key skeletal elements to make the diagnosis, the exact form of these dysplastic lesions is unknown.

Mesomelia

Mesomelic dysplasias include Léri–Weill dyschondrosteosis (LWD), Langer mesomelic dysplasia, and acromesomelic dysplasia Maroteaux type. Mesomelic dysplasias are classified as demonstrating shortening of the upper segment of the skeleton in comparison to the lower segment that is also, but less severely, shortened (Mundlos and Horn, 2014). LWD is an autosomal dominant disease that expresses itself more severely in females. It is characterized by short forearms and short stature with Madelung's deformity (ulna subluxation) of the wrist. A shortened and bowed radius is due to the lack of a distal radial epiphysis and premature fusion of the medial epiphysis (Mundlos and Horn, 2014, p. 240). The radius and ulna begin to separate and a v-shaped cavity remains for the carpus (McAlister and Herman, 2005). A possible case of LWD was identified in a 12-year-old from late Neolithic Switzerland (Fig. 3.3). Lack of the hands, feet and fibulae prevented observation of the full range of deformities, but bilateral shortening and bowing the ulna and right radius suggested mesomelic dysplasia, with LWD the most common form (Milella et al., 2015).

Thanatophoric Dwarfism

This is the lethal form of achondroplasia that usually results in death in utero due to a severely restricted triangular thorax. Thanatophoric dwarfism is a rare inherited disease more common in males with a modern incidence of 0.6 per 10,000 births. It is characterized as type 1 or 2 depending on the severity of the symptoms and pathogenesis. It is caused by mutations in the gene responsible for the growth factor receptors in the fibroblasts and hence, affects the structural integrity of the tissues (Spranger et al., 2002). Type 1 is characterized by extreme rhizomelia, bowed and shortened long bones with flared metaphyses, a "telephone receiver" appearance to the femur, a narrow thorax, a short cranial base with a decreased foramen magnum, a prominent forehead, hypertelorism, and a small vertical diameter to the vertebrae (platyspondyly). In the pelvis, shortened iliac bones display a horizontal inferior margin and small sciatic notches, and the pubic and ischial bodies are broad and short. The ribs are shortened with cupped metaphyseal ends, and the arms display shortened fingers and in some cases, radioulnar synostosis (Resnick and Kransdorf, 2005). In the less severe form or type 2, the long bones are short but straight and individuals display a clover-leaf skull (oxycephaly) (Norris et al., 1994).

A potential case of type 1 thanatophoric dwarfism has been identified in a perinate (c. 38 weeks) from the cemetery of St Hilda's Church (AD, 1813–1815), Newcastle upon Tyne. The appearance of the bones is strikingly similar to that of a modern case (Fig. 3.4). The vertebral bodies are flattened with the lumbar vertebrae tapered anteriorly. The ribs are wider than normal and slightly flared at the

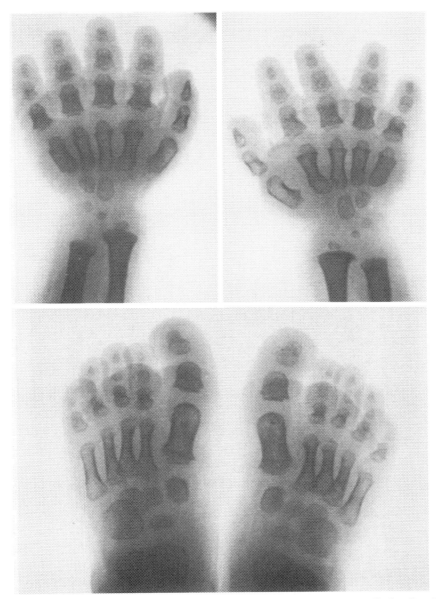

FIGURE 3.2 Clinical radiograph of the hands (above) and feet (below) of a 2.5-year-old boy with acromesomelic dwarfism. There is premature epiphyseal fusion of the metacarpals and metatarsals creating broad and short shafts and short and stubby fingers and toes. *From Borrelli, P., Fasanelli, S., Marini, R., 1983. Acromesomelic dwarfism in a child with an interesting family history. Periatric Radiology 13, 168.*

sternal end, although they do not appear to be reduced in length. The upper limb bones are straight but short and abnormally broad, with an accentuated curvature on the medial aspect. The metaphyseal ends of all of the long bones are flat, angled, and sharp. The short, broad tibiae have an accentuated curve on the lateral aspect. The fibulae have a flat rather than triangular morphology and are curved along the medial aspect. In the pelvis, the ilia are short and broad and the acetabulum has a sharp angular appearance and is orientated anteriorly (Fig. 3.5). The severity of the lesions and flattening of the vertebral bodies may indicate thanatophoric dwarfism type 1, but without the cranial vault commonly associated deformities (i.e., clover-leaf skull) cannot be assessed. Thanatophoric dwarfism is indistinguishable from lethal homozygous achondroplasia that may occur when both parents have achondroplasia (McAlister and Herman, 2005).

Developmental Dysplasia of the Hip and Congenital Hip Dislocation

Developmental (congenital) hip dysplasia results from malformation of the acetabulum in utero (Resnick and Kransdorf, 2005). Congenital dislocation of the hip, by

50 Paleopathology of Children

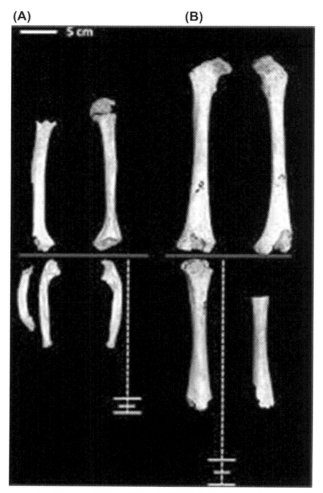

FIGURE 3.3 Upper and lower long bones of a 12-year-old from Schweizerbild, Switzerland (5155 BP, skeleton 6), showing (A) extreme bilateral shortening of the upper segments in comparison to the lower long bones. (B) The radii and ulnae are particularly shortened with enlarged and abnormally bowed shafts. *From Milella, M., Zollikofer, C., Leon, P., 2015. A Neolithic case of mesomelic dysplasia from northern Switzerland. International Journal of Osteoarchaeology 25, 983.*

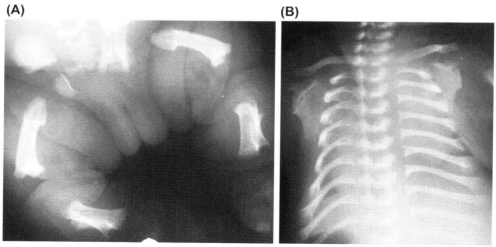

FIGURE 3.4 Clinical radiograph of a newborn with thanatophoric dwarfism showing (A) bowed and shortened long bones with flared metaphyses, with disruption to the cartilage growth plate, and (B) flaring of the vertebral and sternal ends of the ribs. *From the University of Reading, Clinical Radiograph Collection.*

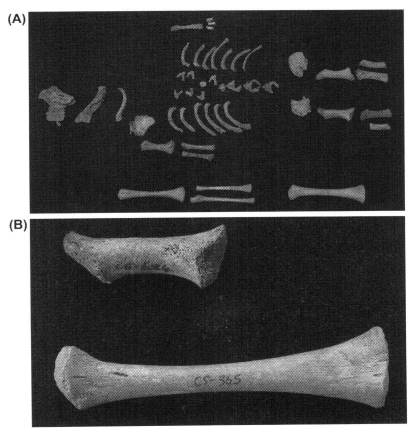

FIGURE 3.5 Possible thanatophoric dwarfism in a perinate from postmedieval St Hildur's Church in Newcastle, England (skeleton 684). (A) There is extreme shortening and broadening of the long bones and (B) "telephone receiver" morphology of the femur (top) compared to a normal femur of a perinate from the same site (below). *Photographs by P. Verlinden courtesy of the University of Sheffield.*

contrast, describes a normally formed hip joint that becomes dislocated during the birth process (Davidson et al., 2008). As the end result will be the same, it is unlikely that we would be able to distinguish between the two forms in skeletal material. Today, developmental dysplasia of the hip (DDH) occurs in around 20 per 1000 live births, and it is more common in females with a ratio of 7:1 (Campion and Benson, 2007). Subluxation and dislocation of the hip is a progressive feature of this disease (Resnick and Kransdorf, 2005). Thirty percent of dysplastic hips will dislocate at birth in children with breech presentation. They may spontaneously reduce within 2 months, only becoming apparent when the child begins to walk with a swaying gait, resulting from the constant dislocation of the hip during weight bearing (Roberts and Manchester, 2007). The left hip is more commonly affected than the right, possibly due to positioning of the neonate at birth, but 10% of DDH cases are bilateral (Campion and Benson, 2007). Dysplastic hips have an extremely variable morphology, but as the acetabulum depends on correct positioning of the femoral head for its normal development, lateral subluxation or dislocation at birth, or due to dysplasia, results in a shallow triangular acetabulum, with no deep cup for the femoral head (Resnick and Kransdorf, 2005). Instead, the anatomical acetabulum fills with fatty material (pulvinar) and the femur develops coxa valga, while femoral head development is delayed (Campion and Benson, 2007). A pseudoarthrosis or "false" joint will form above the true acetabulum. Individuals with developmental hip dysplasia may also have torticollis, spina bifida, sacral agenesis, club foot, or femoral or fibulae aplasia (Davidson et al., 2008). Any condition that causes the femoral head to be displaced from the acetabulum during development will show similarities to DDH and should be considered as a differential diagnosis. Congenital dislocation of the hip, without dysplasia, can result at birth due to infantile pyogenic arthritis, and it is a common finding in cases of myelomeningocele and Down syndrome, where abnormal joint laxity is a feature (Resnick and Kransdorf, 2005). Similarly, a slipped femoral epiphysis (Chapter 5) may occur due to birth trauma or physical abuse in an infant (Davidson et al., 2008).

Congenital hip dislocations, whatever the underlying cause, may have been common in the past as the disorder would not have been corrected at birth, and Walker (1991)

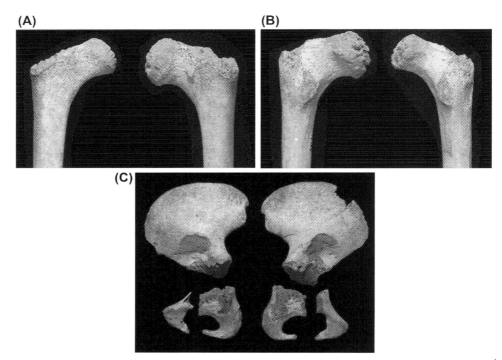

FIGURE 3.6 Possible hip dysplasia in a 6- to 7-year-old from Fishergate House, York, England (AD 1120–1360, skeleton 1246). (A) The left femoral head is enlarged with a bony projection on the anterior aspect at the site of the attachment of the vastus lateralis (quadriceps), which extends the knee; (B) the posterior aspect indicates that the femoral epiphysis was displaced inferior-posteriorly; and (C) pseudoarthroses are evident on the bodies of both ilia, although the left actabulum, visualized best on the ischium, is broader and shallower in comparison to the right. *Photograph courtesy of Rebecca Gowland, University of Durham.*

argues that in DDH shallow hips may have actually made the birth process easier. Although it is unlikely we will be able to determine between developmental hip dysplasia, congenital dislocation, and an infantile slipped femoral epiphysis, Mitchell and Redfern (2008) have provided a classification system for recognizing the defect. The original acetabulum will be triangular or oval, smaller than normal, with the base toward obturator foramen, and apex situated posterior-superiorly. The new or false acetabulum can vary in its morphology from a plaque of bone or a shallow depression, to a fine layer of bone on the cortex. In some cases the original acetabulum may be rounded but not as deep as a normal (Mitchell and Redfern, 2008). Other changes include a greater sciatic notch angle, shorter and broader ilium, flattened femoral head, thinner femoral shaft, a change in position of the trochanter, and asymmetric facets of the spine indicating scoliosis or hemivertebrae (Mitchell and Redfern, 2008). In perinatal material the deformity is likely to go unrecognized as deformities to the acetabulum usually only become evident once the three elements of the pelvis have fused, at around the age of 15 years (Scheuer and Black, 2000). At least three cases have been identified in the archeological context. The youngest case of possible hip dysplasia is in a 6-month-old from medieval Wharram Percy, England, where an abnormally shallow acetabulum on the unfused ilium suggests dislocation would have occurred when the child began to walk (Mays, 2007, p. 186). Holst (2005) identified bilateral congenital hip dislocation in a child from later medieval Fishergate House in York, England (Fig. 3.6). Pseudoarthroses are apparent on both ilia, although the left side is more severely affected.

Metaphyseal Dysplasia (Pyle's Disease)

Metaphyseal dysplasia is a rare inherited disorder that develops in later childhood causing mild joint pain and muscle weakness (Gupta et al., 2008). Osteoclastic dysfunction disrupts bone remodeling causing flared metaphyses described as having the appearance of a wine bottle, known as Erlenmeyer-flask deformity (Fig. 3.7; Gupta et al., 2008). Pyle's disease most commonly affects the distal femur, tibia, and fibula, but there may also be flattening and concavity of the vertebrae, while the pelvis, medial clavicle, and sternal ends of the ribs may be expanded (Resnick and Kransdorf, 2005). Radiographically, the bones are atrophied with a thin cortex, reduced medullary cavity, and the cancellous bone has a cloudy appearance. Sclerotic foci may be evident in the vertebrae, long bones, pelvis, and ribs. The condition may be associated with scoliosis, knock-knees (genu valgum), dental malocclusion, secondary fractures, and thickening of the cranial and facial bones (Gupta et al., 2008; Resnick and Kransdorf, 2005). Several cases of metaphyseal dysplasia have been suggested in the clinical record, but researchers

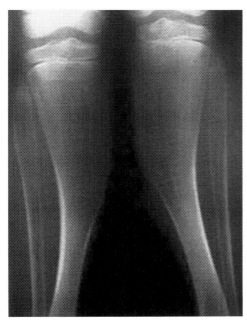

FIGURE 3.7 Clinical radiograph showing bilateral Erlenmeyer-flask deformity in the tibiae of a 12-year-old boy. *From Gupta, N., Kabra, M., Das, C., Gupta, A., 2008. Pyle metaphyseal dysplasia. Indian Pediatrics 45, 324.*

emphasize the importance of distinguishing the lesions from osteomyelitis, trauma, or osteopenia of another cause. In addition, the flask deformity of the distal femur is similar to changes associated with Gaucher's disease (Ortner, 2003, p. 360). Gladykowska-Rzeczycka (1995) argues for two possible nonadult cases in a cemetery from Poland, one based on a single humerus (Fig. 3.8) and the other in a 16- to 18-year-old with hypertrophy of the distal tibiae.

Fibrous Dysplasia

A term coined by Lichtenstein in 1953, fibrous dysplasia refers to an overgrowth of fibrous tissue in bone, and an arrested differentiation of bone cells. It is a noninherited genetic disease caused by gene mutations and is characterized by excessive, abnormal, and imperfect bone growth (Bianco and Wientroub, 2012). Fibrous dysplasia occurs in individuals between the ages 5 and 30 years (Isler and Turcotte, 2003), but the younger the presentation the worse the prognosis (Isler and Turcotte, 2003). Fibrous dysplasia is recognized as a sclerotic well-defined tumor comprising woven bone within an osteoblastic rim and can cause pain, cysts, hemorrhage, and deformities, although it may also be asymptomatic (Khurana and Unni, 2003). Tumors occur at multiple (polystotic) or single (monostotic) sites. If the femoral neck is involved, it can cause a pathological fracture. Trabeculae take on unusual shapes, most commonly forming c-shapes or circles known as "Chinese letters" (Khurana and Unni, 2003). Purely lytic lesions can be seen in children, but a "ground-glass" opacity of the bone is more common (Isler and Turcotte, 2003). Polystotic tumors occur in 20% of cases (Khurana and Unni, 2003) and usually arise in children before puberty. This form usually affects the femur and more rarely, the hands, vertebrae, and feet (Isler and Turcotte, 2003; Khurana and Unni, 2003). Monostotic tumors occur before 30 years of age, affecting the craniofacial bones (33%), more specifically the sphenoid and frontal bones, the tibia and femur (33%), and the ribs (20%) (Darsaut et al., 2001; Isler and Turcotte, 2003). Latent lesions may be reactivated with pregnancy (Khurana and Unni, 2003). In children, differential diagnoses include an endochondroma, Langerhan's cell histiocystosis (eosinophilic granuloma), or an ossifying fibroma.

Craig and Craig (2011) reported a case of monostotic fibrous dysplasia in a 6- to 7-year-old from Spofforth, North Yorkshire (Fig. 3.9). The left facial bones are grossly hypertrophic affecting the mandible, frontal, zygomatic, sphenoid, parietal, and temporal bones, and the margin between the pathological and normal bone is poorly circumscribed. A mass of thick trabeculae occupies the medullary space. On radiograph, the characteristic ground-glass appearance is evident and histology identified metaplastic trabeculae merging with the cortex. In life this child would have had an obvious facial deformity, but they were buried in the usual manner within the cemetery. As fibrous dysplasia can be the result of Albright's syndrome, the epiphyses were checked for signs of precocious puberty, but all were still unfused.

CONGENITAL SYNDROMES

Binder Syndrome (Maxillonasal Dysplasia)

The hypoplastic development of the midface, or Binder syndrome, was first described in 1939 by Noyes. The condition has six distinctive characteristics: an arhinoid face; abnormal nasal bone position; a hypoplastic maxilla; dental malocclusion and projecting central incisors; a reduced or absent nasal spine; and possible absence or hypoplasia of the frontal sinuses (Dyer and Willmot, 2002). Other recognized skeletal features include a flat glabella, pseudo- or true prognathism of the mandible and a decreased anterior cranial base (Mulhern, 2002). Clinically, Binder patients are recognized by a short middle third of the face, broad, flat nose, horizontal nostrils, bulging upper lip, and a marked nasolabial groove, giving the face a concave appearance (Olow-Nordenram and Thilander, 1989). These features become more pronounced with age (Dyer and Willmot, 2002). Around 50% of modern patients with maxillonasal dysplasia also have malformed cervical vertebrae (Mulhern, 2002). As vertebral differentiation and maxilla formation both take place around 5–6 fetal weeks, it has been suggested that there may be a connection with the timing of a stressful event during this period. The exact etiology of the condition is not understood, with both birth trauma and a genetic link put forward as possible factors. There is

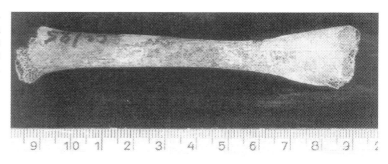

FIGURE 3.8 Humerus of a nonadult with an expanded "flask-shaped" distal metaphysis characteristic of Pyle's disease from Czersk, Poland (12–13th century AD, skeleton C2/85). *From Gladykowska-Rzeczycka, J., 1995. Morbus Pyle (dysplasia metaphysealis congenita) from medieval cemeteries in Poland. Journal of Paleopathology 7 (1), 62.*

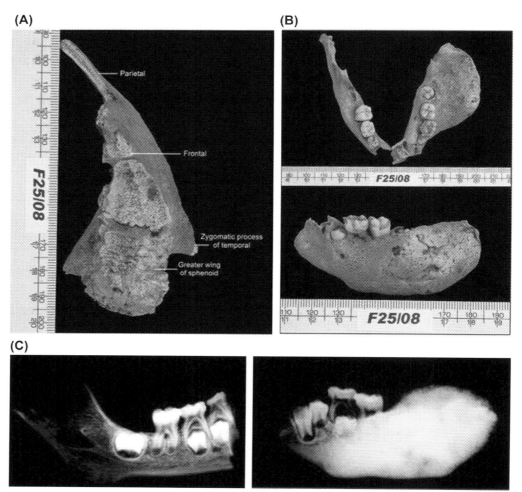

FIGURE 3.9 Mandible of a 6- to 7-year-old from Spofforth in Yorkshire, England (8th- to 12th-century AD, skeleton 177). (A) The left frontal and (B) mandibular ramus are grossly expanded, with irregular and disorganized new bone formation. (C) The radiograph of the mandible shows an unusual pitted or "orange-peel" appearance suggestive of ground-glass opacity. *From Craig, E., Craig, G., 2011. The diagnosis and context of a facial deformity from an Anglo-Saxon cemetery at Spofforth, North Yorkshire. International Journal of Osteoarchaeology 23, 632–634.*

also some evidence that Binder syndrome may be related to maternal alcohol abuse (Ferguson and Thompson, 1985).

Mulhern (2002) reported a possible case of Binder syndrome from a medieval site in New Mexico, in an adolescent female with a restricted nasal aperture, flattened facial bones, and absent nasal spine. The individual also displayed protruding central incisors and a hemififth lumbar vertebra. Comparisons of cranial measurements with modern Binder patients showed similar anterior cranial base and maxillary dimensions to the archeological case (Fig. 3.10). Although Binder syndrome is not uncommon today, this is the first reported paleopathological case. The rhinomaxillary features of leprosy are a potential differential diagnosis.

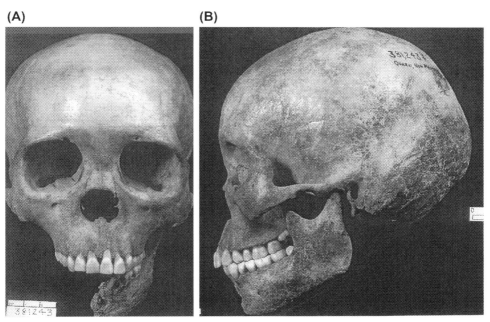

FIGURE 3.10 Skull of a 16- to 17-year-old from Quarai, New Mexico (AD 1375–1450, skeleton 381,243), with a (A) restricted nasal aperture and (B) reduced nasal spine giving the face a sunken appearance. *From Mulhern, D., 2002. Probable case of Binder syndrome in a skeleton from Quarai, New Mexico. American Journal of Physical Anthropology 118, 373, 374.*

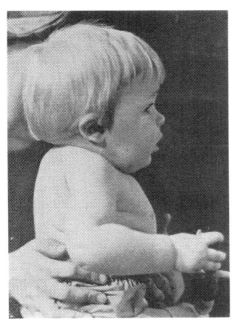

FIGURE 3.11 Child with Klippel–Feil syndrome. Note the reduced neck. *From Noble, T., Frawley, J., 1925. The Klippel-Feil syndrome. Annals of Surgery 82 (5), 728.*

Klippel–Feil Syndrome

First described in 1912 by Klippel and Feil, this syndrome is recognized by a triad of clinical changes; a short neck, low posterior hairline, and limited movement of the neck (Fig. 3.11). The etiology of the condition is not clear, and there are hereditary and sporadic cases in 1 in 30–40,000 live births (Aufderheide and Rodriguez-Martín, 1998). Segmental failure of the spine between the third and eighth week of embryogenesis results in a block of vertebrae, usually in the neck and upper thoracic spine. In 30% of cases there may be other defects that can include: facial asymmetry, occipitalization, scoliosis, cleft or high arch palate, unilateral or bilateral elevation of the scapula, supernumerary digits, upper limb hypoplasia, malformation of the occipital bone, or spina bifida (Aufderheide and Rodriguez-Martín, 1998; Davidson et al., 2008). Clinically, the condition is divided into three types: type 1 involves several cervical and thoracic vertebrae forming one osseous block that usually signals major additional defects (Barnes, 1994). Type 2, probably the most common found in archaeology, involves two or three vertebral segments, usually C2 and C3 followed by C5 and C6. If the thoracic spine is involved, fusion most commonly occurs between T2 and T5. Hemivertebrae and occipitalization may also be present (Pany and Teschler-Nicola, 2007). Type 3 Klippel–Feil involves block cervical vertebra with additional thoracic and lumbar segmental errors (Barnes, 1994).

Klippel–Feil syndrome is widely reported in nonadult paleopathology (Anderson, 1989; Mays, 2007; Pany and Teschler-Nicola, 2007; Shuler and Schroeder, 2013). Anderson (1989) describes axial congenital anomalies, and hence a familial relationship in three child skeletal remains from Homol'Ovi III, part of a Pueblo settlement cluster in Arizona. The first child, an infant, presented fused thoracic spinous processes, and asymmetry of the maxilla and mandible with dental overcrowding, suggesting marked facial asymmetry (Fig. 3.12a). The second child was a perinate

56 Paleopathology of Children

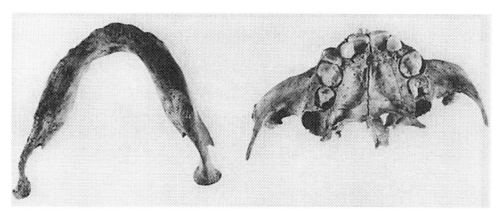

FIGURE 3.12A Asymmetrical mandible and maxilla of the infant from Homol'Ovi III, Arizona. *From Anderson, B., 1989. Immature human skeletal remains from Homol'ovi III. KIVA 54 (3), 235.*

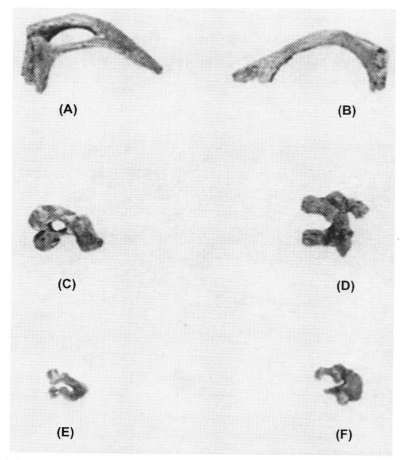

FIGURE 3.12B (A–D) Bicipital and bifurcated ribs, and cervical and thoracic hemiarches in the first of Anderson's perinates. E and F show cervical and thoracic arch fusion in the second perinate from Homol'Ovi III, Arizona. *From Anderson, B., 1989. Immature human skeletal remains from Homol'ovi III. KIVA 54 (3), 238.*

with fused arches of C2 and C3 and two midthoracic vertebral arches, indicating type 2 Klippel–Feil syndrome. The child also had one bicipital and one bifurcated rib. A younger perinate also demonstrated fusion (or nonseparation) of the spinous processes of C2 and C3, and T4 and T5 (Fig. 3.12b). Mays (2007) proposed Klippel–Feil syndrome as a diagnosis for an infant from later medieval Wharram Percy in Yorkshire, UK with occipitalization of the atlas and fusion of two midthoracic vertebrae. A 6-year-old from the same site had ankylosis of C3 and C4 with cleft arches of C4, L4, and L5 that would be consistent with type 3 Klippel–Feil. Pany and Teschler-Nicola (2007) described type 2 Klippel–Feil in an adolescent from a wealthy grave in Gnadendorf, Austria, with fused C2 and C3, and T2 and T3. The teenager also had basilar compression on the occipital, spina bifida, and a possible hearing impairment due to a restricted external auditory meatus. They also displayed a head injury and had undergone surgical intervention.

Pany and Teschler-Nicola (2007) suggest the injury may have contributed to their death by aggravating already existing neurological problems (Fig. 3.13). Fusion of C2–3 and C4–5 with accompanying mandibular deformation was identified in a 9- to 11-year-old from the Newton Plantation in Barbados. The distribution of the lesions and elevated enamel lead levels in the child led Shuler and Schroder (2013) to suggest fetal alcohol syndrome was the cause, perhaps due to maternal consumption of lead tainted rum, a common practice in the enslaved Africans from Barbados.

Dastegue and Gervais (1992) have warned against over diagnosis of this condition and recommended that Klippel–Feil syndrome should only be attributed when both the cervical and thoracic vertebrae are involved. This would mean that fusion of C2 and C3 alone, commonly reported in child skeletal remains, is not sufficient for diagnosis of this syndrome. It is also important to differentiate fusion as the result of trauma or joint disease, from a lack of segmentation. On radiograph, congenitally fused vertebrae have a widened and flattened ("wasp-waist") appearance due to concavity of the anterior and posterior cortex (Guille and Sherk, 2002). In addition to fusion of the vertebral body, the lamina, pedicle, and spinous process should also be fused. The disc space will be narrowed, but in cases of trauma or arthritis there may be early osteophyte formation (Gunderson et al., 1967). Pany and Teschler-Nicola (2007) provide a series of skeletal features associated with Klippel–Feil that may aid diagnosis (Table 3.1).

Down Syndrome (Trisomy 21) and Other Aneuploid Conditions

Since it was first described in 1866 by Langdon Down, this disorder has been recognized as one of the most common congenital syndromes, occurring in around 1 in 800 live births. Rates vary depending on the age of the mother, with the incidence in those aged 25 years reported to be 1 in 1400 births compared to 1 in 46 births in mothers over the age of 46 years (Patton, 2008). Downs is an aneuploid condition, a group of disorders characterized by an abnormal number of chromosomes (e.g., 45 or 47 rather than the normal 46). Down syndrome is caused by an extra copy of chromosome number 21. It falls under the trisomy group as having three chromosomes rather than the usual pair. Down syndrome represents a spectrum of changes including

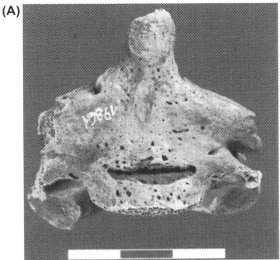

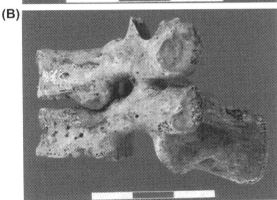

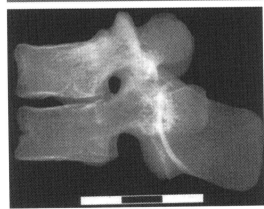

FIGURE 3.13 Klippel–Feil syndrome in a 16- to 18-year-old from Gnadendorf, Hungary (AD 980–1018) showing congenitally fused (A) C2 and C3 and (B) T2 and T3 (with radiograph below). *From Pany, D., Teschler-Nicola, M., 2007. Klippel-Feil syndrome in an early Hungarian period juvenile skeleton from Austria. International Journal of Osteoarchaeology 17 (4), 407, 408.*

mental impairment, hypodontia, and characteristic physical features (Patton, 2008). These include almond-shaped eyes; open-mouthed facial posture; protruding tongue; broad and stocky neck; short, broad, and small hands and feet;

TABLE 3.1 Skeletal Features Associated With Klippel–Feil Syndrome

Diagnostic	Frequent	Rare
C2–C3 fusion	Occipito-atlanto fusion	Hypodontia
C5–C6 fusion	Basilar impression	Os odontoideum
Thoracic fusion	Deafness (abnormal inner ear)	Cervical ribs
Lumbar fusion	Supernumerary C8	Constricted medullary canal
	Cleft lip and/or palate	Dental prognathism
	Scoliosis and/or hemivertebra	Vertical external auditory meatus
	Spina bifida	Upward curving of the occipital bone

After Pany, D., Teschler-Nicola, M., 2007. Klippel-Feil syndrome in an early Hungarian period juvenile skeleton from Austria. International Journal of Osteoarchaeology 17 (4), 406.

shortening and inward curvature of the little finger (clinodactyly); shortening of the shaft of the middle phalanx of the fifth metacarpal; short stature; and a propensity for obesity (Patton, 2008; Starbuck, 2011). In the skull there is brachycephaly with flattening of the occipital and nasal bones, wide-set eyes, and a wide cranial base (Ondarza et al., 1997; Orner, 1972; Suri et al., 2010). The dental changes include delayed eruption of the deciduous and permanent teeth, with abnormal dental positioning in a reduced palate (Patton, 2008), early development of periodontal disease, and a variety of dental anomalies including dental fusion and more commonly, agenesis of the lateral incisors (Reuland-Bosma and van Dijk, 1986). Tan (1971) noted a higher incidence of a retained third fontanelle at the posterior sagittal suture in infants with Down syndrome (58%). This fontanelle normally closes in the seventh fetal month, and its persistence typically signals the presence of other congenital anomalies. The list of skeletal and dental traits reported to occur with greater frequency in Down syndrome is numerous (Table 3.2), and a variety of these abnormalities, in addition to brachycephaly and agenesis of the lateral incisors, should alert researchers to the possibility of Down syndrome in a skeleton. Individuals with the condition may also suffer from numerous infections, including gastrointestinal disorders and persistent serous otitis media leading to hearing loss; heart defects, hip dislocations, and leukemia (Roberts and Manchester, 2007; Sheldon, 1943; Freeman et al., 1998; Davies, 1988). In their study of 25 males and females with Downs from Toronto, Suri et al. (2010) reported hypoplasia of the mesodermal, endochondral, and ectomesenchymal structure of the cranium, with reduced cranial base lengths, thinned cranial vaults, reduced facial height, and a small mandibular ramus. In the teeth they noted hypodontia in 92% of cases with undereruption of the mandibular dentition compared to the maxillary teeth.

The majority of Down syndrome cases result in spontaneous abortion of the fetus, while 20% are stillborn and 40% have heart malformations. Others may only have mild stigmata (Moore, 1988). Clinical studies in Australia have found females to be more prone to heart defects in Down syndrome than males (Glasson et al., 2003). In the 1900s, two-thirds of children with Downs died in childhood, usually before the age of 2 years (Sheldon, 1943), but medical advances and better care have increased the life span into adulthood with people now surviving into their 50s (Patton, 2008, p. 387; Starbuck, 2011). Therefore, in the past we might be most likely to see the condition in nonadult remains. Although the predilection for older mothers might mean there were fewer cases in antiquity where female life expectancy may have been lower (Roberts and Manchester, 2007).

Sonographs of second trimester fetuses hint at the potential to identify Downs in perinates from archeological contexts. These include a shortened femur and humerus when measured against the biparietal diameter and in comparison to the population norm; a shortened iliac length and hypoplasia of the middle phalanx of the fifth digit of the hand (Keeling et al., 1997; Kjaer et al., 1997; Stempfle et al., 1999). While asymmetries in the long bones of perinates may signal the presence of a syndrome, the results are not consistent. Unfortunately, all of these features require a large enough series of well-preserved perinates in the sample to gauge the normal dimensions. While the phalanges of the fingers normally ossify around 24-week gestation, they are so tiny they are unlikely to be excavated, making this identifier impractical, and any evaluation of agenesis impossible. In addition, the accuracy of these measurements to identify Down syndrome is between 40% and 50%, only rising to a more promising 74% when soft tissue features such as a nuchal fold on the neck is included (Benacerraf, 1996). Absence of the nasal bone in the newborn is also common in Down syndrome (Dedick and Caffey, 1953; Keeling et al., 1997; Otaño et al., 2002; Stempfle et al., 1999). Nasal bones should ossify between 15- and 40-week gestation. Otaño et al. (2002) found absence of the bone in

TABLE 3.2 Skeletal and Dental Features Associated With Down Syndrome in the Clinical Literature

Cranial	Dental	Postcranial
Flattened nasal bridge (77%)	Agenesis of maxillary lateral incisor (34%), then the second maxillary or mandibular premolars	Dysplastic middle phalanx of MC5. Lateral margin appears bowed and shorter than medial margin which is longer and curved inwards (clinodactyly). Phalanx is shorter and wider than normal. Most evident in children.
Brachycephaly and hyper-brachycephaly	Agenesis of the deciduous lateral incisors (12%–17%)	Metatarsal primus varus with hallux varus of MT1, with medial displacement of tarsal facets and increased concavity of tarsus.
Retained third fontanelle on the sagittal suture	Microdontia: dimensions of permanent teeth 0.53–2.59 SD below average; deciduous teeth not affected	Patella subluxation.
Persistent metopic suture	Numerous dental anomalies (notching, talon cusp, shoveling, peg-shaped)	Atlanto-axial instability (c.18%), may result on torticollis and spinal cord compression in child.
Reduced cranial sinuses or absence of frontal sinuses	Fused crowns, mandibular lateral incisor to canine, then lateral and central incisors	Hypoplastic or absent 12th rib.
Malformed and/or fused ear ossicles	Wide dental spacing	Increased vertebral height.
Platybasia (flattened occipital bone)	Delayed dental eruption (between 12 and 20 months for deciduous teeth)	Pelvis: widening of the ilium, elongated ischium, decreased acetabular angle.
Open cranial base angle	Early development of periodontal disease without significant calculus	
	Small palate	
	Fluctuating dental asymmetry	

3 of 5 (60%) Down syndrome fetuses compared to 1 in 175 (0.6%) of non-Down cases.

Starbuck (2011) identified eight possible depictions of Down syndrome children in paintings, the earliest dating from AD 1455, and recognized mainly on the basis of a flattened face, depressed nose, drooping eyes, and open-mouthed facial expression. More speculative but no less compelling is the depiction of Downs in ancient figurines and pottery, dating from 1500 BC to AD 1500. To date, five possible cases of Down syndrome have been identified in the archeological record, three of which are children. One is a child around 9 years of age from Breedon-on-the-Hill, England, dating to AD 700–900. The age of the child may be underestimated due to dental delay related to the condition, but it is thought that the association of the site with an early monastery may have aided the survival of the child (Brothwell, 1960). Charlier (2008) suggests Downs as a diagnosis for a 13- to 14-year old from late Bronze Age Rome (1200–850 BC) with slight brachycephaly, a flattened occiput and face, segmentation of the left occipital condyle, thin cranial bones with numerous ossicles, and a metopic suture. There was also evidence for premature arthritis of the temporomandibular joint, rib agenesis, flared iliac crests, and short broad phalanges of the hands and feet. This child was buried outside the normal cemetery area in marshland. The most recent and youngest reported case by Rivolatt et al. (2014) is of a 5- to 7-year-old from 5th- to 6th-century France with a series of cranial features consistent with a diagnosis of Down syndrome. These included brachycephaly, a flattened occipital bone, dental disease, cranial vault thinness, and hypodontia. To aid diagnosis, the authors provide a useful series of cranial measurements. The burial context of the individual was normal for the site, suggesting the child was not treated any differently to the rest of the population (Fig. 3.14). So far none of these cases have been tested using aDNA. Starbuck (2011) concludes by recommending the use of geometric morphometrics to analyze the facial characteristics of Downs.

Two other trisomy aneuploid conditions that may be potentially identified in an infant's remains are Trisomy 13 (Patau syndrome) and Trisomy 18 (Edward's syndrome). Children may survive up to the age of 1 year and have a series of congenital defects. These features include malformations of the lumbosacral and thoracic spine, small and irregular sphenoid bones (Kjaer et al., 1997), and cranial base malformations including extra ossification centers and

60 Paleopathology of Children

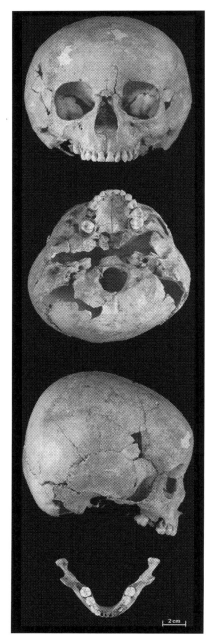

FIGURE 3.14 Anterior, inferior, and lateral views of the skull of the 5- to 7-year-old from Saint-Jean-des-Vignes, France, with possible Down syndrome (5th- to 6th-century AD). Note the brachycephalic vault and flattened occipital bone. The nasal bones were present at excavation. *From Rivollat, M., Castex, D., Hauret, L., Tillier, A.-M., 2014. Ancient Down syndrome: an osteological case from Saint-Jean-des-Vignes, from the 5-6th century AD. International Journal of Paleopathology 7, 9.*

fusion of two or more vertebral bodies. There may also be disproportion in the size of the cervical bodies. It is tempting to suggest a possible diagnosis of aneuploidy in a 38- to 40-week perinate from Andover Road in Winchester, UK, reported by Falys (2010). The perinate had an unfused wing of the pars lateralis resulting in the posterior condylar canal

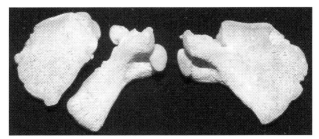

FIGURE 3.15 Left and right partes laterales in a perinate from Andover Road, Winchester, England (7th- to 10th-century AD, skeleton 262). *Photograph taken courtesy of Ceri Falys, Thames Valley Archaeological Services.*

being in two halves (Fig. 3.15). The thickened and regular edge suggests this was a congenital anomaly producing extra ossification centers in the occipital bone, rather than a basilar linear fracture of the occipital.

Osteogenesis Imperfecta

Osteogenesis imperfecta is caused by defective formation of type 1 collagen, affecting many tissues including the ligaments and skin. As osteoid is 90% type 1 collagen (Basal and Steiner, 2009), defects are particularly severe in the skeleton and typified by osteopenia and extreme bone fragility. Also known as "brittle bone disease," this condition is uncommon with an incidence of 1 in 20,000–50,000 live births, although it is likely that mild forms go undetected (Waldron, 2009). Osteogenesis imperfecta has been reported in all populations with an equal sex distribution.

Early accounts of the disease illustrate a fascination with the condition, with an 18th-century commentator describing "a child…borne at term to a woman who had seen an execution upon the wheel…who had all its members broken like those of a thief" (King and Bobechko, 1971, p. 73). In 1943, medical writer Sheldon did not know the cause of the condition but noted that pathological fractures could be delayed by 3–4 years, while in other cases babies had up to 100 fractures at birth. This reflects the variability of skeletal changes that were subsequently divided into two types: "congenita" and "tarda." Today, there are seven different "types" of the disease recognized in the clinical literature (Glorieux et al., 2002; Sillence et al., 1979; Cope and Dupras, 2011). Type I is the most common and mildest form where endosteal growth is normal but intramembranous bone formation is limited, resulting in long thin bones with a thin cortex and sparse trabeculae (Basal and Steiner, 2009). Those with the disease have a normal life expectancy but suffer deafness due to premature otosclerosis. The extreme fragility of their bones leads to frequent fractures as they learn to walk and suffer falls, but fractures decrease with advancing puberty. Fractures heal with abnormal angulations and calluses that may mimic tumors. Dislocations result in the development of pseudoarthroses. Any bone except the skull may be deformed (Basal and Steiner, 2009). Type II (a and c) are lethal forms resulting from new genetic mutations (autosomal dominant). Complications manifest in uterine life with bones fracturing while the child is still in the womb, and during childbirth. Both endochondral and intramembranous bone formation is affected, with compression fractures of the vertebrae and numerous rib fractures. Thin cranial bones with lacunae are common and in the most severe cases, the skull may be represented only by a membranous sac at birth (Caffey, 1945). Type IIb, III, and IV are harder to identify archeologically as diagnosis relies on chemical analysis, but 11% of these children have a triangular-shaped face, a large skull with frontal bossing, platybasia, and basilar impression.

The list of skeletal features seen with osteogenesis imperfecta is extensive and can include multiple fractures, temporal bulging, platybasia with possible hydrocephalus and neuralgia, micrognathia, hypertelorism, growth retardation and dwarfism, shortened upper extremities, scoliokyphosis caused by widening and wedging of vertebrae, a narrow triangular pelvis, "shepherd hook" deformity of the femur, coxa vara, and otosclerosis in young adults (Basal and Steiner, 2009). Avulsion injuries are common as a result of normal muscle pull on weakened joints, telescoping fractures occur, and children may get "popcorn" calcification in the metaphyses or epiphyses, evident as multiple scalloped radiolucent areas on radiograph (Resnick and Kransdorf, 2005). In the dentition, dentinogenesis imperfecta describes brittle and opaque teeth with a blue or brown tinge where the pulp chambers are obliterated by excessive dentine formation (Basal and Steiner, 2009; Waldron, 2009). There is also prognatism, early eruption of teeth, severe dental wear, and eventual tooth loss as the result of defective dental tissues (Ortner, 2003).

A probable case of osteogenesis imperfecta was discovered by forensic anthropologists in a mass grave in Guatemala (Lewis, 2007, p. 170) that demonstrates numerous fractures, dislocations, and pseudoarthroses of the long bones, in addition to malformations of the occipital bone. Wells (1964) was the first to diagnose the condition in archeological material from a single deformed bone of an early medieval adult female at Burgh Castle, Suffolk, while Gray (1969) reported on a now famous case of a 2-year-old mummified child from Speos Artemidos, Beni Hassan in Egypt dating from 1000 BC. The preservation is remarkable, displaying deformity of the skull caused by flattening of vertical axis and widening of the transverse axis ("tam-o-shanter" skull). Recent reanalysis of the skeleton shows that the occipital bone is made up of a complex series of cranial ossicles. The teeth do not show signs of dentinogenesis imperfecta. The long bones have marked anterior-lateral bowing, with disproportionately thick femoral diaphyses and osteopenia. Healed fractures are evident on the ribs and distal humeri, and the vertebral bodies show extreme compression fractures (Fig. 3.16E and F). The age of the child suggests that this was not the lethal form (type 2), but the deformities may be the result of type IIb osteogenesis imperfecta where children may live for several years with the condition. A second case from a later period in Egypt was identified by Cope and Dupras (2011) in the Roman cemetery of Kellis 2, Dakhleh Oasis. The perinate has distinctive bowing of the long bones with possible perimortem fractures of the femur and tibia (Fig. 3.17).

Osteopetrosis (Osteosclerosis Fragilis)

Marble bones were first described by Albers-Schönberg in 1904 with the name "osteopetrosis" later coined by Karschner (1926). It is a rare genetic disorder with an incidence of 1 in 300,000 births (Tolar et al., 2004). Osteopetrosis is caused by a disruption of osteoclastic activity and a reduction in their quantity and quality (Ortner, 2003; Tolar et al., 2004). Dent et al. (1965) have suggested that the underlying cause is an over absorption of calcium from the diet. During primary growth, the calcified cartilage of primary spongiosa are not removed, while the diaphyses are not cut back on the endosteal or periosteal aspects causing gross enlargement (club-shaped) of the metaphyses and thickened dense shafts. The loss of bone plasticity due to an absent medullary cavity results in widespread secondary fractures (Filho et al., 2005). Radiographically, thick bands of radiolucent and radiopaque bone are evident. Foramina fail to enlarge properly during the growth process (Dent et al., 1965) causing additional neurological problems. The condition is divided into four types: type 1, infantile or malignant osteopetrosis, is associated with specific gene mutations. It is the most severe form and is usually fatal in utero. Type 2, childhood osteopetrosis, is an autosomal recessive type with renal tubular acidosis and cerebral calcifications. It is usually recognized by the appearance of multiple pathological fractures and results in short stature and severe mental retardation. This type is also characterized by severe anemia due to loss of the medullary cavity, osteomyelitis, and blindness due to pressure on the optic nerve. Patients do not normally live beyond the age of 20 years (Loría-Cortés et al., 1977). Type 3, or benign osteopetrosis, is usually asymptomatic in children and only visible on radiograph. Fractures and osteomyelitis of the mandible are common in later adulthood. The final form is intermediate osteopetrosis (type 4), which can occur in both adults and children, and may cover the whole spectrum of symptoms, from the most severe to being asymptomatic (Dent et al., 1965; Filho et al., 2005).

Ortner (2003, p. 497, 499) illustrates two clinical cases of osteopetrosis, in a perinate and 4.5-year-old male. Despite the density of the bones that would suggest that affected perinates would survive archeologically, no cases have been identified in an archeological context. This may suggest that osteopetrosis is a relatively recent genetic mutation in humans. Care should be taken not to confuse the radiopaque signs of lead contamination in bone for severe bone density (Molleson et al., 1998).

62 Paleopathology of Children

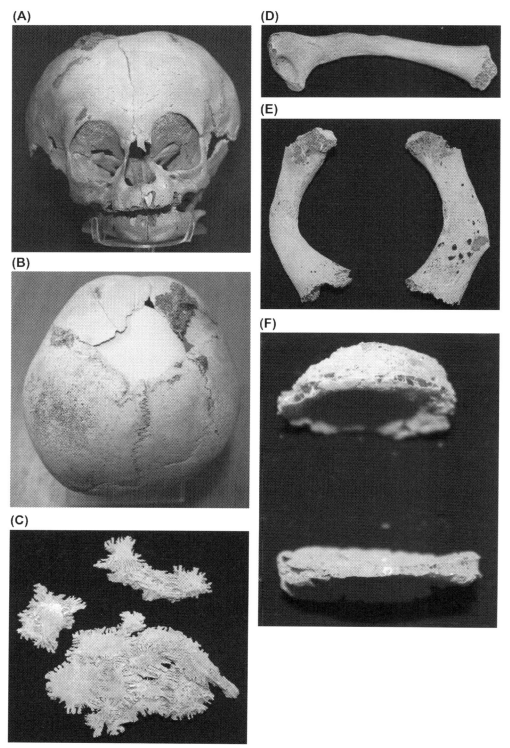

FIGURE 3.16 (A–F) Skeletal changes in the 2-year-old from Speos Artemidos, Beni Hassan in Egypt (1000 BC) with osteogenesis imperfecta. (A) The brachycephalic skull has resulted in elongated orbits and (B) the frontal fontanelle is enlarged and open. (C) Numerous cranial ossicles make up the squama of the occipital bone. In the postcranial skeleton the (D) distal humerus has a healed fracture and (E) the femora are bowed and osteopenic; (F) the thoracic vertebral bodies are also severely compressed. *Photographs taken with the kind permission of the Trustees of The British Museum (specimen number 41603).*

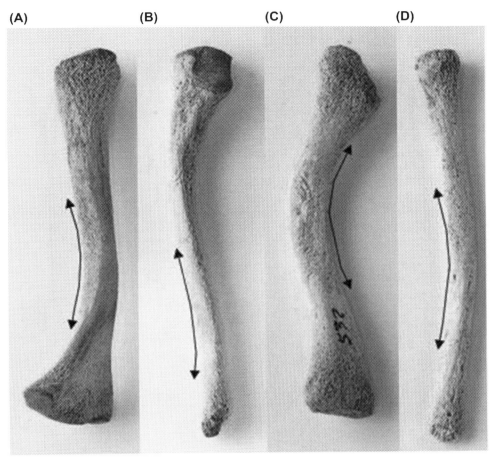

FIGURE 3.17 Osteogenesis imperfecta in a 38-week-old perinate from Kellis 2, Dakhleh Oasis, Egypt (AD 50–450, skeleton 532). Bowing of the (A) humerus, (B) ulna, (C) femur, and (D) fibula. *From Cope, D., Dupras, T., 2011. Osteogenesis imperfecta in the archaeological record: an example from the Dakhleh Oasis, Egypt. International Journal of Paleopathology 1, 193.*

Cerebral Palsy

Cerebral palsy is an umbrella term used to define a series of disorders that result in childhood motor impairment (Badawi et al., 1998). The etiology and pathogenesis of the disorders vary, but to be defined as cerebral palsy, the neuropathy must come from disorders of the brain, usually around birth, rather than through trauma or defects of the spinal cord or muscles (Badawi et al., 1998; Collier, 1924). Today, nearly 500,000 children in the United States live with the disease (Cerebral Palsy Organisation, 2012). By 5 years of age, most cases have become apparent and have either healed spontaneously or become progressively worse (Badawi et al., 1998). In his study of 200 clinical cases of cerebral palsy from Manchester and York in England, Fawcitt (1964) found 57% of sufferers to have abnormal hip joints, 37.5% had coxa valga at over a 140-degree angle, and 38% had subluxation or dislocation of the hip. Some of the children had microcephaly (13%) or varying degrees of cranial asymmetry (1.5%). In the children with hemiplegia, with paralysis of one side of the body, 80% had a shorter femoral and tibial length on the affected side. The degree of shortening was considered less than in the paralysis caused by poliomyelitis, with the greatest length difference noted in the hemiplegia cases being 2.4 cm. Thinned shafts and small epiphyses were also noted but were again, not as severe as that seen in polio (Fawcitt, 1964). In 2009, Megyesi et al. published a warning to forensic anthropologists that individuals with cerebral palsy may appear much younger than their actual age. Their known modern case of a 21- to 23-year-old had a skeletal and dental development age of 11–15 years. There were several skeletal and dental anomalies, including a gracile and undersized skeleton, and delayed epiphyseal fusion. Today, children with cerebral palsy have problems like feeding and swallowing resulting in undernutrition (Megyesi et al., 2009), that may in turn cause delayed maturation, a longer pubertal growth spurt, and retarded skeletal growth (Henderson et al., 2005). Bruxism, resulting in uneven dental wear is also more common in cerebral palsy sufferers (Megyesi et al., 2009).

Two cases of possible cerebral palsy in nonadults have been identified. Hemiplegia in a 14- to 16-year-old with plagiocephaly and septic necrosis and dislocation of the right femur was reported from Salerno in Italy (Valette et al., 2000). The authors argued that the problems with the right hip were caused by alterations to the left hemisphere motor cortex. The second case of possible cerebral palsy was identified in a 1- to 2-year-old from Iron Age Neon U-Loke, Thailand (Tayles, 2001). The diagnosis was made on the basis of careful recording of hand and foot positions in the grave, and the presence of scoliosis, coxa vara of the femur, and abnormal ribs. The most simple form of treatment for muscular contraction would have been splinting to limit the deformity and stretch the muscles (Sharrard, 1967), but it is not known whether individuals in the past would have been treated.

REFERENCES

Albers-Schönberg, H., 1904. Röntgenbilder einer seltenen knockenerkrankung. Munch Med Wochenschr 51, 365–368.

Anderson, B., 1989. Immature human skeletal remains from Homol'ovi III. KIVA 54 (3), 231–244.

Aufderheide, A.C., Rodriguez-Martín, C., 1998. The Cambridge Encyclopedia of Human Paleopathology. Cambridge University Press, Cambridge.

Badawi, N., Watson, L., Petterson, B., Blair, E., Slee, J., Haan, E., Stanley, F., 1998. What constitutes cerebral palsy? Developmental Medicine and Child Neurology 40, 520–527.

Barnes, E., 1994. Developmental Defects of the Axial Skeleton in Paleopathology. University of Colorado Press, Colorado.

Basal, D., Steiner, R., 2009. Osteogenesis imperfecta: recent findings shed new light on this once well-understood condition. Genetics in Medicine 11 (6), 375–385.

Benacerraf, B., 1996. The second-trimester fetus with Down syndrome: detection using sonographic features. Ultrasound Obstetric Gynecology 7, 147–155.

Bianco, P., Wientroub, S., 2012. Fibrous dysplasia. In: Glorieux, F., Pettifor, J., Jüppner, H. (Eds.), Pediatric Bone. Academic Press, London, pp. 589–624.

Borrelli, P., Fasanelli, S., Marini, R., 1983. Acromesomelic dwarfism in a child with an interesting family history. Periatric Radiology 13, 165–168.

Brothwell, D., 1960. A possible case of mongolism in a Saxon Population. Annals of Human Genetics 24 (2), 141–150.

Caffey, J., 1945. Pediatric X-Ray Diagnosis. Year Book Medical Publishers, Inc., Chicago.

Campion, J., Benson, M., 2007. Developmental dysplasia of the hip. Surgery 25 (4), 176–180.

Castro de la Mata, R., Bonavia, D., 1980. Lumbosacral malformations and spina bifida in a Peruvian preceramic child. Current Anthropology 21 (4), 515–516.

Cerebral Palsy Organisation, 2012. Prevalence of Cerebral Palsy. http://cerebralpalsy.org/about-cerebral-palsy/prevalence-of-cerebral-palsy/.

Charlier, P., 2008. The value of palaeoteratology and forensic pathology for the understanding of atypical burials: two Mediterranean examples from the field. In: Murphy, E. (Ed.), Deviant Burial in the Archaeological Record. Oxbow Books, Oxford, pp. 57–70.

Collier, J., 1924. The pathogenesis of cerebral diplegia. Brain: a Journal of Neurology 1 (47), 1–21.

Cope, D., Dupras, T., 2011. Osteogenesis imperfecta in the archaeological record: an example from the Dakhleh Oasis, Egypt. International Journal of Paleopathology 1, 188–199.

Craig, E., Craig, G., 2011. The diagnosis and context of a facial deformity from an Anglo-Saxon cemetery at Spofforth, North Yorkshire. International Journal of Osteoarchaeology 23, 631–639.

Darsaut, T., Lanzino, G., Lopes, M., Newman, S., 2001. An introductory overview of orbital tumours. Neurosurgical Focus Other Titles: NSF 10, 1–9.

Dasen, V., 1990. Dwarfs in Athens. Oxford Journal of Archaeology 9 (2), 191–207.

Dastugue, J., Gervais, V., 1992. The Paleopathology of the Skeleton. Boubée, Paris.

Davies, B., 1988. Auditory disorders in Down's syndrome. Scandinavian Audiology 30 (Suppl.), 65–68.

Davidson, J., Cleary, A., Bruce, C., 2008. Disorders of bones, joints and connective tissues. In: McIntosh, N., Helms, P., Smyth, R., Logan, S. (Eds.), Forfar & Arneil's Textbook of Pediatrics. Elsevier, Edinburgh, pp. 1385–1447.

Dawson, W., 1938. Pygmies and dwarfs in ancient Egypt. The Journal of Egyptian Archaeology 24 (2), 185–189.

Dedick, A., Caffey, J., 1953. Roentgen findings in the skull and chest in 1030 newborn infants. Radiology 61, 13–20.

Dent, C., Smeillie, J., Watson, L., 1965. Studies in osteopetrosis. Archives of Disease in Childhood 40 (7), 7–15.

Dickel, D., Doran, G., 1989. Severe neural tube defect syndrome from the early archaic of Florida. American Journal of Physical Anthropology 80, 325–334.

Down, J., 1866. Observations on the ethnic classification of idiots. Clinical Lecture Reports, London Hospital 3, 259–262.

Dyer, F., Willmot, D., 2002. Maxillo-nasal dysplasia, Binder's syndrome: review of the literature and case report. Journal of Orthodontics 29, 15–21.

East, A., Buikstra, J., 2001. Is the fetus from Elizabeth mound 3, lower Illinois river valley an achrondroplastic dwarf? American Journal of Physical Anthropology 32, 61.

Falys, C., 2010. Human bone. In: Hammond, S., Preston, S. (Eds.), Land Adjacent to 135-7 Andover Road (Winchester Post Excavation Assessment: Unpublished Report).

Fawcitt, J., 1964. Skeletal changes in cerebral palsy children. Annals of Radiology 7 (5–6), 466–471.

Ferguson, J., Thompson, R., 1985. Maxillonasal dyostosis (Binder syndrome) a review of the literature and case reports. European Journal of Orthodontics 7, 145–148.

Filho, A., de Castro Domingos, A., de Freitas, D., Whaites, E., 2005. Osteopetrosis – a review and report of two cases. Oral Diseases 11, 46–49.

Frayer, D., Macchiarelli, R., Mussi, M., 1988. A case of chondrodystrophic dwarfism in the Italian Late Upper Paleolithic. American Journal of Physical Anthropology 75, 549–565.

Freeman, S., Taft, L., Dooley, K., Allran, K., Sherman, S., Hassold, T., Khoury, M., Saker, D., 1998. Population-based study of congenital heart defects in Down syndrome. American Journal of Medical Genetics 80, 213–217.

Gladykowska-Rzeczycka, J., 1995. Morbus Pyle (dysplasia metaphysealis congenita) from medieval cemeteries in Poland. Journal of Paleopathology 7 (1), 57–62.

Glasson, E., Sullivan, S., Hussain, R., Petterson, B., Montgomery, P., Bittles, A., 2003. Comparative survival advantage of males with Down Syndrome. American Journal of Human Biology 15, 192–195.

Glorieux, F., Ward, L., Rauch, F., Lalic, L., Roughley, P., Travers, R., 2002. Osteogenesis imperfecta Type VI: a form of brittle bone disease with a mineralisation defect. Journal of Bone and Mineral Research 17 (1), 30–38.

Gray, P., 1969. A case of osteogenesis imperfecta, associated with dentinogenesis imperfecta, dating from antiquity. Clinical Radiology 20, 106–108.

Guille, J., Sherk, H., 2002. Congenital osseous anomalies of the upper and lower cervical spine in children. Journal of Bone and Joint Surgery 84-A (2), 277–288.

Gunderson, C., Greenspan, R., Glaser, G., Lubs, H., 1967. The Klippel-Feil syndrome, genetic and clinical re-evaluation of cervical fusion. Medicine 46 (6), 491–512.

Gupta, N., Kabra, M., Das, C., Gupta, A., 2008. Pyle metaphyseal dysplasia. Indian Pediatrics 45, 323–325.

Harris, H.A., 1933. Bone Growth in Health and Disease. Oxford University Press, London.

Hawkey, D., 1998. Disability, compassion and the skeletal record: using musculo-skeletal stress markers (MSM) to construct an osteobiography from early New Mexico. International Journal of Osteoarchaeology 8, 326–340.

Hecht, J., Butler, I., 1990. Neurologic morbidity associated with achondroplasia. Journal of Child Neurology 5, 84–97.

Hecht, J., Horton, W., Reid, C., Pyeritz, R., Chakraborty, R., 1989. Growth of the foramen magnum in achondroplasia. American Journal of Medical Genetics 32, 528–535.

Henderson, R., Gilbert, S., Clement, M., Abbas, A., Worley, G., Stevenson, R., 2005. Altered skeletal maturation in moderate to severe cerebral palsy. Developmental Medicine and Child Neurology 47, 229–236.

Holst, M., 2005. Fishergate House artefacts and environmental evidence: the human bone. York Osteoarchaeology (Unpublished Skeletal Report).

Isler, M., Turcotte, R., 2003. Bone tumors in children. In: Glorieux, F., Pettifor, J., Jüppner, M. (Eds.), Pediatric Bone: Biology and Diseases. Academic Press, New York, pp. 703–743.

Karschner, R., 1926. Osteopetrosis. American Journal of Roentgenology 16, 405–416.

Keeling, J., Hansen, B., Kjaer, I., 1997. Pattern of malformations in the axial skeleton in human trisomy 21 fetuses. American Journal of Medical Genetics 68, 466–471.

Keith, A., 1913. Abnormal crania – achondroplastic and acrocephalic. Journal of Anatomy and Physiology 47 (2), 189–206.

Khurana, J., Unni, K., 2003. Pathological diagnosis of common tumours of bone and cartilage. In: Yuehuei, H., Martin, K. (Eds.), Handbook of Histology Methods for Bone and Cartilage. Humana Press, New Jersey, pp. 447–494.

King, J., Bobechko, W., 1971. Osteogenesis imperfecta. An orthopaedic description and surgical review. The Journal of Bone and Joint Surgery 53B (1), 72–89.

Kjaer, I., Keeling, J., Hansen, B., 1997. Pattern of malformations in the axial skeleton in human trisomy 13 fetuses. American Journal of Medical Genetics 70, 421–426.

Klippel, M., Feil, A., 1912. Un Cas d'Absence des Vertebres Cervicales. Nouvelles Iconographie de la Salpetriere 25, 223.

Kozieradzka-Ogunmakin, I., 2011. Multiple epiphyseal dysplasia in an Old Kingdom skeleton: a case report. International Journal of Paleopathology 1, 200–206.

Kozma, C., 2008. Skeletal dysplasia in ancient Egypt. American Journal of Medical Genetics 146A (23), 3104–3112.

Krakow, D., Lachman, R., Rimoin, D., 2009. Guidelines for the prenatal diagnosis of fetal dysplasias. Genetic Medicine 11 (2), 127–133.

Langer, L.O., Beals, R.K., Solomon, I.L., Bard, P.A., Bard, L.A., Rissman, E.M., Rogers, J.G., Dorst, J.P., Hall, J.G., Sparkes, R.S., et al., 1977. Acromesomelic dwarfism: manifestations in childhood. American Journal of Medical Genetics 1, 87–100.

Lewis, M.E., 2007. The Bioarchaeology of Children: Perspectives from Biological and Forensic Anthropology. Cambridge University Press, Cambridge.

Lewis, M., 2016. Childcare in the past. In: Powell, L., Southwell-Wright, W., Gowland, R. (Eds.), Care in the Past Archaeological and Interdisciplinary Perspectives. Oxbow Books, Oxford (in press).

Lichtenstein, L., 1953. Histiocytosis X. Integration of eosinophilic granuloma of bone, "Letterer-Siwe disease" and "Schuller-Christian disease" as related manifestations of a single nosologic entity. AMA Archives of Pathology 56, 84–102.

Loría-Cortés, R., Quesada-Calvo, E., Cordero-Chaverri, C., 1977. Osteopetrosis in children: a report of 26 cases. The Journal of Pediatrics 91 (1), 43–47.

Mays, S., 2007. The human remains. In: Mays, S., Harding, C., Heighway, C. (Eds.), Wharram a Study of a Settlement on the Yorkshire Wolds, XI: The Churchyard York University Archaeological Publications 13. English Heritage, London, pp. 77–192.

McAlister, W., Herman, T., 2005. Osteochondroplasias, dysostoses, chromosonal aberrations, mucopolysaccharidoses, and mucolipidoses. In: Resnick, D., Kransdorf, M. (Eds.), Bone and Joint Imaging. Elsevier Saunders, Philadelphia, pp. 1225–1298.

Megyesi, M., Tubbs, R., Sauer, N., 2009. An analysis of human skeletal remains with cerebral palsy: associated skeletal age delay and dental pathologies. Journal of Forensic Science 54 (2), 270–274.

Milella, M., Zollikofer, C., Leon, P., 2015. A Neolithic case of mesomelic dysplasia from northern Switzerland. International Journal of Osteoarchaeology 25, 981–987.

Mitchell, P., Redfern, R., 2008. Diagnostic criteria for developmental dislocation of the hip in human skeletal remains. International Journal of Osteoarchaeology 18, 61–71.

Molleson, T.I., Williams, C.T., Cressey, G., Din, V.K., 1998. Radiographically opaque bones from lead-lined coffins at Christ Church, Spitalfields, London – an extreme example of bone diagenesis. Bulletin de la Société Géologique de France 3, 425–432.

Moore, K.L., 1988. Essentials of Human Embryology. B.C. Decker Inc, Totonto.

Mulhern, D., 2002. Probable case of Binder syndrome in a skeleton from Quarai, New Mexico. American Journal of Physical Anthropology 118, 371–377.

Mundlos, S., Horn, D., 2014. Limb Malformations. Springer-Verlag, Berlin.

Nehme, A.-M., Riseborough, E., Tredwell, S., 1975. Skeletal growth and development of the achondroplastic dwarf. Clinical Orthopaedics and Related Research 116, 8–23.

Noble, T., Frawley, J., 1925. The Klippel-Feil syndrome. Annals of Surgery 82 (5), 728–734.

Norris, C., Tiller, G., Jeanty, P., Malini, S., 1994. Thanatophoric dysplasia in monozygotic twins. The Fetus 4, 27–32.

Noyes, F., 1939. Case study. Angle Orthodontics 9, 160–165.

Olow-Nordenram, M., Thilander, B., 1989. The craniofacial morphology in persons with maxillonasal dysplasia (Binder syndrome). American Journal of Orthodontics 95 (2), 148–158.

Ondarza, A., Jara, L., Muñoz, P., Blanco, R., 1997. Sequence of eruption of deciduous dentition in a Chilean sample with Down syndrome. Archives of Oral Biology 42 (5), 401–406.

Orner, G., 1972. Eruption of permanent teeth in mongoloid children and their sibs. Journal of Dental Research 52 (6), 1202–1208.

Ortner, D., 2003. Identification of Pathological Conditions in Human Skeletal Remains. Academic Press, New York.

Otaño, L., Aiello, H., Igarzábal, L., Matayoshi, T., Gadow, E., 2002. Association between first trimester absence of fetal nasal bone on ultrasound and Down syndrome. Prenatal Diagnosis 22, 930–932.

Oxenham, M., Tilley, L., Matsumura, H., Nguyen, L., Nguyen, K., Nguyen, K., Domett, K., Huffer, D., 2009. Paralysis and severe disability requiring intensive care in Neolithic Asia. Anthropological Science 117 (2), 107–112.

Pany, D., Teschler-Nicola, M., 2007. Klippel-Feil syndrome in an early Hungarian period juvenile skeleton from Austria. International Journal of Osteoarchaeology 17 (4), 403–415.

Panzer, S., Cohen, M.N., Esch, U., Nerlich, A., Zink, A., 2008. Radiological evidence of Goldenhar syndrome in a paleopathological case from a South German ossuary. HOMO-Journal of Comparative Human Biology 59, 453–461.

Patton, M., 2008. Genetics. In: McIntosh, N., Helms, P., Smyth, R., Logan, S. (Eds.), Forfar & Arneil's Textbook of Pediatrics. Elsevier, Edinburgh, pp. 379–409.

Resnick, D., Kransdorf, M., 2005. Bone and Joint Imaging. Elsevier Saunders, Philadelphia.

Reuland-Bosma, W., van Dijk, J., 1986. Periodontal disease in Down's syndrome: a review. Journal of Clinical Periodontology 13, 64–73.

Rivollat, M., Castex, D., Hauret, L., Tillier, A.-M., 2014. Ancient Down syndrome: an osteological case from Saint-Jean-des-Vignes, from the 5-6th century AD. International Journal of Paleopathology 7, 8–14.

Roberts, C., 2000. Did they take sugar? The use of skeletal evidence in the study of disability in past populations. In: Hurbert, J. (Ed.), Madness, Disability and Social Exclusion. Routledge, London, pp. 46–59.

Roberts, C.A., Manchester, K., 2007. The Archaeology of Disease. Cornell University Press, Cornell.

Sables, A., 2010. Rare example of an early medieval dwarf infant from Brownslade, Wales. International Journal of Osteoarchaeology 20 (1), 47–53.

Scheuer, L., Black, S., 2000. Developmental Juvenile Osteology. Academic Press, London.

Scott, C., 1976. Achondroplastic and hypochondroplastic dwarfism. Clinical Orthopaedics and Related Research 114, 18–30.

Sharrard, W., 1967. Paralytic deformity in the lower limb. Journal of Bone and Joint Surgery 49B (4), 731–747.

Sheldon, W., 1943. Diseases of Infancy and Childhood. J. & A. Churchill Ltd, London.

Shuler, K., Schroeder, H., 2013. Evaluating alcohol related birth defects in the past: skeletal and biochemical evidence from a colonial rum producing community in Barbados, West Indies. International Journal of Paleopathology 3, 235–242.

Sillence, D., Senn, A., Danks, D., 1979. Genetic heterogeneity in osteogenesis imperfecta. Journal of Medical Genetics 16, 101–116.

Spranger, J., Brill, P., Poznanski, A., 2002. Bone Dysplasias: an atlas of genetic disorders of skeletal development. Oxford University Press, Oxford.

Starbuck, J., 2011. On the antiquity of Trisomy 21: moving towards a quantitative diagnosis of Down syndrome in historic material culture. Journal of Contemporary Anthropology 2 (1), 61–89.

Stempfle, N., Huten, Y., Fredouille, C., Brisse, H., Nessmann, C., 1999. Skeletal abnormalities in fetuses with Down's syndrome: a radiographic post-mortem study. Pediatric Radiology 29, 682–688.

Stoll, C., Dott, B., Roth, M.-P., Alembik, Y., 1989. Birth prevalence rates of skeletal dysplasias. Clinical Genetics 35, 88–92.

Suri, S., Tompson, B., Cornfoot, L., 2010. Cranial base, maxillary and mandibular morphology in Down syndrome. The Angle Orthodontist 80 (5), 861–869.

Tan, K., 1971. The third fontanelle. Acta Paediatrica Scandianavia 60, 329–332.

Tayles, N., 2001. Is this a case of cerebral palsy? Paleopathology Newsletter 114, 9–10.

Tilley, L., 2012. The bioarchaeology of care. The SAA Archaeological Record 12 (3), 39–41.

Tolar, J., Teitelbaum, S., Orchard, P., 2004. Osteopetrosis. New England Journal of Medicine 351, 2839–2849.

Valette, A., Capasso, L., Scarsini, B., 2000. A hydrocephalus from the necropolis of Pontecagnano (IX-III Centuries B.C.). In: Thirteenth Biannual European Members Meeting of the Paleopathology Association. Chieti, Italy.

Waldron, T., 2009. Palaeopathology. Cambridge University Press, Cambridge.

Walker, J., 1991. Musculoskeletal development: a review. Physical Therapy 71 (12), 878–889.

Walker, D., 2012. Disease in London, 1st–19th centuries. Museum of London Archaeology, London.

Waters-Rist, A., Hoogland, M., 2013. Osteological evidence of short-limbed dwarfism in a nineteenth century Dutch family: achondroplasia or hypochondroplasia. International Journal of Paleopathology 3 (4), 243–256.

Wells, C., 1964. Bones, Bodies and Disease. Thames and Hudson, London.

Wynne-Davis, R., Walsh, W., Gormley, J., 1981. Achondroplasia and hypochondroplasia: clinical variations and spinal stenosis. The Journal of Bone and Joint Surgery 63B (4), 508–515.

Chapter 4

Dental Disease, Defects, and Variations in Dental Morphology

Chapter Outline

Introduction	67	Hyperdontia (Supernumerary Teeth)	80
Teething	67	Natal and Neonatal Teeth	80
Dental Caries	68	Dental Fusion	81
Deciduous Caries	68	Macrodontia and Microdontia	83
Paleopathology	70	Talon Cusps	83
Recording and Reporting Caries in Children	75	**Dental Trauma**	83
Dental Calculus	76	Dental Modification	84
Periapical Cavitation	77	**Disruption in Dental Development**	84
Periodontal Disease (Periodontitis)	77	Dental Enamel Hypoplasia	84
Antemortem Tooth Loss	78	Turner's and Skinner's Teeth	85
Dental Anomalies	79	**References**	86
Hypodontia	79		

INTRODUCTION

Due to the hard and dense nature of enamel the dentition is usually the best preserved element of archeological human remains. The presence of disease on the deciduous and permanent dentition of nonadults is a largely neglected area of study, despite its potential to reveal information about maternal health, malnutrition, diet, general health, and specific diseases or congenital conditions. The mixed dentition allows the history of dental disease to be reconstructed in more detail than in adults, as for example, caries is known to spread from the deciduous to the permanent teeth. The abnormal structure of teeth may aid in the diagnosis of specific diseases, such as the dental stigmata of congenital syphilis, leprogenic odontodysplasia in leprosy, and dental agenesis and spacing in Down syndrome. Chronic dental conditions such as periodontal disease, antemortem tooth loss, periapical lesions, and abundant calculus occur rarely in children, and their presence may signal more significant pathological conditions. Unlike bone, dental enamel has a limited capacity to remineralize and so any disruption of ameloblasts during the development of the crown provide an almost permanent record of the stress event. Unlike adults, hypoplasia in nonadults are rarely lost as the result of wear and tooth loss. Host factors such as the morphology of the teeth, and the presence of enamel defects, pits and fissures will leave teeth more susceptible to diseases such as caries (Ortner, 2003).

Dental disease causes considerable discomfort for the individual, and can mean intense pain, difficulty in eating, reduced efficiency of the immune system, and even death from infections spreading to the head and neck (Baqain et al., 2004). In children the presence of extensive dental disease can affect speech development (Aligne et al., 2003). In normal circumstances the spread of oral infections into the blood stream (bacteremia) is usually prevented by the body's natural defenses made up of the mucosal epithelium and reticuloendothelial system. These structures act as a phagocytic barrier, although pathogens may be released during dental trauma or extraction (Li et al., 2000). With poor oral health and subsequent accumulation of vast numbers of bacteria, penetration of the phagocytic barrier is more likely. The following sections discuss dental diseases and defects specifically in relation to their development and meaning in a child's remains. More detailed information on the development of the dentition and disease processes in adults can be found in dedicated textbooks (Hillson, 2014; Irish and Scott, 2015).

Teething

The London Bills of Mortality for AD 1775 listed "teeth" as the fourth most common cause of death, affecting 694 individuals (McKinley, 2008). It is likely that for the majority, this described the discomfort of teething that may have been the only physical sign of illness in children who died from infection or fevers of other causes. In 1842, the English Registrar–General's report showed that 4.8% of infants, 7.3% of 1- to 3-year-olds, and 12% of 3- to 4-year-olds died as the result of "teething" (Ashley, 2001). Teething is a dental condition unique to children and Ashley (2001) provides a useful overview of remedies used to soothe children in the past. These included the use of hare's brain as a dental rub from the 1st until the 15th century, when other rubs such as chicken fat, honey, and salt were introduced. In the 6th century AD Aetios of Amida advocated the use of charms to hang over the stomach to ease teething and ward off death. These charms comprised root of colocynth (a poisonous vine) or bramble root in a gold or silver case, or a viper's tooth set in green or gold jasper. The first shed tooth of a colt, set in silver and bone or red coral, was also recommended as a charm by English physician Thomas Phaire in 1545 (Ashley, 2001). Rather than conveying magic, these objects may have worked because the child could suck on and rub the charm on their gums, and it is possible that such charms and materials could be recovered in archeological excavations.

Dental Caries

Dental caries is a multifactorial infectious and transmissible disease characterized by progressive destruction of the crown and root structures due to microbial activity (Ortner, 2003). The main pathogen is *Streptococcus mutans*. Caries normally develops due to the complex interaction of cariogenic oral flora (biofilm) on fermenting dietary carbohydrates over time. However, the host's immune system, genetic susceptibility, diet, tooth structure, biofilm (or dental plaque) pH, oral hygiene, and social status will influence whether a person develops caries. Bacteria within the biofilm metabolize carbohydrates into sugars for energy, producing lactic acid as a by-product. Over time this lowers the pH of plaque to critical levels (below 5.5) and initiates the removal of phosphate and calcium from the dental structures (demineralization) causing a cavity. Once equilibrium is restored, these minerals are then reconstituted into the enamel (remineralization). If demineralization outweighs remineralization, collapse of enamel crystals produces a cavity (caries), a process that can take months or years (Cameron and Widmer, 2008). Saliva plays a critical role in removing substrates, buffering plaque acid, and in providing the calcium and phosphate necessary for the demineralization process. When sufficient time has passed since an acid attack, remineralization will take place leaving the child 'caries inactive' (Cameron and Widmer, 2008, p. 45).

Before the introduction of refined carbohydrates and sugar, natural sugars, and those in cooked starches would have been a risk factor, although caries may have been prevented in some groups due to natural levels of fluoride in the water (Waldron, 2009). With cereal agriculture, the prevalence of caries at the root and cementoenamel junction rose, and with the later introduction of refined sugar, caries became more common in the dental fissures and interproximal surfaces, especially in children (Hillson, 1996). Halcrow et al. (2013) point out that not all carbohydrates have the same cariogenicity. Those with a low molecular weight, such as sucrose, are more easily fermentable and hence more cariogenic. Potatoes and wheat bread, common in Europe, are more likely to lead to caries compared to rice, which is more frequently consumed in Asia (Halcrow et al., 2013).

When examining the nonadult dentition, it is important to consider that different teeth are at risk at different ages, as the teeth erupt into the mouth. It can also take 3 to 4 years for caries to develop once the tooth has erupted (Cameron and Widmer, 2008). In addition, deciduous teeth are more susceptible to caries than permanent teeth (see below), and the presence of hypoplasia, perhaps as the result of poor maternal health increases the risk. Some researchers argue that girls have a higher predisposition to caries than boys, and this may relate to the earlier age of eruption of the teeth in females (Burt, 1981). Coronal and buccal caries of the molars is a particular pattern of disease in children due to the susceptibility of unworn fissures in the teeth, and gradually increases with age. By contrast, root caries is normally a disease of adults (Hillson, 1996). Untreated caries can give rise to lethal complications such as meningitis and cavernous sinus thrombosis, or cause chronic maxillary sinusitis. In the mandible, advanced caries can result in a secondary infection in the jaws (periodontitis) and throat. Childhood caries has also been linked to delayed growth, chronic medical conditions, and cardiovascular disease (Boyce et al., 2010). In Guatemala, children with third degree malnutrition have higher rates of caries than their better nourished peers (Sawyer and Nwoku, 1985), and Miller et al. (1982) found an association between high caries rates and children who failed to thrive. One of the earliest studies into the dental health of children was by Mummery (1869) who argued that dental caries in British children was brought about by too much cerebral activity (i.e., study) that denied their teeth the adequate energy needed to develop normally!

Deciduous Caries

Early childhood caries (ECC), defined as caries in children between the ages of birth and 5 years, is a serious chronic condition in the modern world (Afroughi et al., 2010). Newly erupted deciduous teeth are particularly susceptible to caries due to incomplete maturation, large dental tubules, and thinner enamel that is insufficient to halt the progression of caries (Aligne et al., 2003; Schuurs, 2013).

In addition, the enlarged area around the erupted tooth provides favorable conditions for bacterial colonization (Schuurs, 2013). Child saliva flow rate is slower than in adults and has lower concentrations of secretory immunoglobulin A (IgA). Although IgA is produced after 1 month of life, levels can be impaired by the presence of cortisol in the blood during stress (Boyce et al., 2010). After the formation of white spots, the initial sign of caries that appears after 2–3 weeks of bacterial attack, it takes around 1 year for the outer layer of the enamel to be breached, and 3 years for the lesion to reach the dentine (Fig. 4.1). Lesions on the buccal and lingual surfaces may take longer to reach this florid stage (Schuurs, 2013). The 1-year cavity progression in the deciduous teeth contrasts with the 1.5 years it takes to breach the enamel in the newly erupted permanent teeth, and the 3 years it can take for cavities to appear in the teeth of a 20-year-old (Schuurs, 2013).

Young children can be exposed to oral bacteria and subsequent caries from their mothers, siblings and peers through kisses, or sharing cups and spoons (Darby and Curtis, 2001; Nield et al., 2008). The window of greatest infectivity is calculated to be between 18 and 31 months for caries to spread from mother to child, and the presence of maternal caries is considered the best predictor of caries in 12-year-olds (Schuurs, 2013). Nicotine stimulates the production of *S. mutans*, and mothers who smoke are more likely to suffer from periodontal disease and transmit germs to their children (Aligne et al., 2003). In their study of 3531 American children aged 4–11 years (between 1988 and 1994), Aligne et al. (2003) identified that 53% of children with deciduous caries were exposed to passive smoke. Tobacco smoke is associated with decreased levels of vitamin C and reduced saliva production, which can stimulate the formation of cariogenic bacteria in the mouth. The increased popularity of smoking in Europe and the Americas with industrialization in the 19th century may account for some of the rise in dental disease seen in the children from these periods. While *S. mutans* has generally been considered to be the main pathogen in the development of ECC in children, new research has discovered the pathogen *Scardovia wiggsiae* in the mouths of children with a severe infection, while *S. mutans* was absent (Chandra and Adlakha, 2015; Forsyth Institute, 2011). Afroughi et al. (2010) examined the spread of deciduous caries, demonstrating caries tended to spread to the teeth either side of the original lesion, or to the tooth directly above it. The risk of caries was greater in the maxillary posterior teeth than the anterior or mandibular teeth, and the pattern of decay was usually symmetrical.

There is a strong link between the use of comforters, night bottles, and ECC (Hillson, 1996). Also known as "nursing bottle caries," rampant caries develops on the anterior teeth as drink is sucked up and held under the upper lip allowing sugar and acid to attack the enamel. While today breastfeeding is advocated, feeding at will and

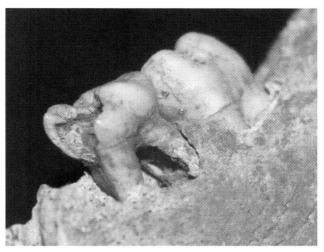

FIGURE 4.1 Large coronal caries on the second deciduous molar of a 5- to 6-year-old from St Oswald's Priory in Gloucester, England (AD 1540–1869, skeleton 251). It takes roughly 3 years for a cavity to reach this advanced stage in deciduous teeth.

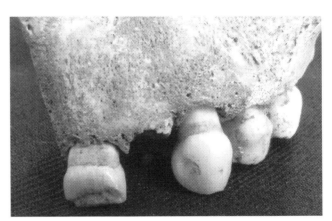

FIGURE 4.2 Caries on the maxillary deciduous central incisor of a 3- to 4-year-old from medieval Whitefriars, Norwich, England (skeleton 10,256). The linear appearance of the lesion suggests the presence of an underlying enamel defect. *Photograph courtesy of Malin Holst, York Osteoarchaeology.*

nocturnal breastfeeding have also been seen as risk factors for ECC due to the buildup of milk around the teeth during periods when saliva flow is reduced (Chandra and Adlakha, 2015). The link between malnutrition and ECC is also well established in the medical literature (Miller et al., 1982), with Clarke et al. (2006) considering ECC a marker of iron-deficiency anemia. Brown et al. (2012) found that 66% of 102 children under treatment for ECC in their London clinic were vitamin D deficient, although they did not have signs of rickets. The link between dental enamel defects and caries formation is well proven (Infante and Gillespie, 1974; Sweeney et al., 1969; Sweeney and Guzman, 1966). The timing of the stress event that causes the hypoplasia affects which teeth are susceptible and at what time (Fig. 4.2). Hence today, the second deciduous molar is the most susceptible as the enamel is normally still forming at 5–6 months of age when children are weaned and at risk of malnutrition and infection.

Paleopathology

Nonadult caries has been identified in early humans, with Trinkaus et al. (2000) reporting a small carious lesion on the first deciduous molar of a middle Paleolithic Neanderthal child from Vaucluse in France. There are numerous studies demonstrating a link between an increase in caries and the adoption of a high carbohydrate diet. A greater prevalence of caries is evident between wheat and maize agriculturalists compared to hunter–gatherers (Larsen et al., 1991), and there is evidence that rice intensification does not produce such a dramatic rise (Halcrow et al., 2013). In their study of caries in nonadults from South Asia, Halcrow et al. (2013) found higher rates of caries in the deciduous teeth (9.9%) compared to the permanent teeth (5.5%). Unrefined rice given to the older children is less cariogenic as it does not stick to the teeth and has a low pH stimulating saliva flow. By contrast, younger children appear to have been fed sticky weaning foods, which may have included mashed banana used by the modern communities. This, in combination with the properties of deciduous teeth seemed to account for the pattern of caries (Halcrow et al., 2013).

The advent of industrialization and widespread availability of refined foods saw a massive increase in the frequency and change in location of caries in English postmedieval populations (Moore and Corbett, 1976). Dental caries rates began to rise from the 15th century when cane sugar (sucrose) imports increased, and the first sugar factory was opened in Britain (AD 1641). These changes meant that the once expensive commodity could be afforded by most of the population. By the end of the 17th century, it is estimated that the population consumed up to 20 pounds of sugar per head per year (Moore and Corbett, 1973, 1975, 1976). Mrs Beeton, a famous household writer of the 19th century England stated that "sugar…should form a large portion of every meal an infant takes in order to promote energy for growth, and pap should be sweetened with sugar" (Beeton, 1861 cited in Miles et al., 2008). New milling methods led to an increase in refined flour, which contributed to the rise in dental disease. Over time the extent of caries as the result of abrasive foods, and located interproximally decreased, while caries of the root increased with softer refined foods. Moore and Corbett (1973, 1975) carried out a detailed study of caries in skeletons from medieval England. In the early medieval period 3.5% (n = 13/370 teeth) of deciduous teeth had caries, compared to 4.5% (n = 30/663 teeth) in the later medieval groups. The most common location was the occlusal surface of the molars (Moore and Corbett, 1973). By the 17th century, the prevalence of deciduous caries had risen to 28.5% (n = 14/49 teeth), and the most common locations now included the interdental areas (Moore and Corbett, 1975). At St Marylebone in postmedieval London, dental caries and calculus increased with the eruption of the permanent dentition, with one child demonstrating caries in a linear position that seemed to track an underlying hypoplastic defect. There was antemortem tooth loss, unusual for children, in 2.7% of the nonadults (Miles et al., 2008). An increase in the prevalence of caries through time was also evident in the nonadults from St Oswald's Priory in Gloucester (Lewis, 2013). In the late medieval period, 0.2% of teeth had caries compared to 6.2% in the postmedieval group. A total of 13% of deciduous teeth were affected compared to just 6.0% of the permanent teeth, suggesting that the maternal stress and the conditions in which the young children from this period were raised made them susceptible to ECC. In 19th century Ontario, Pfeiffer et al. (1989) also remarked on the extent of caries and antemortem tooth loss evident in the children. In addition to access to refined sugar and flour, exposure to tobacco smoke and deficiencies in rickets, scurvy, and iron may also have contributed to this pattern. A peak in postmedieval caries rates in children has also been noted in Croatia (Marin et al., 2005).

The link between ECC and iron-deficiency anemia in modern children inspired O'Sullivan et al. (1989, 1992) to explore the association between caries in the deciduous molars with cribra orbitalia in 221 infants and children from the prehistoric to the later medieval period in England. The highest rates of caries were in the Romano–British and later medieval groups with true prevalence rates of 16.2% and 20.3%, respectively. The lowest rates of caries, at 8.2% were found in the early medieval groups. They reported a significant association between caries and cribra orbitalia and argued that caries was linked to the preeruptive nutritional environment of the children, and poor maternal health. The relationship between dental enamel hypoplasia and caries in nonadults has been explored in several studies. But the relationship is not clear-cut. Garcin et al. (2010) examined dental defects and caries in a 613 nonadults from early medieval Slovakia. They noted that although dental defects were often present in individuals with caries, not all individuals with enamel hypoplasia developed caries. In her study of 38 nonadults (0–15 years) from early Iron Age Sweden, Liebe-Harkort (2012) identified caries in 31.6% of individuals, with rates increasing after the age of 3 years. As the majority of lesions were at the cervical margin rather that the occlusal surface, it was suggested that a transition to the adult diet of starchy foods after weaning, rather than underlying stress, was the main cause of caries.

Of 52 sites that reported true prevalence rates of caries in the deciduous and permanent teeth of nonadults, the majority recorded a higher prevalence in the deciduous teeth at 65% (n = 34). This reflects the clinical pattern that argues for the greater susceptibility of these teeth to decay, but may also suggest that factors such as maternal caries, a high carbohydrate weaning diet, and general malnutrition played a role in the pattern of caries in the past. These sites include children from England (Boulter, 1992; Boylston et al., 1998; Caffell and Holst, 2006, 2007, 2010; Connell et al., 2012; Cox, 1989; Dawson, 2011; James and Miller, 1970; Lewis, 2008, 2013; Mays, 1989, 1991, 1996; Miles et al., 2008; Philips and Leach, 2008; Rahtz et al., 2000; Roffey and Tucker, 2012; Tucker, 2005; Wells, 1982), Continental Europe (Garcin et al., 2010; Liebe-Harkort, 2012; Liebe-Harkort et al., 2010; Lingström and Borrman 1999; Varrela, 1991), North and South America (Hinkes, 1983; Keene, 1986; Powell, 1988), North Africa (Shukrum and Molto, 2009), and Asia (Halcrow et al., 2013; Oxenham and Domett, 2011). This pattern was similar across all periods. True prevalence rates for caries in the deciduous and permanent teeth in samples with over 100 teeth available for observation are presented in Tables 4.1 and 4.2. The lowest rate of deciduous caries is reported for English sites at 2.5% and the highest in Asian sites at 7.6%. The site with the highest recorded rates of deciduous caries was Muang Sema, Thailand at 13.8% (Halcrow et al., 2013). This perhaps reflects differences in the type of weaning foods given to these children - wheat based pap in Europe compared to banana in parts of Asia. For the permanent teeth, again the sites from England had the lowest rates at 1.7% compared to the highest rates of 6.9% in North and South America. The highest rate of dental caries in the permanent teeth was recorded at Iron Age Smorkullen in Sweden (Liebe-Harkort et al., 2010).

Many studies show that the most commonly affected tooth in children is the first molar in both the deciduous and permanent dentition (Boylston et al., 1998; O'Sullivan et al., 1989, 1992; Williams and Curzon, 1985; Lewis, 2013; Prowse et al., 2008) or the posterior dentition in general (James and Miller, 1970; Moore and Corbett, 1973). However, some studies have found a more unusual pattern. In the prehistoric Moundville site, Powell (1988) found that while caries distribution in the permanent teeth of the children reflected the adult pattern, caries in the deciduous teeth while fewer, were more often located anteriorly, perhaps suggesting the use of pacifiers or feeding bottles. Similar examples have been identified in England. A potential case of bottle caries was reported in a 3- to 4-year-old from Late Roman Ancaster, England, displaying widespread (rampant) caries on the lingual and occlusal surfaces of all surviving deciduous teeth (Fig. 4.3; Bonsall et al., 2016). Walker (2012a) describes a case of a 1-year-old from postmedieval Bunhill, London, with caries confined to the central and lateral incisors leading to a periapical abscess of the right lateral incisor. James and Miller (1970) examined the dentitions of 23 children buried at Cuddington Church under Nonsuch Palace, London (AD 1100–1538). Two children, aged 2–5 years had considerable caries on the deciduous molars, and the authors suggest they were ill and required continuous pacification,

TABLE 4.1 True Prevalence Rates (TRP) for Dental Caries in the Deciduous Teeth

	Period	Teeth Observed	Teeth Affected	Deciduous Caries %	Sources
UK Sites					
Cannington, Somerset	Roman	485	3	3.6	Rahtz et al. (2000)
Cirencester, Gloucestershire	Roman	150	4	2.6	Wells (1982)
Great Casterton, Rutland	Roman	262	4	1.5	Philips and Leach (2008)
Poundbury Camp, Dorset	Roman	1041	8	0.7	Lewis (unpublished)
Ancaster, Lincolnshire	Roman	305	18	5.9	Cox (1989)
Empingham II, Rutland	Early medieval	222	2	0.9	Mays (1996)
Raunds Furnells, Northants.	Early medieval	596	4	0.7	Lewis (unpublished)
Chichester, Sussex	Late medieval	457	30	6.5	Lewis (2008)
Blackfriars, Ipswich	Late medieval	123	7	5.7	Mays (1991)
St Gregory's Priory, Canterbury	Late medieval	767	22	2.8	Dawson (2011)
St Helen-on-the-Walls, York	Late medieval	821	5	0.7	Lewis (unpublished)
Taunton, Somerset	Late medieval	683	49	7.1	Dawson (2011)

Continued

TABLE 4.1 True Prevalence Rates (TRP) for Dental Caries in the Deciduous Teeth—cont'd

	Period	Teeth Observed	Teeth Affected	Deciduous Caries % TPR	Sources
Fishergate House, York	Late medieval	595	11	1.8	Holst (2005)
Christ Church Spitalfields, London	Postmedieval	669	38	5.7	Lewis (unpublished)
St Oswald's Priory, Gloucester	Multiperiod	419	14	3.3	Lewis (2013)
Wharram Percy, Yorkshire	Multiperiod	1070	14	1.3	Lewis (unpublished)
Total		**8665**	**223**	**2.5**	
Other European Sites					
Smorkullen, Sweden	Iron Age	221	23	10.4	Liebe-Harkort et al. (2010)
Isola Sacra, Rome, Italy	Roman	556	21	3.8	Prowse et al. (2008)
Turku, Finland	Late medieval	600	20	3.3	Varrela (1991)
Mikulcice, Prague, Czech Rep.	Early medieval	2712	97	2.5	Garcin et al. (2010)
Norroy, Prague, Czech Rep.	Early medieval	366	17	4.6	Garcin et al. (2010)
Prusanky, Prague, Czech Rep.	Early medieval	750	12	1.6	Garcin et al. (2010)
Cherbourg, Prague, Czech Rep.	Early medieval	597	8	1.3	Garcin et al. (2010)
Total		**5802**	**198**	**3.4**	
North and South America					
Moundville, Mississippi	AD 1050–1550	323	32	9.9	Powell (1988)
Grasshopper Pueblo, Arizona	AD 1270–1400	2958	103	3.4	Hinkes (1983)
New York African Burial Ground	Postmedieval	1318	122	9.2	Mack et al. (2009)
Total		**4599**	**257**	**5.5**	
North Africa					
Kellis 2, Egypt	Roman	1116	99	8.9	Shukrum and Molto (2009)
Asia					
Man Bac, Vietnam	Neolithic	270	10	3.7	Oxenham and Domett (2011)
Ban Chiang, Thailand	Prehistoric	159	20	12.6	Halcrow et al. (2013)
Ban Lum Khao, Thailand	Prehistoric	168	11	6.5	Halcrow et al. (2013)
Khok Phanom Di, Thailand	Prehistoric	152	9	5.9	Halcrow et al. (2013)
Mueang Sema, Thailand	Prehistoric	167	23	13.8	Halcrow et al. (2013)
Non Nok Tha, Mongolia	Prehistoric	103	5	4.9	Halcrow et al. (2013)
Total		**1019**	**78**	**7.6**	

perhaps in the form of a piece of honeycomb wrapped in a rag for them to suck. At St Marylebone in postmedieval London 17.4% of all carious lesions occurred in the first permanent incisors of the children. While Miles et al. (2008) do not discount the use of a pacifier as a cause for rampant caries in past populations, they caution that these teeth would also have been more susceptible to caries as they are the first to erupt and hence, are exposed to a cariogenic environment for longer.

More detailed research into the prevalence of child dental caries in different settlement types has begun to emerge. Garcin et al. (2010) found a higher prevalence of

TABLE 4.2 True Prevalence Rates (TPR) for Dental Caries in the Permanent Teeth

	Period	Teeth Observed	Teeth Affected	Permanent Caries %	Sources
UK Sites					
Cannington, Somerset	Roman	827	5	0.6	Rahtz et al. (2000)
Cirencester, Gloucestershire	Roman	310	0	0	Wells (1982)
Great Casterton, Rutland	Roman	170	10	5.9	Philips and Leach (2008)
London Road, Gloucester	Roman	239	6	2.5	Márquez-Grant and Loe (2008)
Poundbury Camp, Dorset	Roman	1302	10	0.7	Lewis (unpublished)
Ancaster, Lincolnshire	Roman	149	1	0.7	Cox (1989)
Empingham II, Rutland	Early medieval	538	2	0.3	Mays (1996)
Raunds Furnells, Northants.	Early medieval	450	2	0.4	Lewis (unpublished)
Chevington Chapel, Northumberland	Late medieval	180	10	5.5	Boylston et al. (1998)
Chichester, Sussex	Late medieval	452	19	4.2	Lewis (2008)
Blackfriars, Ipswich	Late medieval	194	13	6.7	Mays (1991)
St Gregory's Priory	Late medieval	329	0	0	Dawson (2011)
St Helen-on-the-Walls, York	Late medieval	555	8	1.4	Lewis (unpublished)
St Mary's leprosarium, Winchester	Late medieval	157	0	0	Roffey and Tucker (2012)
Taunton, Somerset	Late medieval	385	3	0.7	Dawson (2011)
Fishergate House, York	Late medieval	549	6	1.1	Holst (2005)
Grantham, Lincolnshire	Late medieval	313	3	0.9	Boulter (1992)
Christ Church Spitalfields, London	Postmedieval	320	20	6.2	Lewis (unpublished)
St Oswald's Priory, Gloucester	Multiperiod	486	14	2.6	Lewis (2013)
Wharram Percy, Yorkshire	Multiperiod	647	5	0.8	Lewis (unpublished)
Total		**8552**	**137**	**1.6**	
Other European Sites					
Smorkullen, Sweden	Iron Age	468	82	17.5	Liebe-Harkort et al. (2010)
Turku, Finland	Late medieval	605	41	6.8	Varrela (1991)
Mikulcice, Prague	Early medieval	3011	88	2.9	Garcin et al. (2010)
Norroy, Prague	Early medieval	434	14	1.9	Garcin et al. (2010)
Prusanky, Prague	Early medieval	639	13	2.0	Garcin et al. (2010)
Cherborg, Prague	Early medieval	206	0	0	Garcin et al. (2010)
Bijelo Brdo, Croatia	Early medieval	113	4	4.5	Marin et al. (2005)
Total		**5476**	**242**	**4.4**	
North and South America					
Moundville, Mississippi	AD 1050–1550	798	101	12.6	Powell (1988)

Continued

TABLE 4.2 True Prevalence Rates for Dental Caries in the Permanent Teeth—cont'd

	Period	Teeth Observed	Teeth Affected	Permanent Caries %	Sources
American Indian, Georgia	Precontact	180	0	0	Larsen et al. (1991)
Grasshopper Pueblo, Arizona	AD 1270–1400	830	25	3.0	Hinkes (1983)
Total		1806	126	6.9	
North Africa					
Kellis 2, Egypt	Roman	551	21	3.8	Shukrum and Molto (2009)
Total		551	21	3.8	
Asia					
Shih-San-Hang, Taiwan	Iron Age	2871	19	0.7	Halcrow et al. (2013)
Jomon, Japan	2500 BC-AD 300	427	28	6.5	Temple and Larsen (2007)
North Honshu Yayoi, Japan	2500 BC-AD 300	121	7	5.8	Temple and Larsen (2007)
South Hanshu Yayoi, Japan	2500 BC-AD 300	200	22	10.5	Temple and Larsen (2007)
Tanegashima Yayoi, Japan	2500 BC-AD 300	119	5	4.2	Temple and Larsen (2007)
Man Bac, Vietnam	Neolithic	163	0	0	Oxenham and Domett (2011)
Khok Phanom Di, Thailand	Prehistoric	183	13	7.1	Halcrow et al. (2013)
Total		4084	94	2.3	

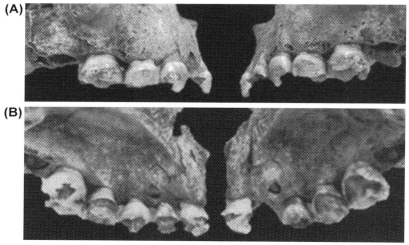

FIGURE 4.3 Severe caries in the anterior deciduous teeth of a 3- to 4-year-old from Ancaster, England (AD 270–410). The severity and location of the lesions suggest the cause was the use of a pacifier or bottle that maintained high levels of sugar in the anterior part of the mouth (see Bonsall et al., 2016). Teeth are viewed from the front (A) and back (B). *Photograph by A. Rohnbogner.*

caries in the children from urban and rural sites than from the coastal sites in the medieval region of Great Moravia (Czech Republic, France), while the rural sample had more severe expressions of caries than the urban sample. In an analysis of 433 nonadults (1–17 years) from 15 urban and rural Romano–British settlements in England, Rohnbogner and Lewis (2016) identified higher rates of caries in the urban sites (1.8%) compared to rural (0.4%) settlements, with children from urban settlements having significantly higher levels of caries in the deciduous dentition (3.0%). It was argued that these differences reflected the influence of the Roman lifestyle in the urban groups, including access to refined flour and high status foods such as honey, as opposed to a more modest diet and coarser food in the countryside.

Recording and Reporting Caries in Children

After a hiatus in the 1990s, the study of dental disease in children from archeological contexts has undergone a recent resurgence. Despite this, many researchers still choose to omit individuals under the age of 20 years from their studies or fail to adequately report the prevalence of lesions (usually caries) in the primary dentition. In other cases, children and unsexed adults are placed in the same category as separate from the rates reported in males and females. Differences in recording and reporting mean that it is difficult to then compare rates in different geographical, ethnic, or subsistence groups to gain some understanding of differences in the factors that influence the development of caries in children. For a detailed review to be carried out, the number of deciduous and permanent teeth available, as well as the number of children with each dentition needs to be reported. Children are more susceptible to caries when their teeth are newly erupted, with caries rates in the primary teeth usually higher than for the permanent teeth, so comparisons within the sample are necessary. Children also have mixed dentition, with teeth coming into occlusion or being shed at different times. Although visible in the skeletonized jaw, teeth that are still contained within the gum will not be susceptible to caries and so need to be counted and removed from true prevalence rates. For example, Keene (1986) divided his sample into a "deciduous group" (6 months–5 years), "mixed dentition group" (6–11 years), and "adolescent group" (12–17 years) allowing the different age groups and dentition types to be compared. As caries is a degenerative disease, the age at which it occurs most frequently should be reported (Halcrow et al., 2013).

That said, studies that merely report the prevalence rate of caries on the number of teeth observed can result in artificially high values. Molars are both most commonly affected by caries, and the most likely teeth to survive the burial environment; hence, a sample with poor preservation of the anterior teeth will have artificially high rates compared to another sample where the preservation of anterior and posterior teeth is equal (Hillson, 1996). In her study of caries in Scottish medieval children, O'Sullivan et al. (1989) reported caries of the molar teeth and anterior teeth separately to take account of this issue, and such an approach that has been employed by other scholars (Buikstra and Ubelaker, 1994; Halcrow et al., 2013; Moore and Corbett, 1973, 1975, 1976). Recording which teeth are affected and on which surfaces may help to discern the time at which children were weaned, and the teeth most susceptible to decay in different populations and time periods. The coexistence of enamel hypoplasia may influence the tooth surface that is affected and also the general susceptibility of each child to developing lesions.

A scheme devised to allow different caries types to be compared has been developed by Moore and Corbett (1971), and adapted by Buikstra and Ubelaker (1994) and Halcrow et al. (2013), and is presented in Table 4.3.

What actually constitutes a carious lesion also needs to be considered. A natural pit on the external surface of the tooth may be indistinguishable from early caries unless viewed internally. As the bacteria can spread through the softer dentine much more easily that the enamel, there is usually an expansion of destruction below the enamel surface producing a "funnel-shaped" lesion (Ortner, 2003, p. 590). Although most researchers favor penetration of the enamel before a carious lesion is identified, rather than scoring the early signs of opacity or straining, even recognition of these lesions can vary between observers (Liebe-Harkort et al., 2010).

TABLE 4.3 Scheme for Recording Dental Caries Type

Code	Caries Type
–	No tooth present, tooth not erupted or observable
0	No lesion present
1	Occlusal surfaces: all grooves, pits, cusps, and the buccal and lingual grooves of the molars
2	Interproximal surfaces: includes the mesial and distal cervical regions
3	Smooth surfaces: buccal (labial) and lingual surfaces other than grooves
4	Cervical: caries originates at a CEJ, except the interproximal regions
5	Root caries: below the CEJ
6	Large caries: cavities have destroyed much of the tooth and cannot be assigned to a particular surface of origin

From Halcrow, S., Harris, N., Tayles, N., Ikehara-Quebral, R., Pietrusewsky, M., 2013. From the mouths of babes: dental caries in infants and children and the intensification of agriculture in mainland southeast Asia. American Journal of Physical Anthropology 150, 412.

There are several methods used for recoding caries; the observed caries rate or caries index is produced by calculating the total number of carious teeth over the total observed presented as a percentage, also known as the true prevalence rate; the decayed, missing, or filled (DMF) index used in modern clinical studies is problematic as it does not take into account individuals having more than one caries on a tooth and is based on the presumption that all 32 permanent (rather than deciduous) teeth are preserved (Hillson, 2001). As with the DMF method, the diseased-missing index assumes that all teeth were lost antemortem as the result of caries and hence, includes resorbed sockets within the count (Hillson, 2001). Similarly, Lukacs' (1995) corrected caries rate (CCR) follows the same principle but calculates CCR in relation to the number of observed teeth with pulp exposure as the result of caries but does not differentiate between anterior and posterior teeth in the final calculation. Hillson (2001) warns that the exfoliation (or shedding) of deciduous teeth means that caries data will be lost when teeth are replaced by permanent teeth. In some cases, it may be desirable to record whether caries occurred more commonly in the maxillary or mandibular dentition, and so, given the complexity of the data, a single caries "index" may not be appropriate. Instead a series of tables and graphs may be necessary to show different categories of lesions, locations, and tooth types.

When reporting dental caries in nonadult populations, the following minimum data is recommended:

- Number of individuals with deciduous dentitions (by age)
- Number of individuals with permanent dentitions (by age)
- Number of individuals with mixed dentitions (by age)
- Number of deciduous teeth observed/in occlusion
- Number of permanent teeth observed/in occlusion
- Number and percentage of occluded deciduous teeth with caries (anterior and posterior)
- Number and percentage of occluded permanent teeth with caries (anterior and posterior)
- Number and percentage of affected teeth with visible underlying enamel hypoplasia

Dental Calculus

Calculus (or tartar) is a hard substance created by mineralized plaque on the surfaces of the tooth. If not removed, plaque will turn into calculus after around 2 weeks. It is predominantly made up of calcium phosphate and survives well in the burial environment. There are two forms of calculus: supra- and subgingival, describing its location on the crown or root of the tooth, respectively (Hillson, 1996). The lingual surfaces of the lower anterior teeth are most commonly affected by calculus deposits as they have the best alkaline environment suitable for its formation. Due to the buildup of calcium phosphates, calculus formation over a carious tooth will halt the progression of the cavity (Waldron, 2009, p. 241). Recent studies of calculus in adult remains have identified fragments of pollen and hair (Weyrich et al., 2015), with advances in biomolecular sequencing proving effective in identifying aDNA of oral pathogens (Warinner et al., 2013). The location of calculus on the teeth may have interesting implications in assessing the lifestyle of the individual. For instance, occlusal calculus indicates a lack of natural wear through chewing, and may be indicative of an abscess or other pathology in the jaw, or perhaps indicate paralysis. A buildup of calculus on the labial aspects of the teeth may indicate a period of invalidity before death (Fig. 4.4). Although considered a degenerative condition that increases with age, dental calculus is seen in nonadult dentitions. For example,

(A)

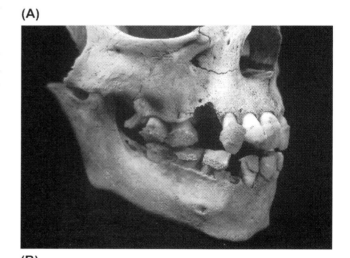

(B)

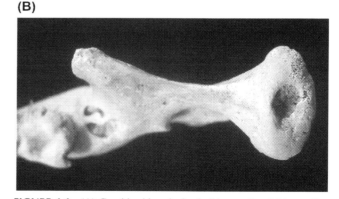

FIGURE 4.4 (A) Considerable calculus buildup on the right mandibular and maxillary teeth of a 10- to 14-year-old from Romano–British Dorchester on Thames, Oxfordshire (skeleton 169). (B) The child has a lytic lesion on the right mandibular condyle indicative of a bone cyst. These are usually benign but malignant cysts are slow growing and are associated with pain on the affected side. It is possible that this may have been the cause for the disuse on the right side of the jaw. *Photograph courtesy of Ceri Falys, Thames Valley Archaeological Service.*

Prowse et al. (2008) recorded dental calculus in 42.3% of the nonadults as young as 2.5 years old from Rome. A total of 16.3% of deciduous teeth were affected, with molars making up 21% of the teeth involved, and the canines and incisors also showing deposits. The authors suggested that the consumption of soft weaning foods contributed to this pattern. Erupting teeth are particularly susceptible to dental infection and dental plaque.

Periapical Cavitation

There are three types of periapical lesion that may be apparent on the alveolar bone: cysts, granulomas, and abscesses. About half of the cavities seen in the jaws are granulomas followed by abscesses and periapical cysts (Waldron, 2009). All result from an infected pulp cavity, where an infection travels down the root canal and emerges at the apical foramen. Low grade infections in the periapical area may become chronic and produce a granuloma, which over time may develop into a cyst. Granulomas are identified as smooth-walled cavities with a diameter typically less than 3 mm (Waldron, 2009). They evolve into cysts when the granulation tissue is replaced by fluid; a cyst has the same smooth-walled appearance but is generally larger than 3 mm (Figs. 4.5 and 4.6). Both granulomas and cysts are benign lesions and are rare in children compared to adults (Dias and Tayles, 1997). Primordial cysts result when a dental follicle fails to develop and undergoes cystic degeneration (Waldron, 2009).

Children are also susceptible to dentigerous cysts that form with a buildup of fluid between the lining of the dental follicle and crown of the developing tooth. They normally occur in the mandible and most often in the third molars (Hillson, 1996). While usually painless, dentigerous cysts may expand and cause enlargement of the jaw (Waldron, 2009). Less severe are eruption cysts that form in the mucosa just as a tooth is about to erupt. They are most common in the mandibular deciduous central incisors and first permanent molars. Clinically they appear as bluish gingival swellings that will eventually resolve (Bodner et al., 2005). A nonadult from St Oswald's Priory, Gloucester, shows a buildup of calculus on the second deciduous molar adjacent to an erupting first molar. The crypt is enlarged when compared to the opposite side, suggesting the presence of an eruption cyst (Fig. 4.7).

If the infection involves pyogenic (pus-forming) bacteria then an acute infection in the form of a periapical abscess may occur. Abscesses usually measure up to 3 mm in diameter and have roughened walls and margins (Dias and Tayles, 1997). In acute cases, the pus tracts through the cortical bone and soft tissue and bursts, resolving the infection. In chronic cases, the abscess will increase to a considerable size, forming a fistula from which the pus will continually drain. In the maxilla, the fistula may extend into the maxillary sinus, causing in secondary sinusitis (Waldron, 2009).

Periodontal Disease (Periodontitis)

Periodontal disease or periodontitis relates to the loss of the supporting structures of the tooth usually as a result of gingivitis from the buildup of plaque bacteria. Children are rarely affected by periodontal disease before puberty (Hillson, 1996), even with an abundance of dental plaque (Manson, 1980). Nevertheless, in a mixed dentition, exfoliating teeth provide a convenient area for plaque retention (Kinane et al., 2001). When it does occur the most common pathogen is *Actinobacillus actinomycetemcomitans* (Waldron, 2009), while viruses and fungi such as *Candida*

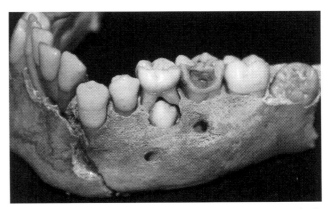

FIGURE 4.5 Small smooth-walled periapical lesion (granuloma) in the mandible of 12- to 14-year-old from St Oswald's Priory in Gloucester, England (AD 1540–1869, skeleton 307). Large caries is evident on the crown of the left first mandibular molar and there is inflammatory pitting of the alveolar bone.

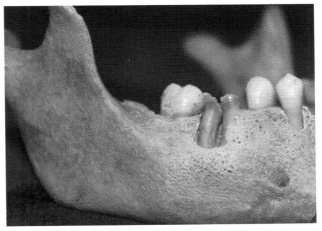

FIGURE 4.6 Large smooth-walled periapical lesion (cyst) on the mandible due to large caries on the right first molar in a 12- to 14-year-old from St Oswald's Priory in Gloucester, England (AD 1540–1869, skeleton 471). Note the pitting indicative of inflammation of the alveolar bone surrounding the lesion.

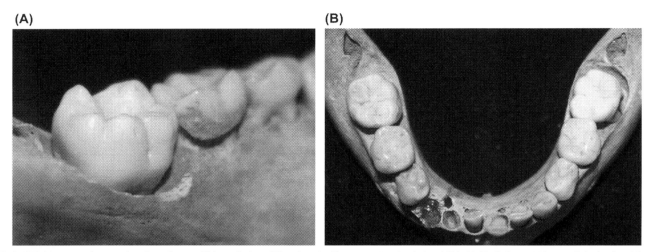

FIGURE 4.7 Eruption cyst in a 5- to 6-year-old from St Oswald's Priory in Gloucester, England (AD 1540–1869, skeleton 416). (A) Calculus is evident on the mandibular, second deciduous molar immediately adjacent to an erupting first permanent molar. (B) The enlarged left crypt when compared to the molar on the right is suggestive of an infection of the susceptible erupting tooth.

albicans are also predisposing factors (Darby and Curtis, 2001). There may be some ethnic predisposition to periodontitis in the deciduous dentition with children of European decent having lower levels than those of Asian, Mexican, or African descent (Jenkins and Papapanou, 2001; Pihlstrom et al., 2005). Scandinavian children are more susceptible to early periodontal conditions than other European groups (Kinane et al., 2001).

Gingivitis can occur in children as the result of infections during dental eruption, dryness from mouth breathing, high gonadotrophic hormone levels at puberty, from vitamin C deficiency and from an infection with the Herpes simplex virus type 1. Primary herpetic gingivostomatitis is a self-limiting infection that occurs in children under 10 years of age and has a peak between the ages of 2 and 4 years (Al-Ghutaimel et al., 2014). The transition from gingivitis to periodontitis may take around 6 months, with only 10%–15% of cases making this transition (Kinane et al., 2001). Both the host and the bacteria release cytokines that initiates the inflammatory process and destruction of the collagen fibers in the alveolar bone (Waldron, 2009).

In clinical studies, periodontal recession is considered to have occurred when the distance between the cementoenamel junction and alveolar crest exceeds 2 mm (Jenkins and Papapanou, 2001). Individuals with periodontitis will loose bone incrementally over the years, and therefore periodontal disease is more readily identified in an adult's remains. Periodontitis usually occurs at puberty in children aged 10–14 years, when there is a documented increase in the number and type of oral microflora not related to oral hygiene that may reflect the hormonal influence on the host's immune response at this time (Darby and Curtis, 2001). Juvenile (aggressive) periodontitis is divided into two forms: localized and generalized. Localized periodontal disease affects two teeth, normally the first permanent molars and the incisors (Al-Ghutaimel et al., 2014). Generalized aggressive periodontal disease is normally seen in adolescents and affects the entire dentition (Al-Ghutaimel et al., 2014). The most severe form is necrosing ulcerating periodontitis seen in young individuals with severe malnourishment, or very poor dental hygiene (Kinane, 2001). Periodontitis will also occur in children with genetic or systemic conditions including leukemia, Langerhans cell histiocytosis, and Down syndrome (Al-Ghutaimel et al., 2014). Children with Down syndrome have a greater susceptibility to periodontitis of the lower anterior teeth, possibly due to defects in the thymus-dependent system (Meyle and Gonzáles, 2001). To date, no specific studies into the prevalence of periodontal disease in nonadults have been carried out, and the condition is generally considered rare.

Antemortem Tooth Loss

It is rarely possible in the archeological record to assess whether a tooth has been lost due to natural causes or as the result of extraction during treatment, and there is little information on dental treatment for children in the past. Normal antemortem tooth loss increases with age and is usually the result of gradual alveolar reduction and secondary cementum deposition; however, teeth may also be lost due to trauma (Hillson, 1996). The number of missing teeth are counted, recorded, and used as part of the recording process. A general rise in the presence of antemortem tooth loss, although still rare, is seen in nonadult skeletons from 19th century contexts (Fig. 4.8).

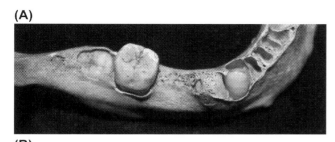

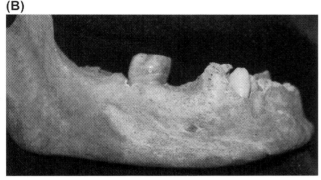

FIGURE 4.8 Antemortem tooth loss of the mandibular second deciduous molar seen from (A) above and (B) the lateral aspect in a 10- to 14-year-old from St Oswald's Priory in Gloucester, England (AD 1540–1869, skeleton 323). The first deciduous molar has been lost postmortem and the second premolar is not erupting.

DENTAL ANOMALIES

Dental anomalies are classified according to the time at which they develop. Numerical anomalies occur during the development of the dental germ, shape anomalies occur during the differentiation phase, and position anomalies occur during dental eruption (Lopes et al., 1991; Schuurs, 2013). Anomalies often occur together and may be related to particular syndromes, for example, supernumerary teeth are related to cleft palate (Lopes et al., 1991), and hypodontia and changes in tooth morphology are regularly seen in Down syndrome. Teeth may also be transposed with the most common appearance being for the maxillary canine to transpose with the first premolar. Over 30 developmental or genetically linked anomalies can be identified in the dentition.

Hypodontia

Hypodontia refers to dentitions with fewer teeth than normal due to agenesis of the dental germ or failure of the dental germ to fully develop (Fig. 4.9). Anodontia refers to a congenital absence of all teeth and oligodontia to the absence of most of the teeth (Schuurs, 2013). Agenesis of a dental germ may result from rubella, birth trauma, endocrine disorders, or can be hereditary. Between 2% and 10% of children of European decent have hypodontia, with girls more commonly affected than boys (Schuurs, 2013). Care should be taken to distinguish true hypodontia, where the tooth has

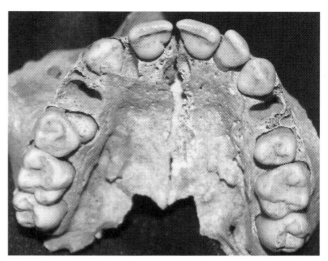

FIGURE 4.9 Hypodontia of the permanent teeth in a 12- to 14-year-old from St Oswald's Priory, in Gloucester, England (AD 1540–1869, skeleton 298). The right maxillary lateral incisor has failed to develop with the canine erupting in its place.

failed to form, from the fusion of two neighboring teeth, or a failure to erupt due to insufficient room in the jaw. The latter will require a radiograph to confirm (Ortner, 2003).

Hypodontia of the deciduous teeth affects less that 1% of children with 50% of cases affecting only one tooth. The most common deciduous teeth to be affected are the maxillary central and lateral incisors. When the canines are affected it usually indicates a genetic disorder such as cleft palate (Schuurs, 2013), and Lopes et al. (1991) reported hypodontia in 33.5% of cleft palate cases compared to 4.5% in the normal population. Hypodontia of the permanent teeth is usually symmetrical, and affects, in order of occurrence, the third molars (<35% of cases), lateral incisors, second premolars, mandibular central incisors, and maxillary first premolars (Ortner, 2003). In hypodontia of the permanent teeth, overall dental development may be delayed by around 1.5 years (Uslenghi and Liversidge, 2006), a factor that needs to be considered when assigning a dental age.

Permanent tooth agenesis often leads to the retention of the overlying deciduous tooth, which may become badly worn and carious. As the normal development of the jaws relies on the formation of the teeth, more severe cases of dental agenesis may also result in abnormalities of the mandible or maxilla (Zivanovic, 1982). Bondarets and McDonald (2000) showed a reduction in anterior facial height of children with agenesis of six or more teeth resulting in a flat or concave facial profile.

Tillier et al. (1998) reported hypodontia in a 9-year-old from Middle Palaeolithic Qafzeh in the Near East with agenesis of the left mandibular second premolar. An early case of dental agenesis was discovered in a 12- to 14-year-old Neanderthal from Malarnaud, France, with hypodontia of the central permanent mandibular incisors. Mack et al. (2009) also reported hypodontia of the left maxillary central incisor in a 4- to 6-year-old with cleft palate, craniostenosis, and rickets from the New York African Burial Ground. A more severe example of oligodontia was reported in an 8- to 9-year-old from El Burgo de Osma Cathedral in Soria, Spain (Fig. 4.10). The child displayed widespread dysplasia and agenesis of the teeth on the right side of the mandible from the lateral incisor to the second molar. The right mandibular ramus was noticeable smaller than the left (Garralda and Herrerin, 2003; Garralda et al., 2002). Anodontia is rare, and there are no known cases in the archeological record probably because it is linked to fatal syndromes (Schuurs, 2013).

Hyperdontia (Supernumerary Teeth)

Hyperdontia normally occurs in the anterior maxillary dentition. Supernumerary teeth are classified according to their location as "normotrophic," occurring within the dental alveolus, or "heterotophic" when they are located in the surrounding jaw, sinuses, or nasal cavity (Ortner, 2003). However, not all heterotrophic teeth are supernumerary. The shape of an additional tooth can vary from a normal morphology, mimicking the original tooth (supplement or eumorphic tooth), to an atypical morphology (Schuurs, 2013). These atypical teeth may display extra cusps (tuberculated) or be more irregular due to tumor-like excessive growth of the dental tissue (odontomatous). Peg-shaped teeth, or mesiodens, are the most common and tend to be located between the central and lateral incisors. Their presence can cause malocclusion, infection, and cyst formation (Rosenzweig and Garbarski, 1965). Hyperdontia is rare in the deciduous dentition, making up 0.5%–1% of cases, whereas up to 3% occur in the permanent teeth (Fig. 4.11). The incidence of supernumerary teeth in modern populations has been estimated at 1.9% (Suzuki et al., 1995), but populations in Alaska have been reported to have a 10% occurrence (Schuurs, 2013). Lopes et al. (1991) recorded an incidence of supernumerary teeth in 16% of individuals with cleft palate.

An example of aheterotrophic supernumerary canine in a 12-year-old from Chicama in Peru was identified by Ortner (2003, p. 599) where an extra canine of normal size and shape (supplement) protrudes from the maxilla above the first premolar. The alveolus for the left canine indicates a tooth that was much smaller than normal. A probable case of anterior unilateral cleft palate and lip from late medieval St Oswald's Priory, Gloucester, demonstrated anterior displacement of the left central incisor with an enlarged supplement tooth taking its position. The lateral incisor has an underdeveloped root and is positioned posterior to the additional tooth but closer to the midline than the normal central incisor (Fig. 4.12).

Wear on the supernumerary tooth shows that it was in occlusion.

Natal and Neonatal Teeth

Natal teeth refer to the premature eruption of the deciduous dentition in utero, while neonatal teeth erupt within a month of birth. Eruption normally occurs in the lower incisors, which may appear normal or be hypoplastic with poorly formed roots. In some countries, children with natal teeth are viewed with suspicion and may be drowned or abandoned to ward off doom, whereas in other cultures, they are seen as a sign of a glorious future. For example, Napoleon and Louise XIV were reported to have had neonatal teeth (Schuurs, 2013).

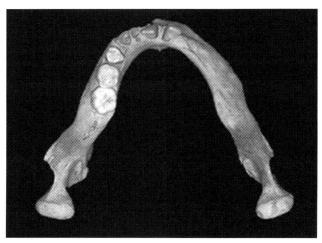

FIGURE 4.10 Oligodontia of the right side of a mandible of an 8- to 9-year-old from El Burgo de Osma, Spain (skeleton 41). *From Garralda, M., Herrerín, J., Vandermeersch, B., 2002. Child pathology in the mendicants' necropolis of El Burgo de Osma Cathedral (Soria, Spain). Bulletins et Mémoires de la Société d'Anthropologie de Paris 14 (3–4), 11.*

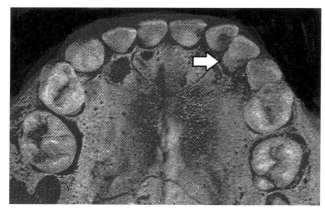

FIGURE 4.11 Extra left lateral deciduous incisor (hyperdontia) in a 2- to 3-year-old from Humic Cemetery, Mos, Hungary. *From Brabant, H., 1967. Palaeostomatology. In: Brothwell, D., Sandison, A., (Eds.), Diseases in Antiquity. Springfield, Charles C. Thomas, p. 541.*

Dental Fusion

Dental fusion usually involves the union of two teeth by the dentine and may involve the crown or the root. A radiograph will assist in assessing whether the pulp chamber is also affected. The etiology of dental fusion is unknown, but it may occur due to a genetic disorder, inflammation, or physical pressure on two adjacent dental germs (Benazzi et al., 2010; Smith and Wojcinski, 2011). Fused teeth may cause delay in eruption and are more common in deciduous teeth (Fig. 4.13). Fused deciduous teeth may precede fused permanent teeth (Schuurs, 2013). A deciduous tooth may also fuse with a supplement supernumerary tooth. It can be

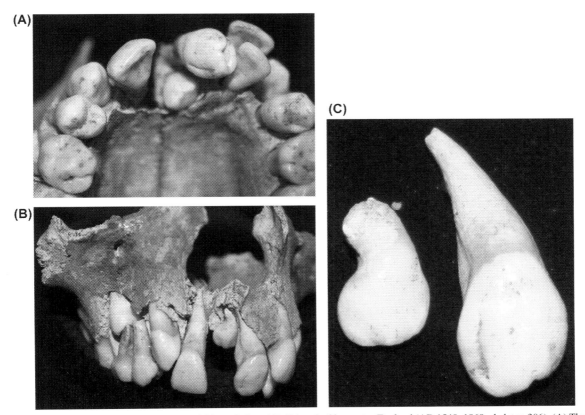

FIGURE 4.12 Supplement tooth in a 6- to 10-year-old from St Oswald's Priory in Gloucester, England (AD 1540–1869, skeleton 306). (A) The anterior palatine roof is absent suggesting cleft palate and lip. (B) The left central and lateral permanent incisors have been displaced by a large supplement tooth and the right central incisor is severely reduced. (C) Close-up of the reduced right central incisor (left) and the supplement tooth (right), which mimics a lateral incisor. Similar protruding supplement teeth have been identified in children with cleft lip and palate.

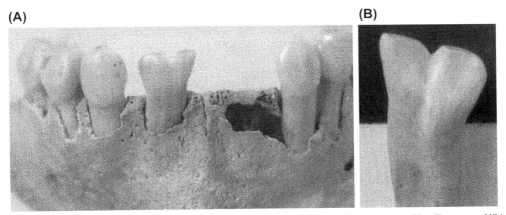

FIGURE 4.13 (A) Fusion of the right central and lateral deciduous incisors in a 3- to 5-year-old from Cherry Site, Tennessee, USA (2500–1000 BC, skeleton 8). (B) Lingual view. *From Smith, M.O., Wojcinski, M.C., 2011. Anomalous double-crowned primary teeth from Pre-Columbian Tennessee: a meta-analysis of hunter–gatherer and agriculturalist samples. International Journal of Paleopathology 1 (3), 176.*

difficult to determine if the anomaly is caused by the union of two separate dental germs or is the result of the abnormal division of a single dental germ.

Twelve of the 15 nonadult cases of fused teeth reported in the archeological record are from the United States with only 3 reported from Europe (Table 4.4). The majority of affected teeth are deciduous mandibular teeth with the lateral incisor and canine affected only slightly more frequently than the central and lateral incisors. Only 3 of the 17 teeth, or 17.6%, are maxillary. While it is more

TABLE 4.4 Cases of Dental Fusion Reported in the Nonadult Literature

Site	Date	Age (Years)	Teeth Affected	Sources
Arroyo Hondo, New Mexico, USA	AD 1300	4–5	Central and lateral incisors, right, deciduous, maxillary	Palkovich (1980, p. 105)
Jemez Valley, New Mexico, USA	–	8–10	Canine and lateral incisor, right, deciduous, mandibular	Ortner Research Slide Collection
Camp Robinson, Nebraska, USA	–	1.5	Central and lateral incisor, right, deciduous, mandibular	Ortner Research Slide Collection
Cherry, Tennessee, USA	2500–1000 BC	5–6	Canine and lateral incisor, right, deciduous, mandibular	Smith and Wojcinski (2011)
Cherry, Tennessee, USA	2500–1000 BC	3–5	Central and lateral incisors, left and right, deciduous, mandibular	Smith and Wojcinski (2011)
Citico, Tennessee, USA	AD 1300–1550	3–4	1. Canine and lateral incisor, left, deciduous, mandibular 2. Canine and lateral incisor, right, deciduous, mandibular 3. Canine and lateral incisor, right, deciduous, maxillary 4. Central and lateral incisors, left deciduous, maxillary	Smith and Wojcinski (2011)
Kays Landing, Tennessee, USA	2500–1000 BC	4–6	Canine and lateral incisor, left, deciduous, mandibular	Smith and Wojcinski (2011)
Oak View Landing, Tennessee, USA	2500–1000 BC	0.5–1	Canine and lateral incisor, right, deciduous, mandibular	Smith and Wojcinski (2011)
Toqua, Tennessee, USA	AD 1300–1550	1–2	1. Central and lateral incisors, left, deciduous, mandibular 2. Central and lateral incisors, left, deciduous, mandibular	Smith and Wojcinski (2011)
Toqua, Tennessee, USA	AD 1300–1550	1–2	Canine and lateral incisor, left, deciduous, mandibular	Smith and Wojcinski (2011)
Toqua, Tennessee, USA	AD 1300–1550	2–2.5	1. Canine and lateral incisor, left, deciduous, mandibular 2. Central and lateral incisors, right, deciduous, mandibular	Smith and Wojcinski (2011)
Toqua, Tennessee, USA	AD 1300–1550	1–2	Canine and lateral incisor, right, deciduous, mandibular	Smith and Wojcinski (2011)
St Martino in Rivosecco, Parma, Italy	14th century	5–6	Central and lateral incisors with supplement, right, deciduous, maxillary	Benazzi et al. (2010)
Wharram Percy, Yorkshire, UK	AD 950–1350	4–5	Central incisor, left, deciduous, mandibular	Mays (2007)
Wharram Percy, Yorkshire, UK	AD 950–1350	4–5	Fused left maxillary central incisor, permanent	Mays (2003)
Caister-on-Sea, Norfolk, UK	Early medieval	5–6	Canine and lateral incisor, right, deciduous, mandibular	Anderson (1990)

common for only two teeth to be involved (double teeth), Benazzi et al. (2010) reported a rare case of fusion of three deciduous teeth in a 5- to 6-year-old from late medieval St Martino, Parma, Italy. The anterior aspect of the maxilla is damaged revealing a peg-shaped mesiodens. This supernumerary tooth has fused to the upper right deciduous lateral and central incisors at both the crown and root. The fused tooth has subsequently been damaged by caries. Although there is postmortem damage obscuring the changes, its possible this is a case of cleft lip.

Macrodontia and Microdontia

Teeth may be unusually small (microdontia) or unusually large (macrodontia). True macrodontia should be differentiated from dental fusion, and microdontia coupled with hypodontia is a common finding in Down syndrome. The morphology of these teeth varies with third molars and lateral incisors in particular being "peg-shaped." Mann et al. (1990) suggest a possible diagnosis of Ekman-Westborg-Julin syndrome for an American–Indian child from Virginia with a series of dental anomalies including macrodontia of the first permanent and second deciduous molars, shovel-shaped central permanent incisors, three-rooted mandibular deciduous molars, dens invaginatus, agenesis of the permanent maxillary canines, and severe enamel defects of the deciduous first molars.

Talon Cusps

Talon cusps are common anomalies identified as supernumerary cusps on the incisors or canines of the deciduous or permanent dentition (Lee et al., 2007; Mellor and Ripa, 1970). They were first identified in 1950 by Bohn in the deciduous teeth of children with cleft lip or palate and have numerous names including: cingulum nodules, dental tubercles, hyperplastic cingulum, medial ridges, lingual cusps, and tuberculum dentale. The term talon cusp is widely used in the paleopathological literature (Stojanowski et al., 2011). The maxillary central incisors are the most common deciduous teeth affected, whereas the lateral maxillary incisors are more often affected in the permanent dentition where they are often associated with additional anomalies such as supernumerary teeth, fused teeth, microdontia, and mesiodens. They may be unilateral or bilateral, but there is no side preference. Talon cusps in the deciduous teeth do not equate to anomalies in their permanent successors (Lee et al., 2007). The appearance of the tubercle is classified according to Hattab et al. (1996) as type 1 (major), type 2 (semitalon), and type 3 (trace talon), with a major talon defined as a well-defined additional cusp that projects over the whole tooth or over half the distance from the cementoenamel junction to the incisal edge of the tooth crown. The anomaly is thought to result from the complex interaction of genetic and environmental factors resulting in hyperactivity of the anterior dental lamina (Lee et al., 2007).

The oldest cases of talon cusps were reported in three nonadults by Stojanowski et al. (2011) from the Windover Pond site, Florida (Fig. 4.14) and the Buckeye Knoll site in Texas, both dating to the Middle archaic period (7500 BP). A permanent talon cusp was found in a mummified child from pre-Columbian Peru by Sawyer et al. (1976) and was later reported in a left lateral deciduous maxillary incisor of an infant from Ban Non Wat in southwest Asia (Halcrow and Tayles, 2010). Mays (2003) studied the anomaly in the lateral maxillary incisor of a 4- to 5-year-old from Wharram Percy, Yorkshire. While major, type 1 talon cusps are obvious in the archeological record, the more subtle forms are likely to be missed. Both Mays (2003) and Halcrow and Tayles (2010) noted the additional presence of double teeth in their individuals. Although comparatively rare, as an epigenetic trait the talon cusp may be a useful tool in tracking broad scale population movement, but issues about its variability and descriptions in the literature make it a challenging area of study (Mays, 2003).

DENTAL TRAUMA

Teeth can be traumatized through a blow to the face, rough play, or biting onto hard material during occupational activity. The maxillary incisors are most commonly affected and males are more likely to experience this type of trauma than females (O'Brian, 1994). Most are confined to cracking of the dental enamel, but if the trauma is severe and the pulp cavity exposed, it may lead to a periapical abscess. Solitary bone cysts may result from trauma that leads to bleeding into the bone and can be recognized with radiography

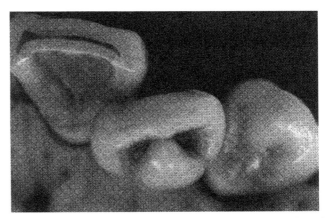

FIGURE 4.14 A type 1 talon cusp in a maxillary left permanent lateral incisor of a 10- to 12-year-old from Windover Pond, Florida (7500 BP, skeleton 75). *From Stojanowski, C., Johnson, K., Doran, G., Ricklis, R., 2011. Talon cusp from two archaic period cemeteries in North America: implications for comparative evolutionay medicine. American Journal of Physical Anthropology 144, 415.*

(Waldron, 2009). Mays (2007) identified dental chipping in the deciduous teeth of two children, a 4- to 5-year-old and a 2.5-year-old from Wharram Percy, England. The first had a fracture of the right deciduous maxillary incisor, and the second child had three affected deciduous first molars, probably from biting down on a hard object. Identification of trauma needs to be distinguished from postmortem damage during curation. True fractures will show rounding of the enamel edges demonstrating subsequent use.

Dental Modification

Dental modification is an ancient practice in the Americas, East Asia, and Africa and involves cutting, filing, and drilling the enamel of the anterior teeth. Inlays of stone and gold may also be observed. In his study of the practice in pre-Hispanic material from the Americas, Romero (1970) provides a chart that is the basis for the classification of these changes. Romero did not report any changes in individuals younger than 18 years. However, dental modification has been reported in nonadults elsewhere. At the slave cemetery at Rupert's Valley, St Helena, 44% of 13- to 18-year-olds (n = 22) had dental modification of their mandibular or maxillary central incisors due to chipping and filing, compared to 10.4% (n = 11) of 7- to 12 year-olds. The youngest child with cultural ablation was 8–10 years old, suggesting the practice may indicate a rite of passage within the group (Witkin, 2011), although Witkin argues that the large number of teenagers without the modification suggests another factor is influencing the practice.

DISRUPTION IN DENTAL DEVELOPMENT

Defects in enamel development and dental morphology as the result of specific conditions including congenital syphilis (mulberry molars, Hutchinson's incisors), leprosy (leprogenic odontodysplasia), osteogenesis imperfecta (amelogenesis imperfecta), and chemotherapy (mercury teeth) are described elsewhere in this book.

Dental Enamel Hypoplasia

Dental enamel hypoplasia are areas of decreased enamel thickness that occur during a disturbance of ameloblast deposition on the developing crowns of permanent and deciduous teeth. Enamel matrix secretion is disrupted due to elevated cortisone levels that inhibit protein synthesis as a result of a stress episode (Rose et al., 1985) and many factors have been associated with their occurrence (Table 4.5). Detailed information on how enamel hypoplasia are recognized and recorded is described elsewhere (Hillson, 2014). Enamel defects in children have the potential to detail specific stressors that may be responsible for their formation, particularly on the deciduous teeth. In their study of 96 modern Finnish children, Aine et al. (2000) identified higher levels of enamel defects in the teeth of children who were born prematurely. Of the premature cohort, 66% and 38% displayed hypoplasia on the deciduous and permanent teeth respectively, compared to 2% and 11% of the full-term children, with 72% (23/32) of the prematurely born children showing hypoplasia in both sets of dentition. Aine et al. (2000) hypothesize that mineral deficiencies at birth are not compensated for in the postnatal period and continue into older childhood, despite supplementation.

Ogden et al. (2007) and Hillson and Bond (1997) discuss wide "plane form" hypoplasia that are produced when a whole band of ameloblasts fail to form (Fig. 4.15). These can result in deep defects exposing the dentine. When they occur during cusp formation result in nodules of enamel similar to mulberry molars of congenital syphilis, often with pitted defects around the edge of the plane

TABLE 4.5 Clinical Features Related to the Formation of Deciduous and Permanent Dental Enamel Defects

Factor	Study
Fever	Kronfield and Schour (1939)
Birth trauma	Kronfield and Schour (1939)
Congenital syphilis	Hillson et al. (1998)
Tuberculosis	Knick (1982)
Low birth weight	Seow (1992)
Severe childhood malnutrition	Sweeney et al. (1971)
Rickets and hypocalcaemia	Kreshover (1960), Levine and Keen (1974), Seow et al. (1984)
Zinc deficiency	Dolphin and Goodman (2002)
Intrauterine undernutrition due to poor maternal diet	Acosta et al. (2003), Noren (1983), Noren et al. (1978)
Prematurity	Aine et al. (2000)

(Hillson, 2014). Ogden et al. (2007) noted a high number of these lesions in postmedieval children from Broadgate in London on both the deciduous and permanent molars and suggested that these "cuspal enamel hypoplasia" represented a more severe form of systemic stress, such as rickets. Ogden et al. (2007) argued for the need to differentiate between the different types of hypoplasia and to record them in association with any systemic conditions. For example, Walker (2012b) provides an example of deep plane form hypoplasia in an 11- to 12-year-old from postmedieval Bunhill, London, with clear evidence of rickets (Fig. 4.16). Hillson (2014, p. 192) discusses the possibility of plane form hypoplasia in deciduous teeth indicating neonatal tetany or respiratory distress. The former has been shown to cause defects on the deciduous canine crowns. Hillson (2014) argues that defects on the first deciduous incisors may indicate stress 1 month after birth, and defects on the lateral deciduous incisors could result from stress between 3 and 4 months after birth and, hence, could be considered perinatal.

Turner's and Skinner's Teeth

In the clinical literature, Turner's teeth describe patches of thinned enamel on the permanent teeth due to overlying caries on the deciduous tooth. They are most common on the permanent premolars as the result of infection in the deciduous molars (Schuurs, 2013). Similar thinned enamel lesions have been reported on the deciduous anterior teeth in archeological populations, most often as isolated patches on the mandibular canine crown (Fig. 4.17; Skinner, 1986; Taji et al., 2000). Skinner and Hung (1986) argue that the midcrown location of the defect suggests mechanical trauma shortly after birth because the labial bulge of the crypt containing the developing canine crown is very thin or absent, making the crown susceptible to even minor trauma (Skinner, 1986). Subsequent localized death of ameloblasts causes the defect (Skinner and Newell, 2003). In the Sudan, where teething problems are treated by lancing the alveolar process over the unerupted tooth with a heated needle, 28% of children receiving the treatment had defects on their deciduous canines compared to 8% in the nontreated group (Rasmussen et al., 1992). Skinner et al. (1994) further reported these pit defects in nutritionally disadvantaged groups and in children born during months of low sunlight and with low levels of retinol (i.e., vitamin A deficiency), which may hinder development of the alveolar bone. Taji et al. (2000) suggest

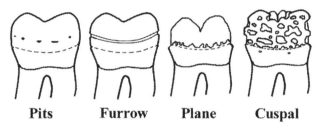

FIGURE 4.15 Diagram showing the different expressions of dental defects in the molars. The *dotted line* indicates the cervical third of the crown that is little affected in all forms. *From Ogden, A., Pinhasi, R., White, W., 2007. Gross enamel hypoplasia in molars from subadults in a 16–18th century London Graveyard. American Journal of Physical Anthropology 133 (3), 964.*

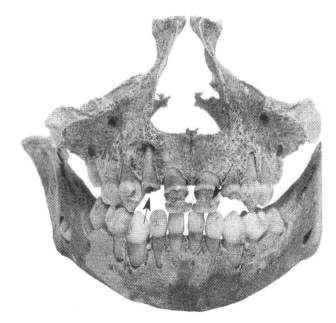

FIGURE 4.16 Severe deep plane enamel hypoplasia on the maxillary deciduous central incisors of an 11-year-old from Bunhill, London (AD, 1833–1853, skeleton 545). Severe caries on the lateral incisors suggests they were also affected. *From Walker, D., 2012b. Disease in London, 1st-19th Centuries, Museum of London Archaeology, London, p. 250.*

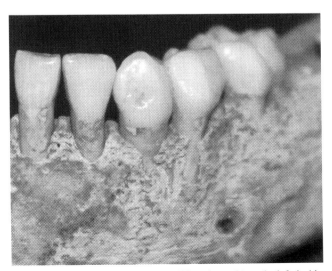

FIGURE 4.17 Pitted enamel defect (Skinner's tooth) on the left deciduous canine of a 4- to 5-year-old from early medieval St Oswald's Priory in Gloucester, England (AD 900–1120, skeleton 484).

genetic predisposition and maternal nutritional status may be linked to their formation (McDonell and Oxenham, 2014; Taji et al., 2000). Halcrow and Tayles (2008) noted a high prevalence of localized pit defects in 40% of infants from prehistoric Thailand suggesting they may be associated with maternal health resulting in low birth weight babies, and noted that the defects leave the child susceptible to caries. As the result of his extensive research, hypoplastic patches on the deciduous canine crowns are often referred to as "Skinner's teeth."

REFERENCES

Acosta, A., Goodman, A., Backstrand, J., Dolphin, A., 2003. Infants' enamel growth disruptions and the quantity and quality of mother's perinatal diets in Solis, Mexico. American Journal of Physical Anthropology 36, 55.

Afroughi, S., Faghihzadeh, S., Khaledim, M., Motlagh, M., 2010. Dental caries analysis in 3-5 years old children: a spatial modelling. Archives of Oral Biology 55, 374–378.

Aine, L., Backström, M., Mäki, R., Kuusela, A., Ikonen, R., Mäki, M., 2000. Enamel defects in primary and permanent teeth of children born prematurely. Journal of Oral Pathological Medicine 29, 403–409.

Al-Ghutaimel, H., Riba, H., Al-Kahtani, S., Al-Duhaimi, S., 2014. Common periodontal diseases of children and adolescents. International Journal of Dentistry 2014, 7.

Aligne, C., Moss, M., Auinger, P., Weitzman, M., 2003. Association of pediatric dental caries with passive smoking. Journal of the American Medical Association 289 (10), 1258–1264.

Anderson, S., 1990. The human remains from Caister-on-Sea. In: Darling, M., Gurney, D. (Eds.), Caister-on-Sea Excavations by Charles Green 1951-1955, pp. 185–190 (Norfolk: East Anglian Archaeology Reports).

Ashley, M., 2001. It's only teething…A report of the myths and modern approaches to teething. British Dental Journal 191, 4–8.

Baqain, Z., Newman, L., Hyde, N., 2004. How serious are oral infections? The Journal of Laryngology & Otology 118, 561–565.

Beeton, I., 1861. Book of Household Management. SO Beeton, London.

Benazzi, S., Buti, L., Kullmer, O., Winzen, O., Gruppioni, G., 2010. Report of three fused primary human teeth in archeological material. International Journal of Osteoarchaeology 20, 481–485.

Bodner, L., Goldstein, J., Sarnat, H., 2005. Eruption cysts: a clinical report of 24 new cases. Journal of Clinical Pediatric Dentistry 28 (2), 183–186.

Bohn, A., 1950. Anomalies of the lateral incisor in cases of harelip and cleft palate. Acto Odontologica Scandinavica 9, 41–59.

Bondarets, N., McDonald, F., 2000. Analysis of the vertical facial form in patients with severe hypodontia. American Journal of Physical Anthropology 111, 177–184.

Bonsall, L., Ogden, A., Mays, S., 2016. A case of early childhood caries (ECC) from late Roman Ancaster, England. International Journal of Osteoarchaeology 26 (3), 555–560.

Boulter, S., 1992. Death and Disease in Medieval Grantham (Ph.D. Thesis) University of Sheffield.

Boyce, W., Den Besten, K., Stamperdahl, J., Zhan, L., Jiang, Y., Adler, N., Featherstone, J., 2010. Social inequalities in childhood dental caries: the convergent roles of stress, bacteria and disadvantage. Social Science and Medicine 71, 1644–1652.

Boylston, A., Coughlan, J., Roberts, C., 1998. Report on the Analysis of Human Skeletal Remains from Chevington Chapel, Northumberland (Calvin Wells Laboratory Unpublished Report). University of Bradford.

Brabant, H., 1967. Palaeostomatology. In: Brothwell, D., Sandison, A. (Eds.), Diseases in Antiquity. Springfield, Charles C. Thomas, pp. 538–550.

Brown, T., Creed, S., Alexander, S., Barnard, K., Hancock, M., 2012. Vitamin D deficiency in children with dental caries – a prevalence study. Archives of Disease in Childhood 97 (103) on-line.

Buikstra, J.E., Ubelaker, D. (Eds.), 1994. Standards for Data Collection from Human Skeletal Remains. Arkansas Archeological Survey, Fayetteville.

Burt, B.A., 1981. The epidemiology of dental caries. In: Silverstone, L.M., Johnson, N.W., Hardie, J.M., Williams, R.A.D. (Eds.), Dental Caries: Aetiology, Pathology and Prevention. Macmillan, London, pp. 18–47.

Caffell, A., Holst, M., 2006. Osteological Analysis, Low Farm, Kirby Grindalythe, North Yorkshire (Unpublished Report). York Osteoarchaeology Ltd.

Caffell, A., Holst, M., 2007. Osteological Analysis, Horncastle, East Lincolnshire (Unpublished Report). York Osteoarchaeology Ltd.

Caffell, A., Holst, M., 2010. Osteological Analysis, The Church of St Michael and St Lawrence, Fewston, North Yorkshire (Unpublished Report). York Osteoarchaeology Ltd.

Cameron A., Widmer R., 2008. Handbook of Pediatric Dentistry. Elsevier Health Sciences, New York.

Chandra, P., Adlakha, V., 2015. Infant oral health. In: Virdi, M. (Ed.), Emerging Trends in Oral Health Sciences and Dentistry. INTECH, Croatia, pp. 151–164.

Clarke, M., Locker, D., Berall, G., Pencharz, P., Kenny, D.J., Judd, P., 2006. Malnourishment in a population of young children with severe early childhood caries. Pediatric Dentistry 28 (3), 254–259.

Connell, B., Gray Jones, A., Redfern, R., Walker, D., 2012. A Bioarchaeological Study of Medieval Burials on the Site of St Mary Spital. Museum of London Archaeology, London.

Cox, M., 1989. The Human Bones from Ancaster (Report 98/89, Unpublished). English Heritage Ancient Monuments Laboratory, London.

Darby, I., Curtis, M., 2001. Microbiology of periodontal disease in children and young adults. Periodontology 2000 (26), 33–53.

Dawson, H., 2011. Unearthing Late Medieval Children: Heath, Status and Burial Practice in Southern England (Ph.D. thesis). University of Bristol.

Dias, G., Tayles, N., 1997. 'Abscess cavity' – a misnomer. International Journal of Osteoarchaeology 7, 548–554.

Dolphin, A., Goodman, A., 2002. The influence of maternal diet on pregnancy-forming enamel zinc concentrations of children from the Solis Valley, Mexico. American Journal of Physical Anthropology 34, 64.

Forsyth Institute, 2011. New Pathogen Connected to Severe Early Childhood Caries Identified. Science Daily. www.sciencedaily.com/releases/2011/02/110228090214.htm.

Garcin, V., Veleminsky, P., Trefny, P., Alduc-Le Bagousse, A., 2010. Dental health and lifestyle in four early medieval juvenile populations: comparisons between urban and rural individuals, and between coastal and inland settlements. Journal of Comparative Human Biology 61, 421–439.

Garralda, M., Herrerin, J., 2003. Pathological mendicant child from the necropolis (XVII-XVIII C. A.D.) of the El Burgo de Osma Cathedral (Soria, Spain). Journal of Paleopathology 15 (1), 33–46.

Garralda, M., Herrerín, J., Vandermeersch, B., 2002. Child pathology in the mendicants' necropolis of El Burgo de Osma Cathedral (Soria, Spain). Bulletins et Mémoires de la Société d'Anthropologie de Paris 14 (3–4), 11.

Halcrow, S., Harris, N., Tayles, N., Ikehara-Quebral, R., Pietrusewsky, M., 2013. From the mouths of babes: dental caries in infants and children and the intensification of agriculture in mainland southeast Asia. American Journal of Physical Anthropology 150, 409–420.

Halcrow, S., Tayles, N., 2008. Stress near the start of life? Localised enamel hypoplasia of the primary canine in late prehistoric mainland Southeast Asia. Journal of Archaeological Science 35, 2215–2222.

Halcrow, S., Tayles, N., 2010. Talon cusp in a deciduous lateral incisor from prehistoric southeast Asia. International Journal of Osteoarchaeology 20 (2), 240–247.

Hattab, F., Yassin, O., Al-Nimri, K., 1996. Talon cusp in permanent dentition associated with other dental anomalies: review of literature and reports of seven cases. ASDC Journal of Dentistry for Children 63, 368–376.

Hillson, S., 1996. Dental Anthropology. Cambridge University Press, Cambridge.

Hillson, S., 2001. Recording dental caries in archaeological human remains. International Journal of Osteoarchaeology 11, 249–289.

Hillson, S., 2014. Tooth Development in Human Evolution and Bioarchaeology. Cambridge University Press, Cambridge.

Hillson, S., Bond, S., 1997. Relationship of enamel hypoplasia to the pattern of tooth crown growth: a discussion. American Journal of Physical Anthropology 104 (1), 89–103.

Hillson, S., Grigson, C., Bond, S., 1998. Dental defects of congenital syphilis. American Journal of Physical Anthropology 107 (1), 25–40.

Hinkes, M., 1983. Skeletal Evidence of Stress in Subadults: Trying to Come of Age at Grasshopper Pueblo. (Ph.D. thesis) University of Arizona, Arizona.

Holst, M., 2005. Fishergate House Artefacts and Environmental Evidence: The Human Bone (Unpublished Skeletal Report). York Osteoarchaeology.

Infante, P.F., Gillespie, G.M., 1974. An epidemiologic study of linear enamel hypoplasia of deciduous anterior teeth in Guatemalan children. Archives of Oral Biology 19, 1055–1061.

Irish, J.D., Scott, G.R., 2015. A Companion to Dental Anthropology. John Wiley & Sons, New York.

James, P.M.C., Miller, W.A., 1970. Dental conditions in a group of medieval English children. British Medical Journal 391–396.

Jenkins, W., Papapanou, P., 2001. Epidemiology of periodontal disease in children and adolescents. Periodontology 2000 (26), 16–32.

Keene, H., 1986. Dental caries prevalence in early Polynesians from the Hawaiian islands. Journal of Dental Research 65 (6), 935–938.

Kinane, D., 2001. Periodontal disease in children and adolescents: introduction and classification. Periodontology 2000 (26), 7–15.

Kinane, D., Podmore, M., Ebersole, J., 2001. Etiopathogenesis of periodontitis in children and adolescents. Periodontology 2000 (26), 54–91.

Knick, S.G., 1982. Linear enamel hypoplasia and tuberculosis in pre-Columbian North America. OSSA 8, 131–138.

Kreshover, S.J., 1960. Metabolic disturbances in tooth formation. Annual of the New York Academy of Sciences 85, 161–167.

Kronfield, R., Schour, I., 1939. Neonatal dental hypoplasia. Journal of the American Dental Association 26, 18–32.

Larsen, C., Shavit, R., Griffin, M., 1991. Dental caries evidence for dietary change: an archaeological context. In: Kelley, M., Larsen, C. (Eds.), Advances in Dental Anthropology. Wiley-Liss, New York, pp. 179–202.

Lee, C.-K., King, N., Lo, E., Cho, S.-Y., 2007. The relationship between a primary maxillary incisor with talon cusp and the permanent successor: a study of 57 cases. International Journal of Paediatric Dentistry 17, 178–185.

Levine, R., Keen, J., 1974. Neonatal enamel hypoplasia in association with symptomatic neonatal hypocalcaemia. British Dental Journal 137, 429–433.

Lewis, M., 2008. The children. In: Magilton, J., Lee, F., Boylston, A. (Eds.). Magilton, J., Lee, F., Boylston, A. (Eds.), Chichester Excavations 'Lepers outside the Gate' Excavations at the Cemetery of the Hospital of St James and St Mary Magdalene, Chichester, 1986-87 and 1993, vol. 10. Council for British Archaeology, York, pp. 174–186 (Research Report, 158).

Lewis, M., 2013. Children of the Golden Minster: St Oswald's Priory and the impact of industrialisation on child health. Journal of Anthropology. http://dx.doi.org/10.1155/2013/959472.

Li, X., Kolltveit, K., Tronstad, L., Olsen, I., 2000. Systemic diseases caused by oral infection. Clinical Microbiology Reviews 13 (4), 547–558.

Liebe-Harkort, C., 2012. Exceptional rates of dental caries in a Scandinavian early Iron Age population – a study of dental pathology at Alvastra, Östergötland, Sweden. International Journal of Osteoarchaeology 22, 168–184.

Liebe-Harkort, C., Ástvaldsdóttir, Á., Tranaeus, S., 2010. Quantification of dental caries by osteologists and odontologists – a validity and reliability study. International Journal of Osteoarchaeology 20, 525–539.

Lingström, P., Borrman, H., 1999. Distribution of dental caries in an early 17th century Swedish population with special reference to diet. International Journal of Osteoarchaeology 9, 395–403.

Lopes, L., Mattos, B., Andre, M., 1991. Anomalies in number of teeth in patients with lip and/or palate clefts. Brazilian Dental Journal 2 (1), 9–17.

Lukacs, J., 1995. The 'Caries Correction Factor': a new method of calibrating dental caries rates to compensate for antemortem loss of teeth. International Journal of Osteoarchaeology 5 (2), 151–156.

Mack, M., Goodman, A., Blakey, M., Mayes, A., 2009. Odontological indicators of disease, diet and nutritional inadequacy. In: Blakey, M., Rankin-Hill, L. (Eds.), Skeletal Biology of the New York African Burial Group Part 1. Howard University Press, New York, pp. 157–168.

Mann, R., Dahlberg, A., Stewert, T., 1990. Anomalous morphologic formation of deciduous and permanent teeth in a 5-year-old 15th century child: a variant of the Ekman-Westborg-Julin syndrome. Oral Surgery, Oral Medicine and Oral Pathology 70, 90–94.

Manson, J., 1980. Periodontics. Kimpton Medical Publishers, London.

Marin, V., Hrvoje, B., Mario Š, Željko, D., 2005. The frequency and distribution of caries in the medieval population of Bijelo Brdo in Croatia (10th-11th century). Archives of Oral Biology 50, 669–680.

Márquez-Grant, N., Loe, L., 2008. The human remains. In: Simmonds, A., Márquez-Grant, N., Loe, L. (Eds.), Life and Death in a Roman City: Excavation of a Roman Cemetery with a Mass Grave at 120–122 London Road, Gloucester. Oxford Archaeological Unit Ltd, Oxford, pp. 29–32.

Mays, S., 1989. The Anglo-Saxon Human Bone from School Street, Ipswich, Suffolk (Ancient Monuments Laboratory Report). English Heritage, London.

Mays, S., 1991. The Medieval Burials from Blackfriars Friary, School Street, Ipswich, Suffolk (Ancient Monuments Laboratory Report). English Heritage, London.

Mays, S., 1996. Human skeletal remains. In: Timby, J. (Ed.), The Anglo-Saxon Cemetery at Empingham II. Oxbow, Rutland. Oxford, pp. 21–34.

Mays, S., 2003. An unusual deciduous incisor in a medieval child. Journal of Paleopathology 15 (3), 159–166.

Mays, S., 2007. The human remains. In: Mays, S., Harding, C., Heighway, C. (Eds.). Mays, S., Harding, C., Heighway, C. (Eds.), Wharram a Study of a Settlement on the Yorkshire Wolds, XI: The Churchyard York University Archaeological Publications, vol. 13. English Heritage, London, pp. 77–192.

McDonell, A., Oxenham, M., 2014. Localised primary canine hypoplasia: implications for maternal and infant health at Man Bac, Vietnam. 4000-3500 years BP. International Journal of Osteoarchaeology 24 (4), 531–539.

McKinley, J., 2008. The 18th Century Baptist Church and Burial Ground at West Butts Street, Poole, Dorset. Wessex Archaeology Ltd., Sailsbury.

Mellor, J., Ripa, L., 1970. Talon cusp: a clinically significant anomaly. Oral Surgery, Oral Medicine and Oral Pathology 29, 225–228.

Meyle, J., Gonzáles, J., 2001. Influences of systemic disease on periodontitis in children and adolescents. Periodontology 2000 (26), 92–112.

Miles, A., Powers, N., Wroe-Brown, R., Walker, D., 2008. St Marylebone Church and Burial Ground in the 18th-19th Centuries. Excavations at St Marylebone School, 1992 and 2004-6. MOLAS Monograph, vol. 46. Museum of London Archaeology Service, London.

Miller, J., Vaughan-Williams, E., Furlong, R., Harrison, L., 1982. Dental caries and children's weights. Journal of Epidemiology and Community Health 36, 49–52.

Moore, W.J., Corbett, E., 1971. The distribution of dental caries in ancient British populations I. Anglo-Saxon period. Caries Research 5, 151–168.

Moore, W.J., Corbett, E., 1973. The distribution of dental caries in ancient British populations II. Iron Age, Romano-British and mediaeval periods. Caries Research 7, 139–153.

Moore, W.J., Corbett, E., 1975. Distribution of dental caries in ancient British populations III. The 17th century. Caries Research 9, 163–175.

Moore, W.J., Corbett, E., 1976. Distribution of dental caries in ancient British populations IV. The 19th century. Caries Research 10, 401–414.

Mummery, J., 1869. On the relations which dental caries, as discovered amongst the ancient inhabitants of Britain, and amongst existing Aboriginal races, may be supposed to hold to their food and social condition. Transactions of the Odontological Society 2, 7–80.

Nield, L., Stenger, J., Kamat, D., 2008. Common pediatric dental dilemmas. Clinical Pediatrics 47 (2), 99–105.

Noren, J., 1983. Enamel structure in deciduous teeth from low-birth-weight infants. Acta Odontologica Scandinavia 41 (6), 355–362.

Noren, J., Magnusson, B., Grahnen, H., 1978. Mineralisation defects in primary teeth in intra-uterine undernutrition. II. A histological and microradiographic study. Swedish Dental Journal 2, 67–72.

O'Brian, M., 1994. Children's Dental Health in the United Kingdom 1993. Her Majesty's Stationary Office, London.

O'Sullivan, E., Williams, S.A., Curzon, M.E.J., 1989. Dental caries and nutritional stress in English archaeological child populations. In: Roberts, C.A., Lee, F., Bintliff, J. (Eds.), Burial Archaeology: Current Research, Methods and Developments. British Series, vol. 211. BAR, Oxford, pp. 167–174.

O'Sullivan, E.A., Williams, S.A., Curzon, M.E.J., 1992. Dental caries in relation to nutritional stress in early English child populations. Pediatric Dentistry 14 (1), 26–29.

Ogden, A., Pinhasi, R., White, W., 2007. Gross enamel hypoplasia in molars from subadults in a 16th-18th century London Graveyard. American Journal of Physical Anthropology 133 (3), 957–966.

Ortner, D., 2003. Identification of Pathological Conditions in Human Skeletal Remains. Academic Press, New York.

Oxenham, M.F., Domett, K., 2011. Palaeohealth at Man Bac. Man Bac: the excavation of a Neolithic site in Northern Vietnam. The Biology 33, 77–93.

Palkovich, A., 1980. Pueblo Population and Society: Arroyo Hondo Skeletal and Mortuary Remains. Arroyo Hondo Archaeological Series, vol. 3. School of American Research, Sante Fe.

Pfeiffer, S., Dudar, J., Austin, S., 1989. Prospect Hill: skeletal remains from a 19th century methodist cemetery, Newmarket, Ontario. Northeast Historical Archaeology 18 (1), 29–48.

Philips, C., Leach, S., 2008. The Human Bone: P1649 Great Casterton, Rutland (HAT 619) (Unpublished report).

Pihlstrom, B., Michalowicz, S., Johnson, N., 2005. Periodontal diseases. Lancet 366, 1809–1820.

Powell, M., 1988. Status and Health in Prehistory. A Case Study of the Moundville Chiefdom. Smithsonian Institution, Washington, DC.

Prowse, T., Saunders, S., Schwarcz, H., Garnsey, P., Macchiarelli, R., Bondioli, L., 2008. Isotopic and dental evidence for infant and young child feeding practices in an Imperial Roman skeletal sample. American Journal of Physical Anthropology 137 (3), 294–309.

Rahtz, P., Hirst, S., Wright, S., 2000. Cannington Cemetery. Society for the Promotion of Roman Studies, London.

Rasmussen, P., Elkhidir Elhassan, F., Raadal, M., 1992. Enamel defects in primary canines related to traditional treatment of teething problems in Sudan. International Journal of Pediatric Dentistry 2 (3), 151–155.

Roffey, S., Tucker, K., 2012. A contextual study of the medieval hospital and cemetery of St Mary Magdalen, Winchester, England. International Journal of Paleopathology 2, 170–180.

Rohnbogner, A., Lewis, M., 2016. Dental caries as a measure of diet, health, and difference in non-adults from urban and rural Roman Britain. Dental Anthropology 29 (3), 16–31.

Romero, J., 1970. Dental mutilation, trephination, and cranial deformation. In: Stewart, T. (Ed.), Handbook of Middle American Indians. Physical Anthropology, vol. 9. University of Texas Press, Texas, pp. 50–67.

Rose, J.C., Condon, K.W., Goodman, A.H., 1985. Diet and dentition: developmental disturbances. In: Gilbert, R., Meilke, J. (Eds.), The Analysis of Prehistoric Diets. Academic Press, Inc., Florida, pp. 281–305.

Rosenzweig, K., Garbarski, D., 1965. Numerical aberrations in the permanent teeth of grade school children in Jerusalem. American Journal of Physical Anthropology 23, 277–284.

Sawyer, D., Allison, M., Pezzia, A., 1976. Talon cusp: a clinically significant anomaly in a primary incisor from pre-Columbian America. Medical College of Virginia Quarterly 12, 64–66.

Sawyer, D., Nwoku, A., 1985. Malnutrition and the oral health of children in Ogbomosho, Nigeria. ASDC Journal of Dentistry for Children 52, 41–45.

Schuurs, A., 2013. Pathology of the Hard Dental Tissues. Wiley-Blackwell, West Sussex.

Seow, K.W., 1992. Dental enamel defects in low birthweight children. Journal of Paleopathology Monographic Publication 2, 321–330.

Seow, W., Brown, J., Tudehope, D., O'Callaghan, M., 1984. Dental defects in the deciduous dentition of premature infants with low birth weight and neonatal rickets. Pediatric Dentistry 6 (2), 88–92.

Shukrum, S., Molto, J., 2009. Child oral health: dental palaeopathology of Kellis 2, Dakhleh, Egypt. A preliminary investigation. In: Lewis, M., Clegg, M. (Eds.), Proceedings of the Ninth Annual Conference of the British Association for Biological Anthropology and Osteoarchaeology. BAR International Series, vol. 1981. Archaeopress, Oxford, pp. 19–30.

Skinner, M., Hadaway, W., Dickie, J., 1994. Effects of ethnicity and birth month on localised enamel hypoplasia of the primary canine. Journal of Dentistry for Children 61, 109–113.

Skinner, M., Hung, J., 1986. Localised enamel hypoplasia of the primary canine. ASDC Journal of Dentistry for Children 53, 197–200.

Skinner, M., Newell, E., 2003. Localized hypoplasia of the primary canine in Bonobos. Orangutangs, and Gibbons. American Journal of Physical Anthropology 102, 61–72.

Skinner, M.F., 1986. An enigmatic hypoplastic defect of the deciduous canine. American Journal of Physical Anthropology 69, 59–69.

Smith, M.O., Wojcinski, M.C., 2011. Anomalous double-crowned primary teeth from Pre-Columbian Tennessee: a meta-analysis of hunter–gatherer and agriculturalist samples. International Journal of Paleopathology 1 (3), 173–183.

Stojanowski, C., Johnson, K., Doran, G., Ricklis, R., 2011. Talon cusp from two archaic period cemeteries in North America: implications for comparative evolutionary medicine. American Journal of Physical Anthropology 144, 411–420.

Suzuki, T., Kusumoto, A., Fujita, H., de Shi, C., 1995. The fourth molar in a mandible found in a Jomon skeleton in Japan. International Journal of Osteoarchaeology 5, 174–180.

Sweeney, E., Cabrera, J., Urrutis, D., Mata, L., 1969. Factors associated with linear hypoplasia of human deciduous incisors. Journal of Dental Research 68, 1275–1279.

Sweeney, E., Guzman, M., 1966. Oral conditions in children from three highland villages in Guatemala. Archives of Oral Biology 11 (7), 687 IN618.

Sweeney, E.A., Saffir, A.J., De Leon, R., 1971. Linear hypoplasia of deciduous incisor teeth in malnourished children American Journal of Clinical Nutrition 24, 29–31.

Taji, S., Hughes, T., Rogers, J., Townsend, G., 2000. Localised enamel hypoplasia of human deciduous canines: genotype or environment? Australian Dental Journal 45 (2), 83–90.

Temple, D., Larsen, C., 2007. Dental caries prevalence as evidence for agriculture and subsistence variation during the Yayoi period in prehistoric Japan: biocultural interpretations of an economy in transition. American Journal of Physical Anthropology 134 (4), 501–512.

Tillier, A.-M., Kaffe, I., Arensburg, B., Chech, M., 1998. Hypodontia of permanent teeth among Middle Palaeolithic hominids: an early case dated to ca. 92 000±5000 years BP at the Qafzeh site. International Journal of Osteoarchaeology 8, 1–6.

Trinkaus, E., Smith, R., Lebel, S., 2000. Dental caries in the Aubesier 5 Neanderthal primary molar. Journal of Archaeological Science 27, 1017–1021.

Tucker, K., 2005. St Stephen's Church, York: The Human Bone (Unpublished Report), York Archaeological Trust.

Uslenghi, S., Liversidge, H.M., 2006. A radiographic study of tooth development in hypodontia. Archives of Oral Biology 51, 129–133.

Varrela, T., 1991. Prevalence and distribution of dental caries in a late medieval population in Finland. Archives of Oral Biology 36 (8), 553–559.

Waldron, T., 2009. Palaeopathology. Cambridge University Press, Cambridge.

Walker, D., 2012a. St Mary Spital in context. In: Connell, B., Gray Jones, A., Redfern, R., Walker, R. (Eds.), A Bioarchaeolgical Study of Medieval Burials on the Site of St Mary Spital. Museum of London Archaeology, London, pp. 149–194.

Walker, D., 2012b. Disease in London, 1st-19th Centuries. Museum of London Archaeology, London.

Warinner, C., Speller, C., Collins, M., 2013. A new era in paleomicrobiology: prospects for ancient dental calculus as a long term record of the human oral microbiome. Philisophical Transactions B 370. Downloaded from: http://rstb.royalsocietypublishing.org/.

Wells, C., 1982. The human burials. In: McWhirr, A., Viner, L., Wells, C. (Eds.), Romano-British Cemeteries at Cirencester. Corinium Museum, Cirencester, pp. 135–202.

Weyrich, L.S., Dobney, K., Cooper, A., 2015. Ancient DNA analysis of dental calculus. Journal of Human Evolution 79, 119–124.

Williams, S., Curzon, M., 1985. Dental caries in a Scottish medieval child population. Caries Research 19 (2), 162.

Witkin, A., 2011. The human skeletal remains. In: Pearson, A., Jeffs, B., Witkin, A., MacQuarrie (Eds.), Infernal Traffic: Excavations of a Libertated African Graveyard in Rupert's Valley, St Helena. Council for British Archaeology, Oxford, pp. 57–98.

Zivanovic, S., 1982. Ancient Diseases. Methuen & Co. Ltd, London.

Chapter 5

Trauma and Treatment*

Chapter Outline

Introduction	91	Rib Fractures	108
Principles of Pediatric Trauma	92	Age-Related Injuries	108
Greenstick Fractures	92	Birth Trauma	108
Plastic Deformation	93	Erb's and Klumph's Palsy (Congenital Brachial Palsy)	109
Buckle Fractures	94	Toddler's Fractures	110
Physeal Fractures	94	Juvenile Osteochondritis Dissecans	110
Long Bone Fractures	96	Slipped Femoral Epiphysis	111
Complications Specific to Child Trauma	96	Other Forms of Trauma	112
Premature Fusion	96	Dislocations	112
Fragment Overlap	97	Dislocations of the Upper Limb	112
Overgrowth	97	Dislocations of the Lower Limb	112
Healing	98	Myositis Ossificans Traumatica (Heterotrophic Ossification)	114
Identifying Postcranial Injuries	100	Burns	114
Callus	101	Treatment: Autopsies and Surgical Intervention	115
Cortical Striations	102	Trepanation	115
Angulation	102	Themes in the Study of Child Trauma	117
Plastic Deformation of the Ulna	102	Violence Associated With Extreme Cultural Conflict	117
Plastic Deformation of the Radius	102	Culturally Sanctioned Ritual Violence	118
Cranial Fractures	102	Caregiver-Induced Violence and Neglect	119
Facial Fractures	103	Activity-Induced Injuries	121
Spinal Injuries	104	Structural Violence	122
Tetanus	106	References	123
Spondylolysis and Spondylolisthesis	106		
Clay-Shoveler's Fractures	107		

INTRODUCTION

Trauma is one of the most common forms of pathology encountered by the paleopathologist. Callus formation, secondary deformities, or infection can make antemortem fractures easy to identify in an adult's remains, and comprehensive reviews are provided in the key textbooks (Almeida and Roberts, 2005; Aufderheide and Rodriguez-Martín, 1998; Larsen, 2015; Ortner, 2003). However, identifying fractures in pediatric bone is more challenging and has received much less attention. The identification of trauma in children differs from adults as the plastic nature of immature bone means fractures are often incomplete (greenstick) and heal rapidly without deformity. In addition, other signatures of trauma such as premature epiphyseal fusion, physeal fractures, and periosteal lesions can be subtle and subject to misdiagnosis. For example, periosteal lesions are usually described as resulting from general inflammation of the periosteum due to trauma, as opposed to a callus overlying a greenstick fracture. The development of new methods to aid in the identification of child trauma in dry bone has begun (Verlinden and Lewis, 2015), but currently rates of accidental nonadult trauma in the past are almost certainly an underestimate. We cannot be sure whether a lack of evidence for child trauma in a past society indicates a strong commitment to child care within that group, or our inability to recognize the subtle signs of injury in these remains (Lewis, 2014). In many cases, evidence for trauma in childhood is gleaned from an adult's remains where trauma was severe enough to cause shortening of a limb (Glencross and Stuart-Macadam, 2000, 2001). Some physical injuries will be invisible to the paleopathologist, including drowning, ingestion of foreign objects, or choking, while others such as burns have yet to be fully explored. Sources from medieval Europe provide a glimpse at the type of trauma some children may have been exposed to. There are many accounts of adolescents in 16th-century England committing suicide

*With contributions from Petra Verlinden.

by hanging themselves (Murphy, 1986) or children sustaining head injuries (Gordon, 1986), being burned, or suffering fractures and dislocations through misadventure (Gordon, 1991; Towner and Towner, 2000). However, the majority of accidental deaths seem to have been caused by drowning (Towner and Towner, 2000). It is becoming increasingly evident that children were also exposed to warfare and physical abuse.

Trauma is culturally defined, and Glencross (2011) emphasizes the importance of examining trauma patterns from a life course perspective, matching age with cultural agency, which dictates when certain activities might take place. The biological and social development of the child will also influence the types of trauma they are exposed to. Up to 2 years of age, children are almost entirely dependent on adults, hence long bone fractures in children before the age of 2 years are suspicious of caregiver-induced violence, whereas in children aged 2–3 years fractures may occur as part of the process of learning to walk and climb (Brown and Fisher, 2004; Wilber and Thompson, 1998). As children develop and become more independent, the child's social and cultural involvement increases, expanding the types of activity that may expose them to accidental injury. Types of injury vary across populations due to socioeconomic conditions, the levels of urbanization, subsistence strategies, technological advances, and cultural practices (Cheng and Shen, 1993). Information on the incidence, type, and pattern of fractures we might expect to identify in children derive from modern clinical literature, which is biased toward the most serious fractures where children are admitted to hospital. In addition, they outline injuries in children performing activities that did not exist in the past (e.g., rugby, skiing, roller-skating, trampolining), and male to female ratios and the age at which fractures occurred may not be relevant in every culture. Caveats also apply for the use of historical accounts. While providing a useful context for the kinds of activities children participated in predisposing them to trauma, data on age, trauma frequency, and gender distributions are mainly based on coroner's records and miracle stories, which are selective in their focus. In recent years, books dedicated to the study of trauma in different societies and periods have been published and focus on the pattern of trauma and violence in adults and children (Knüsel and Smith, 2014; Martin and Anderson, 2014; Martin et al., 2012; Schulting and Fibiger, 2012).

PRINCIPLES OF PEDIATRIC TRAUMA

The pattern and nature of pediatric trauma differs in each child according to their size, anatomy, and the location and extent of growth yet to be achieved. A young child hit by a moving vehicle (e.g., a cart) will sustain much greater injuries than an older child as they are lighter and more likely to become a projectile, sustaining further injury when they hit the ground (Wilber and Thompson, 1998). Furthermore, before the age of 2 years, the ribs are more horizontally positioned than an adult's and do not cover the liver, spleen, or intestines making them more susceptible to serious injury to their vital organs. When an adult falls, they tend to land on their feet, causing fractures of the lower limbs. In a young child, a disproportionately large and heavy cranium means that they are more likely to land on their head as their arms are too short to protect themselves from the impact (Wilber and Thompson, 1998). Hence, injury to a child from a fall or collision is more likely to cause fatal soft tissue damage and perimortem fractures that are difficult to identify. In addition to body proportions, the highly cartilaginous and more plastic nature of pediatric bone influences the types of fracture we may encounter (Resnick and Kransdorf, 2005).

The most common forms of fracture that occur in children are:

1. Greenstick fractures: a partial fracture with bowing of the compressed side and fracture of the tensile side.
2. Plastic deformation: causing unusual bowing without fracture.
3. Torus or buckle fractures: resulting in a bulge of the metaphyses as it fails under compression fractures and,
4. Metaphyseal (physeal) fractures.

Greenstick Fractures

A partial or greenstick fracture that penetrates the cortex but ceases at the medullary cavity is more common in children (Fig. 5.1). The porous nature of the cortex deflects some of the force from the bone surface, while the remaining force is dissipated through transverse cleavage cracks, which limit its progression through the bone. Complete fractures in the long bones of children therefore indicate a much greater degree of force than it would in an adult (Currey and Butler, 1975). The pediatric periosteum is thicker, stronger, and more biologically active than an adult's due to the need for constant remodeling during growth (Wilber and Thompson, 1998). Although firmly attached to the metaphyses through a dense network of fibers (zone of Ranvier), the periosteum is more loosely attached to the diaphyses. Hence, the periosteum is unlikely to rupture during a fracture but instead separates from the bone, remaining intact on the compressed side of the break. Both the nature of break and characteristics of the periosteum lessen the extent of deformity in long bone fractures and allow tissue continuity providing stability for healing (Johnston and Foster, 2001, p. 29). The loose attachment of the periosteum often results in a widespread hematoma and large callus formation along the shaft, but with limited evidence of a fracture line (Wilber and Thompson, 1998). These widespread subperiosteal

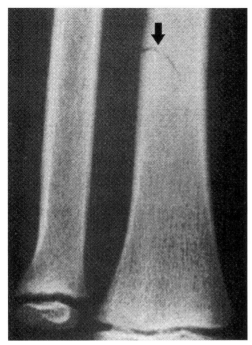

FIGURE 5.1 Clinical radiograph showing a greenstick (partial) fracture of the radius in a child. *From Resnick, D., Goergen, T., 2002. Physical injury: concepts and terminology. In: Resnick, D., (Ed.), Diagnosis of Bone and Joint Disorders. WB Saunders and Company, Philadelphia, p. 2680.*

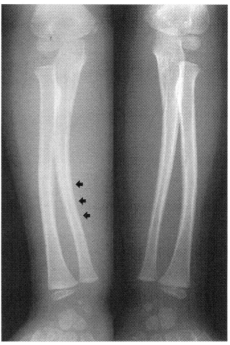

FIGURE 5.2 Clinical radiograph of a 4-year-old with plastic bowing deformity of the ulna due to a fall. *Image provided by Yamamoto (University of Hawaii, Vol 6, Case 16).*

new bone deposits may be mistaken for infection, vitamin C deficiency (scurvy), or bone tumors in paleopathology (Adams and Hamblen, 1991; John et al., 1997). Seven probable examples of greenstick fractures in nonadults have been identified in literature (Brothwell and Powers, 2000; Ghalib, 1999; Mays, 2007a; McKinley, 2008; Verlinden, 2015; Walker, 2012). The youngest child was aged just 9 months (Ghalib, 1999), but there is no discernible pattern in the bones affected, with fractures reported in the femur, tibia, fibula, humerus, radius, and ulna.

Plastic Deformation

Plastic deformation as the result of injury is unique to children due to the highly elastic nature of their bones, allowing greater force to be absorbed before a complete fracture occurs. Acute plastic deformation results from excessive vertical compression force along the shaft of the bone, causing it to bow under the pressure (Fig. 5.2). If the force is removed, the bone returns to normal; but if it persists, the bone will either remain bowed (plastic deformation) with numerous microfractures occurring along the convex aspect, or the bone will suffer a greenstick or complete fracture (Borden, 1974). Resnick (1995) reports that the magnitude of force required to produce plastic deformation can be as much as 100%–150% of the child's own body weight. Such traumatic bowing can be difficult to diagnose even in the clinical setting as changes may be subtle and can occur without the formation of a callus (Borden, 1974; John et al., 1997). Plastic deformation usually occurs in one of the paired bones (i.e., radius and ulna, or tibia and fibula) but is most common in the ulna, resulting in exaggerated mediolateral or anteroposterior bending (Resnick and Kransdorf, 2005; Stuart-Macadam et al., 1998). In the lower leg, plastic deformation of the fibula may occur indirectly when the force penetrating the tibia is absorbed by the interosseous membrane and transmitted to the fibula (John et al., 1997). In young children, rapid remodeling often corrects the deformity, but in children who sustain injuries after 10 years of age the deformity may persist, causing angular deformity and in the arm, a reduction in pronation and supination (Borden, 1974).

Archeological examples of plastic deformation are rare and require comparison with the unaffected side. Walker (2012) identified a bowed fibula in a child from St Mary and St Michael in London, and a plastically deformed ulna was identified in a 14- to 17-year-old from Glen Williams ossuary in Canada (Stuart-Macadam et al., 1998). Further cases have been identified in medieval and Roman England (Fig. 5.3; Clough and Boyle, 2010; Rohnbogner, 2015; Verlinden, 2015). Differential diagnosis should include vitamin D deficiency (rickets), neonatal bowing, osteogenesis imperfecta, and postmortem deformation (Stuart-Macadam et al., 1998). However, in rickets and osteogenesis imperfecta, multiple bones will be bowed.

Buckle Fractures

Buckle (or torus) fractures are caused when there is an insufficient impaction or compression force to cause a complete fracture, but instead the cortex "buckles" (Resnick and Kransdorf, 2005). Unlike greenstick fractures where the cortex fails under tension forces, buckle fractures are caused when the cortex fails under compression, usually at the diaphyseal–metaphyseal junction. The harder diaphyseal bone impacts on the metaphysis causing the cortical fragments to overlap (Light et al., 1984). The bones most commonly affected are the distal radius and humerus. Buckling of the whole shaft circumference is referred to as a "torus" fracture (Pierce et al., 2004), while combined compression and angulation forces may cause one side of the bone to buckle, while the other suffers a greenstick fracture. These are referred to as "lead pipe fractures" (Resnick and Kransdorf, 2005, p. 803). Buckle fractures would be identified macroscopically as a slight bulging of the cortex with a sclerotic area evident on radiograph (Fig. 5.4). To date, no clear cases of a buckle fracture have been identified in a child from an archeological context.

Physeal Fractures

One of the most significant factors in the severity and expression of trauma in children is the presence of the cartilaginous growth plate (or physis) at both ends of the long bones and at one end of the short tubular bones. Today, around 15% of all injuries in children younger than 16 years involve the growth plate as the result of shearing and avulsion forces (80% of cases) or compression forces (20% of cases) (Resnick and Kransdorf, 2005). Injuries that would normally result in joint dislocation in adults will cause fracturing of the metaphyseal margin in children. This is because the joint capsule and ligaments are up to five times stronger than the cartilage growth plate, which is the first to give way under the force (Adams and Hamblen, 1991; Resnick and Kransdorf, 2005). Physeal fractures may involve the cartilage (chondral) alone or affect both the bone and cartilage (osteochondral) within a joint. Fractures can occur at the metaphyseal end with partial detachment of the metaphysis away from the diaphysis (e.g., bucket-handle or corner fractures), or result in avulsion of the entire epiphysis. In the clinical setting, physeal fractures are classified according to the Salter–Harris scheme developed in 1963

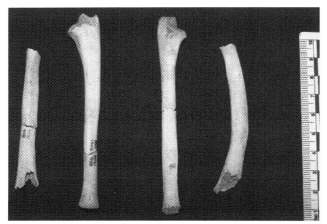

FIGURE 5.3 Plastic deformation of the left radius in a child from St Giles, North Yorkshire, England (skeleton 1506). *Photograph by P. Verlinden. Courtesy of the Biological Anthropology Research Centre, University of Bradford.*

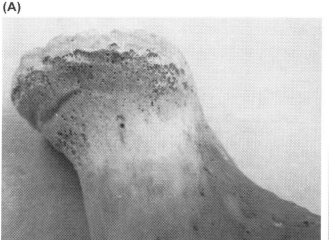
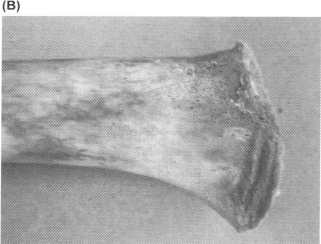

FIGURE 5.4 Buckle fractures of the (A) proximal femur and (B) proximal tibia in a modern 11-year-old from Fredonia, Columbia (CSP 244). The injuries were sustained when the child fell from height. *Photograph courtesy of Judith Arnett, The National Institute of Legal Medicine and Forensic Sciences, Bogotá D. C., Colombia, University of the Andes School of Medicine, Bogotá D. C., Colombia and University of Antioquia, Medellín, Colombia.*

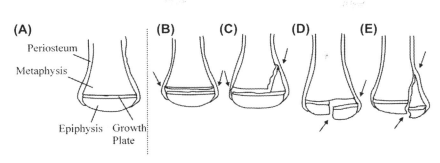

FIGURE 5.5 Schematic drawings depicting (A) normal bone and anatomical features; (B) Salter–Harris I; (C) Salter–Harris II; (D) Salter–Harris III; and (E) Salter–Harris IV fractures. *From Verlinden, P., Lewis, M., 2015. Childhood trauma: methods for the identification of physeal fractures in nonadult skeletal remains. American Journal of Physical Anthropology 157 (3), 412.*

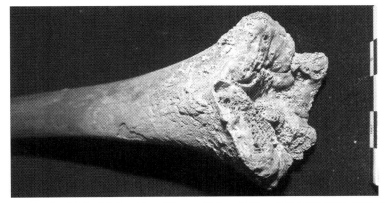

FIGURE 5.6 Growth plate injury of the distal right tibia in a 16- to 17-year-old from St Mary Spital (AD 1250–1400, skeleton 29,075). The metaphysis has become cupped and irregular as the result of central necrosis with normal marginal healing. The new bone formation (cloaking) around the injury is suggestive of periosteal tearing secondary to epiphyseal displacement (Connell et al., 2012). *Photograph by F. Shapland, with the kind permission of the Museum of London.*

(Fig. 5.5). Type I describes the separation of the epiphysis from the diaphysis along the entire germinal layer; type II describes the same injury with the addition of a triangular fragment that remains attached to the periosteum. Type III Salter–Harris fractures run vertically through the epiphysis before abruptly angulating at 90 degrees to exit at the joint surface, while type IV describes a similar oblique fracture through the epiphysis, metaphysis, and diaphysis creating a large triangular fragment. Type I fractures occur most commonly at the distal fibula, type II the distal radius, and hand phalanges; type II the hand phalanges and distal tibia, and type IV is seen most commonly at the distal tibia and distal humerus (Peterson et al., 1994). As physeal fractures are common in the hands and feet of children today, they should be included in any nonadult trauma assessment (Verlinden, 2015).

Physeal injuries rarely cause significant deformity as it is rare for the epiphyses to be displaced (Resnick and Kransdorf, 2005), and rapid remodeling can cause any residual signs of deformity to be lost. Full strength and function of the growth plate can return after just 10 days. Chondral fractures alone will be lost postmortem making identification of many physeal fractures a challenge archeologically. Nevertheless, minimal unilateral periosteal stripping and subsequent new bone formation may be evident for a brief period (O'Connor and Cohen, 1987), and Verlinden and Lewis (2015) have highlighted several macroscopic signs. Metaphyseal and epiphyseal fragmentation may accompany certain physeal fracture types, and damage to the blood supply may cause metaphyseal or epiphyseal necrosis, resulting in partial or complete resorption of these structures. At the metaphysis, this may cause "cupping" of the bone surface, while at the epiphysis this may lead to bifurcation. Periosteal new bone formation may occur around the site of injury due to tearing of the periosteum as the epiphysis becomes dislocated (Fig. 5.6). Finally, peripheral or central growth arrest due to traumatic fusion may result in "joint misalignment" as the unfused normal segment of the epiphysis begins to slant. Radiographic examination can be useful to confirm the presence of a bone bridge when joint misalignment has been identified, and sclerosis of the metaphysis and epiphysis can also be present in cases of fragmentation or necrosis (Verlinden, 2015).

Trauma to the growth plate in archeological material is usually identified by shortening of the long bones in adult skeletal remains. However in England, child cases have been recorded at later medieval Chichester, Sussex (Ortner, 2003), postmedieval London (Lewis, 2002a; Walker, 2012), and early medieval Raunds Furnells in Northamptonshire (Lewis, 2002a). A bucket-handle fracture of the distal tibia was also identified in a 1.5-year-old from Poundbury Camp, Dorset (Lewis, 2010). Verlinden's (2015, p. 202) extensive survey of fractures in archeological sites from England revealed further physeal fractures in children affecting the proximal radius, fibula, femur, distal humerus, tibia, and hand and foot phalanges.

Long Bone Fractures

The most common complete fractures in children today are of the radius and humerus (Rennie et al., 2007; Wilkins and Aroojis, 2001, p. 12), with injuries in those under 18 months often considered indicative of caregiver-induced violence (see below). Today, from the age of 2 years the majority of injuries are the result of the child's increased mobility; for example, falls from furniture, downstairs, or from buildings (Agran et al., 2003). Cheng and Shen (1993) and Cheng et al. (1999) examined the pattern of fractures in over 6000 children of different ages from Hong Kong. The majority of fractures (65%) occurred at the distal radius and the supracondylar aspect of the humerus, followed by the tibial shaft. Fractures to the humerus were most common in the 0- to 7-year-age groups, with the distal radius, hand, tibia, and ankle more commonly affected in 12- to 16-year-olds. During adolescence, female fractures declined, while trauma in males increased dramatically, perhaps due to their propensity for interpersonal violence.

In a study of 0- to 17-year-olds from medieval England (AD 900–1550), 137 fractures were identified in the gray and published literature (Lewis, 2016). The most commonly affected bones were the humerus (n=16), tibia (n=11), feet (n=9), clavicle (n=8), and ribs (n=6). There were only two cases of fractures to the radius. Both children were from London and aged 1–2 years and 6–11 years. The rarity of radial fractures in the archeological record in comparison to the clinical picture may be due to the difficulty in identifying them in young children and the greater likelihood that any injury may result in a more subtle physeal fractures or plastic deformity. Archeological cases of long bone fractures in children are usually identified when they are of similar types to that seen in adults, including spiral fractures (Fig. 5.7), shortening, and secondary osteomyelitis due to an open or complex fracture (Fig. 5.8).

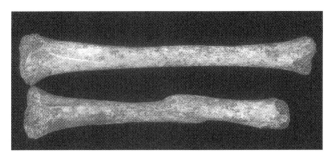

FIGURE 5.7 Spiral fracture of the right tibia in a nonadult. There is overlap of the fractured fragments, and the normal alignment of the proximal and distal metaphyseal ends has been disrupted (provenance unknown).

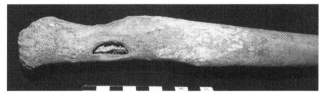

FIGURE 5.8 Fractured left humerus with osteomyelitis as the result of an open fracture in a 16-year-old from St Mary Spital, London (AD 1200–1250, Skeleton 20,370). The sequestrum can be clearly seen through the cloaca. *Photograph by F. Shapland with the kind permission of the Museum of London.*

COMPLICATIONS SPECIFIC TO CHILD TRAUMA

Premature Fusion

Trauma to the metaphysis may result in partial or complete premature epiphyseal fusion and growth arrest due to vascular damage, or the formation of a bony bridge across the growth plate (Rathjen and Birch, 2006). Partial fusion may also lead to disruption and angulation of the joint surface (joint impairment). How much shortening occurs depends on the age of the individual at the time of the trauma, the epiphysis affected, and the amount of longitudinal growth still to occur. In the humerus, only 20% of longitudinal growth from the center of ossification is carried out by the distal growth plate, whereas 80% occurs at the proximal end of the bone (Maresh, 1955). Hence, a fracture and premature epiphyseal fusion of the proximal humerus would cause a greater degree of shortening (growth dysplasia) than similar trauma to the distal end. In theory, detailed knowledge of proportional bone growth could provide evidence of the age at which the fracture occurred. Stuart-Macadam et al. (1998) and Glencross and Stuart-Macadam (2000, 2001) identified healed fractures of the humeral epicondyle, supracondylar buckling, and plastic deformation in adults, providing indirect evidence for childhood trauma (Fig. 5.9). That we are missing the opportunity to identify similar injuries in the children themselves is illustrated by Glencross' (2011) study at the Indian Knoll site. Here only six (CPR=0.27%) fractures were identified in 2200 complete children's bones, compared to 45% (n=35) of fractures in the adults whose injuries were believed to have occurred during childhood.

Humerus varus following trauma, describes a situation where the medial region of the proximal growth plate has retarded or halted growth, while the lateral region develops normally resulting in progressive angular rotation of the humeral epiphysis. This may cause medial metaphyseal radiolucency, medial osseous bridging, or a flattened epiphysis and shortened diaphysis, while functional impairment is minimal (Ellefsen et al., 1994). Differential diagnosis should consider osteomyelitis or skeletal dysplasia as an alternative etiology. Kacki et al. (2013) reported a case of humerus varus following trauma in 6- to 7-year-old from medieval Orléans, France. The right humerus was 2.9 cm shorter than the left, and the proximal surface was flattened and rotated posteriorly, with pitting of the articular surface (Fig. 5.10).

Fragment Overlap

Just as in adults, complete fractures of the long bone may lead to displacement and overlap of the fragments, especially in areas where the spasm of larger muscles cause further displacement. Overlap can occur in any long bone but is more common in the clavicle, femur, and tibia (Allman, 1967; Puttaswamaiah et al., 2006). Complete fractures of the femur can lead to shortening of the affected side by over 2 cm, with the degree of difference increasing as growth progresses (Fig. 5.11; Puttaswamaiah et al., 2006).

Overgrowth

Conversely, where there is considerable separation of the periosteum from the cortex, there may be overgrowth of the affected bone due to stimulation of the growth plate through an increased blood supply at the site of fracture (Hariga et al., 2011). This complication is most common in the femur and may result in a discrepancy between the affected and unaffected bone by as much as 4 cm (Clement

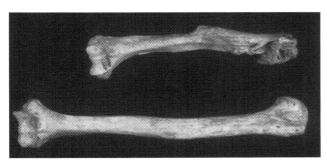

FIGURE 5.9 Shortening of the right humerus in an adult from Raunds Furnells, Northamptonshire, England. There is fusion and necrosis as the result of trauma to the proximal epiphysis during growth. The muscle attachment for the biceps is pronounced, and coupled with the lack of atrophy, indicates the individual carried on using their arm after the injury. *Courtesy of the Biological Anthropology Research Center, University of Bradford.*

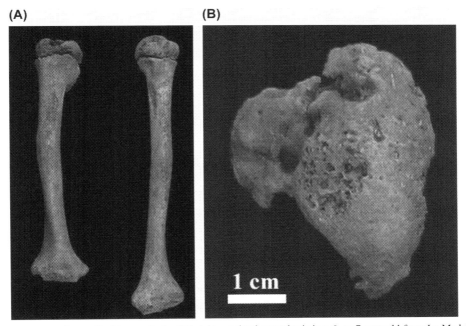

FIGURE 5.10 Humerus varus as the result of trauma to the (A) right proximal metaphysis in a 6- to 7-year-old from La Madeleine, Orléans, France (skeleton T2017). (B) There is necrosis of the surviving humeral epiphysis. *From Kacki, S., Duneufjardin, P., Blanchard, P., Castex, D., 2013. Humerus varus in a subadult skeleton from the medieval graveyard of La Madeleine (Orléans, France). International Journal of Osteoarchaeology 23 (1), 122–123.*

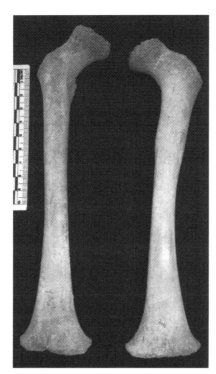

FIGURE 5.11 Proximal fracture of the left femoral diaphysis leading to shortening of the shaft in a 4-year-old from Barton-upon-Humber, Lincolnshire, England (AD 1150–1500, skeleton 906). *Photograph by P. Verlinden.*

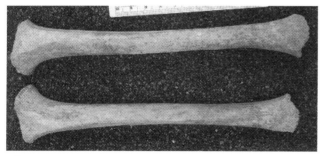

FIGURE 5.12 Overgrowth following a fracture of the left tibia in an 8- to 9-year-old from St Mary Spital, London (AD 1200–1250, skeleton 19,815). *Photograph by P. Verlinden with the kind permission of the Museum of London.*

and Colton, 1986; Stilli et al., 2008). Overgrowth may continue for up to 4 years after fracture in children aged between 5 and 13 years of age, and in 9% of cases overgrowth continues until skeletal maturity (Stephens et al., 1989; Stilli et al., 2008). Contrary to fragment overlap, overgrowth is not a process which is limited to complete fractures, and can occur in buckle and greenstick fractures (Greiff and Bergmann, 1980). An example of overgrowth in a tibia was identified in a child from later medieval London by Verlinden (2015) (Fig. 5.12).

HEALING

The time it takes for a fracture to heal depends on the location and severity of the fracture, the nutritional status of the individual, their age, alignment of fractured ends, the presence of infection, or secondary pathological conditions (Roberts, 2000). In the growing child, rapid healing can cause fractures to go unnoticed, as fracture lines, calluses, and deformities are once again incorporated into the normal dimensions of the bone (Adams and Hamblen, 1991). In some bones, a fracture will heal without a callus ever forming (e.g., terminal phalanges, humerus tuberosity, tibial malleolus) (Caffey, 1945), and in the abused child constant trauma to an area may instead result in layers of periosteal new bone, with neglect and malnutrition further delaying the healing process (O'Connor and Cohen, 1987).

Determining whether a fracture is antemortem, perimortem, or postmortem provides particular challenges for the paleopathologist. Although sustaining an antemortem injury, a child may die in the week before any macroscopic changes such as periosteal new bone formation can become evident. While it is usual to examine the color of the cortical bone in the affected area, fracture outline, fracture angle, and surface appearance to identify a perimortem wound in dry bone, subsequent postmortem damage may disguise these features. Wieberg and Wescott (2008) warn that perimortem injuries and taphonomic damage that occurs before 5 months when the bone is still green (fresh) have similar characteristics (e.g., smooth margins, obtuse and acute angles, v-shaped breaks) that make them indistinguishable. After 5 months the bone begins to dry and more obvious features of postmortem breaks (i.e., jagged edges) appear. A detailed time line of fracture and amputation healing using macroscopic, radiological, and histological techniques on dry bone has been compiled by De Boer et al. (2015) following Barber (1930) and Maat (2008). The authors recommend using histological analysis to provide the most accurate time line and advise reducing the healing times when considering child remains (De Boer et al., 2015; Table 5.1). But the degree of time reduction to be applied is not specified. In infants, a fracture with evidence of periosteal new bone formation has been reported after 4–7 days, with a soft callus forming after 20 days of fracture (O'Connor and Cohen, 1987), similar to the timings reported by De Boer et al. (Table 5.2). In fact, studies of different bones and the use of different terminology to describe the stages of healing means that determining the precise time of fracture occurrence in children is far from clear (Prosser et al., 2005). There is some agreement that in children under 5 years, a hard callus can form in 8 weeks, compared to around 12 weeks in an adolescent or adult (O'Connor and Cohen, 1987). Given these challenges, De Boer et al.'s (2015) table should be used as a rough guide, with the understanding that these are maximum times for nonadult fracture healing.

TABLE 5.1 Healing Features and Time Since Fracture Estimates for Adults

Category of Lesion	Healing Feature	Observation	Time Interval in Adults
Common	Frayed lamellae at the lesion margin	Histology	Before 48 hours
	Absorption of the cortical bone adjacent to lesions	Radiograph	After 4–7 days
	Howship's lacunae at the lesion margin	Histology	After 4–7 days
	Smoothing of the lesion margin	Histology	After 4–7 days
	Start of endosteal and periosteal osteogenesis separate from the cortex	Histology, Radiograph	After 7 days
	Periosteal osteogenesis at a distance from the fracture site		After 7 days
	Clearly visible callus formation	Histology, Radiograph	After 10–12 days
	Aggregation of spiculae into woven bone	Histology, Radiograph	After 12–20 days
	Primary bone tissue deposition	Histology	After 12–20 days
	Osteoporosis of the cortex	Histology, Radiograph	After 12 days
	Margin of the lesion appears more sclerotic	Radiograph	After 12–20 days
	Start of the transition of primary woven bone into secondary lamellar bone	Histology	After 14 days
	Cortical "cutting and closing cones" orientated toward the lesions	Histology	After 14–21 days
	Fields of calcified cartilage at site of callus formation		After 14 days
	Clearly visible periosteal callus	Histology, Radiograph	After 15 days
	Endosteal callus becomes indistinguishable from cancellous bone in the marrow cavity	Histology, Radiograph	After 17 days
	Periosteal callus becomes firmly attached to the cortex	Histology, Radiograph	After 6 weeks
For fractures	First scattered bone tissue, spiculae between lesion ends	Histology, Radiograph	After 4–7 days
	Union by bridging of the cortical bone discontinuity	Histology, Radiograph	After 21–28 days
	Smoothing of the callus outline	Histology	After 2–3 months
	Inadequate immobilization with pseudoarthrosis formation	Histology, Radiograph	After 6–9 months
	Adequate immobilization causing quiescent appearance and subsided healing	Histology, Radiograph	After 1–2 years
For amputations	Visibility of cut marks on surface	Radiograph	Less than 13 days
	Start of "capping" of the medullary cavity	Radiograph	A few weeks
	Complete capping of the medullary cavity	Radiograph	Several months

From De Boer, H., Van Der Merwe, A., Hammer, S., Steyn, M., Maat, G., 2015. Assessing post-traumatic time interval in human dry bone. International Journal of Osteoarchaeology 25 (1), 103.

TABLE 5.2 Timetable of Fracture Healing (Radiographic Features) in Children

Category[a]	Early (e.g., Infant)	Peak	Late
1. Resolution of soft tissue swelling	2–5 days	4–10 days	10–21 days
2. Periosteal new bone	4–10 days	10–14 days	14–21 days
3. Loss of fracture line definition	10–14 days	14–21 days	
4. Soft callus (fiber bone)	10–14 days	14–21 days	
5. Hard callus (lamellar bone)	14–21 days	21–42 days	42–90 days
6. Callus remodeling	3 months	12 months	24 months to epiphyseal closure

[a]Repetitive injuries may prolong categories 1, 2, 5, and 6.
After O'Connor, J., Cohen, J., 2015. Dating fractures. In: Kleinman, P. (Ed.), Diagnostic Imaging of Child Abuse. Second edition. Williams and Wilkins, Baltimore, p. 112.

IDENTIFYING POSTCRANIAL INJURIES

One of the major limitations in the study of nonadult trauma is the difficulty in identifying fractures. Unlike adult trauma, fractures are more likely to occur at the metaphysis or presents as greenstick, buckle, or bowing deformities. Being aware of the most common areas affected by trauma within certain age groups can aid in focusing the analysis, with clavicle or proximal humerus fractures as the result of birth injuries more likely to be encounter in infants, followed by the distal tibia around 2 years of age, and the hand, distal radius and distal humerus in adolescence. Initial identification of possible trauma normally follows comparison with the bone on its opposite side. Length discrepancies are common observations in a nonadult's remains (see Chapter 11). In trauma, they result from fragment overlap, overgrowth, or growth arrest. Determining which bone is causing the discrepancy presents a particular challenge (i.e., whether the changes are due to overgrowth or shortening). The presence of additional features such as an irregular epiphyseal surface or cortical thickening at the site of the fracture may aid diagnosis. Length differences of over 5 mm are considered indicative of a pathological etiology (Hensinger, 1998; Verlinden, 2015). A "tethered" epiphyseal margin in partial fusion will result in an abnormal angle of the joint surface developing, but these deformities depend on the age at which the trauma occurred and the amount of growth still to be achieved. Verlinden (2015) and Verlinden and Lewis (2015) developed a series of clinical features (Table 5.3) and macroscopic traits (Table 5.4) that may help identify nonadult bones that warrant further investigation for potential trauma. While particular traits can be used to indicate specific fracture types, in some cases it will be difficult to distinguish between a well-healed complete fracture and a greenstick or buckle fracture.

TABLE 5.3 Recognition of Fracture Types, by Bone Affected

Bone	Fracture Type	Macroscopic Appearance
Clavicle	Oblique, transverse, plastic bowing	Displaced in 54% cases Exaggerated upward curve in anterior–posterior view
Proximal humerus	Physeal	Partial growth arrest on medial aspect Angulation of epiphysis Irregular "collapsed" appearance of epiphysis
Distal humerus	Subcondylar fracture of the metaphysis	Posterior displacement of the fragment resulting in loss of natural curvature Anterior spur
	Complete and buckle	Varus angulation
	Lateral condyle fracture	Loose fragment displaced Lateral osteophyte (spur) Fishtail injury with partial growth arrest of the trochlear
Radius and ulna	Complete or greenstick fracture of proximal ulna and subsequent dislocation of radius	Ulna may heal without deformity Ulna may have underdeveloped radial notch Dislocated radial head underdeveloped, dome-shaped head, long slender neck
Scaphoid	Buckle fracture Complete	Cortical defect distal to radial articular surface Nonunion with bipartite scaphoid
Metacarpal	Transverse or crush	Widening of base, slight angulation, nonunion, multiple bones
MC5	Boxer's (transverse) fracture of neck	Volar displacement, possible shortening
Distal femur	Physeal	Tenting and cupping of metaphysis Subperiosteal new bone formation Growth arrest Displaced epiphysis
Fibula	Plastic deformity	Exaggeration of natural medial curvature Small area of subperiosteal new bone above hairline fracture
Tibia	Toddler (buckle) fracture	Small area of subperiosteal new bone above hairline fracture Sclerotic area on radiograph Deepened notch for tibial tuberosity

After Verlinden, P., 2015. Child's Play? A New Methodology for the Identification of Trauma in Non-adult Skeletal Remains (Ph.D. thesis). University of Reading, England.

Callus

A callus is normally the main feature used to identify a fracture, although awareness of the different pathological conditions that may mimic a fracture callus is important (Ortner, 2003, p. 204). Unfortunately, the most frequent fracture types encountered in children under 15 years are characterized by subtle or absent calluses (Borden, 1974; Cooper et al., 2004; Light et al., 1984). For example, in a sample of 1022 nonadult individuals from five English medieval cemeteries, only 16% (n = 8/49) of long bone fractures showed a clear callus. The majority of these (n = 5/8 or 63%) were in the adolescent age group (12–17 years). While a callus may be rapidly remodeled, the amount of time required to regain a normal bone outline after fracture is still substantial and can be as long as 18 months (Wilkins, 2005). Even when the external callus has been removed, the bone's interior structure will likely still be remodeling and sclerosis may be evident on radiograph (Fig. 5.13).

TABLE 5.4 List of Macroscopic Traits, With Types of Trauma Likely Indicated

Trait	Fracture Type	Radiograph Required
Callus	Complete, greenstick, buckle	No
Cortical striations	Complete	No
Cortical thickening	Complete, greenstick, buckle	Yes
Angulation	Complete, greenstick, physeal (at metaphysis)	Yes
Bowing	Traumatic bowing	Yes
Length discrepancy	Complete, greenstick, buckle, physeal	Yes
Metaphyseal fragmentation	Physeal (Salter–Harris type II and IV)	No
Metaphyseal necrosis	Physeal (All)	No
Epiphyseal fragmentation	Physeal (Salter–Harris type III and IV)	No
Epiphyseal necrosis	Physeal (All)	No
Joint misalignment	Physeal (All), dislocation	Yes

Adapted from Verlinden, P., Lewis, M., 2015. Childhood trauma: methods for the identification of physeal fractures in nonadult skeletal remains. American Journal of Physical Anthropology 157 (3), 411–420.

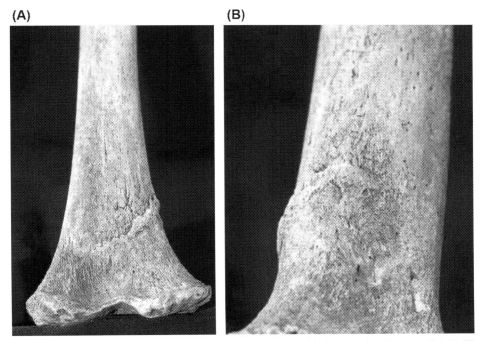

FIGURE 5.13 Greenstick fracture of the right distal femur in a 9-year-old from Pecos Pueblo, New Mexico (Peabody 60,149). The fracture is limited to the lateral aspect of the metaphysis (A) and the callus is minimal (B). *From Ortner, D., 2003. Identification of Pathological Conditions in Human Skeletal Remains, Academic Press, New York, p. 149.*

Cortical Striations

Striations on the cortical surface (Fig. 5.14) have been noted precisely above the location of a fracture in three archeological cases (Verlinden, 2015). Potentially they mark an area of intense periosteal activity that accompanies localized fracture remodeling or bone drift (Gasco and De Pablos, 1997). "Cortical thickening" describes a notable irregularity on the cortical surface due to an abnormal amount of localized lamellar bone distorting the bone's normal shape. These changes may be very subtle and only identified in comparison to the unaffected side.

Angulation

Acute angulations can result from any complete break, while minor angulations may result from greenstick and buckle fractures and traumatic bowing. Although clear radiographic signs are absent immediately after traumatic bowing, clinicians have reported cortical thickening and periosteal activity underlying the concavity during healing. This change can appear up to 10 months after the original injury (Borden, 1975; Sanders and Heckman, 1984). This thickening may be a useful indicator if the macroscopic bowing is very subtle. While angulations should be apparent by comparing one side to another (Fig. 5.15), plastic deformation is harder to define; however clinical methods for identifying traumatic bowing in the ulna and radius are available.

Plastic Deformation of the Ulna

To assess abnormal bowing of the ulna, the posterior aspect of the shaft should be placed on a flat surface and a measurement taken from that surface to edge of the shaft. Curvature with a depth of 3.9 mm or above has been shown to indicate plastic deformation in clinical studies (Lincoln and Mubarak, 1994).

Plastic Deformation of the Radius

Abnormal radial curvature can be assessed by placing the posterior aspect of the radius on a flat surface with the radial tuberosity and interosseous margin pointing upwards. Take a measurement from the distal end of the radius to the base of the radial tuberosity (y), calculate 60% of this length measurement (y/100 × 60), and use this resulting dimension to measure back from the radial tuberosity to a point along the shaft. At this point (x), work out the depth of the maximum curve (r) by taking a measurement from the posterior edge of the radius to the bench. If the depth measurement (x) exceeds 10% of the maximum length measurement (y), then this is an unnatural curve and likely the result of plastic deformation (Firl and Wunsch, 2004).

CRANIAL FRACTURES

Child crania differ from those of adults and adolescents in a number of ways. While the adult cranium is rigid and unyielding, in infants and young children it has an elastic nature and is loosely joined by sutures and fontanels (Pudenz et al., 1961). Thin cranial bones and soft membranous fontanels mean the skull is less able to protect the brain from injury. In addition, the dura mater is more loosely attached to the endocranial surface and susceptible to tearing. This, in combination with wider subarachnoid spaces means children are much more susceptible to subdural hematomas (intracranial bleeding) (Cory et al., 2001). On impact, the infant cranium is more likely to depress inward but not fracture, known as a "ping-pong" injury, or the sutures may separate, defined as a "diastatic fracture." Linear fractures will heal quickly and just as today, fractures to the firmer skull base may go unnoticed (Pudenz et al., 1961). While fractures in children under the age of 2 years are viewed with suspicion of abuse, cranial fractures as the result of falls, or from being accidently dropped by a parent do occur. In a study by Hendrick et al. (1964) of 4465 children under 15 years, the majority of cranial injuries were reported in 4-year-olds, at a time when children are becoming increasingly mobile and interacting with their environment. Children suffered a range of symptoms from drowsiness, headaches, and vomiting, to hematomas, convulsions, brain damage, and death, while

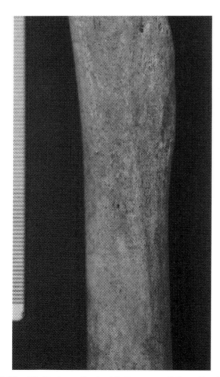

FIGURE 5.14 Vertical cortical striations overlying the fracture site on a nonadult femur. *From Verlinden, P., 2015. Child's Play? A New Methodology for the Identification of Trauma in Non-adult Skeletal Remains (Ph.D. thesis). University of Reading, England, p. 132.*

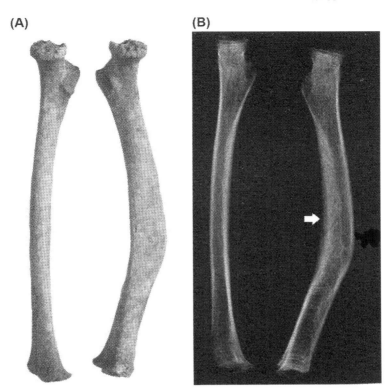

FIGURE 5.15 (A) Greenstick fracture of the left femur viewed from the side in a 6-year-old from Bow Baptist Church, London (AD 1816–1853, skeleton PAY05127). The femur has become acutely angled, and (B) thickening of the cortical bone on the side of the concavity is evident (indicated by an *arrow*) on the radiograph. *After Walker, D., 2012. Disease in London, 1st-19th Centuries, Museum of London Archaeology, London, p. 137.*

neonates suffered from respiratory disorders such as shallow breathing and blue spells (Hendrick et al., 1964). Right-sided linear fractures of the parietal bone were the most common, while concurrent fractures of the clavicle, cervical spine, mandible, and femur were noted in 11.2% of cases. In fatal cases, children died within 24 hours, which would leave little time for any bone repair to become evident.

In archeological contexts, it may be difficult to distinguish linear or depression fractures, suture separation, or bone displacement from postmortem breaks or warping (Crist et al., 1997), and the often fragmentary nature of these crania can prevent detailed observations of pathology. Two of the earliest cases of child head injuries come from the Pleistocene and Middle Paleolithic (Coqueugniot et al., 2012; Wu and Trinkaus, 2015) where both cases are healed depressed fractures. When reexamining the Pleistocene Qafzeh skull using 3D imaging, Coqueugniot et al. (2012) described how the injury on the right frontal bone was compound and extended into the cranium, possibly causing growth delay and a brain injury in this 13-year-old hominin. They suggest that the deliberate ceremonial burial of the child may have been a reflection of the neurological disturbances the child displayed after the trauma. Fibiger (2014) emphasizes that cranial trauma is more likely to be the result of interpersonal violence than postcranial trauma. There are strategic and psychological reasons why someone would target the head and neck, where injuries can be immediately disabling to the victim. Forensic techniques applied to bioarcheological data allow us to distinguish accidental from intentional injury. Accidental cranial trauma is usually linear rather than well-circumscribed; and facial injuries, particularly on the upper left side of the face, tend to indicate violence. In a survey of 32 cases of nonadult cranial trauma from various sites worldwide, Lewis (2014) reported that the majority comprised depressed fractures and 59% (n = 19) were in children aged between 3 and 10 years (Fig. 5.16). A further review of 38 cases showed that the majority were perimortem injuries (n = 32/38 or 84%) with 18% (n = 6) of these children under the age of 5 years. Of the six antemortem cases, five were in children over the age of 6 years, the exception being a 34-week-old perinate with a healed fracture of the orbit (Baxarias et al., 2010). Tung's (2016) review of children killed during the collapse of the Wari Empire suggested children were dispatched by blows to the base of the skull, while kneeling with their hands behind their backs. Perhaps similar violent and organized episodes explain the frequency of perimortem depressed fractures in nonadults.

Facial Fractures

Fractures to the nose, teeth, and mandible have also been reported in nonadult remains. Lewis (2016) identified significantly more facial and rib fractures in the males from urban sites in medieval England compared to their female peers,

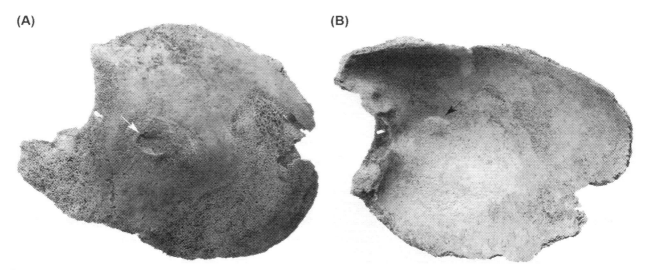

FIGURE 5.16 Depressed perimortem fracture on the right frontal bone of a 10-month-old from postmedieval Bow Baptist Church, London (AD 1863–1853, skeleton 478) (A) seen from the top. (B) The endocranial aspect shows a small indentation. The sharp, well-circumscribed margins of the lesions suggest the bone fractured as opposed to producing a ping-pong injury. *From Walker, D., 2012. Disease in London, 1st-19th Centuries, Museum of London Archaeology, London, p. 100.*

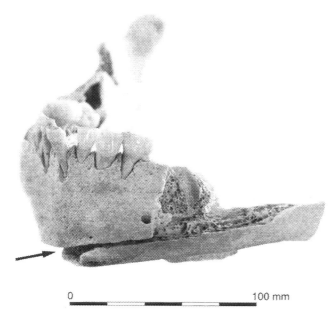

FIGURE 5.17 Perimortem blade injury of the left mandibular body in a 4- to 6-year-old from Romano–British Lankhills, Oxfordshire, England (4th century AD, skeleton 2064). *From Clough, S., Boyle, A., 2010. Inhumations and disarticulated human bone. In: Booth, P., Simmonds, S., Boyle, A., Clough, S., Cool, H., Poore, D. (Eds.), The Late Roman Cemetery at Lankhills, Winchester Excavations 2000-2005. Oxford Archaeology Ltd., Oxford, p. 369.*

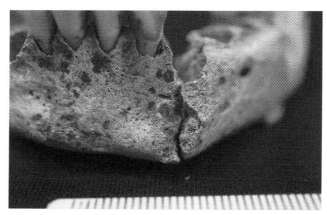

FIGURE 5.18 Fractured mandible with fiber bone callus in a 10- to 11-year-old from the Barbican, York, England (Later medieval, skeleton 2772). *Photograph by P. Verlinden. Courtesy of the University of Sheffield.*

and supporting historical reports of frequent fighting in male adolescents. A blade injury to a mandible was identified in a child from Roman Lankhills, Oxfordshire (Fig. 5.16; Clough and Boyle, 2010), and a fracture to the mandibular body with fractured teeth and callus formation was identified in a 10- to 11-year-old from Barbican, York (Fig. 5.17; Verlinden, 2015). This child had sustained the injury shortly before their death.

Today, fractures to the mandibular condyle are the most common in children under 10 years, with fractures to the mandibular body increasing with advancing age (Thorén et al., 1992). The main cause of mandibular fractures of the condyle, ramus, or body is falls (Namdev et al., 2016; Fig. 5.18).

SPINAL INJURIES

Fractures of the spine are commonly reported in adult skeletal remains but are rarely identified in nonadults. Today, fractures to the spine and ribs in young children are often associated with caregiver violence. Before the age of 10 years the spine has greater flexibility as the result of laxity of the spinal soft tissues, fluidity of the nucleus pulposus, more horizontally placed facets that allow for a higher degree of mobility, a higher cartilage to bone ratio, and the presence of secondary ossification centers (Loder and Hensinger, 2001;

Pathria, 2005). This means multiple fractures are more common than in adults as elastic vertebral discs transmit compression forces as a wave through multiple levels (Loder and Hensinger, 2001). Despite this, compression fractures to the vertebral bodies are unlikely to be identified in dry bone as the fluid nature of the immature nucleus pulpous results in blood being forced into the cancellous bone at the end plates without vertebral collapse (Loder and Hensinger, 2001). Healing of vertebral fractures is also more likely due to stimulation of growth and overgrowth of the vertebral bodies, allowing vertebrae to return to normal, even in cases of multiple compression fractures. It is possible that compression fractures in the youngest individuals may mimic Schmorl's nodes, but further research is needed. After the age of 10 years fractures to a child's spine will follow an adult pattern (Sullivan, 1998).

Spinal fractures are clinically defined by the region affected (i.e., occipito–atlanto–axial, lower cervical, upper thoracic, thoracolumbar, lower lumbar), cause of the injury, and presence or absence of instability (Pathria, 2005). The presence of complex soft tissue structures such as the ligaments and tendons, intervertebral discs and in children, epiphyses at the facets and end plates also need to be considered. Minor fractures are defined as those of a single area or region such as fractures of the spinous process, transverse process, articular facet, or pars interarticularis (spondylolysis). Major injuries involve compression fractures, burst injuries, and fracture dislocations involving the vertebral bodies or more than one area of the spine (Pathria, 2005). Children are likely to sustain spinal cord injuries without any signs on the bony neural elements, which have greater elasticity and are less likely to fracture, even in a serious traumatic event. Hence serious spinal injuries in a child will be hidden in the archeological record unless enough time has elapsed for paralysis to be evident. Difficulties in identifying true vertebral fractures in mild cases that only involve the anterior spine may be addressed by employing techniques used in clinical medicine. For example, Genant et al. (1993) provide images for mild, moderate, and severe "grades" of wedge, biconcave, and crush deformities in the thoracic and lumbar spines, using vertebral height measurements from population means to confirm diagnosis (Ferrar et al., 2005). This method would require the mean height of each vertebra within a sample to be calculated before an abnormal measurement could be identified, not an easy task in those under 10 years when a child's spine is still growing. Systemic conditions such as Gaucher's disease, idiopathic juvenile osteoporosis, tuberculosis, osteogenesis imperfecta, tetanus, leukemia, and neuroblastoma may cause multiple vertebral collapse in children, and in some cases may involve the entire spine (Loder and Hensinger, 2001).

Many factors that cause spinal injuries in children today would not have been present in the past, for example, fractures to the thoracic and lumbar vertebra are usually the result of car accidents, although a smaller number result from falls from heights. Adult injuries tend to occur in the lower cervical and thoracolumbar regions due to the greater degree of

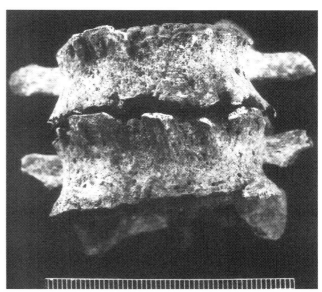

FIGURE 5.19 The reduced height of the vertebral bodies and marginal osteophytes are suggestive of compression fractures of the lumbar vertebrae in this 15-year-old from Romano–British Cannington, Somerset (skeleton 277). *From Brothwell, D., Powers, R., 2000. The human biology. In: Rathtz, P., Hirst, S., Wright, S. (Eds.), Cannington Cemetery. English Heritage, London, p. 221.*

motion in these areas (Pathria, 2005). Cervical fractures are rare in modern populations but are more likely to occur in young children due to the weight of their head and weaker musculature in this region. Breech delivery can cause lower cervical spine and upper thoracic injuries as the result of traction, whereas rotation during cephalic delivery may cause damage to the upper cervical spine (Warner, 2001). Cervical fractures as a whole are more common in male than female children, and the incidence increases with age, with children under 2 years suffering fractures due to birth trauma, and between 3 and 5 years as the result of falls or physical abuse (Sullivan, 1998). Before 10 years of age the most common cervical fractures are of the odontoid process, bilateral spondylolisthesis of C2 (Hangman's fracture), or facet fracture dislocation and burst fractures in the lower cervical spine. Today, such injuries lead to death in the young child and would be hard to identify in skeletal samples.

Adolescents aged 10–18 years may suffer dislocation of the apophyseal vertebral end plates, normally of the lumbar spine (Sullivan, 1998). These may be in the form of soft tissue damage or result from a section of bone being torn away from the posterior aspect of the vertebrae. The cause of these fractures includes lifting weights, shoveling, and hyperextension (Sullivan, 1998). A probable example of this type of injury was identified by Ortner (Smithsonian Institution Research Slide Collection) in a 17-year-old from the medieval hospital of Chichester in Sussex, and Brothwell and Powers (2000) found similar lesions in a 15-year-old from Cannington, England (Fig. 5.19). In infant victims of physical abuse, compression fractures of the vertebral bodies, vertebral subluxation, and avulsion fractures of the spinous processes of the thoracic vertebra are lesions associated with forcible shaking. These generally occur in conjunction with metaphyseal, cranial, and rib fractures rather than in isolation (Pathria, 2005). In many cases it may prove impossible to distinguish compression fractures of the spine in older children from Scheuermann's kyphosis (Chapter 10). In the latter there is normally wedging of thoracic vertebrae and anterior oval depressions of the vertebral surface, but wedging does not always occur, and this circulatory condition may also affect the lumbar spine.

Tetanus

Caused by an infection of the spore *Clostridium tetani* and usually contracted through puncture wounds from dirty objects, tetanus was undoubtedly an infection encountered in the past. However, the skeletal traces of the condition are rarely considered. Tetanus can cause spinal kyphosis as the result of violent convulsions resulting in mild or severe anterior wedging of the thoracic vertebrae, most commonly T3–T7 (Fig. 5.20). There may also be subluxation of the spine. First described in 1907 by Lehndorff, these lesions may be confused with those of Scheuermann's disease (Roberg, 1937). Stronger musculature may be the reason more cases are found in males than females, while children younger than 10 years are considered more susceptible to damage due to the more fragile nature of their spines (Davis and Rowland, 1965; Nte and Gabriel-Job, 2013).

Spondylolysis and Spondylolisthesis

Spondylolysis describes the partial separation of the inferior facets on the neural arch from the vertebral body. The condition usually results from microtrauma in low-grade stress (isthmic spondylolysis) on the lumbar spine as the result of bending and lifting strains (Fredrickson et al., 1984; Waldron, 2009). In rare circumstances it may result from severe acute trauma such as a fall from a height (Wiltse, 1975). An individual may be susceptible to a fatigue fracture due to a congenital fibrous defect of the pars interarticularis (Fredrickson et al., 1984; Leone et al., 2011). The normal occurrence of the lesion in a population is around 6%–8% rising to 63% in individuals involved in certain sporting activities (Leone et al., 2011). In a review of 500 American children between 5 and 18 years Fredrickson et al. (1984) reported an incidence of spondylolysis in 4.4% of children up to the age of 6 years, with rates gradually increasing with age. They noted the lack of pain in the affected individuals and a strong association with spina bifida occulta.

Spondylolysis is normally bilateral (Fig. 5.21) resulting in two separate bone fragments; an anterior segment composed of the vertebral body, pedicals, and transverse process, and a posterior portion comprising the spinous process, inferior articular facets, and laminae (Aufderheide and Rodriguez-Martín, 1998). Although rare, spondylolysis may be unilateral (Fig. 5.22). This fracture most commonly occurs on the fifth lumbar vertebra at any point after a child begins to walk but also occurs on the fourth lumbar. A complication of spondylolysis is spondylolisthesis (Crawford et al., 2015), where the released vertebral body shifts anteriorly causing pain in the legs and lower back (sciatica). Elongation of the pars interarticularis has been noted as a consequence of this slippage (Morita et al., 1995), although Wiltse (1975) suggests the elongation occurs prior to fracture after repeated stress fractures, followed by healing. While spondylolisthesis usually results from trauma, it may also occur in osteogenesis imperfecta and Albers-Schoenberg disease (Wiltse, 1975).

Fibiger and Knusel (2005) carried out an extensive review of spondylolysis in 310 skeletons over 6 years of age from several UK sites. None revealed any examples of spondylolysis in the nonadults. A potential unilateral case was identified in 12-year-old from Chichester, Sussex (Lewis, 2008), with four further cases reported in the later medieval samples of St Helen-on-the Walls, York (n = 1); St Mary Spital, London (n = 2); and St Peter's Church, Barton-upon-Humber (n = 1) (Lewis, 2016).

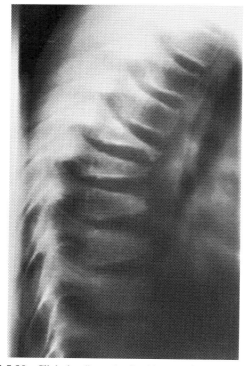

FIGURE 5.20 Clinical radiograph of a 14-year-old with multiple compression fractures and anterior wedging in the thoracic vertebrae as the result of tetanus spasms. *From http://www.isradiology.org/tropical_deseases/tmcr/chapter33/clinical1.htm.*

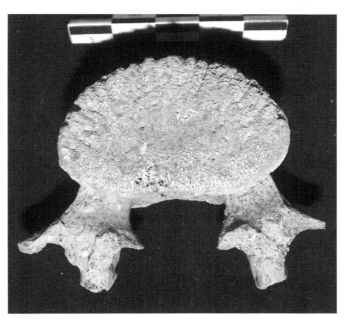

FIGURE 5.21 Bilateral spondylolysis of the fifth lumbar vertebra in a 15-year-old from St Mary Spital, London (AD 1200–1250, skeleton 32,258). *Photograph by F. Shapland with the kind permission of the Museum of London.*

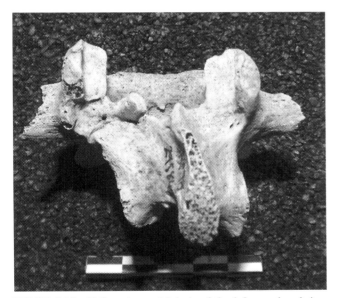

FIGURE 5.22 Unilateral spondylolysis of the left neural arch in a 15-year-old from St Mary Spital, London (AD 1250–1400, skeleton 29,584). *Photograph by F. Shapland with the kind permission of the Museum of London.*

The latter were all in individuals aged 15–16 years and comprised two males and two females. Mays (2007b) attempted to tackle the question of nonadult spondylolysis using the later medieval rural sample from Wharram Percy, Yorkshire. He reported a prevalence of just 0.7% (n = 1/140) in the children compared to 12% in the adult sample. The affected individual was 12 years of age.

The start of strenuous labor in medieval children around 12 years may account for a similar peak in adolescent cases (Mays, 2007b). The lack of evidence for spondylolysis in those less than 12 years in archeological samples is notable given the modern peak of cases around 5 years of age in the clinical literature. It is likely earlier cases are missed in skeletal remains as this is a common area for the bone to break postmortem, and confusion may arise between the age at which the lumbar neural arches are supposed to fuse to the centrum (age 4–5 years) and a pathological fracture. Nevertheless, this does not explain the lack of cases in studies that specifically set out to find the lesion in nonadult remains.

Clay-Shoveler's Fractures

These are oblique vertical avulsion fractures of the spinous process that occur between C6 and T3 with C7 and T1 (Kaloostian et al., 2013). These fractures are rarely seen in children today, although modern cases have noted them in a teenage wrestler, a baseball player and a 14-year-old rock climber (Yamaguchi et al., 2012; Kaloostian et al., 2013). This suggests excessive weight bearing and torsion on the ligaments of the midback is a causative factor. Spinous process fractures are thought to occur when rapidly lifting weights with extended arms, and in individuals unused to physical labor who suddenly exert themselves (Jordana et al., 2006). In the paleopathological literature clay-shoveler's fractures have been particularly associated with shoveling in medieval males (Knüsel et al., 1996).

RIB FRACTURES

In modern clinical medicine, rib fractures in children are commonly associated with caregiver violence when they occur in combination with other injuries (see below). Distinguishing accidental or secondary rib fractures from nonaccidental fractures relies on understanding the location and type of the lesions (Love et al., 2013). Anterior rib fractures are more likely to be associated with accidental injury than the posterior fractures that are thought to be related to squeezing (Love et al., 2013). Secondary fractures of the rib due to generalized bone dysplasia, tumors, or rickets are usually accompanied by general osteopenia (Glass et al., 2002; Pettifor and Daniels, 1997). Kopcsanyi et al. (1969) noted rib fractures in 50% of children with rickets and associated chest infections, calling them "cough" fractures.

Although adult rib fractures are common observations in archeological material (Brickley, 2006b), they are rarely considered in nonadults. While poor preservation can hinder detailed and large scale studies, Brickley (2006b) argues that this should always be attempted due to the valuable information rib fractures can provide. Matos (2009) examined the prevalence of rib fractures in the known collection from Lisbon. Of the 25 individuals with fractures only one nonadult was identified, a 15-year-old female with chronic myocarditis, who had two fractures to the right side of her chest. In a study of 364 nonadults from Roman Poundbury Camp in Dorset, UK, Lewis (2010) identified 12 rib fractures, with half of the cases occurring in children who also had signs of rickets and scurvy. Radiographs later revealed that two children showed osteomas or pseudo-fracture calluses caused by thalassemia (Lewis, 2011), while three children aged 44 weeks, 2 years, and 7 years had no other associated pathology and in the younger children at least, abuse should be considered (Lewis, 2010). The presence of rib fractures in combination with nose and jaw fractures indicated possible interpersonal violence through fighting in a sample of urban medieval male adolescents (10–17 years) from England (Lewis, 2016).

AGE-RELATED INJURIES

Birth Trauma

Birth injury is defined as any condition that adversely affects the fetus during delivery (Gresham, 1975). Injuries may result from compression and traction forces during the birth process, malpresentation, a difficult prolonged labor, and large fetal size. Today, birth trauma is the cause of 2% of neonatal deaths and stillbirths in the United States (Gresham, 1975). Although any bone may be injured, the most typical fractures occur to the clavicle, humerus, proximal femur, and cranium (Brill and Winchester, 1987; Caffey, 1945; Resnick and Goergen, 2002). Clavicle fractures are frequently found

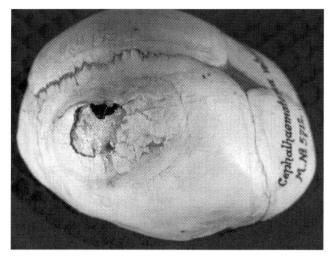

FIGURE 5.23 Birth trauma: ossified hematoma with linear and depressed fractures in a 4-week-old who died in 1840. From the Pathology Museum in Vienna (skeleton FPAM 5712). The ossified bone is extremely fragile and the underlying cortex is pitted. *From Ortner, D., 2003. Identification of Pathological Conditions in Human Skeletal Remains, Academic Press, New York, p. 177.*

in normal deliveries (i.e., 0.2%–2.9% of live births) and are considered to be unpreventable, often healing without any adverse effects (Ahn et al., 2015). Dedick and Caffey (1953) reported fractured clavicles in 1.2% of their 1030 newborns, these were always unilateral and occurred more commonly on the left side. Identifying cranial fractures as a result of birth injury presents more of a challenge for the paleopathologist due to the fragile and fragmentary nature of the perinatal cranium. Linear and depressed fractures may not survive fragmentation in the ground, and if the child dies shortly after birth, perimortem fractures may be indistinguishable from postmortem breaks. In medieval England, the use of a crochet to extract a child from the womb (Eccles, 1977, 1982) may have resulted in perimortem cut marks to the orbits and palatine surface of the maxilla. From the mid-16th century, forceps may have caused crush and linear fractures to the frontal, parietal, or occipital bones (Rushton, 1991) resulting in a hematoma (cephalhematoma) (Sorantin et al., 2006). Caffey (1945) described such injuries as positioned away from midline, a detail that may aid in their differentiation from a congenital meningocele. Ossified hematomas may persist for months or years (Fig. 5.23). The maxilla is also a frequent site for infection in the first few weeks of life due to birth trauma and may be visible as reactive new bone formation around the developing dental germs (Caffey, 1945). New bone formation around erupting teeth and on the cranium is also a sign of scurvy and should be considered as a differential diagnosis. In addition to fractures, breech delivery may cause trauma to the muscles and other soft tissues of the back and lower limbs. Severe muscle damage can result in crush syndrome and be fatal to the child (Ráliš,

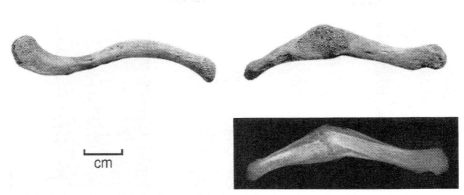

FIGURE 5.24 Fractured right clavicle with a midshaft callus (top right) in an infant from St Martin's Church, Birmingham, England (18th–19th century AD, skeleton 563), shown with the unaffected side (left). The radiograph (bottom right) clearly shows the fracture fragments indicating this was a recent fracture possibly sustained during the birth process. *From Brickley, M., 2006a. The people: physical anthropology. In: Brickley, M., Buteux, S., Adams, J., Cherrington, R. (Eds.), St Martin's Uncovered: Investigations in the Churchyard of St Martin's-in-the-Bull Ring, Birmingham, 2001. Oxbow Books, Oxford, p. 121.*

1975). Damage to the sternomastoid muscle during birth may result in facial asymmetry, or torticollis, which will cause frontal and occipital flattening, a laterally twisted face, dropped orbit, an enlarged mastoid process, and mandibular asymmetry (Skinner et al., 1989).

A healed clavicle fracture in a 4-month-old from Christ Church Spitalfields, London has been interpreted as possible birth trauma (Lewis, 2002b), with four other cases of fractured clavicles reported in infants from England and Italy (Fig. 5.24; Brickley, 2006a; Soren et al., 1995; Verlinden, 2015). Baxarias et al. (2010) identified a healing linear fracture above the left orbit in a 38-week-old infant, suggesting birth trauma caused the injury. In a similar case, Polo-Cerdá et al. (2003) suggested the use of forceps during a basiotripsy as the cause of a perimortem linear cut marks on the parietal and occipital bones of a perinate from 18th-century Castielfabid, Spain. It is not known if the child was dead prompting this procedure or died during this violent extraction process. Soft tissue injuries during birth have also been suggested by Holst (2004), who identified a case of disuse atrophy in the right femur of a 2- to 4-month-old child from Bridlington, UK, which she suggested may have occurred at birth. Skinner et al. (1989) discussed cranial asymmetry from muscular torticollis as the result of breech births in three adult crania from British Columbia. Changes to the distal aspect of the humerus in the tiny remains of a perinate from St Oswald's Priory have been interpreted as an oblique physeal fracture, with posterior displacement of the cartilaginous epiphyses, an injury likely sustained during the birth process (Fig. 5.25; DeLee et al., 1980; Verlinden and Lewis, 2015).

Erb's and Klumph's Palsy (Congenital Brachial Palsy)

Brachial palsy is caused during childbirth as the result of excessive traction and separation of the head and shoulder during a breech delivery. Breech births (where the child

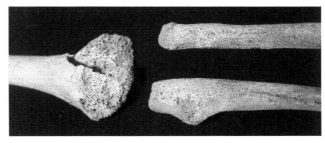

FIGURE 5.25 Probable physeal fracture to the distal metaphysis of the right humerus in a 42-week-old from St Oswald's Priory in Gloucester, England (AD 1120–1230, skeleton 13). The changes to the cortex were initially considered to represent an infection, rather than a fracture callus. The distal humerus is flattened with reactive new bone. The periosteal cloaking is likely due to the localized tearing of the periosteum when the epiphysis became displaced.

presents feet first) are by far the most common form of malpresentation today, accounting for 3%–4% of births at term and 6% of births at 32 weeks. The most common causes of breech birth are advancing maternal age, prematurity, first pregnancy, and fetal anomalies such as hydrocephaly (Simm, 2007). Damage caused during breech births may be fatal, with up to 20% showing some level of handicap by the age of 5 years (Simm, 2007). Damage to fibers from the fifth to sixth cervical roots, which supply the deltoid, spinata, biceps, and brachialis anticus muscles results in paralysis of the upper arm or Erb's palsy (Sheldon, 1943). Less common is damage to the eighth cervical and first thoracic roots, causing lower arm paralysis (Klumpke's palsy). Whole arm paralysis caused by damage to the third to fourth cervical roots is known as Erb–Duchenne–Klumpke palsy (Yates, 1959), but if the whole plexus is torn, bleeding into the spinal column may be fatal. Erb's palsy is reported in between 1.56 and 0.31 per 1000 births, with large babies being more susceptible to injury (Adler and Patterson, 1967). Paralysis is normally unilateral and becomes noticeable a few days after birth when the arm adopts a characteristic position, hanging loosely the shoulder

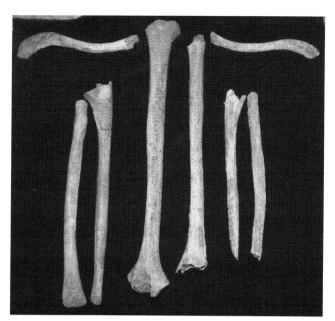

FIGURE 5.26 Disuse atrophy of the left arm (clavicle, humerus, radius, and ulna) in a 10- to 14-year-old from St Oswald's Priory in Gloucester, England (AD 900–1120, skeleton 406). Although the ends of the bones are missing, the lack of infection and involvement of the whole arm is suggestive of birth trauma (Erb's Palsy).

and externally rotated. The condition may resolve in 2 years or, if roots are severely torn, paralysis will be permanent with contracture deformity of the hand and subsequent muscle wasting that may be confused with poliomyelitis (Sheldon, 1943). Adler and Patterson (1967) reported full recovery in 13% of their Erb's palsy infants, while 43% showed elbow deformity into adolescence and early adulthood. Dislocation of the radial head and bowing of the ulna may occur with elbow contracture and would be evident as flattening of the trochlear and anterior angulations of the radial epiphysis. Erb's palsy and other arm injuries associated with childbirth have been suggested in adults (Molto, 2000; Roberts, 1989), and an adolescent from St Oswald's Priory displays disuse atrophy of the left arm that may indicate birth trauma, although poliomyelitis cannot be ruled out as an underlying cause (Fig. 5.26). The hazards associated with vaginal breech delivery may mean that few children survived the process and may account for the rarity of published cases. However, the causes of disuse atrophy are numerous (Chapter 11), making definitive diagnosis difficult in skeletal remains.

Toddler's Fractures

Once children are mobile, climbing and learning to walk, they are more likely to sustain fractures accidentally. A typical fracture in this age group, around 2 years of age, occurs at the distal tibia and is known as the "toddler's fracture." This occurs with external twisting or rotation of the foot while the knee is fixed (Heinrich, 2001). The classic toddler's fracture is subtle and comprises a hairline nondisplaced oblique or spiral fracture of the tibia (Heinrich, 2001; John et al., 1997). These are usually the result of the child tripping, or catching their foot in the bars of their playpen (John et al., 1997). While the distal tibia is the most common site of injury, fractures may also occur on the fibula, femur, and first metatarsal (Resnick and Kransdorf, 2005). Fractures are more common on the right leg and may result in a limp.

Fractures of the foot are typically buckle fractures sustained when the toddler falls or jumps from a height, often resulting in multiple fractures to the base of the metatarsals due to vertical loading and compression forces. Compression fractures of the cuboid may occur when it is forced between the calcaneus and metatarsals after a fall, although these types of lesions are rare and again, very subtle (John et al., 1997). The only sign of foot fractures for the paleopathologist may be new bone formation overlying the site. When the foot is involved, the first metatarsal is the most commonly affected bone, and Owen et al. (1995) suggest the foot's susceptibility to compression forces before 5 years of age is due to the lack of a foot arch.

Juvenile Osteochondritis Dissecans

Juvenile osteochondritis dissecans (JOCD) involves the detachment of a piece of cartilage and possibly the underlying bone at the joint surface. Repetitive stress to the affected area due to vigorous activity is the main contributing factor (Polousky, 2011), causing some to consider posttraumatic subarticular necrosis a better term (Šlaus et al., 2010a). However, other causes include endocrine disorders, familial occurrence, accessory ossification centers, osteonecrosis, and osteochondral fractures (Cahill, 1995; Resnick and Goergen, 2002). JOCD is distinguished from the adult form of the condition as it occurs in individuals with an open growth plate and has a poorer prognosis. The fragment rarely heals or unites without an operative procedure (Cahill, 1995). Distinguishing between JOCD and the less common adult onset form of the condition is unlikely to be possible in skeletal remains once the epiphysis has fused. JOCD is slightly more common in males than females, but this may be a modern reflection of the types of sport the different genders are involved in. The knee is affected in around 90% of cases, most frequently on the medial condyle on the lateral aspect. The convex surfaces of the elbow, ankle, hip, shoulder, and wrist are also vulnerable, in that order (Waldron, 2009). JOCD of the knee is more common in 12- to 19-year-olds than 6- to 11-year-olds (Kessler et al., 2014). After detachment, the fragmented portion may remain in situ, be slightly displaced, or become loose within the joint capsule known as "a joint mouse" (Resnick and Goergen, 2002). Other joint defects may be confused with JOCD especially when they occur on the concave areas of the joint (e.g., the base of MT1), and a porous well-defined margin is needed to diagnose it correctly. In clinical medicine, mapping the location of the lesion is considered

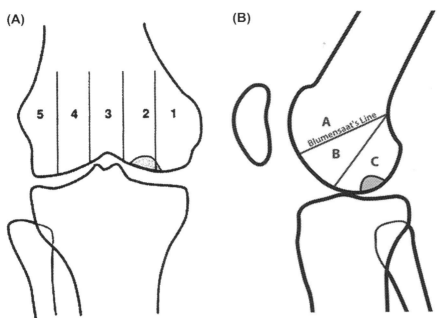

FIGURE 5.27 Diagram to aid in the mapping of the location of juvenile osteochondritis dissecans from the (A) anteroposterior and (B) mediolateral views. Numbers 5–1 indicate locations along the horizontal plane from the lateral to the medial condyles. Letters denote the position of the lesion on the vertical surface of the joint, A, anterior projection; B, lateral projection; C, posterior projection. The shaded lesion on the image is at location 2C. *From Schenik, R., Goodnight, J., 1996. Current concepts review: osteochondritis dissecans. Journal of Bone and Joint Surgery 78 (3), 449.*

important to ascertain the etiology of the defect (Fig. 5.27). Lesions on the lateral aspect of the medial condyle may have a different etiology to those on the medial aspect, as the former is nonweight bearing. Similarly, the size of the lesion may help to determine the underlying cause or severity. An unhealed lesion in an adult may be indicative of a juvenile onset of the condition.

Large scale studies of JOCD in nonadults are rare, although these lesions are frequently mentioned within skeletal reports. In a study of 2549 medieval nonadults aged 7 to 17 years, Lewis (2016) recorded JODC in 38 individuals (0.15%). The distribution of these lesions differed between rural and urban sites, with the urban adolescents having a greater prevalence of the lesion. When the location of urban JOCD was analyzed, males had the lesions most commonly in their shoulders and ankles, while the females had the highest rates of JOCD in their knees (Fig. 5.28). This pattern was attributed to different occupational activities carried out by medieval males and females (Lewis, 2016). In archeological populations, where the location of JOCD is reported, lesions tend to be more common on the distal humerus, followed by the femur, although lesions on the metatarsals, axis, and tibia are also noted (Lewis, 2016; Mays, 1991, 2007a; Šlaus et al., 2010a; Wells, 1974) similar to the pattern seen in modern patients.

Slipped Femoral Epiphysis

A slipped femoral capital epiphysis is characterized as an inferior–medial–posterior displacement of the proximal

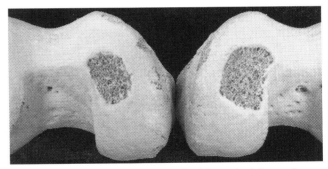

FIGURE 5.28 Bilateral JOCD on the distal femoral epiphyses of a nonadult from late Roman Poundbury Camp in Dorset, England. The base of the lesions is porous and the margins are well defined. The location of the lesion using the Cahill (1995) system is 2B. *Photograph taken with the kind permission of the Museum of Natural History, London.*

epiphysis. The lesion is normally unilateral, and the displaced epiphysis will eventually fuse to the femoral neck in its abnormal position (Resnick and Goergen, 2002). Displacement most commonly occurs between the ages of 10 and 17 years in boys and 8 and 15 years in girls. This relationship to the adolescent growth spurt is thought to be the result of a widened metaphysis that is especially vulnerable to shearing forces. The fracture generally occurs in the metaphyseal side of the growth plate and may result in a new joint (pseudoarthrosis) to accommodate the femoral head on the ilium, while the epiphysis is held in the acetabulum by the ligamentum teres (Ortner and Putschar, 1985). In general, slipped femoral epiphyses occur more often in black individuals, the obese, and very active adolescents (Resnick and Goergen, 2002). A slipped femoral capital epiphysis may also occur after an attempt to reduce a dislocated hip in adolescents (Fiddian and Grace, 1983). Osteoporosis can develop in the femoral neck and head, and there may be buttressing of the neck in the form of reactive new bone. Other complications include varus deformity (inward angulation), a shortened and broadened neck, necrosis (in up to 18% of cases), and early degenerative joint disease (Resnick and Goergen, 2002).

Reports of this type of injury in nonadult remains are rare, probably due to the difficulty in identifying such trauma in an unfused epiphysis. However, Waldron (2007) reported a case of a slipped femoral epiphysis in a 12- to 13-year-old from medieval St Peter's Church in Lincolnshire, England. Another medieval case was reported in a 10- to 14-year-old from Wharram Percy, Yorkshire (Mays, 2007a). Differential diagnoses should include Legg–Calvé–Perthes disease, congenital hip dysplasia, or a fracture to the femoral neck. When considering a differential diagnosis, a slipped femoral epiphysis is characterized by inferior slippage resulting in an absent femoral neck on the superior aspect and a greatly reduce neck inferiorly, subchondral cysts, and a well-defined insertion for the ligamentum teres (Waldron, 2009; Wasterlain and Umbelino, 2013). Deformation and widening of the femoral head and a wide or shallow acetabulum is not a feature of a slipped femoral epiphysis (Wasterlain and Umbelino, 2013).

OTHER FORMS OF TRAUMA

Dislocations

Dislocation refers to a complete loss of normal contact between the bone and articular cartilage components of the joint. Subluxation refers to a partial loss of contact that is more likely to reset spontaneously. There may be corresponding damage to the connective tissue, muscles, ligament nerve, and vascular supply (Ortner, 2003). If left untreated, a false joint (pseudoarthrosis) may develop at the site of displacement. Compression fractures to the rim in the glenoid cavity, acetabulum, humeral, or femoral head have been noted in clinical cases (Hill–Sachs type lesion), although they are more common in adults (Divecha et al., 2012). In all cases, it is important to rule out dislocation or subluxation as the result of a developmental disorder such as congenital dysplasia.

Dislocations of the Upper Limb

Dislocations of the glenohumeral junction are rare in children, although they increase in adolescence. The humerus is normally displaced anteriorly as the result of a fall or fight. Posterior dislocations are normally only seen in modern car accidents or violent assault (Resnick and Goergen, 2002). Cases of nonadult shoulder dislocations are also rare in the archeological record, and it is likely that any dislocations

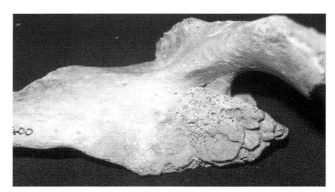

FIGURE 5.29 Possible shoulder dislocation in a 10- to 13-year-old from Barton-upon-Humber, Lincolnshire (AD 1150–1500, skeleton 400). The unfused glenoid cavity is enlarged with a flattened area above the joint indicative of compressions to the outer rim (Hills–Sach deformity). *Photograph by P. Verlinden.*

would have been quickly and easily reduced, although recurring subluxation with ligament laxity could be a feature. One possible case of shoulder dislocation with Hills–Sach deformity of the glenoid cavity was identified in medieval Lincolnshire in a 10- to 13-year-old female (Fig. 5.29).

Nikitovic et al. (2012) reported a dislocated right elbow in a 7- to 8-year-old from Copper Age Croatia (3500–2780 BC). The radial head had dislocated from the ulna resulting in lateral posterior displacement and the development of a medial exostosis on the ulna that acted as a pseudoarthrosis, limiting full movement of the elbow. The lack of a fracture line or underlying deformity ruled out a Monteggia fracture dislocation or congenital malformation. This case likely represents an isolated fracture of the radial head (Monteggia equivalent type I), probably as the result of falling onto an outstretched hand (Stanley and De La Garza, 2001). A similar dislocated right elbow was identified in an adolescent from St Mary Spital, London (Fig. 5.30), and Rohnbogner (2015) reported a fracture to the elbow in a Roman child with gross enlargement of the olecranon (Fig. 5.31).

Dislocations of the Lower Limb

In children, traumatic hip dislocations are rare and make up only 1% of all pediatric fractures (Blasier and Hughes, 2001). Trauma to this area is more likely to result in a slipped femoral epiphysis, although children under 5 years are more susceptible to dislocation after mild trauma due to the shallowness of the acetabulum and fragile epiphyseal junction. As the acetabulum deepens with maturity, more severe force is required for a traumatic injury (Rális and McKibbin, 1973). The majority of dislocations are posteriorly placed. Offierski (1981) classified the force needed for a traumatic injury into three types: mild force as the result of running, tripping, and falling; moderate force from excessive speed or impact, such as cycling, skiing, and football; or severe force as the result of a high energy impact or crushing. The latter would normally be accompanied

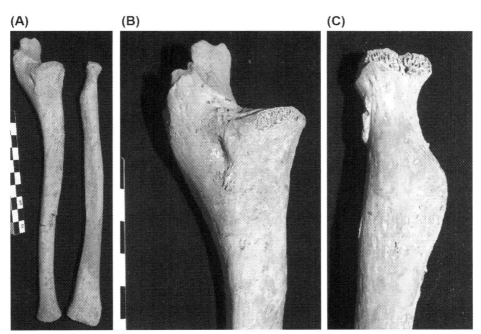

FIGURE 5.30 (A) Posterior dislocation of the right elbow in a 12- to 17-year-old from St Mary Spital, London. (B) The morphology of the ulna suggests a fracture as the cause, (C) but the reduced radial head suggests there may have been an underlying congenital deformity. Both bones show heterotrophic ossification of the ulnar collateral ligament (AD 1400–1540, skeleton 2917). *Photograph by F. Shapland with the kind permission of the Museum of London.*

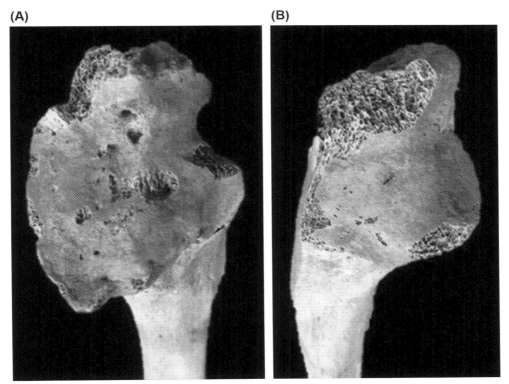

FIGURE 5.31 Dislocated right ulna in a 14-year-old from Romano–British Butt Road (skeleton 299). The left olecranon is grossly enlarged and flattened (A) in comparison to the right (B). *Photograph by A. Rohnbogner.*

by other traumatic injuries such as head or pelvic fractures. Hip dislocations may also occur in conditions where there is known ligament laxity such as Down syndrome. Around 27% of nonadult hip dislocations develop complications, including soft tissue interposition particularly of the acetabulum cartilage ring (posterior acetabular labrum) and avascular necrosis, coxa magna, and osteoarthritis. The threat of avascular necrosis is higher in children due to the vascular barrier created by the growth plate and a reliance on the cervical arteries for the blood supply to the femoral epiphysis (Sulaiman et al., 2014). Reports of hip dislocation should include consideration of the age of death; sex of the individual; destruction to the femoral head; presence, absence, or severity of subperiosteal new bone formation; atrophy; and hip mobility (Blondiaux and Millot, 1991). Blondiaux and Millot (1991) presented a traumatic hip subluxation in an adolescent from Cambrai-Mont des Boeufs, France, based on an innominate with a shallow and enlarged acetabulum and flattening of the superior aspect of the acetabular margin.

Myositis Ossificans Traumatica (Heterotrophic Ossification)

Traumatic myositis ossificans describes rapid abnormal formation of bone within soft tissues, often appearing as a shell of bone containing bone marrow that forms after a fracture, dislocation, or damage to the spinal cord or brain (Pape et al., 2004). These ectopic ossifications may appear in any joint (Balboni et al., 2006) and usually occur between 4 and 8 weeks after injury, with bone maturing in 5–6 months. Complete or partial resorption of this lesion is most often reported in younger individuals (Resnick and Kransdorf, 2005, p. 1348). A radiolucent band between the new bone mass and adjacent cortex provides a differential diagnosis for a tumor arising out of the cortex in the early stages (Resnick and Kransdorf, 2005). Symptoms may vary from localized pain, ankylosis, or the lesion may be asymptomatic. The pathogenesis is not clearly understood, but this abnormal ossification is thought to result from the recruitment and proliferation of osteoprogenitor cells to the site with increased activity of osteoblasts and decreased osteoclastic activity (Balboni et al., 2006).

Burns

Heterotrophic ossification has also been noted in 1%–3% of severe burn cases (second and third degree), most commonly in the hip, shoulder, and elbow (Chen et al., 2009), appearing around 3 months after the injury. After a severe burn, massive amounts of protein-rich fluid are released, and there may be secondary infection of the wound. In addition to soft tissue ossification, periostitis, disuse atrophy, and articular and periarticular changes may occur at the site (Resnick and Kransdorf, 2005). In burns, bone usually forms under the site of trauma, and a period of immobilization is the most common factor in its formation (Chen et al., 2009). Gaur et al. (2003) noted serious restriction in movement of the arm in eight children with severe heterotrophic ossification of the elbow leading to an inability of the children to reach their mouths to eat.

Accidents and death from burning appear commonly in medieval coroner's records from England (Towner and Towner, 2000). Open fires, loose clothing, and the flammable nature of many houses in the past make it likely that children would have sustained such injuries with frequency. That fire and death from burning were a hazard in the distant past is demonstrated by the recovery of three children aged between 8 and 18 years along with two adults from an Iron Age house fire in Denmark (Harvig et al., 2015). The authors suggested that the family died while trying to rescue their valuable animals. While third degree burns would likely have been fatal in the past, it may be possible to identify less severe burns in the archeological record, although this has yet to be fully explored. For example, a 4- to 7-year-old from early medieval Thetford in Norwich, England, demonstrated myositis ossificans on the posterior aspect of the left ilium communicating with the greater trochanter of the femur. It is possible this was caused as the result of trauma or a burn with subsequent immobilization (Fig. 5.32).

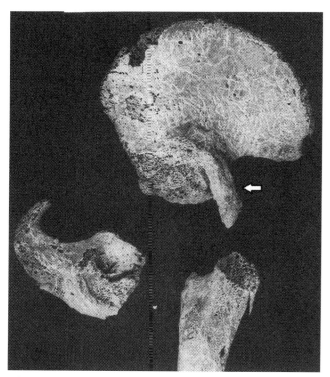

FIGURE 5.32 Myositis ossificans traumatica in the pelvis of a 4- to 7-year-old child from Brandon Road, Thetford, Norwich (skeleton F112). Such lesions may be a sign of burning injuries in archeological remains.

TREATMENT: AUTOPSIES AND SURGICAL INTERVENTION

Transverse cuts to the rib cage and craniotomies have been identified in at least four postmedieval burial sites in England (McKinley, 2008; Miles et al., 2008; Molleson and Cox, 1993; Powers and Miles, 2011). Autopsies were usually confined to opening the crania and the thorax to determine the cause of death, while dissections aimed to more thoroughly examine the entire body for educational purposes (Dittmar and Mitchell, 2015). The most comprehensive survey of medical procedures in skeletal remains was carried out by Dittmar and Mitchell (2015) on 140 individuals dating from AD 1849 to 1913 in England, including 13 juveniles (defined as 3–20 years) and 54 fetuses. The number of child examples demonstrates their importance in the development of medicine and medical instruction during the 19th century and corresponds to the rise in pediatrics during this time (Lomax, 1996).

Waldron and Rogers (1987) identified amputations performed on the legs of four children in an 18th- to 19th-century Gloucester Infirmary. This included the amputation of a child's right thigh, perhaps due to the presence of an osteosarcoma or osteomyelitis, although the recovered bones appear normal. Three embryotomies have been identified in perinatal material, two dating to the Romano–British period. The Poundbury Camp perinate was decapitated and has extensive cut marks throughout (Fig. 5.33; Molleson and Cox, 1988), while an embryotomy was suggested as the cause of a cut mark on the femur of a perinate from Yewdon Roman Villa in Buckinghamshire (Mays et al., 2012). A possible 19th century embryotomy was identified in L'Aquila, Italy (Capasso et al., 2016), showing a dissected skull and severe jumbling of the bones in a wrapped and mummified 29-week-old fetus. The remains could only be observed on radiograph and so the presence of additional cut marks is unknown. Redfern (2007) reported a hand amputation in a Romano–British child believed to have occurred as the result of a perimortem accident, while Powers and Miles (2011) reported a lower leg amputation in an adolescent from postmedieval London with the leg subsequently becoming osteomyelitic (Fig. 5.34).

Trepanation

Trephination is the surgical procedure in which a hole is created in the skull by the removal of circular piece of bone, while a trepanation is the opening created by this procedure (Stone and Miles, 1990). Trephinations are the most common type of procedure encountered in archeological material (Ortner, 2003) and appear to have been performed for a variety of medical, cultural,

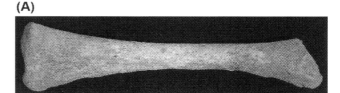

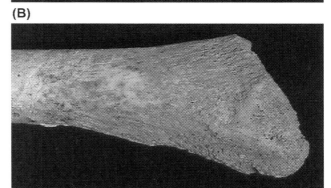

FIGURE 5.33 (A) One of a series of perimortem cut marks in a late Roman perinate. Cuts to the proximal femur made to remove the leg from the hip during a possible embryotomy, (B) with close-up view. The perinate was recovered from Poundbury Camp in Dorset (skeleton 1414). *Photographs taken with the kind permission of the Natural History Museum, London.*

or spiritual reasons. Five methods of trephination have been identified; scraping, bore and saw, sawing, drilling, and gouging (Arnott et al., 2005), with differences in the amount and depth of bone being removed. Ortner (2003, p. 172) suggests that trephinations carried out to treat cranial trauma are likely to be the largest as they involved removing the fractured fragment from the wound. Death can occur due to poor technique resulting in injury to the brain, secondary brain damage as the result of bleeding, or infection. In cases where the lesion appears to be unhealed, it is not possible to determine whether death resulted from the procedure or whether the procedure was carried out postmortem. In Northern Peru, the cranium of a 7-year-old with a scraped trepanation was discovered in a sample of 18 adult skulls suggesting that children were not differentiated from adults in the use of this procedure (Nystrom, 2007). In fact, around 13 trepanations have been reported in nonadult remains and most have accompanying pathological lesions. An 8-year-old from Cinnos Cerros, Peru, exhibited a circular fracture to the right partial bone with a radiating fracture extending to the base of the skull. A large unhealed sawing-type trephination was performed above the trauma suggesting an attempt to treat the child (Ortner, 2003, p. 173). In pre-Columbian Ancon, Peru, a 4- to 5-year-old with artificial cranial modification displayed a depressed penetrating lesion on the occipital bone interpreted as a healed scraped trepanation. This seems

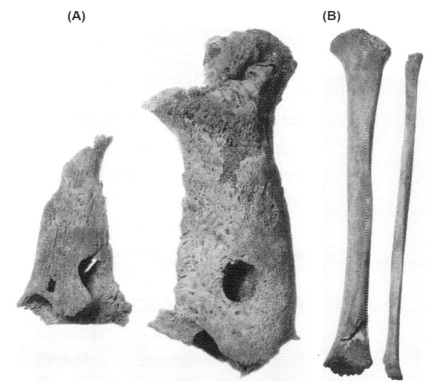

FIGURE 5.34 Lower legs of a 14-year-old from Bow Baptist Church, London (AD 1816–1853; skeleton 281). The right leg (A) was amputated and the remaining tibia and fibula fragments developed osteomyelitis. (B) Shows the unaffected left side. *From Walker, D., 2012. Disease in London, 1st-19th Centuries, Museum of London Archaeology, London, p. 155.*

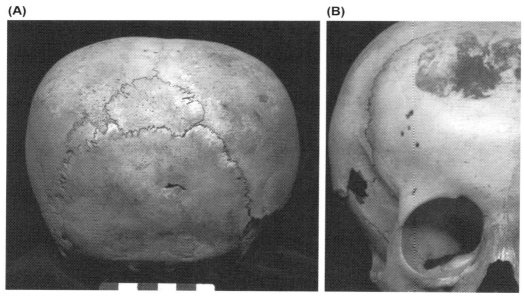

FIGURE 5.35 Skull of a 5-year-old from Ancon, Peru (AD 650–1200, skeleton 56) with a healing scraped trepanation on the (A) right aspect of the occipital bone and (B) perimortem drill holes on the right frontal bone. *From Kato, K., Shinoda, K., Kitagawa, Y., Manabe, Y., Oyamada, J., Igawa, K., Vidal, H., Rokutanda, A., 2007. A possible case of prophylactic supra-inion trepanation in a child cranium with an auditory deformity (pre-Columbian Ancon site, Peru). Anthropological Science 115, 229.*

to have been followed years later by five small perimortem drill holes on the right aspect of the frontal bone (Fig. 5.35). On the same side, the child has a restricted external auditory canal suggesting congenital atresia that may have led them to be deaf, hard of hearing or showing deformities of the external ear (Kato et al., 2007).

Elsewhere, Mogle and Zias (1995) suggest a partial scraped trephination was carried out on an 8- to

9-year-old from Israel dating to 2200 BC. It is suggested the procedure was an attempt to treat severe subperiosteal hemorrhaging as the result of scurvy. The lesion is located at the bregma but does not penetrate the inner surface of the skull, suggesting the target lesion was ectocranial. While a hemorrhaging lesion due to scurvy may explain the intervention, none of the signature signs of scurvy were identified, but the child was unusually edentulous. Possible hydrocephalus was suggested as the reason for a trepanation of the right frontal bone in a 5- to 6-year-old from Fidenae in Rome (Mariani-Costanitini et al., 2000). The profile of the opening (sloping inward) indicates a chisel was used to carefully remove a roundel of bone without damaging the meninges. Pitting at the margins suggest the child survived for a few days after the procedure. Both studies highlight the more hazardous nature of carrying out a trephination on a child. Mogle and Zias (1995) suggest the location at the bregma in their child was particularly complex, as the sutures were unfused and the three cranial plates prone to movement, while Mariani-Costanitini et al. (2000) argue the choice of gouging was following Galen who stated cutting rather than drilling was the safest method in cases where the skull bones are thin, as in their child. A further trepanation was discovered on an isolated child cranium from Neolithic Prague in the Czech Republic (Smrčka et al., 1998). A large unhealed trepanation is present on the left side of the skull crossing the parietal and occipital bones. It appears to have been made to remove a roundel of bone. This 4- to 5-year-old also had a lytic defect on the right parietal bone, which appears to be a second attempt at trephination although a neoplasm was not ruled out. An 8- to 9-year-old from Late Antique Period Shirakavan (1st century BC to 3rd century AD) in Armenia had a drilled trepanation resulting in a funnel-shaped lesion on their right parietal, although no reason for the procedure was evident, and the lack of healing suggests this may have been a postmortem ritual practice (Khudaverdyan, 2011). Finally, five cases of trepanations in children from the Avar period (AD 568–811) in Hungary have been identified, one of which was connected to a head injury and the youngest was aged around 3 years. Evidence suggests the practice spanned the transition between the Avar and Hungarian conquests in the region (László, 2016).

THEMES IN THE STUDY OF CHILD TRAUMA

As Pérez (2012, p. 14) states: "violent acts often exemplify intricate social and cultural dimensions and are frequently themselves defined by these same social contexts" and therefore, violence should never be reduced to an analysis of the trauma itself, but interpreted within its cultural and social context. Children were often victims or participants of violence in the past; violence resulting from climate change and pressure for resources, sporting contests, domestic abuse, veneration of the dead, warfare, and raids (Lewis, 2014; Mays, 2014). Mays (2014) considers that a child's special status as a liminal member of society may act to both spare them and make them susceptible to violence. Being outside politics and feuds that dominate violence in war may protect them from victimization, while their very status as liminal beings may single them out for sacrifice. When examining the nature and meaning of trauma in a nonadult sample, Gaither (2012) called for three types of violence to be considered: violence associated with extreme cultural conflict, culturally sanctioned ritual violence, and likely caregiver-induced violence. This clarification of terminology provides a useful basis for our understanding of a child's involvement with violence in the past. It is useful also to consider patterns of trauma that indicate activity-induced injuries as the result of play or through work. This adds another dimension to our study of trauma and reminds us that young people also had an active role to play in the past, rather than seeing them as merely passive victims of violence.

Violence Associated With Extreme Cultural Conflict

Infants and children have been recovered from mass graves in Paleolithic Sudan, Mesolithic Bavaria, and Neolithic Germany (Whittle, 1996, p. 170; Thorpe, 2003; Wahl and Trautmann, 2012). There is also a link between the proportion of women and the proportion of children in these graves, suggesting that in prehistoric conflicts, where the women were killed, the children were too (Mays, 2014). While Novak and Kopp's (2003) analysis of the 19th century massacre at Mountain Meadows Utah indicates that children under 8-year-old were mostly unharmed by their attackers, cranial trauma in the Chanka group in Andahuaylas, Peru (AD 600–1400), showed that children with skull modifications were targeted, suggesting genocide of a single cultural group (Kurin, 2012). Numerous examples of embedded projectiles, perimortem injuries, and evidence of scalping in children as young as 4 years suggest they were not spared during violent raids on their settlement, or during civil war and were also taken as captives (Fig. 5.36). This appears to have been a global and multiperiod phenomenon (Brødholt and Holck, 2012; Ferllini, 2014; Kjellström, 2014; Lambert, 2014; Meyer et al., 2009; Pfeiffer and Van der Merwe, 2004; Schug et al., 2012; Šlaus et al., 2010b; Smith, 2003; Standen and Arriaza, 2000; Tung and Knudson, 2010). A 13-year-old male with chipped teeth and perimortem depressed cranial fractures from a pit in Chalcolithic Israel (4500–3200 BC) is suggestive of face-to-face combat and indicates the minimum age at which males may have became warriors in this society (Dawson et al., 2003). In contrast to the prehistoric periods, Mays' (2014) review of historic periods revealed that only adolescents were included in war graves, while noncombatants were, perhaps, spared.

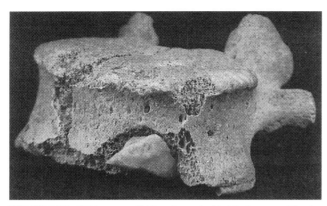

FIGURE 5.36 White quartz lithic point embedded in the second lumbar vertebra of a 16- to 17-year-old from Maderas Enco, Chinchorro, Chile (4000 BP, skeleton C1). *From Standen, V., Arriaza, B., 2000. Trauma in the Preceramic coastal populations of Northern Chile: violence or occupational hazards? American Journal of Physical Anthropology 112, 242.*

In her study of 215 nonadults from Neolithic Europe, Fibiger (2014) identified 13 head injuries (6%), which peaked in the 8- to 12-year-olds who showed both multiple and single wounds. The top of the head was the most common location for an injury, suggesting the assailant was taller or at least elevated above the victim. The cases of child head trauma were recovered from mass graves within settlements rather than regular cemetery contexts, suggesting that their deaths occurred during particular violent events. Fibiger (2014) surmises that children were considered easy targets because, not only would they be a significant loss to the village, they could also not be allowed to live to reap their revenge when they were older. An assessment of the age at which trauma patterns change in nonadults from any given group may help elucidate the age at which children changed from being victims to participants in violence in the past.

Culturally Sanctioned Ritual Violence

Veneration of the dead is complex and includes honoring certain deceased community members, or aiding the soul in its journey through the afterlife. Interpreting veneration is difficult as practices vary and often include acts of violence (Anderson, 2012). Remains of sacrificial victims may be dismembered, dispersed, or burned making their identification challenging. While any member of a community may be sacrificed, children were often selected for a belief in their liminal status or purity, meaning they were often considered the most effective mediators between humans and deities (Ardren, 2011; Ceruti, 2015). Klaus (2014) offers several examples from the Lambayeque Valley in Peru where children and adolescents were among victims of sacrificial offerings, dispatched through decapitations, throat slitting, and chest opening.

In Argentina, once the southern province of the Inca Empire, the *capacocha* ceremony (15th–16th century AD) involved the sacrifice of the young offspring of nobles to the sun and other Inca deities. Child sacrifices were made for many reasons; to celebrate a new ruler, in response to a natural disaster, as fertility and health offerings, or to consecrate special construction projects (Ceruti, 2015). They were sacrificed on mountaintops with the minimum of trauma (by a blow to the head, buried alive, or asphyxiated) to ensure nothing incomplete was dedicated to the gods (Ceruti, 2004, 2015). Isotopic evidence suggests the children came from across the Inca Empire, and that they were elevated in social status, fed a specialized diet, and prepared for their high-altitude pilgrimage with drugs (Andrushko et al., 2011; Wilson et al., 2007). Crandall and Thompson (2014) analyzed sacrificial victims from La Cueve de Los Muertos Chiquitos, Durango, Mexico, dating between AD 571 and 1168. In addition to the religious and cultural systems that dictated the practice, they examined the bodies of the children themselves, considering their age, the presence of disease, and exploring ideas of personhood and liminality. Of the 31 individuals identified at the site, 81% (n = 25) were infants and children and the majority were below 6 months of age. Intriguingly, it appeared that the youngest individuals who had signs of scurvy were afforded more elaborate burials than those without a visible pathology. The authors hypothesize that these children were already ill, and were selected as they were perceived as closer to the afterlife than their healthy peers. Early signs of scurvy indicates that they were fed a specialized diet in preparation for their death, just as with the Inca children. Or, taking a more functional approach, perhaps adults were more willing to sacrifice the sickest portion of their community, who may die anyway, over the more healthy babies (Crandall and Thompson, 2014). Tung and Knudson's (2010) analysis of seven nonadult crania recovered from the Wari Era site of Conchopata (AD 600–1000) in Peru identified perimortem holes at bregma as well as in the ascending rami of the mandible, and cut marks to the phalanges. They suggest that, similar to the adults, the heads and fingers of these children were used as trophies, perhaps after a sacrifice. The children were aged between 3 and 8 years, suggestive of an age at which their identity changed from child to adult in the minds of the Wari.

The majority of evidence for child sacrifice comes from Central and South America, but whether the European tophet infant burials of Carthage were the result of sacrifice remains a matter of debate (Schwartz et al., 2010; Smith et al., 2011). European Iron Age bog bodies are seen to represent sacrificial victims and 10% of these were children (Mays, 2014). Mays (2014) cites an 8- to 9-year-old boy dating to the 348–311 BC who was tied up and stabbed in the neck before being deposited in the peat bog. Wall et al. (1986) reported on a remarkable series of disarticulated remains of at least five children excavated from the basement rooms of a house in Knossos with cut marks on 35.7% of the bones. The distribution of the remains indicated that the bodies were already decomposing when they were thrown into the basement. Elsewhere on the site, a child's remains were recovered from a drain. Wall et al. (1986) suggested that the site was used as a ritual area where children were killed and dismembered. Palkovitch (2012) provides one possible interpretation for the similar discovery of three mutilated bodies of children aged between 3 and 4 years in a rubbish filled room from 14th century Arroyo Hondo, Rio Grande, New Mexico. She suggests they may have been considered a threat to the community who clubbed them and broke their teeth to damage their bodies so they could not be taken over by evil spirits or witches. As children under 6 years they would have been perceived as vulnerable liminal beings in Puebloan cosmology and still linked to the underworld.

Caregiver-Induced Violence and Neglect

Clearly violence toward children was a sanctioned part of life in some past communities; often forming part of the matrix of a society, with children also considered legitimate targets during conflict. Identifying physical abuse meted out on a single individual by a caregiver provides greater challenges. Often lesions associated with abuse are perimortem and may be difficult to identify in the thin crania and small bones of infants, and a series of lesions are required to make a definitive diagnosis. The limited evidence for abuse in past populations may suggest that this is a practice particular to modern societies (Walker, 1997), but the situation is likely to be more complex. It is possible that the paucity of evidence is the result of victims being disposed of in clandestine burials rather than cemetery sites (Waldron, 2000), or that the practice of swaddling by many societies caused a different pattern of injuries than we would expect from modern forensic cases (De Mause, 1974; Knight, 1986). Today, physical child abuse tends to occur close to home, with the majority of deaths in boys under 3 years of age as victims of violence from their mother, taking the form of blunt and sharp force injuries (Schmidt et al., 1996). This is not necessarily the pattern we should expect to see in the past. Walker (1997) argues that different social circumstances may mean that older children, rather than infants were most susceptible to abuse, usually by their employers.

Waldron (2000) identified several references to intentional abuse in children from the historical records, including the comment by Arab Physician Rhazes (AD 854–925) that not all child trauma was accidental; a warning from Soranus (c. AD 98–138) that angry wet-nurses may drop their charges; and an Old Norse children's song from the 17th century that referred to children being struck against a wall if they cried too much. A reassessment of the case of an English mother who lost four children as the result of neonatal convulsions in the 1660s suggests these may have been the earliest recorded cases of whiplash injury (Williams, 2001). Child physical abuse is seen to reflect a high level of stress within the community as the result of overcrowding, poverty, or parental consumption of alcohol, and when the male is the perpetrator, maternal and child abuse coincide (Handwerker, 2001). Illegitimate and disabled children are also at greater risk of attack (Bethea, 1999), while Ross et al. (2009) suggest toddlers may be vulnerable as they become more defiant and self-assertive. The psychological impact of suffering abuse from a caregiver can result in a repeated pattern of abuse through generations (Servaes et al., 2016). All of these factors may have contributed to a pattern of abuse in the past. However, as Gaither (2012) argues, evidence for abuse in the archeological record needs to be considered within each cultural context. For example, Roman society relished violent sports; and this attitude to violence is reflected in their attitudes to child rearing, which commonly involved the use of physical punishment that members of Roman society would not have recognized as "abuse" (Rawson, 2003). In addition, the greater likelihood of childhood infection or metabolic disease in producing periosteal lesions, and potentially lower rates of high impact accidental injuries (due to a lack of automobiles, trampolines, etc.) are likely to alter the significance, frequency, and nature of lesions we may expect to indicate intentional injury in past populations (Gaither, 2012). Stunted growth as the result of chronic malnutrition is another indicator used to identify possible cases of child neglect in clinical contexts (Cardoso and Magalhães, 2011; Wehner et al., 1999). For the paleopathologist, retarded growth is a common expectation in nonadults, particularly those growing up in impoverished or conflict-ridden environments. But it is exactly these environments that provide the circumstances for abuse in modern society. While it may be possible to identify individual children who fall below the average height (or 50th percentile) of other nonadults in the sample, we cannot know that they represent the same generation of children, or be able to eliminate all other underlying conditions that may result in their growth delay.

Nevertheless, forensic anthropology has provided us with a comprehensive series of lesions that may signal physical abuse (Buckley and Whittle, 2008) and these serve as a starting point for any investigation. In particular, multiple fractures at different stages of healing, in combination with subperiosteal new bone formation are considered highly indicative of abuse, especially if the fractures occur in the ribs (Table 5.5). The frequency at which these lesions occur in children who are known to have suffered abuse differs and the mechanism, type, and pattern of trauma needs to be assessed to separate intentional from accidental injury and rule out underling conditions such as osteogenesis imperfecta, rickets, or in the youngest individuals, birth trauma (Carty, 1993; Heldrich, 2011; Servaes et al., 2016). For example, multiple, depressed,

TABLE 5.5 Skeletal Lesions Commonly Associated With Physical Child Abuse

Type of Lesion	Location	Cause	Comments	Sources
Fractures	Ribs	Anterior–posterior compression or direct blunt force trauma	First rib considered most severe and potentially pathognomonic Fracture at costovertebral angle Fracture at costochondral junction Bilateral fractures Callus formation 1–2 weeks posttrauma Multiple stages of healing	Wilber and Thompson (1998), Starling et al. (2002), Kleinman et al. (1995), Carty (1993), and Servaes et al. (2016)
	Long bones (particularly femur, tibia, humerus)	Twisting, pulling, bending, or shearing forces Falling awkwardly Warding off blows Shaking with limbs hanging	More common in children under 3 years Metaphysis affected in 89% cases "bucket-handle" lesions at metaphysis Midshaft fractures Impaction or buckle fractures at the metaphyses (usually distal femur and proximal tibia)	Kleinman et al. (1995), Brogdon (1998), Thomas et al. (1991), and Rao and Carty (1999)
	Cranium	Blunt force trauma	Multiple fractures that cross sutures Bilateral complex fractures Basilar fractures (complex, stellate, depressed) Depressed occipital fractures Fractures of different ages	Wilber and Thompson (1998), Crist et al. (1997), and Rao and Carty (1999)
	Hand and foot phalanges	Twisting, pulling, or compression force Crushing digits	Linear, oblique or spiral fractures May cause bone displacement Suspicious in nonambulatory infants	Brogdon (1998)
	Spine	Hyperflexion and extension of the spine due to violent shaking Lesions of the spine are rare	Usually affects thoracic and lumbar vertebrae Fracture of neurocentral synchondrosis, but trauma to growth plates will be difficult to observe before fusion. Compression fractures Fractured spinous process Fractures and dislocation of the spine may lead to kyphosis	Cullen (1975), Hobbs (1989), Vialle et al. (2006), and Rao and Carty (1999)
	Clavicle	Blunt force trauma, compression, torsion, and bending forces	Usually acromial end oblique, greenstick, or linear fracture	Brogdon (1998), Resnick and Goergen (2002), and Carty (1993)
	Scapula	Blunt force trauma (compression)	Compression fracture to scapula blade Fracture of acromion or coracoid process	Brogdon (1998), Carty (1993), and Servaes et al. (2016)
	Dentition	Fractured or necrosed teeth	But also common as accidental injuries and through play	Abel (2011)
	Innominates	Fractured sacroiliac joint, illum	Rare In severe trauma, unlikely to occur in isolation	Brogdon (1998) and Abel (2011)
New bone formation	Cranium (ecto- and endocranial) Mastoid process, superior manubrium	Blunt force trauma causing subperiosteal bleeding Repetitive trauma Rough handling causing periosteal tearing	May take 10–14 days for subperiosteal new bone to appear	Saternus et al. (2000), Walker (1997), and Hobbs (1989)
	Sternal end of clavicle		Attachment of the sternocleidomastoid	Carty (1993)
	Proximal humerus		Underlying the brachial plexus Diaphyseal lesions usually extend beyond metaphysis Usually bilateral	Carty (1993) and Abel (2011)
	Proximal aspect of linear aspera (femur)		Attachment of gluteus maximus Diaphyseal lesions usually extend beyond metaphysis Usually bilateral	Carty (1993) and Abel (2011)

and bilateral cranial fractures that cross sutures are suggestive of high impact injuries pointing to intentional abuse (Rao and Carty, 1999), whereas accidental cranial injuries tend to be unilateral, linear, and contained within the suture lines (Kahana and Hiss, 1999). Recurring fractures would suggest that the child was exposed to a continuous cycle of abuse (Martin and Harrod, 2015). Long bone shaft fractures are considered indicative of abuse in children less than 18-months-old who are not yet mobile (Brown and Fisher, 2004; Coffey et al., 2005; Strait et al., 1995), and generally present as spiral and metaphyseal fractures of the humerus, femur, and tibia (Brogdon, 1998; Coffey et al., 2005; Resnick and Goergen, 2002). In their study of 215 abused children, Thomas et al. (1991) concluded that any humeral fracture, with the exception of the common supracondylar fractures, were the result of abuse. By contrast, femoral shaft fractures were often caused by a running child tripping and falling and were not indicative of abuse in walking age children (Schwend et al., 2000).

Rib fractures are the most common lesion associated with child abuse in modern cases, especially when they occur in combination with other injuries. In a survey of 165 postcranial fractures from suspected child abuse cases, Kleinman et al. (1995) identified rib fractures in 31 (51%) cases. Posterior rib fractures are considered more indicative of abuse than anterior fractures due to squeezing of the chest, and fractures of the first rib tend to occur at the subclavian groove where it is weakest. The type of fracture (i.e., transverse, buckle, oblique) may also aid in understanding the type of injury sustained, with buckle fractures associated with anterior and posterior compression to the chest (Love and Symes, 2004). Fractures of the first rib and pelvis are seen in the most severe cases (Starling et al., 2002; Wilber and Thompson, 1998) and are caused by compression forces to the chest, violent shaking, or slamming the child down onto a hard surface (Strouse and Owings, 1995; Love et al., 2013). While there are bones that are most commonly affected, it is clear from the clinical literature that almost any bone may be affected in physical abuse.

As early as 1978, Kerley attempted to catalog the pattern of abuse using the forensic evidence from three infants recovered from clandestine graves. In each case, fractures at various stages of healing were evident on the mandibular ramus, clavicle, and ribs with fractures also evident on the radius and ulna of one infant. Blondiaux et al. (2002) were the first to suggest physical abuse in the archeological record, in a 2-year-old from Roman Lisieux-Michelet, France, who had sustained several head injuries and rib fractures in addition to suffering rickets. Since then, several other possible cases have been identified. Wheeler et al. (2007) reported on a 2- to 3-year-old with multiple trauma and widespread subperiosteal reactions from Kellis 2 in the Dakhleh Oasis. The child had fractures to both humeri, clavicles, ribs, and plastic deformation to the right ilium. Given the pattern of trauma with various stages of healing, the authors suggest caregiver induced violence is the most probable cause. Also from the Roman period, Lewis (2010) identified a tibial bucket-handle fracture in an infant from Romano–British Poundbury Camp. While the tibial injury may be a toddler's fracture, at 18 months, this injury would be suspected as nonaccidental in a child of that age today. Gaither (2012) carried out a systematic review of the type of trauma in 242 nonadults from Puruchuco-Huaquerones in Peru, applying modern clinical signatures of intentional injury to see if caregiver-induced violence could be identified. Eleven (4.5%) of the children displayed a series of lesions including fractures to the humerus, femur, spine and ribs, bilateral cranial trauma, and endocranial new bone formation that suggested probable caregiver abuse. Cook et al. (2014) report on a case of probable physical abuse in an older individual, a 14- to 15-year-old female from Hopewell Pete Klunk mound in Midwest America. She had sustained trauma to her face that had left her blind in one eye, before being fatally wounded with a blow to the head some time later. It is unclear whether the long-term abuse was suffered at the hands of the elderly male she was buried with, who may have been her caregiver, or reflected her general low status within the community.

A 1- to 2-year-old child from St Oswald's Priory in Gloucester, England, illustrates the difficulty in interpreting caregiver-induced violence in archeological samples. The child has a partially healed transverse midshaft fracture to the right humerus (Fig. 5.37). Diaphyseal fractures of the humerus are considered particularly suspicious of abuse cases in modern contexts (Thomas et al., 1991), and the child is also the only one in the nonadult sample (n=144) with active rickets (Lewis, 2013). Shaft fractures associated with rickets are rarely reported in the paleopathological literature but are recognized in clinical practice in advanced cases, although they tend to occur in the lower arm (Servaes et al., 2016). It is possible that the child was crawling and could have fallen resulting in an accidental injury, but individuals suffering from rickets are often less mobile. While it is possible rickets weakened the bone resulting in a fracture, the presence of this disease in a single child may also signal ongoing neglect. On balance, the absence of any other fractures, for example, of the ribs (the lower skeleton was not preserved), means that no firm conclusions can be drawn.

Activity-Induced Injuries

Evidence for the impact of physical labor and other activities on the skeleton of a developing child is a recent theme in nonadult trauma studies. Osteochondritis dissecans was identified in a 12-year-old from 11th to 12th century Giecz in Poland, as was a compression fracture of the spine of a

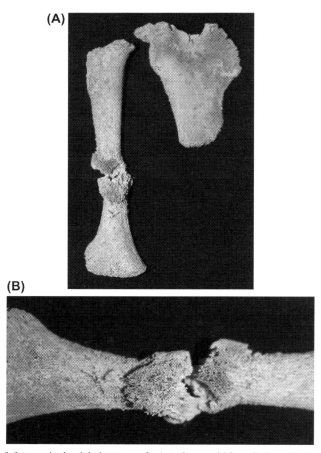

FIGURE 5.37 (A) Transverse midshaft fracture in the right humerus of a 1- to 2-year-old from St Oswald's Priory in Gloucester, England (AD 1120–1230, skeleton 376). The child also displayed evidence for rickets. (B) Note the fiber bone fracture callus indicating the injury was sustained shortly before the child died.

16- to 18-year-old. Both were considered to be the result of activity. Jimenez-Brobeil et al. (2007) noted numerous fractures in children living in the mountainous region of Bronze Age Iberia with fractured clavicles and humeri that were considered the result of falls in the rugged terrain. The children were aged between 3 and 8 years, and it was suggested these represented summer accidents when children were more likely to stray from home and spend more time outside exploring their environment. A similar rugged terrain was considered the cause of a fractured arm in an 8-year-old from Semna in the Sudan, perhaps while carrying water back to the settlement. A fractured skull in a child from the same site was interpreted as the result of a slingshot injury in a playing accident (Alvrus, 1999). Klaus (2012) suggests early cases of degenerative joint disease in children serve as examples of structural violence where children were exploited as laborers. The high occurrence of injuries to the spine and joints (i.e., spondylolysis, JOCD, degenerative changes, compression fractures) in individuals aged between 10 and 17 years, particularly from urban sites served to illustrate the affect of strenuous activity on the developing bodies of adolescents from medieval England (Lewis, 2016).

Structural Violence

Another recent area in the study of trauma in past populations is the existence of "structural violence." This describes where unequal power, restricted access to resources, and systematic oppression meted out through the denial of needs is reflected and sustained through culturally sanctioned violence (Galtung, 1969; Martin and Harrod, 2015). This often subtle form of oppression is multigenerational and normalized by those who experience and exert it (Farmer, 2004; Klaus, 2012). Klaus (2012) emphasizes the special role children play in the interpretation of structural violence. For example, fetal health may be affected through the stresses experienced by their mother, and infection and malnutrition in the child, while not direct evidence for trauma, provide a multigenerational experience of structural violence when coupled with markers of childhood stress in the adults. Tung (2016) examined patterns of violence and the diet of children living in the tumultuous Late Intermediate Period (AD 1000–1400) of the post-Wari Peruvian Andes. They demonstrated a sharp rise in violent cranial trauma in children under 12 years in the post-Wari period, suggesting that they were singled out for lethal violence in community raids, perhaps systematically. Isotopic evidence signalled a decrease in maize consumption in the children and indicated that competition for dwindling resources as the result of drought may have caused the rise in conflict and denial of resources for some members of the community. Following the Spanish conquest of the Inca Empire in AD 1532, Gaither and Murphy (2012) demonstrated a rise in fatal head injuries in the nonadults from Puruchuco-Huaquerones, Peru, immediately after the invasion. They argue that the inability of the community to shield their children from violence underlines how profoundly the Spanish conquest affected the social fabric of the indigenous community. When exploring structural violence in the past, Martin and Harrod (2015) emphasize the need to look beyond simply describing trauma in the skeletal sample, advocating a multifaceted approach that combines archeological, paleopathological, and ethnohistorical evidence.

REFERENCES

Abel, S., 2011. Non-accidental injury. In: Ross, A., Abel, S. (Eds.), The Juvenile Skeleton in Forensic Abuse Investigations. Humana Press, New York, pp. 61–77.

Adams, J., Hamblen, D., 1991. Outline of Fractures. Churchill-Livingstone, London.

Adler, J., Patterson, R., 1967. Erb's palsy. Long-term results of treatment in eighty-eight cases. Journal of Bone and Joint Surgery. American Volume 49 (6), 1052–1064.

Agran, P., Winn, D., Anderson, C., Trent, R., Walton-Haynes, L., Thayer, S., 2003. Rates of pediatric injuries by 3-month intervals in children 0 to 3 years of age. Pediatrics 111 (6), 683–692.

Ahn, E., Jung, M., Lee, Y., Ko, S., Shin, S., Hahn, M., 2015. Neonatal clavicular fracture: recent 10 year study. Pediatrics International 57 (1), 60–63.

Allman, F., 1967. Fractures and ligamentous injuries of the clavicle and its articulation. Journal of Bone and Joint Surgery. American Volume 49 (4), 774–784.

Almeida, A., Roberts, I., 2005. Bone involvement in sickle cell disease. British Journal of Haematology 129 (4), 482–490.

Alvrus, A., 1999. Fracture patterns among the Nubians of Semna South, Sudanese Nubia. International Journal of Osteoarchaeology 9, 417–429.

Anderson, C., 2012. Victims of violence? A methodological case study from precolonial Northern Mexico. In: Martin, D., Anderson, C. (Eds.), Bioarchaeological and Forensic Perpsectives on Violence. Cambridge University Press, Cambridge, pp. 83–100.

Andrushko, V., Buzon, M., Gibaja, A., McEwan, G., Simonetti, A., Creaser, R., 2011. Investigating a child sacrifice event from the Inca heartland. Journal of Archaeological Science 38, 323–333.

Ardren, T., 2011. Empowered children in classic Maya sacrificial rites. Childhood in the Past 4, 133–145.

Arnott, R., Finger, S., Smith, C., 2005. Trepanation. CRC Press, New York.

Aufderheide, A.C., Rodriguez-Martín, C., 1998. The Cambridge Encyclopedia of Human Paleopathology. Cambridge University Press, Cambridge.

Balboni, T., Gobezie, R., Mamon, H., 2006. Heterotopic ossification: pathophysiology, clinical features, and the role of radiotherapy for prophylaxis. International Journal of Radiation Oncology, Biology and Physics 65 (5), 1289–1299.

Barber, C., 1930. The detailed changes characteristic of healing bone in amputation stumps. Journal of Bone and Joint Surgery 12 (2), 353–359.

Baxarias, J., Fontaine, V., Garcia-Guixé, E., Dinarés, R., 2010. Perinatal cranial fracture in a second century BC case from Ilturo (Cabrera de Mar, Barcelona, Spain). In: XVIII European Meeting of the Paleopathology Association, p. 22 Vienna, Austria.

Bethea, L., 1999. Primary prevention of child abuse. American Family Physician 59 (6), 1577–1597.

Blasier, R., Hughes, L., 2001. Fractures and traumatic dislocations of the hip in children. In: Beaty, J., Kasser, J. (Eds.), Rockwood and Wilkins' Fractures in Children, fifth ed. Lipencott Williams and Wilkins, Philadelphia, pp. 913–939.

Blondiaux, G., Blondiaux, J., Secousse, F., Cotten, A., Danze, P.-M., Flipo, R.-M., 2002. Rickets and child abuse: the case of a two year old girl from the 4th century in Lisieux (Normandy). International Journal of Osteoarchaeology 12 (3), 209–215.

Blondiaux, J., Millot, F., 1991. Dislocation of the hip: discussion of eleven cases from Mediaeval France. International Journal of Osteoarchaeology 1 (3–4), 203–207.

Borden, S., 1974. Traumatic bowing of the forearm in children. Journal of Bone and Joint Surgery. American Volume 56 (3), 611–616.

Borden, S., 1975. Roentgen recognition of acute plastic bowing of the forearm in children. American Journal of Roentgenology 125 (3), 524–530.

Brickley, M., 2006a. The people: physical anthropology. In: Brickley, M., Buteux, S., Adams, J., Cherrington, R. (Eds.), St Martin's Uncovered: Investigations in the Churchyard of St Martin's-in-the-Bull Ring, Birmingham, 2001. Oxbow Books, Oxford, pp. 90–151.

Brickley, M., 2006b. Rib fractures in the archaeological record: a useful source of sociocultural information? International Journal of Osteoarchaeology 16, 61–75.

Brill, P.W., Winchester, P., 1987. Differential diagnosis of child abuse. In: Kleinmann, P. (Ed.), Diagnostic Imaging of Child Abuse. Williams and Wilkins, Baltimore, pp. 221–241.

Brødholt, E., Holck, P., 2012. Skeletal trauma in the burials from the royal Church of St. Mary in medieval Oslo. International Journal of Osteoarchaeology 22 (2), 201–218.

Brogdon, B., 1998. Child abuse. In: Brogdon, B. (Ed.), Forensic Radiology. CRC Press, New York, pp. 281–314.

Brothwell, D., Powers, R., 2000. The human biology. In: Rathtz, P., Hirst, S., Wright, S. (Eds.), Cannington Cemetery. English Heritage, London.

Brown, D., Fisher, E., 2004. Femur fractures in infants and young children. American Journal of Public Health 94 (4), 558–560.

Buckley, H., Whittle, K., 2008. Identifying child abuse in skeletonised subadult remains. In: Oxenham, M. (Ed.), Forensic Approaches to Death, Disaster and Abuse. Australian Academic Press, Brisbane, pp. 123–132.

Caffey, J., 1945. Pediatric X-Ray Diagnosis. Year Book Medical Publishers, Inc., Chicago.

Cahill, B., 1995. Osteochondritis dissecans of the knee: treatment of juvenile and adult forms. Journal of the American Academy of Orthopaedic Surgeons 3 (4), 237–247.

Capasso, L., Sciubba, M., Hua, Q., Levchenko, V., Viciano, J., D'Anastasio, R., Bretuch, F., 2016. Embryotomy in the 19th century of central Italy. International Journal of Osteoarchaeology 26 (2), 345–347.

Cardoso, H., Magalhães, T., 2011. Evidence of neglect from immature human skeletal remains: an auxological approach from bones and teeth. In: Ross, A., Abel, S. (Eds.), The Juvenile Skeleton in Forensic Abuse Investigations. Humana Press, New York, pp. 125–150.

Carty, H., 1993. Fractures caused by child abuse. Journal of Bone and Joint Surgery. British Volume 75, 849–857.

Ceruti, C., 2004. Human bodies as objects of dedication at Inca mountain shrines (north-western Argentina). World Archaeology 36 (1), 103–122.

Ceruti, M., 2015. Frozen mummies from Andean mountaintop shrines: bioarchaeology and ethnohistory of Inca human sacrifice. BioMed Research International:439428. http://dx.doi.org/10.1155/2015/439428.

Chen, H., Yang, J., Chuang, S., Huang, C., S Y, 2009. Heterotopic ossification in burns: our experience and literature reviews. Burns 35 (6), 857–862.

Cheng, J., Shen, W., 1993. Limb fracture pattern in different pediatric age groups: a study of 3,350 children. Journal of Orthopaedic Trauma 7 (1), 15–22.

Cheng, J., Ying, S., Lam, P., 1999. A 10-year study of the changes in the pattern and treatment of 6,493 fractures. Journal of Pediatric Orthopedics 19, 344–350.

Clement, D., Colton, C., 1986. Overgrowth of the femur after fracture in childhood. The Journal of Bone and Joint Surgery. British Volume 68 (4), 534–536.

Clough, S., Boyle, A., 2010. Inhumations and disarticulated human bone. In: Booth, P., Simmonds, S., Boyle, A., Clough, S., Cool, H., Poore, D. (Eds.), The Late Roman Cemetery at Lankhills, Winchester Excavations 2000-2005. Oxford Archaeology Ltd., Oxford, pp. 339–403.

Coffey, C., Haley, K., Hayes, J.T., Groner, J., 2005. The risk of child abuse in infants and toddlers with lower extremity injuries. Journal of Pediatric Surgery 40, 120–123.

Connell, B., Gray Jones, A., Redfern, R., Walker, D., 2012. A Bioarchaeological Study of Medieval Burials on the Site of St Mary Spital. Museum of London Archaeology, London.

Cook, D., Thompson, A., Rollins, A., 2014. Death and the special child: three examples from the ancient midwest. In: Thompson, J., Alfonso-Durruty, M., Crandall, J. (Eds.), Tracing Childhood Bioarchaeological Investigations of Early Lives in Antiquity. University of Florida Press, Gainesville, pp. 17–35.

Cooper, C., Dennison, E.M., Leufkens, H.G., Bishop, N., van Staa, T.P., 2004. Epidemiology of childhood fractures in Britain: a study using the general practice research database. Journal of Bone and Mineral Research 19 (12), 1976–1981.

Coqueugniot, H., Dutour, O., Arensburg, B., Duday, H., Vandermeersch, B., Tillier, A.-M., 2012. Earliest cranio-encephalic trauma from the Levantine Middle Palaeolithic: 3D reappraisal of the Qafzeh 11 skull, consequences of pediatric brain damage on individual life condition and social care. PLoS One 9 (7), e102822.

Cory, C., Jones, M., James, D., Leadbeatter, S., Nokes, L., 2001. The potential and limitations of utilising head impact injury models to assess likelihood of significant head injury in infants after a fall. Forensic Science International 123, 89–106.

Crandall, J., Thompson, J., 2014. Exploring the identity of sacrificed infants and children at la Cueva de Los Muertos Chiquitos, Durango, Mexico (AD 571-1168). In: Thompson, J., Alfonso-Durruty, M., Crandall, J. (Eds.), Tracing Childhood Bioarchaeological Investigations of Early Lives in Antiquity. University of Florida Press, Gainesville, pp. 36–57.

Crawford, C.H., Ledonio, C.G., Bess, R.S., Buchowski, J.M., Burton, D.C., Hu, S.S., Lonner, B.S., Polly, D.W., Smith, J.S., Sanders, J.O., 2015. Current evidence regarding the etiology, prevalence, natural history, and prognosis of pediatric lumbar spondylolysis: a report from the scoliosis research society evidence-based medicine committee. Spine Deformity 3 (1), 12–29.

Crist, T.A., Washburn, A., Park, H., Hood, I., Hickey, M., 1997. Cranial bone displacement as a taphonomic process in potential child abuse cases. In: Haglund, W., Sorg, M. (Eds.), Forensic Taphonomy: The Postmortem Fate of Human Remains. CRC Press, New York, pp. 319–336.

Cullen, J.C., 1975. Spinal lesions of battered babies. Journal of Bone and Joint Surgery. British Volume 57 (3), 364–366.

Currey, J., Butler, G., 1975. The mechanical properties of bone tissue in children. The Journal of Bone and Joint Surgery. American Volume 57 (6), 810–814.

Davis, P., Rowland, H., 1965. Vertebral fractures in west Africans suffering from tetanus. A clinical and osteological study. Journal of Bone & Joint Surgery, British Volume 47 (1), 61–71.

Dawson, L., Levy, T., Smith, P., 2003. Evidence of interpersonal violence at the Chalcolithic village of Shiqmim (Israel). International Journal of Osteoarchaeology 13, 115–119.

De Boer, H., Van Der Merwe, A., Hammer, S., Steyn, M., Maat, G., 25 (1), 2015. Assessing post-traumatic time interval in human dry bone. International Journal of Osteoarchaeology 98–109.

DeLee, J., Wilkins, K., Rogers, L., Rockwood, C., 1980. Fracture-separation of the distal humeral epiphysis. Journal of Bone and Joint Surgery. American Volume 62 (1), 46–51.

De Mause, L., 1974. The History of Childhood. The Psychohistory Press, New York.

Dedick, A., Caffey, J., 1953. Roentgen findings in the skull and chest in 1,030 newborn infants. Radiology 61, 13–20.

Dittmar, J., Mitchell, P., 2015. A new method for identifying and differentiating human dissection and autopsy in archaeological human skeletal remains. Journal of Archaeological Science Reports 3, 73–79.

Divecha, H., Desai, N., Sheikh, M., Sochart, D., 2012. Traumatic anterior hip dislocation in an adolescent with an associated femoral head "Hill-Sachs" type lesion. Journal of Trauma and Treatment 12, 114–115.

Eccles, A., 1977. Obstetrics in the 17th and 18th centuries and its implications for maternal and infant mortality. Bulletin for the Society of the Social History of Medicine 20, 8–11.

Eccles, A., 1982. Obstetrics and Gynaecology in Tudor and Stuart England. Croom Helm, London.

Ellefsen, B., Frierson, M., Raney, E., Ogden, J., 1994. Humerus varus: a complication of neonatal, infantile and childhood injury and infection. Journal of Pediatric Orthopedics 14, 479–486.

Farmer, P., 2004. An anthropology of structural violence. Current Anthropology 45 (3), 305–325.

Ferllini, R., 2014. Recent conflicts, deaths and simple technologies. The Rwandan case. In: Knusel, C., Smith, M. (Eds.), The Routledge Handbook of the Bioarchaeology of Human Conflict. Routledge, London, pp. 641–655.

Ferrar, L., Jiang, G., Adams, J., Eastell, R., 2005. Identification of vertebral fractures: an update. Osteoporosis International 16 (7), 717–728.

Fibiger, L., 2014. Misplaced childhood; interpersonal violence and children in Neolithic Europe. In: Knusel, C., Smith, M. (Eds.), The Routledge Handbook of the Bioarchaeology of Human Conflict. Routledge, London, pp. 127–145.

Fibiger, L., Knusel, C., 2005. Prevalence rates of spondylolysis in British skeletal populations. International Journal of Osteoarchaeology 15, 164–174.

Fiddian, N., Grace, D., 1983. Traumatic dislocation of the hip in adolescence with separation of the capital epiphysis. Journal of Bone and Joint Surgery. British Volume 65 (2), 148–149.

Firl, M., Wunsch, L., 2004. Measurement of bowing of the radius. Journal of Bone and Joint Surgery. British Volume 86 (7), 1047–1049.

Fredrickson, B., Baker, D., McHolick, W., Lubicky, J., 1984. The natural history of spondylolysis and spondylolisthesis. Journal of Bone and Joint Surgery. American Volume 66 (5), 699–707.

Gaither, C., 2012. Cultural conflict and the impact on non-adults at Puruchuco-Huaquerones in Peru: the case for refinement of the methods used to analyse violence against children in the archeological record. International Journal of Paleopathology 2, 69–77.

Gaither, C., Murphy, M., 2012. Consequences of conquest? The analysis and interpretation of subadult trauma at Puruchuco-Huaquerones, Peru. Journal of Archaeological Science 39, 467–478.

Galtung, J., 1969. Violence, peace, and peace research. Journal of Peace Research 6 (3), 167–191.

Gasco, J., De Pablos, J., 1997. Bone remodeling in malunited fractures in children. Is it reliable? Journal of Pediatric Orthopaedics B 6 (2), 126–132.

Gaur, A., Sinclair, M., Caruso, E., Perettii, G., Zaleske, D., 2003. Heterotopic ossification around the elbow following burns in children: results after excision. Journal of Bone and Joint Surgery 85 (8), 1538–1543.

Genant, H.K., Wu, C.Y., van Kuijk, C., Nevitt, M.C., 1993. Vertebral fracture assessment using a semiquantitative technique. Journal of Bone and Mineral Research 8 (9), 1137–1148.

Ghalib, D., 1999. Subadult health in a northeastern Arkansas middle Mississipian site. The Arkansas Archaeologist 38, 69–99.

Glass, R., Norton, K., Mitre, S., Kang, E., 2002. Pediatric ribs: a spectrum of abnormalities. Radiographics 22, 87–104.

Glencross, B., 2011. Skeletal injury across the life course: towards understanding social agency. In: Agarwal, S., Glencross, B. (Eds.), Social Bioarchaeology. Wiley-Blackwell, Chichester, pp. 390–409.

Glencross, B., Stuart-Macadam, P., 2000. Childhood trauma in the archaeological record. International Journal of Osteoarchaeology 10, 198–209.

Glencross, B., Stuart-Macadam, P., 2001. Radiographic clues to fractures of distal humerus in archaeological remains. International Journal of Osteoarchaeology 11, 298–310.

Gordon, E., 1986. Child health in the middle ages as seen in the miracles of five English saints, AD 1150-1220. Bulletin of the History of Medicine 60, 502–522.

Gordon, E., 1991. Accidents among medieval children as seen from the miracles of six English saints and martyrs. Medical History 35, 145–163.

Greiff, J., Bergmann, F., 1980. Growth disturbance following fracture of the tibia in children. Acta Orthopaedica Scandinavica 51 (1–6), 315–320.

Gresham, E., 1975. Birth trauma. Pediatric Clinics of North America 22 (2), 317–328.

Handwerker, W.P., 2001. Child abuse and the balance of power in parental relationships: an evolved domain-independent mental mechanism that accounts for behavioral variation. American Journal of Human Biology 13, 679–689.

Hariga, H., Mousny, M., Docquier, P.-L., 2011. Leg length discrepancy following femoral shaft fracture in children: clinical considerations and recommendations. Acta Orthopaedica Belgica 77 (6), 782.

Harvig, L., Kveiborg, J., Lynnerup, N., 2015. Death in flames: human remains from a domestic house fire from early Iron Age, Denmark. International Journal of Osteoarchaeology 25, 701–710.

Heinrich, S., 2001. Fractures of the shaft of the tibia and fibula. In: Beaty, J., Kasser, J. (Eds.), Rockwood and Wilkins' Fractures in Children, fifth ed. Lipencott Williams and Wilkins, Philadelphia, pp. 1077–1120.

Heldrich, C., 2011. Birth trauma. In: Ross, A., Abel, S. (Eds.), The Juvenile Skeleton in Forensic Abuse Investigations. Humana Press, New York, pp. 49–60.

Hendrick, E., Harwood-Hash, D., Hudson, A., 1964. Head injuries in children: a survey of 4465 consecutive cases at the hospital for sick children, Toronto, Canada. Clinical Neurosurgery 11, 46–65.

Hensinger, R., 1998. Complications of fractures in children. In: Green, N., Swiontkowski, M. (Eds.), Skeletal Trauma in Children. WB Saunders Company, Philadelphia, pp. 121–147.

Hobbs, C., 1989. ABC of child abuse: fractures. British Medical Journal 298, 1015–1018.

Holst, M., 2004. Osteological Analysis. Bempton Lane, Bridlington (Unpublished Report). York Osteoarchaeology Ltd.

Jimenez-Brobeil, S., Oumaoui, I., Du Souich, P., 2007. Childhood trauma in several populations from the Iberian Peninsula. International Journal of Osteoarchaeology 17 (2), 189–198.

John, S., Moorthy, C., Swischuk, L., 1997. Expanding the concept of the toddler's fracture. Radiographics 17 (2), 367–376.

Johnston, E., Foster, B., 2001. The biologic aspects of children's fractures. In: Beaty, J., Kasser, J. (Eds.), Rockwood and Wilkins' Fractures in Children. Lipencott Williams and Wilkins, Philadelphia, pp. 21–48.

Jordana, X., Galtés, I., Busquets, F., Isidro, A., Malgosa, A., 2006. Clay-shoveler's fracture: an uncommon diagnosis in palaeopathology. International Journal of Osteoarchaeology 16 (4), 366–372.

Kacki, S., Duneufjardin, P., Blanchard, P., Castex, D., 2013. Humerus varus in a subadult skeleton from the medieval graveyard of La Madeleine (Orléans, France). International Journal of Osteoarchaeology 23 (1), 119–126.

Kahana, T., Hiss, J., 1999. Forensic radiology. The British Journal of Radiology 72, 129–133.

Kaloostian, P., Kim, J., Calabresi, P., Bydon, A., Witham, T., 2013. Clay-Shoveler's fracture during indoor climbing. Orthopedics 36 (3), 381–383.

Kato, K., Shinoda, K., Kitagawa, Y., Manabe, Y., Oyamada, J., Igawa, K., Vidal, H., Rokutanda, A., 2007. A possible case of prophylactic supra-inion trepanation in a child cranium with an auditory deformity (pre-Columbian Ancon site, Peru). Anthropological Science 115, 227–232.

Kerley, E., 1978. The identification of battered-infant skeletons. Journal of Forensic Sciences 23, 163–168.

Kessler, J., Nikizad, H., Shea, K., Jacobs, J., Bebchuk, J., Weiss, J., 2014. The demographics and epidemiology of osteochondritis dissecans of the knee in children and adolescents. The American Journal of Sports Medicine 42 (2), 320–326.

Khudaverdyan, A., 2011. Trepanation and artificial cranial deformations in ancient Armenia. Anthropological Review 74, 39–55.

Kjellström, A., 2014. Interpreting violence: a bioarchaeological perspective of violence from medieval central Sweden. In: Knusel, C., Smith, M. (Eds.), The Routledge Handbook of the Bioarchaeology of Human Conflict. Routledge, London, pp. 237–250.

Klaus, H., 2012. The bioarchaeology of structural violence: a theoretical model and case study. In: Martin, D., Harrod, R., Pérez, V. (Eds.), The Bioarchaeology of Violence. University Press of Florida, Tallahassee, pp. 29–62.

Klaus, H., 2014. A history of violence in the Lambayeque valley: conflict and death from the late pre-Hispanic apogee to European colonization of Peru (AD 900-1750). In: Knusel, C., Smith, M. (Eds.), The Routledge Handbook of the Bioarchaeology of Human Conflict. Routledge, London, pp. 389–414.

Kleinman, P., Marks, S., Richmond, J., Blackbourne, B., 1995. Inflicted skeletal injury: a postmortem radiologic-histopathologic study in 31 infants. American Journal of Radiology 165, 647–650.

Knight, B., 1986. The history of child abuse. Forensic Science International 30, 135–141.

Knüsel, C., Smith, M. (Eds.), 2014. The Routledge Handbook of the Bioarchaeology of Human Conflict. Routledge, London.

Knüsel, C.J., Roberts, C., Boylston, A., 1996. Brief communication: when Adam delved…an activity related lesion in three human skeletal populations. American Journal of Physical Anthropology 100, 427–434.

Kopcsanyi, I., Laczay, A., Nagy, L., 1969. Cough fractures of ribs in infants with dyspnoea. Acta Paediatrica Academiae Scientiarum Hungaricae 10 (2), 93–98.

Kurin, D., 2012. Cranial trauma and cranial modification in post-imperial Andahuaylas, Peru. In: Martin, D., Anderson, C. (Eds.), Bioarchaeological and Forensic Perspectives on Violence. Cambridge University Press, Cambridge, pp. 236–260.

Lambert, P., 2014. Violent injury and death in a prehistoric farming community of southwestern Colorado: the osteological evidence from Sleeping Ute Mountain. In: Knusel, C., Smith, M. (Eds.), The Routledge Handbook of the Bioarchaeology of Human Conflict. Routledge, London, pp. 308–332.

Larsen, C.S., 2015. Bioarchaeology: Interpreting Behavior from the Human Skeleton. Cambridge University Press, Cambridge.

László, O., 2016. Detailed analysis of a trepanation from the late Avar Period (turn of the 7th–8th centuries) and its significance in the anthropological material of the Carpathian Basin. International Journal of Osteoarchaeology 26 (2), 359–365.

Lehndorff, H., 1907. Deformitäten der Wirbelsäl und der rippen im verlaufe eines schweren tetanus. Wiener Medizinische Wochenschrift 67 (1), 2477.

Leone, A., Cianfoni, A., Cerase, A., Magarelli, N., Bonomo, L., 2011. Lumbar spondylolysis: a review. Skeletal Radiology 40 (6), 683–700.

Lewis, M., 2002a. The impact of industrialisation: comparative study of child health in four sites from medieval and post-medieval England (850-1859 AD). American Journal of Physical Anthropology 119 (3), 211–223.

Lewis, M., 2002b. Urbanisation and Child Health in Medieval and Post-medieval England: An Assessment of the Morbidity and Mortality of Non-adult Skeletons from the Cemeteries of Two Urban and Two Rural Sites in England (AD 850–1859). Archaeopress, Oxford.

Lewis, M., 2008. The children. In: Magilton, J., Lee, F., Boylston, A. (Eds.)Magilton, J., Lee, F., Boylston, A. (Eds.), Chichester Excavations 'Lepers Outside the Gate' Excavations at the Cemetery of the Hospital of St James and St Mary Magdalene, Chichester, 1986-87 and 1993, vol. 10, pp. 174–186 York: Council for British Archaeology Research Report, 158.

Lewis, M., 2010. Life and death in a civitas capital: metabolic disease and trauma in the children from late Roman Dorchester. Dorset. American Journal of Physical Anthropology 142, 405–416.

Lewis, M., 2011. Thalassaemia: its diagnosis and interpretation in past skeletal populations. International Journal of Osteoarchaeology 21 (2), 685–693.

Lewis, M., 2013. Children of the Golden Minster: St Oswald's Priory and the impact of industrialisation on child health. Journal of Anthropology: 959472. http://dx.doi.org/10.1155/2013/959472.

Lewis, M., 2014. Sticks and stones: exploring the nature and significance of child trauma in the past. In: Knusel, C., Smith, M. (Eds.), The Routledge Handbook of the Bioarchaeology of Human Conflict. Routledge, London, pp. 39–63.

Lewis, M., 2016. Work and the adolescent in medieval England (AD 900-1550). The osteological evidence. Medieval Archaeology 60 (1), 138–171.

Light, T., Ogden, D., Ogden, J., 1984. The anatomy of metaphyseal torus fractures. Clinical Orthopaedics and Related Research 188, 103–111.

Lincoln, T., Mubarak, S., 1994. "Isolated" traumatic radial head dislocation. Journal of Pediatric Orthopedics 14 (4), 454–457.

Loder, R., Hensinger, R., 2001. Fractures of the thoracic and lumbar spine. In: Beaty, J., Kasser, J. (Eds.), Rockwood and Wilkins' Fractures in Children. Lipencott Williams and Wilkins, Philadelphia, pp. 847–880.

Lomax, E.M.R., 1996. Small and Special: The Development of Hospitals for Children in Victorian Britain. Wellcome Institute for the History of Medicine, London.

Love, J., Symes, S., 2004. Understanding rib fracture patterns: incomplete and buckle fractures. Journal of Forensic Sciences 49 (6), 1153–1158.

Love, J.C., Derrick, S.M., Wiersema, J.M., Pinto, D.C., Greeley, C., Donaruma-Kwoh, M., Bista, B., 2013. Novel classification system of rib fractures observed in infants. Journal of Forensic Sciences 58 (2), 330–335.

Maat, G., 2008. Dating of fractures in human dry bone tissue. The Berisha case. In: Kimmerle, E., Baraybar, J. (Eds.), Skeletal Trauma: Identification of Injuries Resulting from Human Rights Abuse and Armed Conflict. CRC Press, Boca Raton, pp. 245–254.

Maresh, M.M., 1955. Linear growth of long bones of extremities from infancy through adolescence. American Journal of Diseases in Children 89 (3), 725–742.

Mariani-Costantini, R., Catalano, P., Gennaro, D., Tota, D., Angeletti, L., 2000. New light on cranial surgery in ancient Rome. Lancet 355, 305–307.

Martin, D., Anderson, C. (Eds.), 2014. Bioarchaeological and Forensic Perspectives on Violence. Cambridge Universty Press, Cambridge.

Martin, D., Harrod, R., 2015. Bioarchaeological contributions to the study of violence. Yearbook of Physical Anthropology 156 (59), 116–145.

Martin, D., Harrod, R., Pérez, V. (Eds.), 2012. The Bioarchaeology of Violence. University Press of Florida, Tallahassee.

Matos, V., 2009. Broken ribs: paleopathological analysis of costal fractures in the human identified skeletal collection from the Museu Bocage, Lisbon, Portugal (Late 19th to Middle 20th centuries). American Journal of Physical Anthropology 140 (1), 25–38.

Mays, S., 1991. The Medieval Burials from Blackfriars Friary, School Street, Ipswich, Suffolk. Ancient Monuments Laboratory Report. English Heritage, London.

Mays, S., 2007a. The human remains. In: Mays, S., Harding, C., Heighway, C. (Eds.). Mays, S., Harding, C., Heighway, C. (Eds.), Wharram a Study of a Settlement on the Yorkshire Wolds, XI: The Churchyard York University Archaeological Publications, vol. 13. English Heritage, London, pp. 77–192.

Mays, S., 2007b. Spondylolysis in non-adult skeletons excavated from a medieval rural archaeological site in England. International Journal of Osteoarchaeology 17 (5), 504–513.

Mays, S., 2014. The bioarchaeology of the homicide of infants and children. In: Thompson, J., Alfonso-Durruty, M., Crandall, J. (Eds.), Tracing Childhood Bioarchaeological Investigations of Early Lives in Antiquity. University of Florida Press, Gainesville, pp. 99–122.

Mays, S., Robson-Brown, K., Vincent, S., Eyers, J., King, H., Roberts, A., 2012. An infant femur bearing cut marks from Roman Hambleden, England. International Journal of Osteoarchaeology 24 (1), 111–115.

McKinley, J., 2008. The 18th Century Baptist Church and Burial Ground at West Butts Street, Poole, Dorset. Wessex Archaeology Ltd., Sailsbury.

Meyer, C., Brandt, G., Haak, W., Ganslmeier, R., Meler, H., Alt, K., 2009. The Eulau eulogy: bioarchaeological interpretation of lethal violence in Corded Ware multiple burials from Saxony-Anhalt, Germany. Journal of Anthropological Archaeology 28, 412–423.

Miles, A., Powers, N., Wroe-Brown, R., Walker, D., 2008. St Marylebone Church and Burial Ground in the 18th-19th Centuries. Excavations at St Marylebone School, 1992 and 2004-6. MOLAS Monograph 46. Museum of London Archaeology Service, London.

Mogle, P., Zias, J., 1995. Trephination as a possible treatment for scurvy in a middle Bronze Age (ca. 2200 BC) skeleton. International Journal of Osteoarchaeology 5, 77–81.

Molleson, T., Cox, M., 1988. A neonate with cut bones from Poundbury Camp, 4th century AD, England. Bulletin of the Royal Society of Anthropology and Prehistory 99, 53–59.

Molleson, T., Cox, M., 1993. The Spitalfields Project, Volume II – The Middling Sort. York: Council for British Archaeology Research Report. 86.

Molto, J., 2000. Humerus varus deformity in Roman period burials from Kellis 2, Dakhleh, Egypt. American Journal of Physical Anthropology 113 (1), 103–109.

Morita, T., Ikata, T., Katoh, S., Miyake, R., 1995. Lumbar spondylolysis in children and adolescents. Journal of Bone and Joint Surgery. British Volume 77 (4), 620–625.

Murphy, T.R., October 1, 1986. "Woful childe of parents rage": suicide of children and adolescents in early modern England, 1507-1710. The Sixteenth Century Journal 259–270.

Namdev, R., Jindal, A., Bhargava, S., Dutta, S., Singhal, P., Grewal, P., 2016. Patterns of mandible fracture in children under 12 years in a district trauma center in India. Dental Traumatology 32 (1), 32–36.

Nikitovic, D., Janković, I., Milhelić, S., 2012. Juvenile elbow dislocation from the prehistoric site of Josipovac-Grvinjak, Croatia. International Journal of Paleopathology 2, 36–41.

Novak, S., Kopp, D., 2003. To feed a tree in Zion: osteological analysis of the 1857 Mountain Meadows massacre. Historical Archaeology 37 (2), 85–108.

Nte, A., Gabriel-Job, N., 2013. Tetanus with multiple wedge vertebral collapses: a case report in a 13 year old girl. Nigerian Journal of Paediatrics 40 (2), 189–191.

Nystrom, K., 2007. Trepanation in the Chachapoya region of northern Peru. International Journal of Osteoarchaeology 17 (1), 39–51.

O'Connor, J., Cohen, J., 1987. Dating fractures. In: Kleinman, P. (Ed.), Diagnostic Imaging of Child Abuse, second ed. Williams and Wilkins, Baltimore, pp. 103–113.

Offierski, C., 1981. Traumatic dislocation of the hip in children. Journal of Bone & Joint Surgery. British Volume 63 (2), 194–197.

Ortner, D., 2003. Identification of Pathological Conditions in Human Skeletal Remains. Academic Press, New York.

Ortner, D.J., Putschar, W.G.J., 1985. Identification of Pathological Conditions in Human Skeletal Remains. Smithsonian Institution Press, Washington.

Owen, R., Hickey, F., Finlay, D., 1995. A study of metatarsal fractures in children. Injury 26 (8), 537–538.

Palkovitch, A., 2012. Community violence and everyday life: death at Arroyo Hondo. In: Martin, D., Harrod, R., Pérez, V. (Eds.), The Bioarchaeology of Violence. University Press of Florida, Tallahassee, pp. 111–120.

Pape, H., Marsh, S., Morley, J., Krettek, C., Giannoudis, P., 2004. Current concepts in the development of heterotopic ossification. The Journal of Bone and Joint Surgery. British Volume 86 (6), 783–787.

Pathria, M., 2005. Physical injury: spine. In: Resnick, D., Kransdorf, M. (Eds.), Bone and Joint Imaging. Elsevier Saunders, Philidelphia, pp. 879–904.

Pérez, V., 2012. The politicization of the dead: violence as performance, politics as usual. In: Martin, D., Harrod, R., Pérez, V. (Eds.), The Bioarchaeology of Violence. University Press of Florida, Tallahassee, pp. 13–28.

Peterson, H.A., Madhok, R., Benson, J.T., Ilstrup, D.M., Melton III, L.J., 1994. Physeal fractures: Part 1. Epidemiology in Olmsted county, Minnesota, 1979-1988. Journal of Pediatric Orthopedics 14 (4), 423–430.

Pettifor, J., Daniels, E., 1997. Vitamin D deficiency and nutritional rickets in children. In: Feldman, D., Glorieux, F., Pike, J. (Eds.), Vitamin D. Academic Press, New York, pp. 663–678.

Pfeiffer, S., Van der Merwe, N., 2004. Cranial injuries in stone age children from the Modder river mouth, western Cape Province, South Africa. South African Archaeological Bulletin 59 (180), 59–65.

Pierce, M., Bertocci, G., Vogeley, E., Moreland, M., 2004. Evaluating long bone fractures in children: a biomechanical approach with illustrative cases. Child Abuse and Neglect 28 (5), 505–524.

Polo-Cerdá, M., Miquel-Feucht, M., Villalaín-Blanco, J., 2003. Study of a foetus whose death was caused by basiotrispsy, found in Castielfabid (Valencia-Spain) in partial state of mummification. In: Lynnerup, N., Andreasen, C., Berglund, J. (Eds.), Mummies in a New Millenium Proceedings of the 4th World Congress on Mummy Studies Nuuk, Greenland. Greenland National Museum and Archives and Danish Polar Center, Nuuk, Greenland, pp. 197–200.

Polousky, J., 2011. Juvenile osteochondritis dissecans. Sports Medicine and Arthroscopy Review 19 (1), 56–63.

Powers, N., Miles, A., 2011. Nonconformist identities in 19th century London: archaeological and osteological evidence from the burial grounds of Bow baptist chapel and the catholic mission of St. Mary and Michael, Tower Hamlets. In: King, C., Sayer, D. (Eds.), The Archaeology of Post-Medieval Religion. The Boydell Press, Woodbridge, pp. 233–248.

Prosser, I., Maguire, S., Harison, S., Mann, M., Sibert, J., Kemp, A., 2005. How old is this fracture? Radiological dating of fractures in children: a systematic review. American Journal of Radiology 184, 1282–1286.

Pudenz, R., Todd, E., Shelden, C., 1961. Head injuries in infants and young children. California Medicine 94 (2), 6–71.

Puttaswamaiah, R., Chandran, P., Sen, R., Kataria, S., Gill, S.S., 2006. Deformities in conservatively treated closed fractures of the shaft of the femur in children. Acta Orthopaedica Belgica 72 (2), 147.

Rális, Z., 1975. Birth trauma to muscles in babies born by breech delivery and its possible fatal consequences. Archives of Disease in Childhood 50 (4), 4–13.

Rális, Z., McKibbin, B., 1973. Changes in shape of the human hip joint during its development and their relation to its stability. Journal of Bone and Joint Surgery. British Volume 55 (4), 780–785.

Rao, P., Carty, H., 1999. Non-accidental injury: review of the radiology. Clinical Radiology 54 (1), 11–24.

Rathjen, K., Birch, J., 2006. Physeal injuries and growth disturbances. In: Beaty, J., Kasser, J. (Eds.), Rockwood and Wilkins' Fractures in Children. Lippincott Williams and Wilkins, Philadelphia-Baltimore, pp. 99–131.

Rawson, B., 2003. Children and Childhood in Roman Italy. Oxford University Press, Oxford.

Redfern, R., December 2007. An investigation of a possible perimortem limb amputation in a post-medieval subadult from the Isle of Wight, England. Paleopathology Newsletter 140, 6–10.

Rennie, L., Court-Brown, C.M., Mok, J.Y., Beattie, T.F., 2007. The epidemiology of fractures in children. Injury 38 (8), 913–922.

Resnick, D. (Ed.), 1995. Diagnosis of Bone and Joint Disorders. W.B. Saunders Company, Philadelphia.

Resnick, D., Goergen, T., 2002. Physical injury: concepts and terminology. In: Resnick, D. (Ed.), Diagnosis of Bone and Joint Disorders. WB Saunders and Company, Philadelphia, pp. 2627–2789.

Resnick, D., Kransdorf, M., 2005. Bone and Joint Imaging. Elsevier Saunders, Philadelphia.

Roberg, O., 1937. Spinal deformity following tetanus and its relation to juvenile kyphosis. Journal of Bone and Joint Surgery 19 (3), 603–629.

Roberts, C., 1989. The Human Remains from 76 Kingsholm, Gloucester (Unpublished Report). University of Bradford, Bradford.

Roberts, C., 2000. Trauma in biocultural perspective: past present and future work in Britain. In: Cox, M., Mays, S. (Eds.), Human Osteology in Archaeology and Forensic Science. Greenwich Medical Media Ltd, London, pp. 337–356.

Rohnbogner, A., 2015. Dying Young: A Palaeopathological Analysis of Child Health in Roman Britain (Ph.D. thesis). University of Reading, England.

Ross, A., Abel, S., Radisch, D., 2009. Pattern of injury in child fatalities resulting from child abuse. Forensic Science International 188, 99–102.

Rushton, J., 1991. The secret 'iron tongs' of midwifery. The Historian 30, 12–15.

Salter, R., Harris, W., 1963. Injuries involving the epiphyseal plate. Journal of Bone and Joint Surgery 45 (3), 587–622.

Sanders, W.E., Heckman, J.D., 1984. Traumatic plastic deformation of the radius and ulna. Clinical Orthopaedics and Related Research 188, 58–67.

Saternus, K.-S., Kernbach-Wighton, G., Oehmichen, M., 2000. The shaking trauma in infants – kinetic chains. Forensic Science International 109, 203–213.

Schenik, R., Goodnight, J., 1996. Current concepts review: osteochondritis dissecans. Journal of Bone and Joint Surgery 78 (3), 439–483.

Schmidt, P., Grass, H., Madea, B., 1996. Child homicide in Cologne (1985-94). Forensic Science International 79, 131–144.

Schug, G.R., Gray, K., Mushrif-Tripathy, V., Sankhyan, A., 2012. A peaceful realm? Trauma and social differentiation at Harappa. International Journal of Paleopathology 2, 136–147.

Schulting, R., Fibiger, L. (Eds.), 2012. Sticks, Stones and Broken Bones: Neolithic Violence in a European Perspective. Oxford University Press, Oxford.

Schwartz, J., Houghton, F., Macchiarelli, R., Bondioli, L., 2010. Skeletal remains from Punic Carthage do not support systemic sacrifice of infants. PLoS One 5 (2), e9177.

Schwend, R.M., Werth, C., Johnston, A., 2000. Femur shaft fractures in toddlers and young children: rarely from child abuse. Journal of Pediatric Orthopedics 20 (4), 475–481.

Servaes, S., Brown, S.D., Choudhary, A.K., Christian, C.W., Done, S.L., Hayes, L.L., Levine, M.A., Moreno, J.A., Palusci, V.J., Shore, R.M., 2016. The etiology and significance of fractures in infants and young children: a critical multidisciplinary review. Pediatric Radiology 46 (5), 591–600.

Sheldon, W., 1943. Diseases of Infancy and Childhood. J. & A. Churchill Ltd., London.

Simm, A., 2007. Fetal malpresentaion. Obstetrics, Gynaecology and Reproductive Medicine 17 (10), 283–288.

Skinner, M., Barkley, J., Carlson, R., 1989. Cranial asymmetry and muscular torticollis in prehistoric northwest coast natives from British Columbia (Canada). Journal of Paleopathology 3 (1), 19–34.

Šlaus, M., Cicvara-Pećina, T., Lucijanić, I., Pećina, M., Stilinović, D., 2010a. Osteochondritis dissecans of the knee in a subadult from a medieval (ninth century AD) site in Croatia. Acta Clinica Croatica 49, 189–195.

Šlaus, M., Novak, M., Vyroubal, V., Bedić, Ž., 2010b. The harsh life on the 15th century Croatia-Ottoman Empire border: analysing and identifying the reasons for the massacre in Čepin. American Journal of Physical Anthropology 141, 358–372.

Smith, M., 2003. Beyond palisades: the nature and frequency of late prehistoric deliberate trauma in the Chickamauga Reservoir of East Tennessee. American Journal of Physical Anthropology 121, 303–318.

Smith, P., Avishai, G., Greene, J., Stager, L., 2011. Aging cremated infants: the problem of sacrifice at the Tophet of Carthage. Antiquity 85 (329), 859–874.

Smrčka, V., Marik, I., Dockalova, M., Svensonova, M., 1998. Congenital deficiency of the tibia at the medieval monastic cemetery in Olomouc (Czech Republic). Journal of Paleopathology 10 (3), 111–120.

Sorantin, E., Brader, P., Thimary, F., 2006. Neonatal trauma. European Journal of Radiology 60, 199–207.

Soren, D., Fenton, T., Birkby, W., 1995. The late Roman infant cemetery near Lugnano in Teverina, Italy: some implications. Journal of Paleopathology 7 (1), 13–42.

Standen, V., Arriaza, B., 2000. Trauma in the Preceramic coastal populations of Northern Chile: violence or occupational hazards? American Journal of Physical Anthropology 112, 239–249.

Stanley, E., De La Garza, J., 2001. Monteggia fracture-dislocation in children. In: Beaty, J., Kasser, J. (Eds.), Rockwood and Wilkins' Fractures in Children, fifth ed. Lipencott Williams and Wilkins, Philadelphia, pp. 529–562.

Starling, S., Heller, R., Jenny, C., 2002. Pelvic fractures in infants as a sign of physical abuse. Child Abuse and Neglect 26, 475–480.

Stephens, M., Hsu, L., Leong, J., 1989. Leg length discrepancy after femoral shaft fractures in children. The Journal of Bone and Joint Surgery. British Volume 71 (4), 615–618.

Stilli, S., Magnani, M., Lampasi, M., Antonioli, D., Bettuzzi, C., Donzelli, O., 2008. Remodelling and overgrowth after conservative treatment for femoral and tibial shaft fractures in children. La Chirurgia Degli Organi di Movimento 91, 13–19.

Stone, J.L., Miles, M.L., 1990. Skull trepanation among the early Indians of Canada and the United States. Neurosurgery 26 (6), 1015–1020.

Strait, R., Siegal, R., Shapiro, R., 1995. Humeral fractures without obvious etiologies in children less than 3 years of age: when is it abuse? Pediatrics 97 (4), 667–671.

Strouse, P., Owings, C., 1995. Fractures of the first rib in child abuse. Radiology 197, 763–765.

Stuart-Macadam, P., Glencross, B., Kricun, M., 1998. Traumatic bowing deformities in tubular bones. International Journal of Osteoarchaeology 8, 252–262.

Sulaiman, A., Munajat, I., Mohd, E., 2014. Outcome of traumatic hip dislocation in children. Journal of Pediatric Orthopedics B23 (2), 204–205.

Sullivan, J., 1998. Fractures of the spine in children. In: Green, N., Swiontkowski, M. (Eds.), Skeletal Trauma in Children. WB Saunders Company, Philadelphia, pp. 343–367.

Thomas, S.A., Rosenfield, N.S., Leventhal, J.M., Markowitz, R.I., 1991. Long-bone fractures in young children: distinguishing accidental injuries from child abuse. Pediatrics 88 (3), 471–476.

Thorén, H., Iizuka, T., Hallikainen, D., Lindqvist, C., 1992. Different patterns of mandibular fractures in children. An analysis of 220 fractures in 157 patients. Journal of Cranio-maxillofacial Surgery 20 (7), 292–296.

Thorpe, I., 2003. Anthropology, archaeology, and the origin of warfare. World Archaeology 35 (1), 145–165.

Towner, E., Towner, J., 2000. Developing the history of unintentional injury: the use of coroners' records in early modern England. Injury Prevention 6, 102–105.

Tung, T., 2016. Patterns of violence and diet among children during a time of imperial decline and climate change in the ancient Peruvian Andres. In: VanDerwarken, A., Wilson, G. (Eds.), The Archaeology of Food and Warfare. Springer International Publishing, Switzerland, pp. 193–228.

Tung, T., Knudson, K., 2010. Childhood lost: abductions, sacrifice, and trophy heads of children in the Wari Empire of the ancient Andes. Latin American Antiquity 21 (1), 44–66.

Verlinden, P., 2015. Child's Play? A New Methodology for the Identification of Trauma in Non-adult Skeletal Remains (Ph.D. thesis). University of Reading, England.

Verlinden, P., Lewis, M., 2015. Childhood trauma: methods for the identification of physeal fractures in nonadult skeletal remains. American Journal of Physical Anthropology 157 (3), 411–420.

Vialle, R., Mary, P., Schmider, L., le Pointe, H.D., Damsin, J.-P., Filipe, G., 2006. Spinal fracture through the neurocentral synchondrosis in battered children: a report of three cases. Spine 31 (11), E345–E349.

Wahl, J., Trautmann, I., 2012. The Neolithic massacre at Talheim: a pivotal find in conflict archaeology. In: Schulting, R., Fibiger, L. (Eds.), Sticks, Stones and Broken Bones: Neolithic Violence in a European Perspective. Oxford University Press, Oxford, pp. 77–100.

Waldron, T., 2000. Hidden or overlooked? Where are the disadvantaged in the skeletal record? In: Hurbert, J. (Ed.), Madness, Disability and Social Exclusion. Routledge, London, pp. 29–45.

Waldron, T., 2007. St Peter's, Barton-upon-Humber, Lincolnshire, Vol 2. The Human Remains. Oxbow Books, Oxford.

Waldron, T., 2009. Palaeopathology. Cambridge University Press, Cambridge.

Waldron, T., Rogers, J., 1987. Iatrogenic palaeopathology. Journal of Paleopathology 1 (3), 117–129.

Walker, D., 2012. Disease in London, 1st-19th Centuries. Museum of London Archaeology, London.

Walker, P.L., 1997. Skeletal evidence for child abuse: a physical anthropological perspective. Journal of Forensic Sciences 42 (2), 196–207.

Wall, S., Musgrave, J., Warren, P., 1986. Human bones from a late Minoan IB house at Knossos. The Annual of the British School at Athens 81, 333–388.

Warner, W., 2001. Cervical spine injuries in children. In: Beaty, J., Kasser, J. (Eds.), Rockwood and Wilkins' Fractures in Children. Lipencott Williams and Wilkins, Philadelphia, pp. 809–846.

Wasterlain, S., Umbelino, C., 2013. Legg-Calvé-Perthes disease and slipped femoral epiphyses in th skeletal remains of a medieval necropolis of Santa Maria (Sintra, Portugal). Cadernos do GEEvH 2 (2), 27–39.

Wehner, F., Schieffer, M., Wehner, H.-D., 1999. Percentile charts to determine the duration of child abuse by chronic malnutrition. Forensic Science International 102, 173–180.

Wells, C., 1974. Osteochondritis dissecans in ancient British skeletal material. Medical History 18 (4), 365–369.

Wheeler, S., Beauchesne, P., Wiliams, L., Molto, J., 2007. Fractured childhood: a case of probable child abuse from the Kellis 2 cemetery, Dakhleh Oasis, Egypt. In: 72nd Annual Meeting of the Society of American Archaeologists. Texas, Austin.

Whittle, A., 1996. Europe in the Neolithic: The Creation of New Worlds. Cambridge University Press, Cambridge.

Wieberg, D., Wescott, D., 2008. Estimating the timing of long bone fractures: correlation between the postmortem interval, bone moisture content, and blunt force trauma fracture characteristics. Journal of Forensic Sciences 53, 1028–1034.

Wilber, J., Thompson, G., 1998. The multiply injured child. In: Green, N., Swiontkowski, M. (Eds.), Skeletal Trauma in Children, second ed. W.B. Saunders Company, Philadelphia, pp. 71–102.

Wilkins, K., Aroojis, A., 2001. The present status of children's fractures. In: Beaty, J., Kasser, J. (Eds.), Rockwood and Wilkins' Fractures in Children. Lipencott Williams and Wilkins, Philadelphia, pp. 3–20.

Wilkins, K.E., 2005. Principles of fracture remodeling in children. Injury 36 (1), S3–S11.

Williams, A., 2001. Too good to be true? Thomas Willis – neonatal convulsions, childhood stroke and infanticide in seventeenth century England. Seizure 10, 471–483.

Wilson, A.S., Taylor, T., Ceruti, M., Chavez, J., Reinhard, J., Grimes, V., Meier-Augenstein, W., Cartnell, L., Stern, B., Richards, M., et al., 2007. Stable isotope and DNA evidence for ritual sequences in Inca child sacrifice. Proceedings of the National Academy of Sciences 104 (42), 16456–16461.

Wiltse, L., 1975. Spondylolisthesis. Western Journal of Medicine 122 (2), 152–153.

Wu, X., Trinkaus, E., 2015. Neurocranial trauma in the late archaic human remains from Xujiayao, Northern China. International Journal of Osteoarchaeology 25, 245–252.

Yamaguchi Jr., K., Myung, K., Alonso, M., Skaggs, D., 2012. Clay-Shoveler's fracture equivalent in children. Spine 37 (26), E1672–E1675.

Yates, P., 1959. Birth trauma to the vertebral arteries. Archives of Disease in Childhood 34, 436–441.

Chapter 6

Infectious Diseases I: Infections of Nonspecific Origin

Chapter Outline

Introduction	131	Chronic Sinusitis	137
Subperiosteal New Bone Formation	131	Otitis Media and Mastoiditis	140
Infective Osteitis	133	Endocranial Lesions	141
Osteomyelitis	134	Infantile Cortical Hyperostosis	145
Infantile Osteomyelitis	136	References	147
Brodie's Abscess	136		
Spinal Osteomyelitis	137		

INTRODUCTION

Nonspecific infections refer to those for which a precise pathogen or cause (etiology) is unknown. This category of lesions includes periostitis, osteitis (or nonsuppurative osteomyelitis), and osteomyelitis. In archeological cases, when the lesions affect a single bone or have no particular distribution, it is difficult to identify the actual cause of the infection. Nevertheless, all three processes can occur in particular areas of the skeleton as part of a specific disease complex (i.e., treponemal disease, leprosy, or tuberculosis). Understanding the mechanisms, cause, and patterning behind the development of these lesions in adults and children is one of the foundations of paleopathological study. The majority of the infections that can be identified in the skeleton are chronic with a bacterial or fungal origin. However, there is a growing body of evidence that viral disease such as rubella and smallpox can leave subtle traces on the skeleton or result in conditions such as osteomyelitis, congenital defects, and juvenile arthritis. The potential for the identification of these conditions will also be discussed in Chapter 7.

SUBPERIOSTEAL NEW BONE FORMATION

The periosteum is a fibrous sheath that surrounds all the bones of the skeleton, with the exception of the endocranial surface of the skull and the area of the joints covered by hyaline cartilage. The sheath has two layers, with the outer layer consisting of white fibrous tissue with a few fat cells, and the inner layer being made up of a dense network of fine elastic fibers (Williams and Warwick, 1980).

This inner layer retains its osteogenic capacity throughout life. Subperiosteal new bone formation is recognized as the deposition of a new layer of bone under an inflamed periosteum as a result of injury, hemorrhage, or infection. As new bone formation can be stimulated by stretching, tearing, or contact with the periosteum in many circumstances, the term 'periostitis', with the suffix 'itis' denoting inflammation is no longer considered accurate unless the underlying cause is understood (Weston, 2008).

The periosteum is bound to the cortex by Sharpey's fibers. The need for rapid and constant intramembranous transverse growth means that these fibers are more loosely attached to the cortex, less numerous and shorter in children, leaving the periosteum more susceptible to rupture (Caffey, 1945). Compression and stretching of blood vessels by a buildup of blood, pus, granulation tissue, neoplasms, or through trauma causes elevation of the fibrous outer layer of the periosteum. After a sufficient period of time the bone tissue directly under the periosteum dies. Repair of the blood vessels results in an increased blood flow to the area and initial resorption (pitting) followed by new bone formation on the normal cortical surface (Weston, 2008). New bone formation may also occur with the transformation of fibroblasts into osteogenic cells or, on the areas of bone related to constantly inflamed lymph nodes (Harisinghani et al., 2000). Initially, the bone deposited is disorganized and has a porous appearance referred to as "woven" (or fiber) bone, representing an active phase of formation. Later, the new bone layer becomes remodeled with concentric layers of bone organized within a system of Haversian canals (or osteons); this smooth "lamellar" bone is continuous with the original cortex, and its presence is diagnostic of an event that occurred and healed well before the person's death. A mix of woven and lamellar bone is interpreted as indicating a chronic, recurring, and active infection. Infective suppurative periostitis caused by the accumulation of infective organisms on the subperiosteal surface may result in an extension of the infection into the cortex (osteitis), or the cortex and medullary cavity (osteomyelitis) (Resnick and Kransdorf, 2005).

The diagnosis of subperiosteal new bone formation as a pathological process in nonadult skeletal remains is particularly challenging. In the long bones of children under 4 years of age, appositional (normal) growth involves the deposition of immature disorganized bone on the cortical surface. This new bone is macroscopically identical to the fiber bone deposited as a pathological response. In addition, on clinical radiograph features such as double contours, cupping, and spurring, which are the characteristics of new bone formation in response to an infection, rickets, or metaphyseal fractures, can occur as the result of body (or bone) positioning during radiography (Gleser, 1949). Gleser (1949) warned that increased formation and mineralization of the long bones during the normal growth process may mimic signs of congenital syphilis, scurvy, and rickets in infants. Shopfner (1966) examined the radiographic appearance of the long bones of 335 healthy premature and full-term infants and noted "normal" periosteal new bone in 35% of cases. The new bone was invariably bilateral and present on the femur, humerus, tibia, ulna, and radius in that order of frequency. While the new bone was concentric in most bones, the tibia was most commonly affected on the medial aspect. The bone deposits were thick, but not multilayered, and appeared on radiograph as double contours, before becoming incorporated into the underlying cortex. In a later study, De Silva et al. (2003) argued that normal or "physiological periostitis" in infants was mainly confined to the diaphysis (Fig. 6.1). East (2003) examined a small number of known age perinates from Mexico and Tennessee and noted that every individual exhibited some form of new bone formation calling into the question the presence of infection. Shopfner (1966) could not explain why some infants showed periosteal new bone formation while others did not and suggested it would only be apparent in children undergoing the most rapid growth. It seems likely that this "physiological subperiosteal new bone" would be even more apparent in dry bone specimens than in clinical radiographs. It could be argued that if physiological periostitis in living infants signals that they were experiencing a growth "spurt," common sense would dictate that a sick child on the brink of death is unlikely to be undergoing rapid growth. However, this does not account for fatal accidents where growth would have proceeded normally before death. Ortner (2003) asserts that before the age of 4 years, the presence of woven periosteal new bone should be expected as part of the normal growth process.

Early studies considered pathological new bone as the result of an infection to present as a unilateral, isolated patch of bone rising above the original cortex (Anderson and Carter, 1994; Buckley, 2000; Mensforth et al., 1978; Walker, 1997). More recently, it has been recognized that these types of lesions may also represent subtle fracture calluses in children (Lewis, 2014, Fig. 6.2). Microscopic features (e.g., polsters, grenzstreifen, and sinuous lacunae) may help to distinguish normal deposits from pathological ones, although they are unlikely to enable us to identify the specific cause of the lesion (Weston, 2009). In an infant's remains, difficulties in distinguishing pathology from growth has meant postnatal conditions such as birth trauma, child abuse, primary hypertrophic osteoarthropathy, syphilis, hypervitamintosis A, and infantile cortical hyperostosis (ICH) are rarely considered, despite their clinical frequency in newborns (Lewis, 2000). Until we can develop diagnostic strategies to differentiate the normal growth process from a pathological response, we remain unable to fully explore the prevalence of these conditions in past populations. For now, diffuse, symmetrical, and

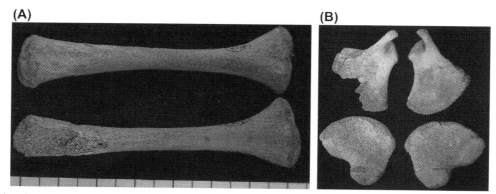

FIGURE 6.1 Perinatal new bone formation. (A) A fine porous layer of new bone covers the anterior aspect of the humeral diaphyses in this perinate. It is currently not possible to determine whether this deposit is the result of rapid growth (i.e., physiological periostitis) or indicates a pathological process. (B) Thicker more patchy bilateral deposits of gray woven bone are present on the ilia and scapulae of this perinate. While the thicker and less diffuse nature of new bone on the scapula bodies is more suggestive of a lesion, it is still symmetrical.

thin deposits of fiber bone that spare the metaphyses should be treated with caution in infant remains.

Perhaps due to the difficulties discussed above, studies that explore the frequency of nonspecific infections in nonadult skeletons are rare. More often, evidence for subperiosteal lesions in older children are discussed under the heading of nonspecific stress. Weston (2012) cautioned against this practice, emphasizing that the way in which glucocorticoids respond to stress inhibits bone mineralization and therefore periosteal new bone formation. Hence, these lesions may be caused by many factors, but a physiological stress response is unlikely to be one of them.

INFECTIVE OSTEITIS

Osteitis is a term used to describe involvement of the bone cortex, either as an isolated phenomenon or as a prequel to osteomyelitis. Also known as nonsuppurative osteomyelitis or Garré's sclerosing osteomyelitis, these terms denote the lack of abscess formation (Resnick and Kransdorf, 2005). Osteitis results in a thickened cortex causing a diminished medullary cavity. It may develop along with subperiosteal new bone formation, or the cortex may remain smooth over an enlarged area of bone. Osteitis is a descriptive term rather than a specific diagnosis in the clinical literature, and radiographs are essential to differentiate infection from a tumor or fracture callus, or to rule out osteomyelitis. Garré's sclerosing osteomyelitis is a rare disease in children and adolescents and occurs mostly in boys with an average age of 10 years (Styczyński et al., 2002). It is a mild and chronic infection causing sclerosis and thickening of the cortex with small granulations. Lesions are common in the proximal tibia where thickening is normally limited to one side of the shaft, and in the mandible and maxilla (Fig. 6.3). In the jaws, infection from dental caries is considered to be the most likely source of infection (Gumber et al., 2016), but the etiology of the disease is often unknown (Styczyński et al., 2002). *Staphylococcus aureus* and *Staphylococcus albus* are the most common pathogens associated with the condition. Garré's sclerosing osteomyelitis has a distinctive layered appearance on radiograph due to a successive buildup of subperiosteal new bone. ICH, hypervitaminosis A, syphilis, leukemia, treponemal disease, Ewing's sarcoma, and metastatic neuroblastoma are differential diagnoses (Gumber et al., 2016). Chronic recurrent multifocal osteomyelitis is a condition seen in children and adolescents of unknown etiology. In 40% of cases pustules are also present on the palms and soles of the hands and feet. The condition is symmetrical and diffuse, commonly affecting the distal femur and tibia, with or without hypertrophy of the clavicle and sclerosis on the medial aspect (Resnick and Kransdorf, 2005, p. 1444). The age of onset is between 5 and 10 years, although the condition has been reported in infants. Despite its name, the main feature of the condition is osteitis (Resnick and Kransdorf, 2005, p. 736). The location at the distal end of the femur and

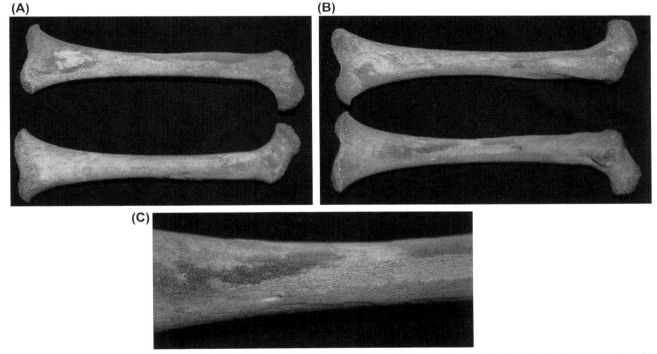

FIGURE 6.2 Active subperiosteal new bone formation on the (A) lateral aspect and (B) posterior femoral shafts of a 4- to 5-year-old from St Oswald's Priory in Gloucester, England (AD 1120–1230, skeleton 136). A close-up view (C) shows a thick deposit of active bone overlying a fine and paler layer of remodeling bone. The age of the child supports the diagnosis of pathological new bone formation, despite the bilateral nature of the lesions. The cause is unknown and the new bone may be the result of infection, bleeding, trauma to the periosteum or a fracture callus in response to a greenstick fracture.

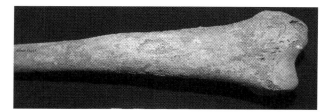

FIGURE 6.3 Osteitis of the distal right femur in a 16- to 17-year-old from St Mary Spital, London (AD 1400–1540, skeleton 20,634). There is hypertrophy without abscess formation and active subperiosteal new bone formation on the cortical surface. The femur has taken on a flasklike appearance. This individual has been diagnosed with treponemal disease. *Photograph by F. Shapland taken with the kind permission of the Museum of London.*

"flasklike" appearance of the deformity means that Pyle's disease, Brodie's abscess (see below), treponemal disease and Gaucher's disease are differential diagnoses. Unilateral shaft enlargement and clavicle involvement should aid in a more accurate diagnosis.

OSTEOMYELITIS

Osteomyelitis is a term that describes purulent infection of the bone and marrow that occupies the medullary cavity and bone ends. Osteomyelitis can result from fungal infections, TB, sickle cell anemia, smallpox, chickenpox, typhoid fever, and congenital syphilis, but it is rarely possible to identify the specific cause of the infection (Schmit and Glorion, 2004). More common and easier to identify is osteomyelitis as the result of an open fracture. Osteomyelitis occurs due to the direct spread of an infection from an adjacent fracture or lesion or, an infection may reach the medullary cavity indirectly via the bloodstream (i.e., hematogenously) (Resnick and Kransdorf, 2005; Steinbach, 1966). Pathogens rely on a wealth of iron to achieve their full growth and replication potential (Ulijaszek, 1990), and due to the greater quantity of red (blood forming) marrow nonadult bone provides the ideal environment for their spread and survival. For this reason hematogenous osteomyelitis is the most frequent form seen in children. The most common pathogens are *S. aureus* (85% of cases), followed by *Streptococcus pyogens* and *Haemophilus influenzae* (Schmit and Glorion, 2004), and *Pseudomonas aeruginosa*, which is found in the soil and causes infections usually as the result of puncture wounds on the foot (Blickman et al., 2004). Deep animal bites can also introduce infection, commonly in the hand, arm, and leg with 5% of dog bites and 20%–50% of cat bites resulting in an infection, normally with *Pasteurella multocida* (Resnick and Kransdorf, 2005, p. 724). In England, Anderson and Carter (1995) reported a case of osteomyelitis in the hand ("dactylitis") affecting two metacarpals of a 3- to 5-year-old child from early medieval Canterbury in Kent. The authors suggest the child developed osteomyelitis as the result of a dog bite (Fig. 6.4).

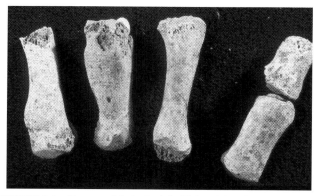

FIGURE 6.4 Osteomyelitis in the left third and fourth metacarpals of a 3- to 5-year-old from St Gregory's Priory in Canterbury, England (AD 1084–1537, skeleton 1201). *From Anderson, T., Carter, A.R., 1995. An unusual osteitic reaction in a young medieval child. International Journal of Osteoarchaeology 5, 193.*

Osteomyelitis can be divided into two forms, pyogenic (pus-producing) and nonpyogenic. Pyogenic osteomyelitis is described as acute, subacute, or chronic depending on the intensity of the inflammation (Steinbach, 1966). Acute osteomyelitis is the most common in children with symptoms occurring within weeks of onset, presenting as edema and suppuration of the affected area (Lew and Waldvogel, 2004). The infection is normally confined to the metaphysis, lifting the periosteum and penetrating the periosteal membrane. Joint involvement can cause subluxations, avascular necrosis, a slipped epiphysis, pathological fractures, and premature epiphyseal closure (Blickman et al., 2004). If the infection spreads hematogenously then death can result from septicemia before the chronic form of the disease can develop. Chronic osteomyelitis evolves over months and years presenting as a low-grade infection. Subcortical scalloping and new bone formation is recognized after 7–10 days from the onset of infection (Blickman et al., 2004). As inflammation ensues through the medullary cavity, Haversian system of the cortex, adjacent tissues and extends along the growth plate to the periosteum, the buildup of exudate causes interosseous pressure, vascular compression, and subsequent tissue necrosis (Fig. 6.5). The infection pierces the periosteum giving rise to surface abscesses. The shredding of the periosteum away from the cortex causes the creation of a new sheath of bone (involucrum) with the necrotic original cortex (sequestrum) gradually expelled through a draining sinus or "cloaca" (Steinbach, 1966). It can take 2–3 weeks for the sequestrum to become visible and it acts as a source of continuous infection (Steinbach, 1966). Profuse involucrum formation is a common feature in the child (Trueta, 1959) as the more loosely attached periosteum is stripped from the entire length of the shaft resulting in enlargement (hypertrophy) of the affected bone. Conversely, the porous nature of the growing metaphysis means that osteomyelitis may also be

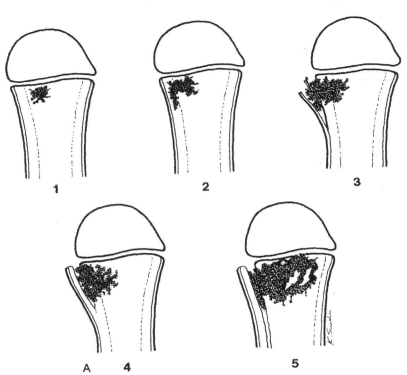

FIGURE 6.5 Pathogenesis of hematogenous osteomyelitis in the child. (1) Infection focused within the medulla at the metaphysis; (2) infection spreads laterally invading the cortex; (3) cortical involvement elevates the periosteal membrane; (4) a shell of new bone begins to form (involucrum); (5) the involucrum increases with continued infection. *From Resnick, D., Kransdorf, M., 2005. Bone and Joint Imaging, third ed. Elsevier Saunders, Philadelphia, p. 171.*

present without the formation of an involucrum or a readily identifiable cloaca, as pus is leached through the bone easily without subsequent vascular pressure and bone necrosis (Turlington, 1970). Overgrowth of the long bone at the site of the infection is stimulated by hypervascularization and has been reported in 21% of child cases (Trueta, 1959). Overgrowth can account for as much as 2 cm growth (Fig. 6.6), although any discrepancy with the unaffected side may be compensated for by angular deformities that reduce the length (Shapiro, 2001), or by premature closure of the epiphysis (Caffey, 1945).

Rasool (2001) reported that 71% of primary osteomyelitic infections occurred at the tibial diaphysis in the 24 child cases he examined and this may be due to the vulnerability of this bone to trauma in the child. The highly vascularized nature of the metaphyses, coupled with small end capillaries at the growth plate, allow for localized infections to take hold (Steinbach, 1966). Secondary hematogenous spread of osteomyelitis is determined by the rate and timing of growth in individual bones, with the knee frequently affected (Ortner, 2003). There is some debate about the protective quality the cartilaginous growth plate affords in preventing the spread of infection from the metaphysis to the epiphysis. When the epiphysis is involved, it is usually the result of a primary focal infection, whereas secondary infections due to a spread from the metaphysis are rare (Shapiro, 2001). While the central portion of the growth plate may act as a barrier, the periphery communicates with the metaphysis, periosteum and surrounding muscles via arterial branches that may facilitate the spread of infection. Abscesses at the epiphyseal and metaphyseal margin are often only visible on X-ray as depressions, that will be difficult to identify in dry bone, particularly if any part of this area is broken postmortem (Ogden, 1979). In the shoulder and hip the metaphysis forms part of the articular surface, allowing for the spread of infection into the joint capsule (Blickman et al., 2004). Such a spread can have serious consequences for the developing child, with septic arthritis, necrosis, and dislocation of the joint and shortening of the limb due to premature epiphyseal fusion all potential complications (Blickman et al., 2004).

Trueta (1959) reported hematogenous osteomyelitis in 7% of infants and 80% of children in the preantibiotic era. Given the low occurrence of osteomyelitis reported in children from archeological contexts, these figures are surprising. Death from septicemia before the disease could become chronic may account for this discrepancy. For example, in their study of hospital records from Portugal between 1923 and 1929, Santos and Suby (2012) reported that 76% of child deaths were attributed to acute osteomyelitis. However, this figure may be artificially high as the children represented the most severe cases in need of a surgical procedure to treat the

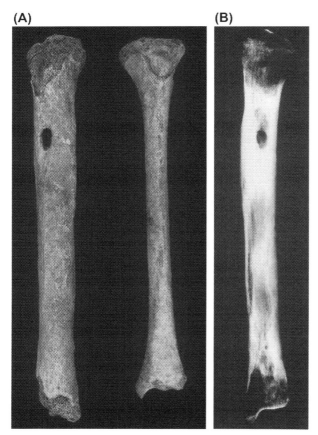

FIGURE 6.6 Chronic osteomyelitis of the right tibia in a 16- to 17-year-old from early medieval Eccles in Kent, England (skeleton L2a). The involucrum (A) covers the whole expanse of the shaft with a large cloaca evident on the anterior aspect. Overgrowth and hypertrophy of the affected bone is clearly evident next to the unaffected side (on the right). (B) On X-ray multiple foci of infection are evident as radiolucent areas.

condition. The only trace of bone lesions reported in these hospital records was in a 12-year-old girl who had an area of radiodensity on the femoral shaft, overlain by a macroscopic layer of periosteal new bone, a subtle involucrum.

Ortner and Hunter (1981) were the first to present a case of multifocal osteomyelitis in a 7-year-old from pre-Columbian Maryland (AD 900–1300). Lytic lesions are evident on the right proximal humerus, both proximal ulnae, one left metacarpal and both tibiae. In some areas the lesion had penetrated the metaphysis and extended into the epiphysis. The left tibia had sustained a fracture and was 1 cm longer than the right. This suggests that the fracture had been open (complex) and the site of the initial infection which then spread hematogenously. The overgrowth was initiated by the highly oxygenated environment that ensued. Ortner (2003) later described three further cases in children aged between 6 and 9 years from different sites in North and Central America. In one case, osteomyelitis is thought to have spread from a dental abscess. In the others, the hyperemia caused by hypervascularity to the infected site had again resulted in overgrowth of the infected bone. Ortner (2003, p. 202) uses the presence of a Harris line in the unaffected bone to estimate that the 9-year-old child from La Oroya in Peru had suffered the condition for at least 4 years before their death. Prior to this, Canci et al. (1991) described probable hematogenous osteomyelitis in a 5-year-old from Bronze Age Toppo Daguzzo in Italy. All the surviving bones were affected, with the fibula showing the most extensive changes with several necrotic areas visible on radiograph. The authors concluded that the fibula was the most probable site of the initial infection, and that the child may have survived for up to 6 months after its spread.

Infantile Osteomyelitis

In the fetal period and early infancy, the metaphysis and epiphysis are linked by transphyseal vessels that travel through the growth plate making secondary and extensive spread of infection more likely (Shapiro, 2001). The ends of the vessels eventually form a loop around 12–18 months ending the link across the growth plate (Fig. 6.7; Stephen et al., 2012). This development provides the clinical differentiation between infantile and child hematogenous osteomyelitis (Trueta, 1959). The clinical features of infantile osteomyelitis include multiple bone involvement, profuse involucrum formation, and joint involvement resulting in growth deformity, disuse atrophy, limb shortening, or dislocation of the joint (Ogden, 1979). The maximum reported amount of shortening is 19 cm (Shapiro, 2001). Septic arthritis is most common in the distal femoral epiphyses in neonates, and in infants affects the hip (Tom Smith's disease), shoulder, or knee (Shapiro, 2001; Smith, 1874). Osteomyelitis may drain spontaneously and heal, but usually death occurs and the mortality rate can be as high as 45% (Trueta, 1959). To date, no cases of nonspecific infantile osteomyelitis have been identified in the archeological record, although several cases of multiple lesions thought to be associated with osteomyelitis in TB, or congenital syphilis have been described in young children.

Brodie's Abscess

Brodie's abscess is a feature of subacute or chronic osteomyelitis and forms either because the infection is not particularly virulent or the individual is relatively healthy (Griffiths, 1987). A Brodie's abscess is common in children especially in boys (Waldron, 2009), and normally forms in the metaphysis of the distal tibia or distal femur. In young children they may appear within the epiphyses. The lesion is typically elongated with a length three to four times greater than its width. On radiograph, this circumscribed lesion is recognized as a translucent area surrounded by a sclerotic margin. There is a lack of sequestra formation, but a channel extending from the metaphysis into what would have been the growth plate may aid in the diagnosis (Resnick and Kransdorf, 2005;

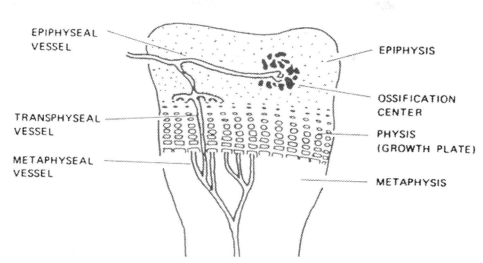

FIGURE 6.7 Diagram showing a transphyseal vessel linking the epiphysis and diaphysis across the growth plate in early infancy, allowing for the spread of infection. *From Stephen, R., Benson, M., Nade, S., 2012. Misconceptions about childhood acute osteomyelitis. Journal of Child Orthopeadics 6, 354.*

Waldron, 2009, p. 718). The affected bone may be slightly enlarged due to periosteal reaction, but the changes can be subtle and may go unnoticed. In more chronic cases, the infection may spread extensively through the bone resulting in osteitis (Steinbach, 1966). In Shapiro's (2001) study of modern Brodie's abscesses, an extension of the infection into the epiphysis did not cause growth problems, even in children under 10 years of age who still had considerable growth yet to be achieved. However, this may be because the infection was treated medically and we cannot know what impact it may have had in the past prior to chemotherapy. When located within the cortex, a differential diagnosis of a Brodie's abscess is an osteoid osteoma, although an osteoma will be typically smaller than 2 cm. Campillo (2006) described a Brodie's abscess of the humerus in a 3-to 4-year old from the late Roman period. A potential case of Brodie's abscess was identified in the distal tibia of a 14-year-old from Barton-on-Humber, England (Fig. 6.8), and at Trinitatas Church, Sweden. The latter case was bilateral and the abscess showed communication between the epiphysis and metaphysis.

Spinal Osteomyelitis

Staphylococcal lesions of the spine are the most common between the ages of 10–15 years as the developing vertebrae are particularly susceptible to infection. Infection from the urinary tract may pass into the spine via the paravertebral venous plexus (Steinbach, 1966) or lumbar infections may track along the psoas muscle to the pelvis. The main consideration when diagnosing this condition is differentiating it from Pott's disease of tuberculosis (TB). Pyogenic osteomyelitis of the spine differs to TB in that it more commonly affects the neural arches, pedicles and processes, and although vertebrae may collapse, they do not produce the

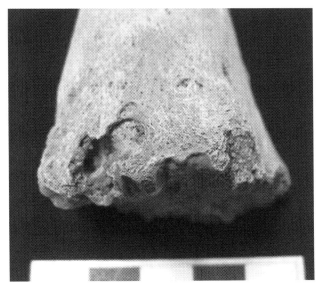

FIGURE 6.8 Possible Brodie's abscess on the lateral anterior aspect of the left tibial metaphysis in a 14-year old from St Peter's Church Barton-on-Humber, England (AD 1300–1700, Skeleton 1010). The lytic lesion is longer than it is wide, and extends towards the growth plate. Note the remodeled base of the lesion. *Photograph taken by P. Verlinden.*

marked gibbus of Pott's disease (Steinbach, 1966). However, not all TB affected spines will result in fusion. Although uncommon, osteomyelitis as the result of typhoid condition is also reported in the spine (Rozansky et al., 1948).

CHRONIC SINUSITIS

New bone formation and ossifications within the paranasal sinuses are indicative of chronic sinusitis as a result of inflammation of the mucous membrane (Rushton et al.,

1994; Tovi et al., 1992). The four paired paranasal sinuses are located in the ethmoid, sphenoid, maxillary, and frontal bones and are air-filled spaces that develop after birth (Allen, 1961). The maxillary sinuses are the largest of these structures. At birth the maxillary antrum appears as a slit-like cavity. The first phase of growth occurs from birth to 3 years of age and the second between 6 and 12 years. In the first phase, growth is horizontal and posterior, while in the second stage growth proceeds inferiorly toward the maxillary dentition. By 3 years the floor of the sinus has reached the area of the hard palate and by 8 years the maxillary sinus has reached 68% of its length and 55% of its height (Alberti, 1976), allowing for visualization and pathological assessment to be carried out in skeletal remains. The frontal sinus reaches almost adult dimensions by 8 years (Fig. 6.9; Maresh, 1940). Early studies on animals have shown that removal of the teeth, birth trauma, or chronic infection within the paranasal sinuses can restrict their development (Maresh, 1940). Potentially, asymmetry of the sinuses may be indicative of early trauma or infection, although, in normal development the maxillary sinuses can vary greatly in size (Maresh, 1940). The internal surface of the sinuses is covered by the mucous membrane that provides communication between the sinuses and the nose. The lining is populated by tiny hairs (cilia) that pulsate at 1000 beats per minute and act like a conveyor belt, removing trapped particulate matter from the sinus and through the sinus opening (ostium) where it is swallowed (Wald, 1985).

In adults, the ostium is elevated from the sinus floor meaning that any blockage of the opening, drying out of the cilia, or swelling of this lining inhibits the function of the cilia and causes a buildup of fluid that may become infected. Trapped bacteria are attacked by white blood cells but are hindered by the low oxygen levels and die, producing exudate that allows the bacteria to thrive and continue to lower the level of oxygen in the sinus (Lundberg and Engquist, 1983).

Maxillary sinusitis in children may be purulent or nonpurulent (dry), acute, or chronic (Wald et al., 1981). Before the age of around 8 years, wide ostia and shallow sinuses mean that they are less likely to retain pus during an infection and the purulent form is rare in this age group (Rachelefsky et al., 1988). The affected child may suffer a persistent cough, wheezing, constant nasal discharge, headaches, and fever, or they may be asymptomatic (DeMuri and Wald, 2012; Wasson, 1932). Although rare, complications of a chronic infection include a subperiosteal abscess of the orbit, an intracranial abscess, meningitis, and subdural empyema (Arruda and Platts-Mills, 1994; DeMuri and Wald, 2012). Sinusitis as a result of upper respiratory tract infections is particularly prevalent, and today is common in children attending nursery school, where close contact with a large number of children allows respiratory infections to be easily transmitted. Clement et al. (1989) diagnosed nasal and sinus infections in 64% of children under the age of 9 years and remaining high at 65% until 14 years. In archeological populations, high rates of respiratory infection have

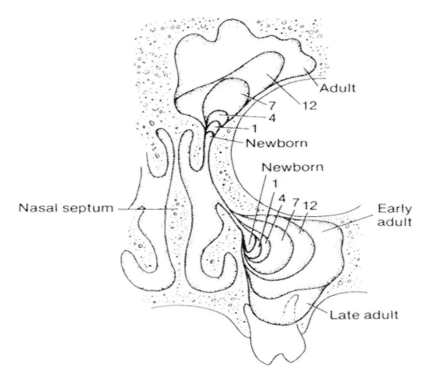

FIGURE 6.9 Development of the frontal (above) and maxillary (below) sinuses. Numbers refer to the ages of development in years.

been linked to chronic exposure to smoke, crowded dwellings, high population density, poor hygiene, and the existence of other respiratory infections (Lewis et al., 1995; Merrett and Pfeiffer, 2000). It is likely that in the past, children would have been equally susceptible to respiratory infections and sinusitis.

The main pathogens associated with sinus infections are *Streptococcus pneumoniae*, *H. influenzae*, and *Moraxella catarrhalis* (Wald et al., 1981). Allergies such as hay fever and asthma are other well recognized contributing factors for the development of acute and chronic sinusitis in children. An allergic mucosa is prone to infection due to a reduced immune function (Corren and Rachelefsky, 1994) and nasal polyps may develop in the lining causing further obstruction and inhibiting drainage of the sinus (Rachelefsky et al., 1988). Acute bacterial sinusitis is known to occur in 80% of modern children after a viral respiratory infection (DeMuri and Wald, 2012), with other predisposing factors including obstruction by a foreign body in the nose (Litton, 1971) or congenital conditions such as cystic fibroses, Gaucher's disease, deviated septum, cleft palate, and Down syndrome (Arruda and Platts-Mills, 1994; Schwartz et al., 1988; Wald, 1985). Infiltration of pathogens into the sinuses in leprosy is well documented (Barton, 1979; Hauhnar et al., 1992) and upper respiratory tract infections such as otitis media, bronchitis, and rhinitis can exacerbate sinus infection. One of the most important factors in the development of chronic sinusitis is their close physical relationship with the maxillary dentition, with larger sinuses allowing protrusion of the molar roots (and more rarely, premolars and canines) into the cavity (Alberti, 1976). These roots may be covered in a bony cap (Ericson and Welander, 1964) and the spread of infection from dental caries or an abscess is a frequent complication. For example in 1928, Berry found 89% of his adult maxillary sinusitis cases were related to the presence of carious and abscessed teeth. There is some debate in the clinical literature about the role of periodontal disease in sinus infections, but this association is considered rare (Dayal et al., 1976; Lane and O'Neal, 1984). In their archeological study, Panhuysen et al. (1997) found a strong correlation between dental disease and the development of maxillary sinusitis. Today, good dental hygiene means that dental disease is rare in the development of childhood sinusitis, but the role of dental disease should be considered in any study of sinusitis in past populations.

Calcified bodies in the mucosa of people with chronic maxillary sinuses was first noted by Ide et al. (1981). These have been interpreted as the "cobweb-like" lesions noted in the sinuses in archeological material, often overlying more recent new bone formation on the sinus wall (Fig. 6.10; Lewis, 2002). In children, the limited size of the developing sinuses until around 8 years makes visualizing any pathology problematic, and developing teeth may prevent the use of the endoscope where the antra are intact. For

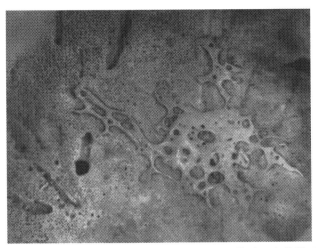

FIGURE 6.10 Cobweb-like lesion on the sinus wall of an individual from Raunds Furnells in Northamptonshire, England (AD 980–1100). The lamellar bone lesion lies over an area of active new bone formation. The structure of the overlying lesions is suggestive of ossified mucous membrane in response to inflammation.

this reason many population-based studies focus only on adults (Roberts, 2007). In other studies, the limited number of children affected or nonadult antra preserved prohibited further study (Panhuysen et al., 1997; Sundman and Kjellström, 2013a,b). Boocock et al. (1995) provide a grading scheme for scoring a variety of lesions found in the sinuses, which was later modified by Merrett and Pfeiffer (2000). The interpretation of large pits on the sinus floor as inflammatory lesions, however, is problematic in nonadult studies. The example provided by Boocock et al. (1995, p. 486, Figure 1) is of an individual aged around 17-year-old whose molars would have just finished developing, but between 6 and 12 years of age, the antra develop inferiorly as they expand to accommodate the developing permanent dentition, and are fed by the palatine nerves (Lewis et al., 1995). For this reason, large pits are not an uncommon feature of dry bone sinuses in children and care should be taken not to over diagnose the condition. Wells (1977) first reported maxillary sinusitis in a 12-year-old from Romano–British Owlesbury, however, the appearance of the large pits at the base of the atrium and the age of child mean that these lesions may be representative of normal growth.

Sundman and Kjellström (2013a) have argued that the bone changes of sinusitis do not have time to develop in a child's remains, but despite this several convincing cases have been identified in the literature. Connell et al. (2012) describe a severe case of bilateral frontal sinusitis in a 12- to 15-year-old from St Mary Spital in London, with draining sinuses on the frontal bone (Fig. 6.11). It was suggested that the adolescent developed the condition as an apprentice working in a poorly ventilated area. Strouhal (1999) describes a 12-year-old from Egypt with a depressed fracture of the frontal bone and a draining sinus leading from the

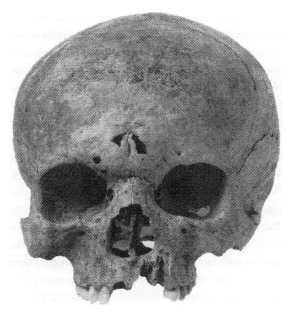

FIGURE 6.11 Frontal sinusitis in a 12- to 17-year-old from St Mary Spital, London (AD 1200–1250, skeleton 3263). *From Connell, B., Gray Jones, A., Redfern, R., Walker, D., 2012. A Bioarchaeological Study of Medieval Burials on the Site of St Mary Spital, Museum of London Archaeology, London, p. 155.*

antrum to the orbit. In adults, air pollution associated with industrial environments provide a popular area of research for archaeologists, beginning with Wells' (1977) study (Lewis et al., 1995; Merrett and Pfeiffer, 2000; Roberts, 2007; Krenz-Niedbała and Lukasik, 2016), although odontogenic sinusitis continues to complicate research into environmental factors (Panhuysen et al., 1997). Today, children are considered more prone to the dual effects of environmental air pollution and more localized parental smoking (Cogswell et al., 1987; Horiuchi et al., 1981; Ross and Fleming, 1994), both factors that may also have affected children in the past with the introduction of tobacco. Merrett and Pfeiffer (2000) examined the sinuses of 93 infants and children from the Uxbridge Ossuary in Ontario (AD 1400), a population exposed to significant air pollution in their homes. They found sinus lesions without evidence for dental infection in 26.7% of nonadults below 12 years, with an increase in sinus infections during adolescence (12–19 years) at 45%. Merrett and Pfeiffer (2000) concluded that respiratory infections were the most prominent cause of childhood sinusitis, with dental disease complicating the picture in adulthood, and that maxillary sinusitis in children and adolescents may be a useful indicator of endemic respiratory distress. Lewis (2002) reported maxillary sinusitis in 9.6% of the sinuses of 0- to 17-year olds from medieval and postmedieval England, and lesions once again showed an increase with age (Fig. 6.12). Eighty percent were free from dental disease. Much higher crude prevalence rates were recorded by Liebe-Harkort (2012) who diagnosed

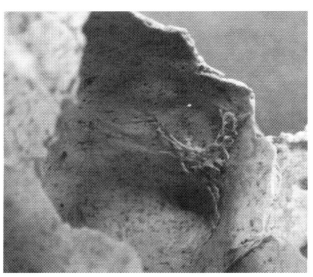

FIGURE 6.12 Spicules indicative of ossification of the mucosa in chronic maxillary sinusitis on the walls of the maxillary antra of an 8- to 10-year-old from later medieval St. Helen-on-the-Walls, York, England (skeleton 5518).

maxillary sinusitis in 45% of 1-to 14-year olds (n = 9/20) from medieval Sweden and identified one case of frontal sinusitis (CPR 25%). Liebe-Harkort (2012) suggests that a compromised immune system may have contributed to the high rates of respiratory infection and that this was also reflected in the large number of deaths under 8 years in the Swedish sample. Previous studies of German children from the Neolithic, Bronze Age, and medieval periods identified a prevalence of frontal sinusitis in 8.3%, 4%, and 16.7%, respectively (Liebe-Harkort, 2012).

OTITIS MEDIA AND MASTOIDITIS

The middle ear comprises the Eustachian tube, tympanic cavity, and ear ossicles. The tympanic cavity is connected to the antrum above the pneumatized cells of the mastoid process. Acute otitis media normally results from the invasion of bacteria via the Eustachian tube into the tympanic cavity, although viral and fungal infections such as herpes and influenza may also be implicated (Flohr and Schultz, 2009). Inflammation of the mucous membrane and changes to the underlying bone structure will often affect both the middle ear (otitis media) and the mastoid process (mastoiditis). Otitis media is primarily a disease of children, usually occurring under the age of 4 years as the result of *S. pneumoniae* or *H. influenzae* infections (Aufderheide and Rodriguez-Martín, 1998; Verhoeff et al., 2006). Infected skin cells in the middle or outer ear (cholesteatoma) block drainage and cause erosion of the ossicles and subsequent mastoiditis (Mays and Holst, 2006). In chronic cases of otitis media, swelling of the Eustachian tube and pus buildup can drain through the tympanic membrane causing new bone formation, lytic lesions and in some cases, fusion (otosclerosis) of the stapes, incus and/or malleus (Dalby et al., 1993). The infection may heal spontaneously or continue to recur into adulthood. Middle ear disease can have serious complications including pain, dizziness, and deafness. The tracking of pus from the middle ear to the brain can result in death of the child. Today, nearly 80% of children experience some form of otitis media before the age of 6 years, making acute and suppurative otitis media one of the most common childhood conditions in the modern world. Recurrent infections result in tinnitus, hearing loss, and meningitis (Verhoeff et al., 2006). The anatomy of the Eustachian tube has been associated with the development of a chronic infection. Children have short horizontal tubes, and the under development of the Eustachian tube in Down syndrome and cleft palate makes these individuals particularly susceptible to chronic infection (Verhoeff et al., 2006). Infections on the mastoid processes, auditory ossicles, and tympanic walls have all been identified in archeological contexts (Flohr et al., 2014), although Flohr et al. (2014) caution against pseudo-new bone formation in the tympanic canal.

Mastoiditis is the leading complication of acute otitis media. It occurs when the infection tracks into the adjoining air cells. In the preantibiotic era, 20% of otitis media cases evolved into mastoiditis (Kiple, 2003), which had a mortality rate of 2 per 100,000 children. Today, 55% cases occur in children under 5 years of age. The child develops swelling and redness behind the ear, headaches, and fever. Complications include meningitis, cerebral abscess, vascular thrombosis, neck abscesses, deafness, and vertigo (Özkaya et al., 2011). In chronic ear disease of childhood, the mucous membrane of the mastoid may lose its ability to proliferate resulting in an asymmetrical, unpneumatized, or hypocellular mastoid process (Flohr and Schultz, 2009). As pneumatization of the mastoid process only occurs before 7 years of age (Scheuer and Black, 2004, p. 84), this method can be used to identify chronic infections in early childhood. In archeological contexts, mastoiditis is recognized as osteoclastic resorption of the pneumatized cells and in older individuals, complete infilling of the cells (density) with reactive new bone formation (Flohr and Schultz, 2009) or, by noting asymmetric mastoid processes. Flohr and Schultz (2009) argue for the more frequent use of endoscopy and scanning electron microscopy to examine temporal bones for these conditions.

Although archeological research into otitis media and mastoiditis has been largely confined to adult skeletal remains, ear ossicles are at their full size in newborns and, with the exception of the incus, do not remodel in life (Scheuer and Black, 2004, p. 84). Hence, any infection in nonadults should be just as evident as in adult skeletal remains, bearing in mind that analysis of otitis media relies on the recovery and curation of these of tiny ear ossicles. Similarly, changes in the mastoid process air cells should be evident from at least 7 years. Cases of these potentially serious conditions in children have mainly been reported as case studies, although a

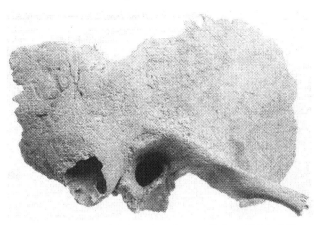

FIGURE 6.13 Mastoiditis in an 8- to 9-year-old from 10th to 14th century Cedynia, Poland (skeleton 1082). The air cells have been completely destroyed by the infection. *From Krenz-Niedbała, M., Lukasik, S., 2016. Skeletal evidence for otitis media in medieval and post-medieval children from Poland, Central Europe. International Journal of Osteoarchaeology. http://dx.doi.org/10.1002/oa.2545, Figure 4.*

few larger scale studies have included nonadults in the analysis (Bruintjes, 1990; Dalby et al., 1993; Krenz-Niedbała and Lukasik, 2016). Campillo (2006) notes otitis media with an internal draining fistula in a 12-year-old from Neolithic Girona in Spain. Tillier et al. (2002) reported on a case of otitis media and mastoiditis in a 13-year-old from Qafzef cave in Israel, with a cloaca in the mastoid process. A possible case of osteomyelitis of the mastoid process was also identified at Chichester, England (Lewis, 2008). Bruintjes (1990) found lytic lesions in 64% of the 28 nonadult ear ossicles he examined (0–20 years) compared to only 47% in the adult group. Three cases of children with otosclerosis have also been identified from archeological sites in England, with the youngest child aged 2 years (Dalby et al., 1993). In a rare large study, Krenz-Niedbała and Lukasik (2016) examined the ossicles and mastoid processes of 99 children from medieval and postmedieval Poland (Figs. 6.13 and 6.14). They provide a grading scheme for scoring bone changes on the ear ossicles. Of 168 ear ossicles, 33.9% showed lesions and prevalence was higher in younger children, and those residing in the urban areas. They noted difficulties in examining the stapes due to its delicate structure and the more common involvement of the incus, especially the long process.

ENDOCRANIAL LESIONS

The presence of blastic endocranial lesions in nonadult skeletal remains has been recorded in many different periods and geographical locations. These features appear as diffuse or isolated layers of new bone on the original cortical surface, expanding around meningeal vessels; as "hair-on-end" extensions of the diploë or, as "capillary" impressions extending into the inner lamina of the cranium. Although commonly found on the occipital bone, outlining

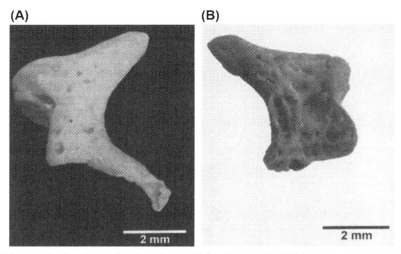

FIGURE 6.14 (A) Porous lesions on the right incus of an 8- to 9-year-old from late medieval Slaboszewo, Poland. The left incus (B) has much more severe changes and additional lesions on the mastoid process indicate the child suffered bilateral otitis media and left sided mastoiditis. *From Krenz-Niedbała, M., Lukasik, S., 2016. Skeletal evidence for otitis media in medieval and post-medieval children from Poland, Central Europe. International Journal of Osteoarchaeology. http://dx.doi.org/10.1002/oa.2545, Figure 5.*

the cruciate eminence, endocranial lesions have also been recorded on the parietal and frontal bones, and appear to follow the areas of venous drainage. The exact etiology of these lesions, however, is still open to debate (Brothwell, 2003; Cecconi et al., 2007; Lewis, 2004). The various expressions are divided into four specific types (Lewis, 2004; Fig. 6.15):

1. Inflammatory pitting
2. Deposits of white or gray fiber bone
3. Capillary formations (new bone organized with/around vascular structures)
4. "Hair-on-end" formation; in some cases, the "hair-on-end" lesions may become "frosted" or thickened and remodeled

The meninges is the term for the three fibrous membrane layers that separate the brain from the cranial vault known as; the dura mater, the arachnoid, and the pia mater. The dura mater is the outermost and thickest of the layers and is continuous with the periosteum lining the vertebral column (Williams and Warwick, 1980). The middle arachnoid layer bridges the sulci on the cortical surface and, as the name suggests, has a "weblike" structure. The innermost layer of the meninges, the pia mater, is the most fragile layer, which turns inward and provides a partition between the brain and the spinal cord (Agur, 1991). Between the dura mater and arachnoid layers is the subdural space into which hemorrhage may occur. Between the arachnoid and pia mater layers is the subarachnoid space, which contains cerebrospinal fluid. Similar to the periosteum, the dura mater has two layers; the outer osteogenic layer closest to the cranial vault and an inner fibrous layer (Fig. 6.16). In the infant, cerebrospinal fluid is absorbed along the dural plexus of the dura mater and enters the venous system, performing the function of arachnoid granulations that only develop in later childhood (Mack et al., 2009). New bone on the endocranial surface would suggest disruption of the venous drainage system, inflammation of the meninges, a tumor or ossification of a subdural hematoma.

Koganei (1912) was the first to describe endocranial lesions and identified pitted and grooved lesions, in addition to "weblike" deposits on the internal surfaces of the frontal, parietal, and occipital bones, which sometimes communicated with the inner diploë. Koganei (1912, p.120–121) found that lesions occurred more often in adults and more commonly on the frontal bone. He even described peeling off a layer of fibrous exudate, superior to a hyperemic dura, to reveal a "rough" skull surface, believed to be the result of a "chronic infection of the skull plates." Nearly seventy years later, Mensforth et al. (1978) described healed and active vascularized "periosteal reactions" on the endocranial surfaces in 645 of the Libben children aged between 11 months and 2 years. They argued against the lesions being extensions of porotic hyperostosis from the ectocranial surface but supported the view that they were the result of an inflammatory reaction. Schultz (1984, 1989, 1993a,b, 1994, 2001) systematically recorded these lesions in a number of nonadult remains throughout Europe, using histological analysis to understand the mechanism behind their appearance. Schultz concluded that "hair-on-end" lesions, described as "calcified plaques on pedicles," represented ossified soft tissue as the result of inflammation, that fiber bone deposits indicated active bleeding of the meninges, and that the vascular or "capillary" type of lesion was suggestive of healing. Hershkovitz et al. (2002) suggested respiratory diseases such as TB caused deep vascular lesions, which they termed "serpens endocranial symmetrica." Others

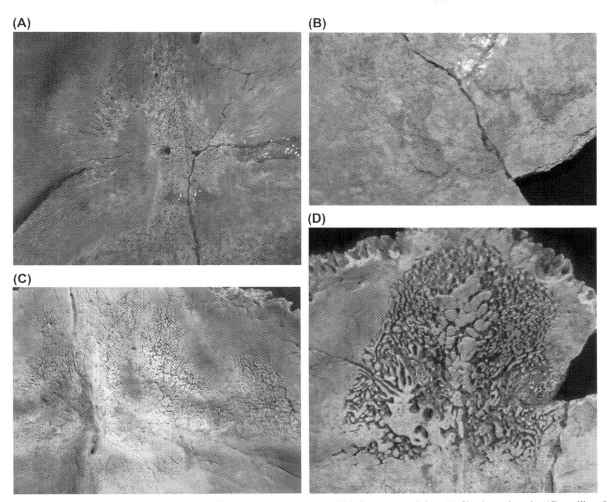

FIGURE 6.15 Different classifications of endocranial lesions in nonadult crania: (A) inflammatory pitting, (B) fiber bone deposits, (C) capillary formations, and (D) "hair-on-end" lesions.

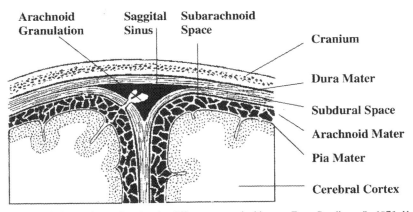

FIGURE 6.16 Coronal section through the meninges showing the different anatomical layers. *From Bradbury, S., 1973. Hewer's Textbook of Histology for Medical Students, Heinemann Medical Books Ltd., London, p. 171.*

have described the appearance of tuberculoid endocranial lesions as isolated lytic "corn-sized" impressions (Jankauskas and Schultz, 1995; Teschler-Nicola, 1997; Teschler-Nicola et al., 1998). Various other etiologies have been suggested for these lesions including chronic meningitis, trauma (epidural hematoma), anemia, neoplasia, scurvy, rickets, lead poisoning, and venous drainage disorders. All may cause inflammation and/or hemorrhage of the meningeal vessels (Griffith, 1919; Kreutz et al., 1995; Patterson, 1993; Schultz, 1993b, 2001).

Meningitis may involve the dura mater (pachymeningitis) or the arachnoid and pia layers (leptomeningitis). Acute leptomeningitis usually produces purulent exudate in the subarachnoid space and cerebral swelling, congestion of the vessels, hemorrhage (McGee et al., 1992, p. 1836), and the ossification of "small-grained, scalelike soft tissue" (Schultz, 1993a, p. 195). Acute leptomeningitis may have killed the child too rapidly for bone lesions to occur in the past, but children with the chronic form of meningitis in the early 20th century were reported to survive for a month or even a year, and often fell into a coma before they died (Griffith, 1919), long enough to produce new bone formation. As pediatric bone is more vascular it responds more readily to hyperemic or inflammatory stimuli and therefore, we are more likely to see changes more quickly than we would expect to in an adult's remains. Meningitis has numerous etiologies, both primary and secondary, but usually results from a bacterial infection in childhood (Rosenthal et al., 1988). Infections may be secondary to otitis media, syphilis, typhoid fever, gastroenteritis, measles, whooping cough, mumps, measles, TB, and pneumonia (Hutchinson and Moncrieff, 1944; Kim-Farley, 1993). TB is the most common cause of chronic leptomeningitis with a spread of infection directly from the petrous portion of the skull or the spine (Cappell and Anderson, 1971, p. 625). While the new bone may result from inflammation of the dura mater in TB, research suggests that lesions are more likely to be small granulomas (cortical foci), similar to arachnoid granulations (Chapter 7). This fits with paleopathological studies that point to corn-sized impressions in dry bone. In congenital syphilis, the base of the skull may be particularly affected, causing hydrocephalus and distension of the scalp veins, and spastic paralysis, mental defects, fits and pituitary disorders can occur (Sheldon, 1943). Cook and Buikstra (1979) identified endocranial lesions in 27% of their Lower Illinois Valley nonadults and found an association between these lesions, periostitis, dental defects, and a lower life expectancy. They suggested meningitis secondary to endemic treponematosis as a causative factor, although these lesions are rarely reported in other paleopathological cases. Examination of the endocranial surface in cases where treponemal disease is suspected will allow this link to be explored more fully.

Subdural hematomas occur from the disruption of delicate bridging veins extending from the surface of the brain to the dura matter, with blood and fluid draining into the sagittal sinus. As blood accumulates within the subdural space, the brain is displaced adding increasing traction to the bridging veins, which hemorrhage with subsequent trauma (Kleinman, 1987). After the bleeding has ceased, the blood clot is surrounded by a fibrous, vascularized membrane, which later becomes detached from the dura, and usually extends bilaterally to the posterior parietal region, or to the floor and anterior/middle cranial fossa (Caffey, 1945).

Occasionally, these hematomas may ossify (Kleinman, 1987). Subdural bleeding is a common and serious outcome in the first 2 years of life as the result of accidental and nonaccidental cranial trauma. In 1974, Caffey described subdural and bilateral intraocular bleeding in habitually shaken babies resulting from whiplash. In the early 20th century, death from an epidural hematoma at childbirth usually occurred in the first 24 hours (Griffith, 1919) and may have resulted from increased and prolonged pressure on the cranium. In 2002, Blondiaux et al. reported successive plaquelike deposits on the endocranial surface of a nonadult from 4th century Normandy suspected of having suffered child abuse. Epidural hematomas usually originate from an arterial source after a cranial fracture, and therefore, are often fatal. However, in cases where there are small bleeds they are recorded as being indistinguishable from subdural hematomas (Kleinman, 1987). Extradural hematomas result from cranial fractures, with subsequent separation of the dura from the cranium up to the connective tissue forming the suture, but may occur without evidence of fracture in children (Cappell and Anderson, 1971). Nevertheless, the presence of any trauma to the cranial vault should be noted when recording endocranial lesions. Schultz (1989) found endocranial lesions in up to 22% of Bronze Age children from five sites in Central Europe and Anatolia and recorded an increase in their frequency between the Bronze Age and medieval period. Schultz (2001) suggested that cranial trauma, resulting in an epidural hematoma and meningitis as a result of hydrocephalus were the cause of these lesions, and that the increase may be the result of population growth and sociopolitical change.

Endocranial new bone formation on the parietal bones, with skull thickening and bony projections along areas of sinus drainage have been noted in cases of vitamin A deficiency (Wolbach and Bessey, 1941); however, it is scurvy as the result of vitamin C deficiency that has received the most attention in endocranial research. Minor trauma to weakened meninges may result in slow hemorrhage stimulating osteoblastic activity and an ossified hematoma (Cecconi et al., 2007). Various other causes have been suggested for endocranial lesions in archaeological contexts. Holliday (1993) found them under a large lytic lesion of the occipital bone in an infant that she ascribed to cradle boarding and Janovic et al. (2012) suggested a neurological cause, with developmental anomalies of the blood vessels irrigating the brain causing tortuous vascular lesions.

Research into the nature and distribution of endocranial lesions suggest that gray fiber bone deposits are very common around the cruciate eminence of infant occipital bones at a time when the skull is undergoing rapid growth. Capillary and "hair-on-end" lesions tend to occur in older children where the lesions are also more widespread, suggesting that perhaps the lesions identified in the younger infants are nonpathological in origin (Lewis, 2004). The fine gray bone located along the cruciate eminence may be the result of continued thickening of the occipital bone in that area. Conversely, Mitchell (2006) states that lesions confined to the occipital bones argues against growth, as growth would result in new bone formation spread evenly across all of the vault bones. Mitchell (2006) identified new bone on the occipital bones in 14% of children younger than 2 years of age at Parvum Geranium in Israel. He suggested that pus or blood inside the skull resulting from trauma or infection would naturally come to rest at the occipital when the children lay on their backs. It is important that we consider the growth mechanisms of the cranial vault when describing these lesions. This includes perinates, where intramembranous ossification of the vault occurs through expansion in a spicular pattern, and it is possible this may still be visible at birth. Until we can differentiate between new bone as the result of growth and deposits caused by pathology we will be limited in our ability to trace infantile disease. We need to be consistent in the way we record the lesions. Recording needs to take into account lesion distribution, type, and the age of individuals affected, in addition to the presence of other skeletal lesions that may suggest a specific pathology.

INFANTILE CORTICAL HYPEROSTOSIS

ICH or Caffey's disease is an uncommon condition and denotes a series of lesions comprising painful swelling of soft tissues, irritability, fever, and massive subperiosteal bone formation (Raza et al., 2011). The specific etiology of ICH is still unknown. Modern cases are thought to result from a latent transplacental viral infection (Caffey, 1945), a genetic defect, hypervitamintosis A, trauma, arterial abnormality, or an allergic reaction of collagen (Resnick and Kransdorf, 2005). The condition has both a familial and sporadic etiology, heals spontaneously, and usually has its onset and resolution in infancy. More recently, a novel collagen mutation (COL1A1) has been implicated in cases of ICH (Cerruti-Mainardi et al., 2011). There is a rare but more severe prenatal form of the condition that appears in the 24th week of intrauterine life causing marked angulations of the long bones and thick deposits of new bone on the shafts, lung hypoplasia, and prematurity (Barba and Freriks, 1953; Hochwald and Osiovich, 2011). Postnatal ICH is known throughout the world, which affects all ancestral groups, and has equal prevalence in boys and girls (Resnick and Kransdorf, 2005). The affected child may suffer from painful pseudoparalysis, pleurisy, and anemia (Resnick and Niwayama, 1988). The condition may persist over several months and manifests as a localized tender lump usually on the mandible, clavicle, or rib (Resnick and Kransdorf, 2005). Lesions may be symmetrical, but in the long bones are often asymmetrical, sparing the epiphyses. New cases are rarely reported after 5 months (Caffey, 1945), but in some instances active cases have continued into the second or third year of life (Swerdloff et al., 1970). Recurring forms of the disease can result in interosseous bridging of the radius and ulna and between the ribs, dislocation of the radial head, mandibular asymmetry, bowing of the tibiae, and other severe deformities (Caffey, 1945; Barba and Freriks, 1953; Blank, 1975). Cases of recurrent ICH have been reported in individuals up to 19 years of age (Keipert and Campbell, 1970; Swerdloff et al., 1970).

As the name suggests, cortical hyperostosis is the hallmark of the disease with bones becoming double or three times their normal width (Resnick and Kransdorf, 2005). In the early stages of the condition, the periosteum becomes thickened and cellular, with the loss of the outer fibrous layer causing it to merge with the surrounding tissues. Osteoid is then deposited around the sheath and into the tissues. Profuse layers of new bone give the shaft a thickened appearance, while the medullary cavity retains its normal proportions. As the condition stabilizes, the periosteum reestablishes its fibrous layer and the new layer of bone becomes incorporated into the original cortex. Remodeling begins from the endosteal surface, causing the medullary cavity to widen and the bones to become more fragile (Caffey, 1945). The skeletal distribution of the condition varies in the clinical literature, with early studies noting lesions on the long bones (Barba and Freriks, 1953), clavicle, scapula (Caffey and Silverman, 1945; Neuhauser, 1970), skull (Neuhauser, 1970), ribs (Barba and Freriks, 1953; Caffey and Silverman, 1945), hands, and feet (Caffey and Silverman, 1945), while later papers cite bone changes on the mandible as being the most common (Blank, 1975; Finsterbush and Husseini, 1979; Swerdloff et al., 1970). Currently, lesions are considered indicative when they appear on the mandible, clavicle, and long bones (Couper et al., 2001). Although rarely fatal, ICH should be explored in cases of infant bones with widespread profuse new bone formation. Congenital syphilis, osteogenesis imperfecta, and hypophosphatasia should be considered as differential diagnoses.

In 1988, Rogers and Waldron reported two probable cases of ICH, one in a Romano–British infant, and the other in a 1-year-old from Anglo-Saxon England. Despite poor preservation, the skeletons exhibited porotic hyperostosis, mandibular lesions, and limited subperiosteal new bone formation. A remarkable 57 cases of ICH were suspected at Roman Poundbury Camp, Dorset, and it was suggested as secondary to recovery from smallpox (Farwell and Molleson, 1993). Reassessment with new diagnostic criteria revealed TB, rickets, scurvy, and thalassemia to be the most likely causes of the various bone changes in these individuals (Lewis, 2010, 2011a,b). Bagousse and Blondiaux (2001) reported on fetal remains from Lisieux in France found within the pelvic area of a female and an infant from same area. Both showed profuse new bone on the surviving long bones, but the infant's tibiae and skull were the most severely affected. The inflammatory pitting of the mandible and an enlarged frontal bone in a Romano–British child from Stanton Field in England led Lewis and Gowland (2009) to suggest a diagnosis of infantile cortical hyperostosis, although scurvy could not be ruled out (Fig. 6.17). Whatever the cause of the lesions, the unusual inhumation of the child in a cremation cemetery and next to a potential spring, suggests special treatment for a child who would have been visibly ill. The confusion surrounding the etiology and manifestation of ICH in the medical literature seems to be reflected in paleopathology, with ICH seemingly used as a "catchall" to describe widespread lesions on an infant's remains. Future research into the skeletal manifestations of the disease is needed. However, the nonfatal nature of the disease means that those children who may have

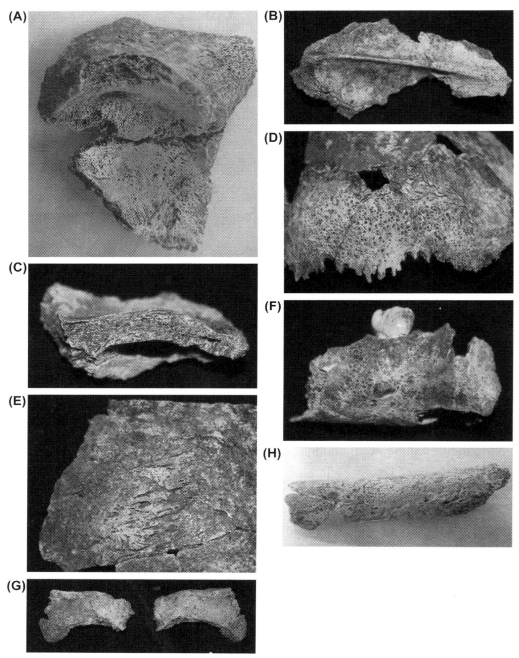

FIGURE 6.17 Possible infantile cortical hyperostosis in a 1.5-year-old from Stanton Field in Bath, England (1st century AD, skeleton 107). There is severe cortical hyperostosis of the (A) orbits and (B) frontal bone with (C) layering of trabecular bone on cross section. The cranial bones exhibit (D) porotic hyperostosis and (E) new bone formation on the ectocranial surface. Inflammatory pitting is present on the (F) mandibular body and (G) greater wings of the sphenoid bone. (H) A thin layer of active new bone is evident on the femoral shaft.

developed the condition could recover completely, leaving no traces of the disease behind.

REFERENCES

Anderson, T., Carter, A.R., 1995. An unusual osteitic reaction in a young medieval child. International Journal of Osteoarchaeology 5, 192–195.

Agur, A.M.G., 1991. Grant's Atlas of Anatomy. Williams & Wilkins, Baltimore.

Alberti, P., 1976. Applied surgical anatomy of the maxillary sinus. Otolaryngologic Clinics of North America 9 (1), 3–20.

Allen, B., 1961. Applied anatomy of paranasal sinuses. Journal of the American Osteopathic Association 60, 978–983.

Anderson, T., Carter, A.R., 1994. Periosteal reaction in a new born child from Sheppey, Kent. International Journal of Osteoarchaeology 4, 47–48.

Arruda, L.K., Platts-Mills, T.A.E., 1994. Sinusitis. Current Opinion in Infectious Diseases 7, 368–373.

Aufderheide, A.C., Rodriguez-Martín, C., 1998. The Cambridge Encyclopedia of Human Paleopathology. Cambridge University Press, Cambridge.

Bagousse, A.-L., Blondiaux, J., 2001. Hyperostoses corticales foetal et infantile à Lisieux (IVe s.): retour à Costebelle. Centre Archaéologique du Var, pp. 60–64.

Barba, W.P., Freriks, D.J., 1953. The familial occurrence of infantile cortical hyperostosis in utero. Journal of Pediatrics 42 (2), 141–150.

Barton, R., 1979. Radiological changes in the paranasal sinuses in lepromatous leprosy. Journal of Laryngology and Otology 93, 597–600.

Berry, G., 1928. Dental caries in paranasal sinus infections. Archives of Otolaryngology 8 (6), 698–706.

Blank, E., 1975. Recurrent Caffey's cortical hyperostosis and persistent deformity. Pediatrics 55 (6), 856–860.

Blickman, J., Van Die, C., De Rooy, J., 2004. Current imaging concepts in pediatric osteomyelitis. European Radiology 14 (4), L55–L64.

Blondiaux, G., Blondiaux, J., Secousse, F., Cotten, A., Danze, P.-M., Flipo, R.-M., 2002. Rickets and child abuse: the case of a two year old girl from the 4th century in Lisieux (Normandy). International Journal of Osteoarchaeology 12 (3), 209–215.

Boocock, P., Roberts, C., Manchester, K., 1995. Maxillary sinusitis in medieval Chichester, England. American Journal of Physical Anthropology 98 (4), 483–496.

Bradbury, S., 1973. Hewer's Textbook of Histology for Medical Students. Heinemann Medical Books Ltd., London.

Brothwell, D., 2003. On the need for a more systematic evaluation of endocranial vault abnormality. Journal of Paleopathology 15 (1), 13–21.

Bruintjes, T., 1990. The auditory ossicles in human skeletal remains from a leper cemetery in Chichester, England. Journal of Archaeological Science 17, 627–633.

Buckley, H., 2000. Subadult health and disease in prehistoric Tonga, Polynesia. American Journal of Physical Anthropology 113, 481–505.

Caffey, J., 1945. Pediatric X-Ray Diagnosis. Year Book Medical Publishers, Inc., Chicago.

Caffey, J., Silverman, W.A., 1945. Infantile cortical hyperostosis. Preliminary report on a new syndrome. American Journal of Roentgenology and Radium Therapy 54 (1), 1–16.

Campillo, D., 2006. Paleoradiology IV: infections. Journal of Paleopathology 18 (1), 21–42.

Canci, A., Tarli, S.M.B., Repetto, E., 1991. Osteomyelitis of probable haematogenous origin in a Bronze age child from Toppo Daguzzo (Basilicata, Southern Italy). International Journal of Osteoarchaeology 1, 135–139.

Cappell, D.F., Anderson, J.R., 1971. Muir's Textbook of Pathology. Edward Arnold, London.

Cecconi, E., Mallegni, F., D'Anastasio, R., 2007. Endocranial lesions in a subadult of the cemetery of San Sebastiano's Church, Saluzzo, Piedmont, Italy (XV century). Journal of Paleopathology 19 (1–3), 11–18.

Cerruti-Mainardi, P., Venturi, G., Spunton, M., Favaron, E., Zignani, M., Provera, S., Dallapiccola, B., 2011. Infantile cortical hyperostosis and COL1A1 mutation in four generations. European Journal of Pediatrics 170, 1385–1390.

Clement, P.A., Bijiloos, J., Kaufman, L., Lauwers, L., Maes, J.J., Van Der Veken, P., Zisis, G., 1989. Incidence and etiology of rhinosinusitis in children. Acta Otorhinolaryngologica 43 (5), 523–543.

Cogswell, J.J., Mitchell, E.B., Alexander, J., 1987. Parental smoking, breast-feeding and allergic respiratory infection in development of allergic diseases. Archives of Diseases in Childhood 62, 338–344.

Connell, B., Gray Jones, A., Redfern, R., Walker, D., 2012. A Bioarchaeological Study of Medieval Burials on the Site of St Mary Spital. Museum of London Archaeology, London.

Cook, D.C., Buikstra, J.E., 1979. Health and differential survival in prehistoric populations: prenatal dental defects. American Journal of Physical Anthropology 51, 649–664.

Corren, J., Rachelefsky, G., 1994. Interrelationship between sinusitis and asthma. Immunology and Allergy Clinics of North America 14 (1), 171–184.

Couper, R., McPhee, A., Morris, L., 2001. Imomethacin treatment of infantile cortical periostosis in twins. Journal of Paediatrics and Child Health 37, 305–308.

Dalby, G., Manchester, K., Roberts, C.A., 1993. Otosclerosis and stapedial footplate fixation in archaeological material. International Journal of Osteoarchaeology 3, 207–212.

Dayal, V., Jones, J., Noyek, A., 1976. Management of odontogenic maxillary sinus disease. Otolaryngologic Clinics of North America 9 (1), 213–222.

De Silva, P., Evans-Jones, G., Wright, A., Henderson, R., 2003. Physiological periostitis; a potential pitfall. Archives of Diseases in Childhood 88, 1124–1125.

DeMuri, G., Wald, E., 2012. Acute bacterial sinusitis in children. The New England Journal of Medicine 367 (12), 1128–1134.

East, A., 2003. Normal periosteal bone growth and skeletal pathology in documented fetuses, University of New Mexico, Maxwell Museum documented collection and University of Tennessee documented collection. American Journal of Physical Anthropology 32, 115.

Ericson, S., Welander, U., 1964. Sinographic examination of the maxillary sinus in cases of chronic periapical osteitis. Ofentologisk Tidskrift 72, 119–131.

Farwell, D.E., Molleson, T.I., 1993. Excavations at Poundbury 1966-80 Volume II: The Cemeteries. Dorset Natural History and Archaeological Society, Dorset.

Finsterbush, A., Husseini, N., 1979. Infantile cortical hyperostosis with unusual clinical manifestations. Clinical Orthopaedics and Related Research 144, 276–279.

Flohr, S., Kerdorf, U., Jankaukas, R., Puschel, B., 2014. Diagnosis of stapedial footplate fixation in archaeological human remains. International Journal of Palaeopathology 6, 10–19.

Flohr, S., Schultz, M., 2009. Mastoiditis – paleopathological evidence of a rarely reported disease. American Journal of Physical Anthropology 138 (3), 266–273.

Gleser, K., 1949. Double contour, cupping and spurring in roentgenograms of long bones in infants. American Journal of Roentgenology and Radium Therapy 61 (4), 482–492.

Griffith, J., 1919. The Diseases of Infants and Children. W.B. Saunders and Company, London.

Griffiths, H.J., 1987. Basic Bone Radiology. Appleton-Century, Norwalk, USA.

Gumber, P., Sharma, A., Sharma, K., Gupta, S., Bhardwaj, B., Jakhar, K.K., 2016. Garre's sclerosing osteomyelitis – a case report. Journal of Advanced Medical and Dental Sciences Research 4 (2), 78.

Harisinghani, M.G., McLoud, T.C., Shepard, J., Ko, J.P., Shroff, M.M., Mueller, P.R., 2000. Tuberculosis from head to toe 1. Radiographics 20 (2), 449–470.

Hauhnar, C.Z., Mann, S., Sharma, V.K., Kaur, S., Mehta, S., Radotra, B., 1992. Maxillary antrum involvement in multibacillary leprosy: a radiologic, sinuscopic, and histologic assessment. International Journal of Leprosy and Other Mycobacterial Diseases 60, 390–395.

Hershkovitz, I., Greenwald, C., Latimer, B., Jellema, S.-B., Eshed, V., Dutour, O., Rothschild, B., 2002. Serpens Endocrania Symmetrica (SES): a new term and a possible clue for identifying intrathoracic diseases in skeletal populations. American Journal of Physical Anthropology 118 (3), 201–216.

Hochwald, O., Osiovich, H., 2011. Prenatal Caffey disease. Israel Medical Association Journal 13, 113–114.

Holliday, D., 1993. Occipital lesions: a possible cost of cradleboards. American Journal of Physical Anthropology 90, 283–290.

Horiuchi, H., Kaneko, S., Endo, T., 1981. An epidemiological study of the relationship between air pollution and nasal allergy. Rhinology 1, 161–167.

Hutchinson, R., Moncrieff, A., 1944. Lectures on Diseases of Children. Edward Arnold and Co., London.

Ide, F., Sano, R., Shimura, H., Miyata, G., Kusuhara, S., Ohnuma, H., Miyake, T., Nakajima, T., 1981. Unusual calcified bodies in the submucosal connective tissue of the maxillary sinus. The Journal of Nihon University School of Dentistry 23 (4), 188–194.

Jankauskas, R., Schultz, M., 1995. Meningeal reactions in a late medieval-early modern child population from Alytus, Lithuania. Journal of Paleopathology 7 (2), 106.

Janovic, A., Milovanovic, P., Sopta, J., Rakocevic, Z., Filipovic, V., Nenezic, D., Djuric, M., 2012. Intracranial arteriovenous malformations as a possible cause of endocranial bone lesions and associated neurological disorder. International Journal of Osteoarchaeology 25 (1), 88–97.

Keipert, J.A., Campbell, P.E., 1970. Recurrent hyperostosis of the clavicles: an undiagnosed syndrome. Australian Paediatric Journal 6, 97–104.

Kim-Farley, R.J., 1993. Mumps. In: Kiple, K. (Ed.), The Cambridge World History of Human Disease. Cambridge University Press, Cambridge, pp. 887–889.

Kiple, K. (Ed.), 2003. The Cambridge Historical Dictionary of Disease. Cambridge University Press, Cambridge.

Kleinman, P., 1987. Skeletal trauma: general considerations. In: Kleinman, P. (Ed.), Diagnostic Imaging of Child Abuse, second ed. Williams and Wilkins, Baltimore, pp. 5–27.

Koganei, H., 1912. Cribra cranii und cribra orbitalia. Mitt Med Fak Toyko 10, 113–154.

Krenz-Niedbała, M., Lukasik, S., 2016. Skeletal evidence for otitis media in medieval and post-medieval children from Poland, Central Europe. International Journal of Osteoarchaeology. http://dx.doi.org/10.1002/oa.2545.

Kreutz, K., Teichmann, G., Schultz, M., 1995. Palaeoepidemiology of inflammatory processes of the skull: a comparative study of two early medieval infant populations. Journal of Paleopathology 7 (2), 108.

Lane, J., O'Neal, R., 1984. The relationship between periodontitis and the maxillary sinus. Journal of Periodontology 55 (8), 477–481.

Lew, D.P., Waldvogel, F.A., 2004. Osteomyelitis. Lancet 364 (9431), 369–379.

Lewis, M., 2000. Non-adult palaeopathology: current status and future potential. In: Cox, M., Mays, S. (Eds.), Human Osteology in Archaeology and Forensic Science. Greenwich Medical Media Ltd., London, pp. 39–57.

Lewis, M., 2002. Urbanisation and Child Health in Medieval and Post-medieval England: An Assessment of the Morbidity and Mortality of Non-adult Skeletons from the Cemeteries of Two Urban and Two Rural Sites in England (AD 850–1859). British Archaeological Research Report 339, Archaeopress, Oxford.

Lewis, M., 2004. Endocranial lesions in non-adult skeletons: understanding their aetiology. International Journal of Osteoarchaeology 14, 82–97.

Lewis, M., 2008. The children. In: Magilton, J., Lee, F., Boylston, A. (Eds.). Magilton, J., Lee, F., Boylston, A. (Eds.), Chichester Excavations 'Lepers Outside the Gate' Excavations at the Cemetery of the Hospital of St James and St Mary Magdalene, Chichester, 1986-87 and 1993, vol. 10. Council for British Archaeology, York, pp. 174–186. Research Report, 158.

Lewis, M., 2010. Life and death in a Civitas Capital: metabolic disease and trauma in the children from late Roman Dorchester. Dorset. American Journal of Physical Anthropology 142, 405–416.

Lewis, M., 2011a. Thalassaemia: its diagnosis and interpretation in past skeletal populations. International Journal of Osteoarchaeology 21 (2), 685–693.

Lewis, M., 2011b. Tuberculosis in the non-adults from Romano-British Poundbury Camp, Dorset, England. International Journal of Paleopathology 1 (1), 12–23.

Lewis, M., 2014. Sticks and stones: exploring the nature and significance of child trauma in the past. In: Knusel, C., Smith, M. (Eds.), The Routledge Handbook of the Bioarchaeology of Human Conflict. Routledge, London, pp. 39–63.

Lewis, M., Gowland, R., 2009. Infantile Cortical Hyperostosis: cases, causes and contridictions. In: Lewis, M., Clegg, M. (Eds.), Proceedings of the Ninth Annual Conference of the British Association for Biological Anthropology and Osteoarchaeology. BAR International Series 1981, Archaeopress, Oxford, pp. 43–51.

Lewis, M., Roberts, C.A., Manchester, K., 1995. Comparative study of the prevalence of maxillary sinusitis in later medieval urban and rural populations in northern England. American Journal of Physical Anthropology 98 (4), 497–506.

Liebe-Harkort, C., 2012. Cribra orbitalia, sinusitis and linear enamel hypoplasia in Swedish Roman Iron Age adults and subadults. International Journal of Osteoarchaeology 22, 387–397.

Litton, W., 1971. Acute and chronic sinusitis. Otolaryngologic Clinics of North America 4 (1), 25–37.

Lundberg, C., Engquist, S., 1983. Pathogenesis of maxillary sinusitis. Scandinavian Journal of Infectious Disease 39, 53–55.

Mack, J., Squier, W., Eastman, J.T., 2009. Anatomy and development of the meninges: implications for subdural collections and CSF circulation. Pediatric Radiology 39 (3), 200–210.

Maresh, M.M., 1940. Paranasal sinuses from birth to adolescence. American Journal of Diseses in Children 60, 55–78.

Mays, S., Holst, M., 2006. Palaeo-otology of cholesteaoma. International Journal of Osteoarchaeology 16, 1–15.

McGee, J.D., Isaacson, P., Wright, N., 1992. Oxford Textbook of Pathology. Oxford University Press, Oxford.

Mensforth, R.P., Lovejoy, O.C., Lallo, J.W., Armelagos, G.J., 1978. The role of constitutional factors, diet and infectious disease in the etiology of porotic hyperostosis and periosteal reactions in prehistoric infants and children. Medical Anthropology 2 (1), 1–59.

Merrett, D.C., Pfeiffer, S., 2000. Maxillary sinusitis as an indicator of respiratory health in past populations. American Journal of Physical Anthropology 111 (3), 301–318.

Mitchell, P., 2006. Child health in the Crusader period inhabitants of Tel Jezreel, Israel. Levant 38, 37–44.

Neuhauser, E.B.D., 1970. Infantile cortical hyperostosis and skull defects. Postgraduate Medicine 48 (6), 57–59.

Ogden, J., 1979. Pediatric osteomyeltitis and septic arthritis: the pathology of neonatal disease. The Yale Journal of Biology and Medicine 52, 423–448.

Ortner, D., 2003. Identification of Pathological Conditions in Human Skeletal Remains. Academic Press, New York.

Ortner, D.J., Hunter, S., 1981. Hematogenous osteomyelitis in a Precolumbian child's skeleton from Maryland. Museum Applied Science Center for Archaeology 1 (8), 236–238.

Özkaya, H., Akcan, A., Aydemir, G., 2011. Mastoiditis in childhood: review of the literature. African Journal of Microbiology Research 5 (33), 5998–6003.

Panhuysen, R.G.A., Coenen, V., Bruintjes, T.D., 1997. Chronic maxillary sinusitis in medieval Maastricht, The Netherlands. International Journal of Osteoarchaeology 7, 610–614.

Patterson, K.D., 1993. Meningitis. In: Kiple, K. (Ed.), The Cambridge World History of Human Disease. Cambridge University Press, Cambridge, pp. 875–880.

Rachelefsky, G.S., Katz, R.M., Siegel, S.C., 1988. Chronic sinusitis in the allergic child. Pediatric Clinics of North America 35 (5), 1091–1101.

Rasool, M., 2001. Primary subacute haematogenous osteomyelitis in children. The Journal of Bone and Joint Surgery. British Volume 83 (1), 93–98.

Raza, A., Ijaz, I., Naz, F., Butt, T., 2011. Caffey's disease in an infant. Journal of the College of Physicians and Surgeons Pakistan 21 (10), 634–636.

Resnick, D., Kransdorf, M., 2005. Bone and Joint Imaging, Elsevier Saunders, Philadelphia.

Resnick, D., Niwayama, D. (Eds.), 1988. Diagnosis of Bone and Joint Disorders, W.B. Saunders Company, Philadelphia.

Roberts, C., 2007. A bioarchaeological study of maxillary sinusitis. American Journal of Physical Anthropology 133 (2), 792–807.

Rogers, J., Waldron, T., 1988. Two possible cases of infantile cortical hyperostosis. Paleopathology Newsletter 63, 9–12.

Rosenthal, J., Dagan, R., Press, J., Sofer, S., 1988. Differences in the epidemiology of childhood community-acquired bacterial meningitis between two ethnic populations cohabiting in one geographical area. Paediatric Infectious Disease Journal 7 (9), 630–633.

Ross, A.M., Fleming, D.M., 1994. Incidence of allergic rhinitis in general practice. British Medical Journal 308, 897–900.

Rozansky, R., Ehrenfeld, E.N., Matoth, Y., 1948. Paratyphoid osteomyelitis: report of two cases. British Medical Journal 2, 297–298.

Rushton, V., Theaker, E., Whitehouse, R., Taylor, P., 1994. Radiological appearance of clinical inflammatory sinus disease with bone destruction. The significance of contrast enhancement. Dentomaxillofacial Radiology 23, 33–36.

Santos, A., Suby, J., 2012. Skeletal and surgical evidence for acute osteomyelitis in non-adult individuals. International Journal of Osteoarchaeology 25 (1), 110–118.

Scheuer, L., Black, S., 2004. The Juvenile Skeleton. Elsevier, London.

Schmit, P., Glorion, C., 2004. Osteomyelitis in infants and children. European Radiology 14, 44–54.

Schultz, M., 1984. The diseases in a series of children's skeletons from Ikiz Tepe, Turkey. In: Capecchi, V., Rabino Massa, E. (Eds.), Proceedings of the Fifth European Meeting of the Paleopathology Association, Siena, Italy. Tipografia Senese, Siena, pp. 321–325.

Schultz, M., 1989. Causes and frequency of diseases during early childhood in Bronze Age populations. In: Capasso, L. (Ed.), Advances in Palaeopathology. Marino Solfanelli Editore, Chieti, pp. 175–179.

Schultz, M., 1993a. Initial stages of systemic bone disease. In: Grupe, G., Garland, A.N. (Eds.), Histology of Ancient Human Bone: Methods and Diagnosis. Springer-Verlag New York Inc., New York, pp. 185–203.

Schultz, M., 1993b. Vestiges of Non-specific Inflammation in Prehistoric and Historic Skulls: A Contribution to Palaeopathology. Anthropolggische Beitrage, Aesch.

Schultz, M., 1994. Comparative histopathology of syphilitic lesions in prehistoric and historic human bones. In: Dutour, O., Palfi, G. (Eds.), The Origin of Syphilis in Europe: Before of After 1493?. Universite de Provence, France, pp. 63–67.

Schultz, M., 2001. Palaeohistopathology of bone: a new approach to the study of ancient diseases. Yearbook of Physical Anthropology 44, 106–147.

Schwartz, M., Weycer, J., McGavran, M., 1988. Gaucher's disease involving the maxillary sinuses. Archives of Otolaryngology Head and Neck Surgery 114 (2), 203–206.

Shapiro, F., 2001. Pediatric Orthopedic Deformities: Basic Science, Diagnosis and Treatment. Academic Press, New York.

Sheldon, W., 1943. Diseases of Infancy and Childhood. J. & A. Churchill Ltd., London.

Shopfner, C.E., 1966. Periosteal bone growth in normal infants. A Preliminary Report 97 (1), 154–163.

Smith, T., 1874. On the Acute Arthritis of Infants. St Bartholomew's Hospital Reports, vol. 10, pp. 189–204.

Steinbach, H., 1966. Infections in bones. Seminars in Roentgenology 1 (4), 337–369.

Stephen, R., Benson, M., Nade, S., 2012. Misconceptions about childhood acute osteomyelitis. Journal of Child Orthopeadics 6, 353–356.

Strouhal, E., 1999. Ancient Egypt and tuberculosis. In: Palfi, G., Dutour, O.Deak, O. (Eds.), Tuberculosis: Past and Present. Golden Book Publishers, Hungary, pp. 453–460.

Styczyński, J., Biliński, P., Lasek, W., Gajewska-Guryn, A., Wysocki, M., Balcar-Boroń, A., 2002. Garré type periostitis ossificans: effective antibiotic therapy case report and literature review. Clinical Practice Review 3 (1), 46–50.

Sundman, E., Kjellström, A., 2013a. Chronic maxillary sinusitis in medieval Sigtuna, Sweden: a study of sinus health and effects on bone preservation. International Journal of Osteoarchaeology 23, 447–458.

Sundman, E., Kjellström, A., 2013b. Signs of sinusitis in times of urbanisation in Viking age early medieval Sweden. Journal of Archaeological Science 40, 4457–4465.

Swerdloff, B.A., Ozonoff, M.B., Gyepes, M.T., 1970. Late recurrence of infantile cortical hyperostosis (Caffey's disease). American Journal of Roentgenology 108, 461–467.

Teschler-Nicola, M., 1997. Differential diagnosis of tuberculosis: the diagnostic value of endocranial features. In: ICEPT Proceedings of the Evolution and Palaeoepidemiology of Tuberculosis. Tuberculosis Foundation, Szegred.

Teschler-Nicola, M., Gerold, F., Prodinger, W., 1998. Endocranial features in tuberculosis. In: Twelfth European Meeting of the Paleopathology Association, p. 92 Prague.

Tillier, A., Arensburg, B., Duday, H., 2002. The Qafzeh 11 adolescent: a case of otitis media in the Levantine Middle Paleolithic. In: 14th European Meeting of the Paleopathology Association, Coimbra, 28-31 August, 2002. Universidade de Coimbra. Departamento de Antropologia, Coimbra, Portugal.

Tovi, F., Benharroch, D., Gatot, A., Hertzanu, Y., 1992. Osteoblastic osteitis of the maxillary sinus. The Laryngoscope 102, 426–430.

Trueta, J., 1959. The three types of haematogenous osteomyelitis. Journal of Bone and Joint Surgery 41B, 671–680.

Turlington, E.G., 1970. Chronic sclerosing nonsuppurative osteomyelitis. Transactions of the Fourth International Conference of Oral Surgery 120–124.

Ulijaszek, S.J., 1990. Nutritional status and susceptibility to infectious disease. In: Harrison, G.A., Waterlow, J.C. (Eds.), Diet and Disease in Traditional and Developing Societies. Cambridge University Press, Cambridge, pp. 137–154.

Verhoeff, M., van der Veen, E., Rovers, M., Sanders, E., Schilder, A., 2006. Chronic suppurative otitis media: a review. International Journal of Otorhinolaryngology 70, 1–12.

Wald, E.R., 1985. Epidemiology, pathophysiology and etiology of sinusitis. Pediatric Infectious Disease 4 (6), 51–54.

Wald, E.R., Milmoe, G.J., Ad, B., Ledesma-Medina, J., Salamon, N., Bluestone, C.D., 1981. Acute maxillary sinusitis in children. The New England Journal of Medicine 304 (13), 749–754.

Waldron, T., 2009. Palaeopathology. Cambridge University Press, Cambridge.

Walker, P.L., 1997. Skeletal evidence for child abuse: a physical anthropological perspective. Journal of Forensic Sciences 42 (2), 196–207.

Wasson, V., 1932. Sinusitis in childhood. Archives of Disease in Childhood 7, 277–286.

Wells, C., 1977. Disease of the maxillary sinus in antiquity. Medical and Biological Illustration 27, 173–178.

Weston, D., 2008. Investigating the specificity of periosteal reactions in pathology museum specimens. American Journal of Physical Anthropology 137 (1), 48–59.

Weston, D., 2012. Nonspecific infection in paleopathology. In: Grauer, A. (Ed.), A Companion to Paleopathology. Wiley Blackwell, Chichester, pp. 492–512.

Weston, D.A., 2009. Brief communication: paleohistopathological analysis of pathology museum specimens: can periosteal reaction microstructure explain lesion etiology? American Journal of Physical Anthropology 140 (1), 186–193.

Williams, P.L., Warwick, R., 1980. Gray's Anatomy. Churchill Livingston, Edinburgh.

Wolbach, S., Bessey, O.A., 1941. Vitamin A deficiency and the nervous system. Archives of Pathology 32, 689.

Chapter 7

Infectious Diseases II: Infections of Specific Origin

Chapter Outline

Smallpox (Osteomyelitis Variolosa)	151	Rhinomaxillary Syndrome	167
Rubella	152	Dentition	167
Poliomyelitis	153	Hands and Feet	169
Tuberculosis	155	Periostitis and Osteomyelitis	170
Cranium	156	Paleopathology	171
Mandible	158	Treponemal Diseases	172
Scapula	158	Yaws	175
Spine	158	Endemic Syphilis (Bejel, Treponarid)	176
Ribs	160	Congenital Syphilis	176
Joints	160	Early Onset Congenital Syphilis	178
Long Bones	161	Late Onset Congenital Syphilis	179
Hands and Feet	162	Dentition	179
Paleopathology	162	Paleopathology	182
Leprosy	164	References	185
Infantile Leprosy	164		
Pathogenesis in Children	166		
Nerve Damage	167		
Skeletal Manifestations	167		

SMALLPOX (OSTEOMYELITIS VARIOLOSA)

Smallpox is caused by the variola virus and comes in two forms: variola major that has a 25%–30% mortality rate and variola minor with fewer and less serious clinical signs and a death rate of 1% (Crosby, 2003). Symptoms of smallpox include high fever, headache, back and muscle pain and in children, convulsions and vomiting (Bancroft, 1904). Survivors of the infection develop long-term immunity, therefore smallpox requires highly populated areas with a ready supply of unexposed hosts. In smallpox endemic areas these are usually infants and children (Crosby, 2003). Osteomyelitis variolosa was coined by Chiari (1893) to describe the lesions he saw in a smallpox outbreak in Prague during 1891. It commonly affects the elbows (80%), the wrists (20%), and ankles (18%) and in 50% of cases affects multiple sites (Cockshott and MacGregor, 1959; Jackes, 1983). Bancroft (1904, p. 333) noted purulent inflammation of the elbow joint in the third week of the disease in two children from his large sample of 1200 cases from Boston during the 1902 epidemic. Davidson and Palmer (1963) reviewed 82 cases of smallpox in children aged between 9 months and 14 years and indicated that 2%–5% of children would develop osteomyelitis variolosa. It occurred more frequently in the mild form developing 5–28 days after infection. Davidson and Palmer (1963) described osteomyelitis variolosa as different to the phyogenic form of osteomyelitis. The earliest stage of infection is a radiolucent band caused by destruction of the metaphysis, followed by displacement of the epiphysis and a sheath of periosteal new bone often extending along the whole diaphyseal length (Fig. 7.1). This bone formation was described as gross and florid with irregular thickness along the length of the shaft that appeared to have been "dipped in a thick creamy paint" (Davidson and Palmer, 1963, p. 690). Clinically, smallpox is considered the underlying cause of osteomyelitis when the elbows are affected symmetrically, and when all three bones of the elbow are involved or, if there is bilateral involvement of the ankle (distal tibia and fibula). Ankylosis of the affected joints is common, with premature fusion and destruction of the epiphyses causing shortening of the affected limb, arthritis, and deformation due to weight bearing (Davidson and Palmer, 1963; Musgrave et al., 1913; Silverman, 1976).

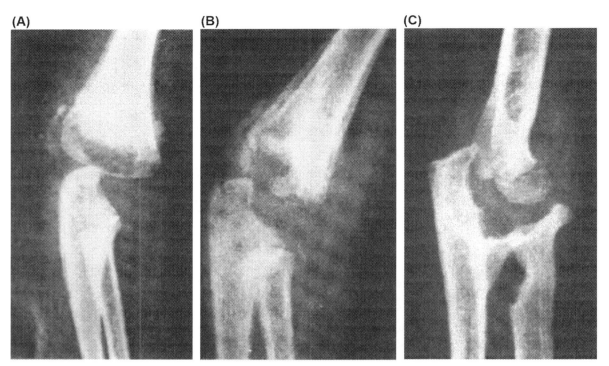

FIGURE 7.1 Changes to the elbow in osteomyelitis variolosa. (A) In the acute stage, (B) 3 weeks after infection there is periosteal new bone formation and destruction of the joint, and (C) flail joint changes are apparent after 2 years. *From Cockshott, W.P., Osteomyelitis Variolosa. Zeitschrift fur Tropenmedizin und Parasitologie 1965, Vol. 16, No. 2, pp. 199-206 ref.15.*

There is some suggestion that smallpox was present in ancient Egypt and was responsible for some of the pandemics that swept the Roman Empire in the 2nd–3rd century AD. But descriptions of the infection are not definitive. Smallpox is thought to have spread from the Old to the New World in the 1500s carried by European invaders (Crosby, 2003). A virulent strain of the disease was reported between the 17th and 18th century causing a rise in fatal cases with one in five people believed to have suffered from it in the United Kingdom (Duncan et al., 1993). Eighty percent of these victims were less than 10 years old (Crosby, 2003). Given the likelihood of children surviving variola minor in the past, it is possible some cases of osteomyelitis in nonadult skeletons are due to this disease. The earliest paleopathological case of possible smallpox was reported by Darton et al. (2013). They describe a 15- to 17-year-old from medieval Aube, France, with bilateral changes to the elbows. There was ankylosis of the right elbow, while the left had an enlarged olecranon and destruction of the radius and distal humerus. These lesions are strikingly similar to those illustrated by Silverman (1976) (Fig. 7.2). The authors argue that the bilateral expression of the disease makes tuberculosis (TB) or pyogenic osteomyelitis a less likely diagnosis. In 18th-century London, a 4-year-old displayed bilateral osteomyelitis of the distal humeri with destruction of the joint surfaces and a cloak of periosteal new bone. The child was recovered from a mass grave, possibly relating to a smallpox epidemic (Miles et al., 2008). In the New World, Ortner (2003, p. 336) reported bilateral osteomyelitis of the elbows in a 12-year-old from 18th-century Alaska considered to be osteomyelitis variolosa. The child also displayed a frontal lesion that Ortner suggests was related to skin lesions. Smallpox had been introduced to Alaska by Russian merchants.

RUBELLA

Congenital rubella, resulting from a spread of the rubella virus from an infected mother in the first trimester, would have had serious consequences for the survival of a newborn in the past. The main outcome of this infection is a spontaneous abortion or stillbirth, and these young perinates are likely to enter the archeological record without any pathological changes that would point to the cause of their death. Live born babies suffer congestive heart failure, low birth weight, and difficulty in feeding (Cooper et al., 1969) affecting their long-term survival. Interestingly, Rudolf et al. (1965) reported that 45.3% of perinates with exposure to maternal rubella displayed bone lesions between the ages of 1 and 8 weeks after birth. These were described as wide radiolucent bands, and "beaklike projections" at the metaphyseal ends of the long bones during healing, coupled with enlarged anterior fontanelles (Rudolf et al., 1965, p. 430). Periosteal new bone is rare in rubella. Blickman et al. (2004) describe a "celery-stalk" appearance to the shaft with widening at the metaphyseal ends and longitudinal

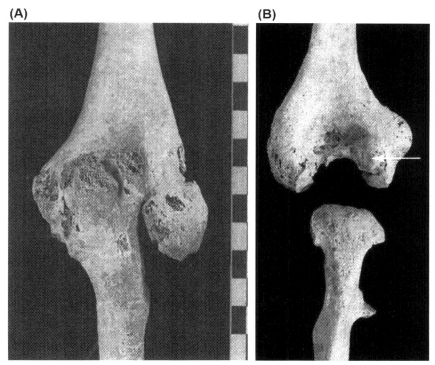

FIGURE 7.2 Possible osteomyelitis variolosa in the (A) left and (B) right elbows of an adolescent from Aube, France (AD 1022–1155, skeleton 833). The arrow indicates destructive changes to the joint surface on the humerus. *From Darton, Y., Richard, I., Truc, M.-C., 2013. Osteomyelitis variolosa: a probable medievel case combined with unilateral sacroilitis. International Journal of Paleopathology 3, 289, 291.*

thickened bands running from the midshaft to the metaphysis, most commonly at the knee (Fig. 7.3). These lesions are similar to those seen in osteopathia striata (Chapter 11). Reed (1969) identified the cause of the bands as a disruption in the proliferation of fibroblasts and osteoblasts as a direct effect of the rubella virus. Rubella's capacity to inhibit cell multiplication had already been noted in other organs of the body (Naeye and Blanc, 1965). These poorly defined zones of calcification on radiograph are similar to those caused by active rickets or congenital syphilis, meaning they may be misdiagnosed. Once virus excretion has ceased, bone lesions can disappear in several months (Sekeles and Ornoy, 1974). Children who survive the infection often suffer long-term consequences such as deafness and cerebral palsy (Cooper et al., 1969). A follow-up study of 376 children born to mothers during the rubella epidemic in New York in 1964 showed 252 were deaf, 182 had heart disease, 46 developed cerebral palsy, and 85 children had died by the age of 4 years (Cooper et al., 1969).

Three perinates aged between 3 and 6 months were identified with unusually large fontanelles in South Africa dating to the 20th century, leading Steyn et al. (2002) to suggest rubella as a possible differential diagnosis. There were no postcranial changes. Although rubella lesions are rare and transient in the perinatal period, it should be considered as a cause of perinatal mortality, and as a differential diagnosis in early rickets cases.

POLIOMYELITIS

Polio is caused by a ribonucleic acid enterovirus spread via the fecal–oral route. Women who contract poliomyelitis during the first trimester are at risk of a miscarriage or may transmit the disease to the child during childbirth (Siegal and Greenberg, 1956). The virus replicates in the throat and intestinal tract before invading the lymphatic system and bloodstream (Waldron, 2009). In the majority of cases, the disease is asymptomatic, or it causes mild flulike symptoms that resolve quickly. In 1% of cases the virus enters the central nervous system destroying the motor nerve cells causing paralysis. Polio meningitis and hydrocephalus are also likely outcomes of central nervous system involvement in children. Writing in 1943, Sheldon reported polio to be most common in children aged 2–5 years with the majority of cases occurring in the summer months.

The extent and severity of polio paralysis depends on the nerves and muscle groups affected, and the age at which the disease was contacted (Singh et al., 2013). In the most severe cases, bulbar–spinal polio of the brain stem causes paralysis of the diaphragm making it impossible to breathe without an artificial respirator (Singh et al., 2013). Clearly in the past this form would have been fatal. Relatively few cases of polio result in permanent paralysis. A small number of intact motor nerve cells may allow for continued muscle action and eventual recovery

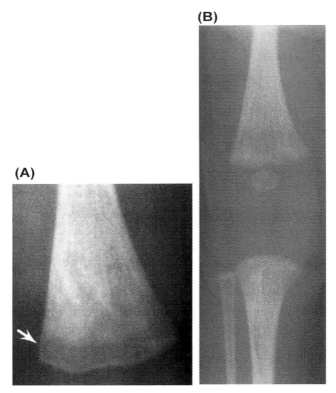

FIGURE 7.3 Rubella infection in two neonates. Clinical radiographs show (A) a thick radiolucent band at the distal end of the femur, and (B) longitudinal striations giving the bones a "celery-stalk" striated appearance. *From Resnick, D., Kransdorf, M., 2005. Bone and Joint Imaging, Elsevier Saunders, Philadelphia, p. 779.*

from paralysis, with around 50% of sufferers reported to recover after 6 months of initial paralysis, 75% recovering after 1 year, and 95% after 2 years (Bukh, 1968; Sharrard, 1955). The prognosis of recovery from paralysis is better when proximal muscles are affected or only one muscle group is involved (Bukh, 1968).

Spinal paralysis results from infection of the ventral horn of the spinal cord, usually causing asymmetrical paralysis of the leg. Scoliosis as the result of polio paralysis was noted in 30% of polio cases in 1941. The deformity usually occurred within a year of the infection but could take up to 15 years to fully develop (James, 1956). Unilateral paralysis of the lateral trunk muscles causes curvature of the thoracic area of the spine, either confined to the upper thoracic region or extending from T1 to T11 or T2 to L2. Scoliosis of T1 or T2 causes the most severe deformities affecting the position of the head and neck. There is compensatory cervical lordosis and rotation of the associated ribs. On the convex side of the curvature, ribs become aligned vertically and are crowded. Lower spinal paralysis of T6–L1 causes tilting of the pelvis, a deformity that is most severe in children who develop polio before the age of 5 years (James, 1956).

In the limbs, paralysis of one leg is common especially in those under 5 years (Regan, 1918; Singh et al., 2013). The lower leg and foot are the most likely areas to become permanently paralyzed. Hence polio is recognized as the second most common cause of talipes cavus due to paralysis of the *triceps surae*. Talipes cavus refers to a high arched foot and an exaggerated talocalcaneal angle (Brewerton et al., 1963). Talipes equinovarus, where the foot is also twisted out of position, is a further complication. Long-term paralysis of the femur results in coxa valga of the femoral head due to delayed development of the trochantic growth plate in the absence of muscle stimuli, while the femoral neck continues to lengthen longitudinally in line with the shaft (Resnick and Kransdorf, 2005, p. 1036). The femoral shaft becomes laterally rotated and there is underdevelopment of the innominate on the affected side with compensatory changes to the sacroiliac joint on the opposite side (Resnick and Kransdorf, 2005). Also in this area, hip dislocation may result when there is paralysis of the gluteal muscles, while the flexor muscles are unaffected, causing severe flexion and adduction (Sharrard, 1967). In a study of women suffering from postpolio paralysis in Norway between 1967 and 1998, Veiby et al. (2007) noted higher rates of preeclampsia, proteinuria, and urinary tract infections in the mothers. Their paralysis meant they were not able to aid in the delivery, while spinal and pelvic deformities as the result of long-term paralysis caused birth obstructions. Both factors resulted in the increased use of forceps and caesarean sections. Perinatal deaths were more common, and the children who did survive often had a low birth weight as the result of reduced placental function in the mothers.

Limb shortening as the result of polio paralysis has been reported in 78%–97% of children who suffered paralysis for between 5 and 17 years (Barr, 1948; Ratliff, 1959). Hence, differences in length between one limb bone and another, in the absence of trauma or infection to a joint, should raise suspicions of postpolio paralysis. In children, the extent of length discrepancy between limbs depends on the age at which they were affected, and it is considered most acute if suffered before the age of 10. While rapid growth may mean that limb discrepancy between the affected and normal side would be more exaggerated than in an adult, should the child die shortly after limb paralysis occurs then any differences would be less pronounced. If their paralysis is reversed, rapid growth also means that their bones are more likely to return to their normal dimensions rendering the disease invisible to the paleopathologist. This is providing that the child recovered at an age with enough growth time left for the bone length to catch up before the epiphyses fused. But how much limb discrepancy should we expect to see? The amount of shortening has been reported to be up to 5 inches once both limbs have ceased growing, although up to 2 inches is considered more usual (Ratliff, 1959). In his review, Ratliff (1959) noted that several clinical cases actually reported *lengthening* of the paralyzed leg at least 2 years after the onset of the disease, but that this discrepancy was rarely more than half an inch, and the discrepancy was temporary. Even when only the lower leg was affected with paralysis, shortening of both the femur and tibia was common. Based on these reports, Thompson (2014) argues the importance of measuring all of the limb bones for length discrepancies even when only one bone shows evidence for atrophy. Ratliff (1959) found no clear association between the severity of the paralysis and degree of shortening in his cases (n=225 children) and reported premature epiphyseal closure only in 0.1% of cases. Where it does occur, premature fusion of the metatarsals and the knee is the most common finding, with Currarino (1966) reporting it in 7.6% (metatarsals) and 1.2% (knee) of his 250 patients from Dallas. Ratliff (1959) was suspicious that premature epiphyseal closure only occurred because children were treated surgically, and questioned whether the use of splints contributed to limb lengthening. If this is true then premature fusion and lengthened may not be an appropriate diagnostic feature in the archeological record.

The first clinical case of paralysis due to poliomyelitis was described in 1734 by Salzmann (Rida, 1962), with polio finally recognized as a distinct disease in 1840 by Jakob Heine. The poliovirus was isolated in 1908 (Singh et al., 2013). There are no records of polio epidemics before the 19th century when in the 1830s three small epidemics were reported in England, the United States, and St Helena (Wyatt, 2003). The disease rapidly became one of the most dreaded childhood diseases, often referred to as "infantile paralysis." Archeological evidence suggests that it was a disease that affected the human populations from many geographical regions at a much earlier date. The first case of polio was suggested in the Egyptian mummy of an elderly male dated to 3700 BC (Mitchell, 1900), and another potential case of polio is illustrated in an Egyptian Stele from 1580-1350 BC (Rida, 1962). Cases of asymmetry linked to polio are normally only described in adult skeletons (Gladykowska-Rzeczycka and Smiszkiewicz-Skwarska, 1998; Kozłowski and Piontek 2000; Lieverse et al., 2008; McKinley, 1993; Novak et al., 2014; Roberts and Cox, 2003; Roberts et al., 2004; Thompson, 2014; Wells, 1982). However, Winkler and Grosschmidt (1987) ascribe the death of a full-term fetus (c. 40 weeks) in early medieval Austria to scoliosis and secondary alterations of the pelvis in the mother due to long-term polio paralysis. A similar double burial of a female and her full-term perinate was described by Thompson (2014) in 19th century Mississippi.

TUBERCULOSIS

TB is a chronic infectious disease of overcrowding, be it in a thriving agricultural community or the unsanitary environments of rapid industrialization. Poor housing and nutrition, close contact with infected animals and humans, poverty, climate, and occupation have all been cited as causative factors (Roberts and Buikstra, 2003). The close proximity of infected individuals and a depressed immune status is required for the disease to take hold. TB is most commonly the result of infection from *Mycobacterium tuberculosis* in humans, although other members of the *M. tuberculosis* complex (MBTC) may be involved, including *Mycobacterium africanum*, *Mycobacterium canetti*, *Mycobacterium bovis*, *Mycobacterium microti*, *Mycobacterium pinnipedii*, and *Mycobacterium caprae* (Müller et al., 2014). TB can affect the lungs (pulmonary TB), lymph nodes (tuberculous adenitis), skin (scrofula), and intestine (gastrointestinal TB) and in fewer cases, the bones and joints (Resnick and Kransdorf, 2005). TB has three forms: primary, miliary, and secondary. Primary TB from a site of initial inoculation is the most common form in children (Leung et al., 1992), with secondary TB resulting from a reactivation of a latent infection, usually occurring in adolescents (Marais et al., 2004). Miliary TB is a frequent complication in children and results from an extension of primary caseating lesions into the pulmonary vessels leading to the hematogenous or lymphatic spread of infection into the lungs and distant sites (Shingadia and Novelli, 2003). Cystic TB, either as solitary or multiple lytic lesions (Jüngling's disease) is a rare childhood form of TB osteomyelitis (Harisinghani et al., 2000; Rasool et al., 1994).

Accounts from the early 1900s show that death from primary TB in infancy was common, but as the child aged, their ability to survive the condition into its chronic stages was greatly improved. Recovery from TB meningitis, however, was rare (Griffith, 1919). The identification of TB in nonadult remains is significant as they represent the pool from which a large proportion of infected adults will arise. Because children are usually infected by adults, child cases indicate the continual transmission of TB within a community (Walls and Shingadia, 2004). Children are more likely to develop primary TB after exposure than adults, and modern estimates put the likelihood of infection after exposure at 5%–10% for adults, 15% for adolescents (14+ years), 24% for 1- to 5-year-olds, and 43% for infants (Walls and Shingadia, 2004). There may also be an underlying genetic susceptibility to the development of clinical TB after exposure (Levin and Newport, 2000). The disease will normally be evident between 1 and 6 months after infection and in modern populations, the ages between birth and 5 years, 15–30 years, and 60 years plus are the age groups with the highest frequencies of the disease (Roberts and Buikstra, 2003). There is some debate about the existence of congenital TB, with Jordan and Spencer (1949) reporting advanced tubercles in the spleen of a 30-day-old newborn removed from his infected mother immediately after birth. Although rare, it is suggested that transmission from the mother to the child can occur via the placenta, the umbilical vein, or due to the fetus ingesting bacteria through infected amniotic fluid (Cantwell et al., 1994; Lorin, 1983). Ingestion of infected fluid causes gastrointestinal lesions, whereas a hematogenous transmission results in foci in the liver and lungs (Cantwell et al., 1994). Children may also be infected shortly after birth through infected breast milk (Roberts and Buikstra, 2003). In 1918, pregnancy was shown to exacerbate pulmonary TB in the mother, who often died while giving birth. While most children appeared healthy, some babies were miscarried, stillborn, or died shortly after birth (Holt, 1909; Norris and Landis, 1918). Today, TB in pregnant women increases the risk of perinatal death, premature birth, retarded intrauterine growth, and low birth weight; although this picture is complicated by the coexistence of HIV in modern reports (Sugarman et al., 2014).

Nearly 30 million people suffer from TB today, and between 1% and 3% develop skeletal lesions (Rankin and Tuli, 2009), although others report a higher incidence of 3%–5% (Resnick, 1995). This figure may be higher in children whose blood-filled growing bones attract the bacilli. For example, in her study of medical records the Stannington children's sanatorium in Northumbria, Bernard (2002) found the majority of the children were admitted with pulmonary TB, and that the bones and joints were affected in 12% of cases. As the most common mode of transmission of TB is by inhalation of airborne droplets from an infected person or animal, a primary infection in the lungs is most common. In 1943, 61%–67% of children dying from TB in London had the pulmonary form of the disease (Sheldon, 1943). The highest incidence was in children between the ages of 2 and 3 years, and the most susceptible had suffered from either whooping cough or measles, which were thought to have led to a reactivation of a primary TB infection. A secondary hematogenous spread to the gastrointestinal tract is uncommon, as it requires a greater period of time for lesions to manifest (Shingadia and Novelli, 2003) although a secondary spread to the stomach may occur due to swallowing of infected sputum from pulmonary TB (Sharma and Bhatia, 2004). Gastrointestinal TB is usually the result of a primary infection with *M. bovis* through infected meat and milk (Sheldon, 1943; Spiro, 1995) and is responsible for around 20% of bone and joint changes in children (Griffith, 1919). Much of what we know about the prevalence of TB in children is based on post-1950s data where the natural progression of the disease is hindered by chemotherapy. The expression of the disease in skeletons from the preantibiotic era is likely to have been more severe. Marais et al. (2004) provide valuable insight into such a group of children (under 15 years) during the 1920s and 1950s. They noted that primary infection with TB in children less than 2 years typically resulted in miliary TB within 12 months, with joint involvement common between 1 and 3 years of age. Primary infection between the ages of 2 and 10 years rarely resulted in miliary TB. After 10 years, primary infection led to more adult-type involvement of the spine. The skeletal expression of TB in the different areas of the skeleton and their differential diagnoses are outlined below.

Cranium

Cranial involvement due to a direct extension of an infection from the orbit or paranasal sinuses, or indirectly through a hematogenous or lymphatic route is rare, comprising only 0.5% of bone lesions. Fifty percent of these cases occur in children under 10 years (Malhotra et al., 1992; Rajeshwari and Sharma, 1994; Tata, 1978). This childhood predilection may be linked to the presence of blood-rich hemopoietic marrow in the diploë (Ortner, 2003). Conversely, the lack of cancellous bone in the skull before 1 year accounts for the limited cases seen in infants (Malhotra et al., 1992). "Punched-out" lesions penetrate both tables of the cranium and usually affect the frontal and parietal bones as single isolated lesions (Meng and Wu, 1942). They have a "moth-eaten" appearance, with round foci measuring up to 2 cm, and they are greater in diameter on the endocranial surface (Figs. 7.4 and 7.5; Klaus et al., 2010; Ortner, 2003). The lateral side of the orbit, zygomatic and nasal bones, and maxilla may also be involved (Meng and Wu, 1942). Otitis media secondary to TB can result in destructive lesions on the petrous bone and mastoid process (Ortner, 2003).

TB meningitis is a serious complication in the childhood disease. It can occur within 3 months of exposure to the bacillus and often proves fatal (Griffith, 1919;

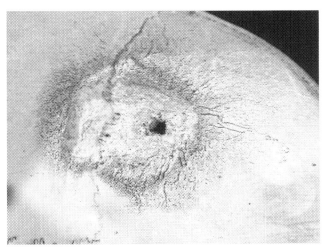

FIGURE 7.4 The endocranial appearance of a tuberculous lesion in a 10-year-old female showing active "stellate" new bone formation around a lytic central focus (skeleton AMN 2439). *From Ortner, D., 2003. Identification of Pathological Conditions in Human Skeletal Remains, Academic Press, New York, p. 252.*

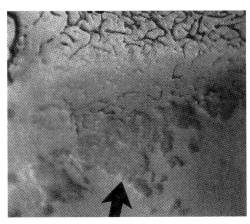

FIGURE 7.6 Demarcated erosive lesions on the endocranial surface of an individual with tuberculosis. *From Hershkovitz, I., Greenwald, C., Latimer, B., Jellema, S.-B., Eshed, V., Dutour, O., Rothschild, B., 2002. Serpens Endocrania Symmetrica (SES): a new term and a possible clue for identifying intrathoracic diseases in skeletal populations. American Journal of Physical Anthropology 118 (3), 204.*

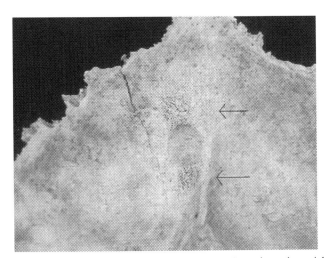

FIGURE 7.5 Possible tuberculous lesion (*arrows*) on the endocranial surface of the parietal bone in a 4- to 5-year-old from Taunton in Sussex, England (AD 1150–1539, skeleton 2077), with a lytic area surrounded by active new bone formation. *From Dawson, H., Robson Brown, K., 2012. Childhood tuberculosis: a probable case from late medieval Somerset, England. International Journal of Paleopathology 2, 34.*

Wallgren, 1948). Meningitis is a common complication of untreated miliary TB (Cruz and Starke, 2007) but may also result from a spread of a primary infection directly from the petrous portion of the skull or the spine (Cappell and Anderson, 1971, p. 625). Children aged 4 and under account for 80% of TB meningitis cases (Walls and Shingadia, 2004), which if survived, can result in neurological complications including blindness, deafness, and mental retardation (Walls and Shingadia, 2004). Given the severity of the condition, it may be argued that skeletal signatures of TB meningitis in nonadult skeletons would be unlikely.

However, in the preantibiotic era children were reported to have suffered meningitis for up to a week before falling into a coma and dying 4–5 days later (Sheldon, 1943). Lorber (1958) reported 129 cases of TB meningitis in Sheffield, where intracranial calcifications and ossifications occurred between 18 months and 3 years after the onset of the disease. However, these children were receiving treatment for meningitis, and it is not possible to know whether the resulting calcifications would occur in nontreated cases. Where miliary TB was the cause of meningitis, it is unlikely that the postcranial skeleton will show any signs of the disease, as this acute infection usually spreads from a primary soft tissue lesion in the lung or intestine (Griffith, 1919).

Research into the identification of tuberculous meningitis in the archeological context indicates that lesions are likely in the form of small granulomas (cortical foci), remnants of solitary tubercles producing lesions similar to arachnoid granulations (Hershkovitz et al., 2002; Jankauskas, 1999; Jankauskas and Schultz, 1995; Lewis, 2004; Lorber, 1958; Meng and Wu, 1942; Teschler-Nicola et al., 1998). Hershkovitz et al. (2002) noted erosive lesions on the endocranial surfaces of 36% of individuals documented to have suffered from TB compared to 10% in those who died of other causes (Fig. 7.6). In Teschler-Nicola et al.'s (1998) study of 111 skeletons from Vienna where the cause of death was due to TB, 73% had "corn-size" depressions thought to be the residues of calcified tubercles. These findings are supported by the work of Pálfi et al. (2000) who identified endocranial lesions in an infant and a child aged 10–12 years in France. No other lesions were present but they both tested positive for TB aDNA. But the evidence is not clear cut. In their Portuguese sample of 66 nonadults, Santos and Roberts (2001, p. 44) only found one case of "slight" endocranial lesions, but this was in an individual reported to be nontuberculous.

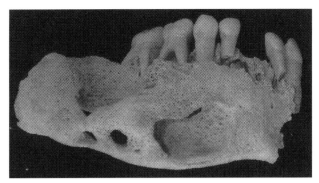

FIGURE 7.7 Possible tuberculous osteomyelitis in the mandible of a 3- to 4-year-old from late Roman Poundbury Camp in Dorset, England (skeleton 636). This child also had widespread new bone formation on the long bones. *Photograph taken with the kind permission of the Natural History Museum, London.*

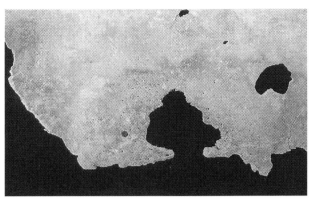

FIGURE 7.8 Abscess formation on the scapula body of a 12-year-old from Poundbury Camp in Dorset, England (skeleton 501). There is inflammatory pitting around the lesion and the anterior aspect had a profuse deposit of fiber bone along the margin. This individual also had lesions indicative of TB on the pelvis. *Photograph taken with the kind permission of the Natural History Museum, London.*

Mandible

Osteomyelitis of the mandible is rare due to the limited cancellous bone in this region, but has been reported in around 2% of skeletal TB cases in adults and children (Fig. 7.7). It normally results from a hematogenous spread of a pulmonary infection (Imamura et al., 2004). Primary TB of the mandible is associated with localized trauma to the site or the invasion of infection via a carious tooth (Gupta and Singh, 2007; Imamura et al., 2004). One study reported mandibular TB more frequently (60% of cases) in children under the age of 15 years (Meng, 1940). A possible differential diagnosis is actinomycosis, a bacterial disease located in the oral cavity. Actinomycosis commonly affects the mandible, but the lesions are described as multiple small resorptive foci (Resnick and Kransdorf, 2005; Rothschild et al., 2006). Associated with agricultural workers, today actinomycosis is not common in children under 15 years of age, and hematogenous spread to the rest of the skeleton is rare (Puzzilli et al., 1977). When it does occur, the spine, ribs, and sacrum are affected with small lytic lesions surrounded by reactive bone sclerosis (Aufderheide and Rodriguez-Martín, 1998).

Scapula

Osteomyelitis of the scapula is an unusual presentation of skeletal TB, with only four cases reported in the clinical literature. It is most common where the disease is endemic (Resnick and Kransdorf, 2005; Singh et al., 2009). A 12-year-old from 5th-century Poundbury Camp in Dorset demonstrated pitting and profuse new bone formation around a lytic lesion on the scapula that may be attributed to TB present at the site (Fig. 7.8).

Spine

Today, 50% of all skeletal TB infections are estimated to involve the spine (Moon, 1997), with spinal TB reported in 16% of children under 4 years and 48% under 15 years of age (Antunes, 1992). Hematogenous spread of the bacillus leads to abscesses on the anterior portion of the vertebrae, where there is greater vascularization (Antunes, 1992) eventually resulting in collapse and a kyphotic deformity (Pott's disease, Fig. 7.9). Unlike in adults, where infection begins in the center of the vertebral body and works its way into the intervertebral disk, in children the disc's vascular supply is the greatest and the infection may start in the disc and extend into the vertebral body (Buikstra, 1976a). As segmentary arteries often branch to the adjacent vertebra, spread of infection from one vertebra to another is common, and involvement of the posterior arch may result (Antunes, 1992). Although involvement of the neural arches is not a common feature of TB, Kelley and El Najjar (1980) noted it in the skeletons of modern individuals who had died from TB. Involvement of the cervical spine is less common than for the rest of the spine (Moon, 1997; Rajeshwari and Sharma, 1994) but may be present with the absence of any other vertebral involvement (Mathur and Bais, 1997). Children are more susceptible to instability of the spine, and vertebral displacement and risk of cord compression can result in limb paralysis (Moon, 1997). TB spinal osteomyelitis is characterized by lytic lesions with minimal bone formation (involucrum) and bone necrosis (sequestrum). In 1961, Morse listed the features he considered should be used to distinguish Pott's disease from other conditions that may affect the spine:

1. 1–4 vertebrae affected
2. Bone destruction
3. Angular kyphosis
4. Neural arch involvement is rare
5. Extravertebral cold abscesses are frequent
6. Limited bony regeneration

Buikstra (1976b) argued that this definition was too narrow and that involvement of the joints should also be considered. She also argued that age was important and we might expect to see TB in adolescents and young adults who have the highest modern incidence and mortality from the disease. Although it is children below 10 years who have the most frequent and varied bone changes. In addition, recovery from spinal collapse includes spontaneous spinal fusion, particularly in children and can involve as many as 12 vertebrae rather than the stated 1–4. Secondary neural arch involvement with vertebral collapse is also common and Matos et al. (2009) reported it in 20% of documented cases of TB. Further, Ortner and Bush (1993) suggest that a distinction should be made between reactive bone formation and bone repair in TB cases. Osteophytes are generally considered more indicative of brucellosis when coupled with spinal collapse due to the limited bone remodeling usually seen in TB. However, Haas et al. (2000) suggest osteophytes are an early indicator of spinal TB and identified them in cases diagnosed using aDNA. There is a danger that TB will be over diagnosed if all spinal lytic lesions and spinal collapse is defined as "Pott's disease" without proper detailed description or consideration of the variety of differential diagnoses (Fig. 7.10).

Lytic lesions in the spine can have numerous etiologies. One of the most challenging diseases to distinguish from TB based on spinal lesions is brucellosis (undulant fever). Scheuermann's kyphosis is another condition that should be considered when lytic lesions are present in the spines of older children. This disease is characterized by anterior wedging of the thoracic and lumbar vertebrae (commonly T1–2 and T12–L1), anterior–superior destruction and repair of the vertebral bodies, kyphosis and possible fusion of the anterior aspects of the spine (Resnick and Kransdorf, 2005). Destruction of the spine can also occur in neoplastic diseases that affect children (e.g., Hodgkin lymphoma, Ewing sarcoma, and leukemia) but these lytic lesions tend to be more discrete and regular and affect other areas of

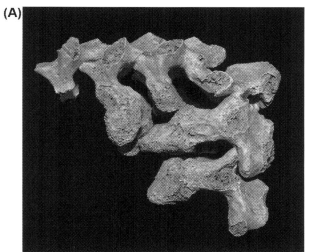
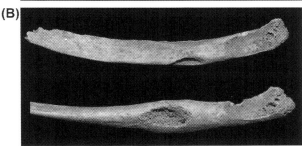

FIGURE 7.9 Pott's kyphosis in the thoracic vertebrae (A) of a 9- to 10-year-old from 4th century AD Pécs, Hungary (skeleton L/74). The child also had lytic lesions on the ribs (B). *From Hlavenková, L., Teasdale, M., Gábor, O., Nagy, G., Beňuš, R., Marcsik, A., Pinhasi, R., Hajdu, T., 2015. Childhood bone tuberculosis from Roman Pécs, Hungary. HOMO-Journal of Comparative Human Biology 66 (1), 29.*

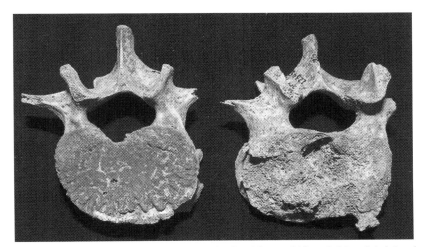

FIGURE 7.10 Lytic lesions on the superior aspect of a lower thoracic vertebra in a 15-year-old from St Mary Spital, London (AD 1250–1400, skeleton 22,345). The spine has not collapsed and an anterior osteophyte may be indicative of healing, but brucellosis or phyogenic osteomyelitis should be considered as differential diagnoses. *Photograph by F. Shapland with the kind permission of the Museum of London.*

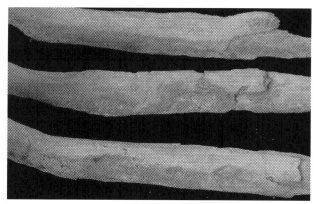

FIGURE 7.11 Profuse active subperiosteal new bone formation (grade 3) on the visceral aspects of the ribs in a 9- to 10-year-old from late Roman Poundbury Camp, Dorset, England (skeleton 228). These lesions are indicative of a chronic respiratory infection, possibly tuberculosis. *Photograph taken with the kind permission of the Natural History Museum, London.*

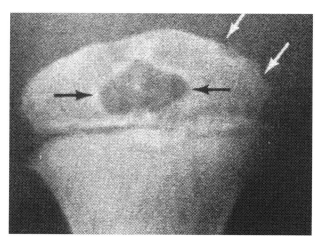

FIGURE 7.12 Tuberculosis in the epiphysis of a 3-year-old with sclerotic margins (*black arrows*) and lytic lesions on the external aspect of the epiphysis (*white arrows*). *From Caffey, J., 1945. Pediatric X-Ray Diagnosis, Year Book Medical Publishers, Inc., Chicago, p. 673.*

the skeleton (Hershkovitz et al., 1998; Matos et al., 2009). Non-TB infectious involvement of the spine is uncommon, with pyogenic osteomyelitis of the vertebrae representing only 1% of all osteomyelitis locations. When it does occur, it usually affects a single lumbar vertebra (Antunes, 1992). Coccidioidomycosis, a fungal disease restricted to the western United States and Central and South America, can result in granuloma development and lytic destruction of the joints and collapse of the spine (Capoor et al., 2014; Kelley and El-Najjar, 1980). It is advised that any spinal collapse be described as angular kyphosis, while the most likely cause is explored (Buikstra, 1976b; Matos et al., 2009).

Ribs

New bone formation and lytic lesions on the visceral (internal) surfaces of the ribs is more common in pulmonary TB than any other condition (Eyler et al., 1996) and may represent an early sign of the disease before spinal lesions have had time to manifest (Fig. 7.11; Wilbur et al., 2009). However, similar rib lesions that occur along the line of pleural membrane attachment have been identified in modern autopsied individuals with chronic upper respiratory tract infections such as pneumonia or bronchitis (Roberts et al., 1994). Several studies have examined whether TB most commonly affects the sternal or vertebral ends of the ribs, but the results are inconclusive (Matos and Santos, 2006; Santos and Roberts, 2001). Subperiosteal new bone formation on the visceral surfaces of the ribs are not recorded in clinical TB cases, although enlargement of the ribs has been noted (Eyler et al., 1996). Lesions have been graded according to appearance by Nicklisch et al. (2012):

0 = no changes.

1 = slight periosteal reaction, streaky, or nodular without discernible new bone formation.

2 = slight (mild/patchy) new bone formation.

3 = severe (diffuse and profuse) new bone formation.

4 = Lytic lesions present.

Joints

In children, widespread hemopoietic marrow, and vascularization at the growth plates means that TB lesions of the skeleton are more widespread, and involvement of the hip, knee, and ankle joints (especially the calcaneus) is common (Walls and Shingadia, 2004). The initial site of infection is in the synovial fluid extending into the epiphysis and metaphysis (Hayes, 1961). As epiphyses are not routinely radiographed in archeological samples these early lesions may be easily missed (Fig. 7.12; Lewis, 2007). The joints may be affected bilaterally or unilaterally with equal frequency (Teklali et al., 2003; Teo and Peh, 2004). As with the spine, lesions are characterized by minimal bone formation and necrosis with marked osteoporosis in the affected limb. Tuberculous granulomata (localized masses of granulation tissue) destroy the joint cartilage and underlying bone, causing necrosis and pus formation, with the end result being fibrous or bony fusion (Shapiro, 2001). Cystic TB causes a honeycomb appearance of the metaphyses (Harisinghani et al., 2000; Rasool et al., 1994). A probable case of cystic TB was identified in a well-preserved 4- to 5-year-old from Predynastic Egypt, with angular kyphosis, dactylitis, and widespread lytic lesions (Fig. 7.13). TB was not only diagnosed on the strength of these lesions but also indirectly when aDNA confirmed TB in an older child from the same site (Crubézy et al., 1998; Dabernat and Crubézy, 2010).

After the spine, the hip joint is the most common area affected in child TB cases and may cause dislocation and

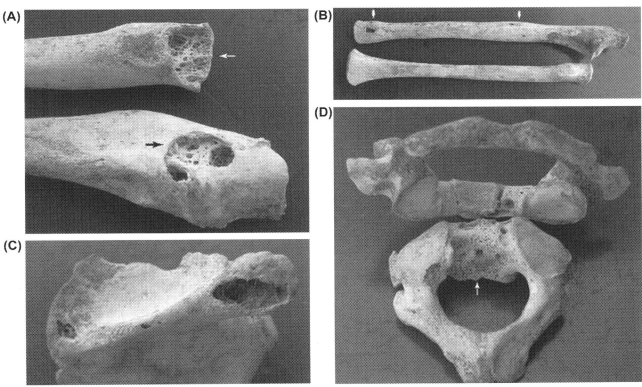

FIGURE 7.13 Lytic lesions indicative of cystic tuberculosis in the (A) proximal radius and ulna, (B) ulna diaphysis, (C) acromion of the scapula, and (D) axis of a 4- to 5-year-old from Adaima, Egypt (3500-2700 BC, skeleton 500). *From Dabernat, H., Crubézy, E., 2010. Multiple bone tuberculosis in a child from predynastic upper Egypt (3200 BC). International Journal of Osteoarchaeology 20 (6), 719–730.*

atrophy of the hip and fibrous ankylosis (Campbell and Hoffman, 1995). One study from the 1930s suggests a peak in hip involvement in children aged 4–6 years (Sorrel and Sorrel-Dejerine, 1932). The ilium may be involved directly through a primary infection of the gastrointestinal tract or a spread of infection from the spine. In the latter, the infection perforates the anterior longitudinal ligaments in the spine and spreads into the paravertebral muscles, such as the psoas muscle (forming a psoas abscess). From there, infection extends along the muscle plane to the ilium and the greater trochanter of the femur creating smooth cavitations (Ortner, 2003).

Long Bones

Although less frequent, the bone shaft may become infected through a primary focus of infection in the nutrient canals or through the infected metaphysis (Caffey, 1945). When this occurs, bone thickening under the inflamed periosteum, usually of the femur or tibia, is considered a common radiographic sign (Hayes, 1961). Stiffness of the joint followed by skin abscesses, joint dislocation, muscle wasting, and limb shortening are additional clinical symptoms of skeletal involvement (Teklali et al., 2003). Limb lengthening of up to 3 cm is a complication of TB affecting the knee as a result of stimulation of the growth plate (Kant et al., 2014).

Santos and Roberts (2001) identified active widespread subperiosteal new bone formation on the long bones, scapulae, tarsals, and metatarsals of 7- to 21-year-olds who died from TB in Coimbra, Portugal, in the preantibiotic era (1904–36). Not reported in the clinical literature, such lesions would probably have been too subtle to have been noted on radiographs and would not have been examined on autopsy (Santos and Roberts, 2001). It is possible these lesions represent a form of hypertrophic osteoarthropathy (HOA), a condition most commonly caused by pulmonary TB in children (Cavanaugh and Holman, 1965). The syndrome is characterized by soft tissue clubbing of the digits, seen on radiograph as shortening of the distal phalanges (Ddungu et al., 2006), and bilateral involvement of the joints (Assis et al., 2011). It manifests as bilateral hypertrophic new bone formation on the tibiae, fibulae, radii, and ulnae, although it may also affect the hands and feet. The usual expression is a dense, lumpy surface thickest at the midshaft, and tapering off toward the metaphysis (Fig. 7.14). The epiphyses, spine, and skull are normally unaffected (Assis et al., 2011). The new bony layer is clearly distinct from the underlying cortex, although in long standing cases there may be resorption. Bronchiectasis, congenital heart

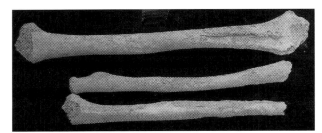

FIGURE 7.14 Profuse active subperiosteal new bone formation on the right humerus, radius, and ulna shafts of an 11- to 12-year-old from late Roman Poundbury Camp in Dorset, England (skeleton 900). *Photograph taken with the kind permission of the Natural History Museum, London.*

disease, a collection of pus in the pleural cavity (empyema), lung abscesses, bronchial cancer, and cystic fibrosis are differential diagnoses (Kelly et al., 1991). Widespread active new bone formation on the long and flat bones could also be indicative of hemorrhage as the result of vitamin C deficiency.

Hands and Feet

Involvement of the short bones of the hand and foot, although rare is a more common manifestation in children. Dactylitis, where the entire finger is inflamed, can result in profuse new bone formation on the metacarpals and phalanges (Fig. 7.15). In TB, a cystic form, spina ventosa (ventosa meaning "puffed full of air") can occur (Feldman et al., 1971; Jensen et al., 1991) with the development of an expanded center encased by an involucrum. If healing occurs, the digits may be shortened due to destruction of the growth plate (Harisinghani et al., 2000). Dactylitis can also occur in yaws, leprosy, sickle cell anemia, and osteomyelitis (Jensen et al., 1991).

Paleopathology

It is not known when TB first became a parasite of humans, but the human form is believed to have increased during the Neolithic period where it was spread from bovine TB with the widespread adoption of agriculture. More recent research suggests that TB was also carried by feral animals and was present in bison during the late Pleistocene, and sea lions in the Holocene. Hence, it may have been present in human populations at a much earlier date (Bos et al., 2014; Roberts and Buikstra, 2003). Factors that result in high levels of TB are complex, often interlinked, and in some cases impossible to measure. This list includes physiological and psychological stress, climate, age, sex, ethnicity, poverty, and migration (Roberts and Buikstra, 2003). In the past, it was children who were most susceptible to the gastrointestinal form of the disease (Griffith, 1919). One of the major causes was the use of cow's milk for infant feeding. During its height (AD 1850–1860)

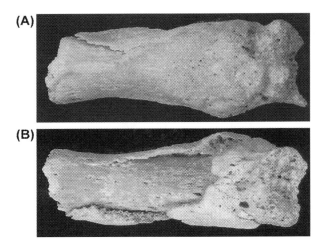

FIGURE 7.15 Profuse sheath of new bone formation characteristic of dactylitis on the metacarpal of a 12-year-old with tuberculosis from late Roman Poundbury Camp in Dorset, England (skeleton 506). Both the anterior (A) and posterior (B) aspects are shown. *Photograph taken with the kind permission of the Natural History Museum, London.*

milk was produced in urban cowsheds or on the outskirts of towns. Reports of adulterated and infected milk were common, as the transportation of milk from the countryside could take up to 24 hours in unrefrigerated conditions before being stored, uncovered in shops or in the home (Atkins, 1992). By the 1870s, improvements in sanitation in the urban centers led to a decline in TB. It remained a problem in the rural areas that did not benefit from the new reforms and as late as 1931, even after strict rules had been applied to the storage and supply of milk, 6.7% of "fresh" milk in England was still infected with bovine TB (Atkins, 1992; Cronjé, 1984).

Despite the high incidence of skeletal TB in children reported in the clinical literature, the paucity of TB in nonadult skeletons has been attributed to poor skeletal preservation, segregated burial, or death before skeletal changes could manifest (Roberts and Buikstra, 2003, p. 50). There may also be other factors. Holloway et al. (2011) reviewed cases of TB identified in 221 archeological sites spanning 7250 BC–AD 1899. They suggest that the distribution of lesions has changed over time, from mainly spinal lesions to a combination of spinal and extraspinal lesions, so earlier dated cases may be more subtle in their expression. Children in the past may have died of meningeal TB before any obvious changes to the spine and joints could manifest. For example, a review of the Coimbra University Hospital records (AD 1919–1928) showed that 73% of infants and 51% of 1- to 10-years-olds died of meningeal TB. Pott's disease was only evident in 2.9% of cases, and was absent in infants, while joint involvement occurred in only 2.4% of cases. Twenty-one percent of the children died from widespread TB of the intestines and other soft tissues. Of the 11- to 20-year-olds, 10% died of meningitis, 2.3% had bone involvement, and 0.6% had Pott's disease

(Santos, 2015). The low numbers of individuals displaying Pott's disease was of note given this is one of the most common skeletal signs used in paleopathology. It serves to highlight the importance of examining the ribs and endocranial surfaces for sign of meningeal or pulmonary TB infections (Santos, 2015). The pattern of widespread soft tissue infection in adolescents reflects current thinking on the impact of a maturing immune system on the spread of *M. tuberculosis*. Marais et al. (2005) argue that the transition from containment of an infection characteristic in the immune system of under 5 year olds to destruction in older children allows TB to spread more readily to the lungs in an oxygen-rich microenvironment. Hence, we may only see more characteristic lytic lesions in the bones of older children. As there are no features that are considered pathognomonic of TB in dry bone, differential diagnosis is always required (Wilbur et al., 2009). For children, this may include brucellosis, bronchitis, pneumonia, Scheuermann's disease (juvenile kyphosis), scurvy, primary HOA, actinomycosis, or hematogenous osteomyelitis of unspecified cause.

Based on skeletal presentation alone, the youngest identified case of TB is in the mummified remains of an infant from Les Mesa de Los Santos, Colombia with calcified pleura (Arateco, 1998). Derry (1938, p. 197) reported a case of Pott's disease in a 9-year-old from Early Dynastic Dakka, Egypt with destruction and fusion of T10–L2 into an "irregular mass." Other cases, however, have been in older children. Allison et al. (1981) suggested TB in the mummified remains of a 14-year-old from precontact Peru, when a calcified nodule was identified on the chest radiograph. Pfeiffer (1984) noted that of the individuals showing lytic lesions of the spine and sacrum 15th–16th century Uxbridge, Ontario, the most severe changes were in the children. She suggests that warfare, overcrowding, and a poor diet may have contributed to the usually high prevalence of TB in this particular Iroquoian sample. One of the earliest dated cases of TB in Europe is of a 15-year-old male discovered in a cave in Neolithic Liguria, Italy. Lytic destruction and collapse of the spine from T11 to L1 had led to severe kyphosis. The gracile nature of the skeleton compared to two other Neolithic adolescents led Formicola et al. (1987) to suggest the infection had been long standing, and that the teenager's regular burial and survival suggested his acceptance within the community. In their review of TB in the New World, Roberts and Buikstra (2003) listed 20 cases of children with possible TB. Less certain are individuals with isolated lesions identified on the extra spinal bones. Ortner (1979) suggested a likely diagnosis of TB in a child with a lytic lesion on the left sphenoid bone, which showed similarities to a pathological specimen with the disease. Santos and Roberts (2001) identified skeletal lesions in 72% of 7- to 21-year-olds from Portugal (1904–36), this high frequency of skeletal lesions is explained by the introduction of new diagnostic criteria of widespread subperiosteal new bone formation on the skeleton. These criteria were included in a study of nonadults from Poundbury Camp in Roman Britain, where TB had previously not been noted in the children. This absence had been used to argue that TB was a rare and perhaps newly introduced condition to Roman England (Lewis, 2011). Lewis (2011) identified 7 (4.2%) cases of probable TB in children aged between 2 and 15 years. The nonadults displayed a variety of lesions from widespread subperiosteal new bone formation, profuse, and lytic visceral rib lesions, osteomyelitis of the mandible and scapula, lytic lesions of the spine, and dactylitis of the hand and foot phalanges. Interestingly, clear lytic lesions only occurred in children who were around 12 years of age. Further evidence that TB was actually a significant childhood disease in Roman Britain is suggested by the identification of four additional cases from other sites (Clough and Boyle, 2010; Müller et al., 2014; Rohnbogner, 2015). A rare case of cervical spine involvement in TB was identified in an 8-year-old with associated Pott's disease from medieval Isle of May, Scotland (Willows, 2015).

Biomolecular analysis is being increasingly used to identify skeletons with more subtle traces of tuberculous infection, and allow for the specific strain of TB (MTB complex) to be isolated. Arriaza et al. (1995) provided direct evidence for TB in a 12-year-old from Arica, Chile. The child had numerous cloacae on the anterior aspects of the cervical and lumbar vertebra bodies, spinal collapse of the thoracic spine, with neural arch involvement, and visceral rib lesions. In addition, new bone formation was evident of the humeri and femora. Of additional interest was the inclusion of a belt around the child's lower back that may have been used to compensate for the spinal collapse and provide some relief. The first positive identification of *M. bovis* in human remains was made in Iron Age Siberia in a 15- to 17-year-old with visceral rib lesions suggesting a pulmonary route for the infection (Murphy et al., 2009). DNA is helping us understand the large degree of skeletal variation we might expect in children with TB, and cases that would have been overlooked are now being identified. TB aDNA was isolated in a child with lytic and blastic lesions of a single vertebra (Klaus et al., 2010), and TB joint involvement was identified in a well-preserved skeleton of a 12- to 14-year-old from medieval Spain. There were lytic lesions on both recently fused proximal tibial epiphyses, but no other lesions that would have allowed TB to be determined macroscopically (Baxarias et al., 1998). Endocranial lesions were the only clue to TB in the case presented by Pálfi et al. (2000), and visceral rib lesions were the only elements with indicative lesions in a 16-year-old from Romano–British Kingsholm (Müller et al., 2014). More arrestingly in Lithuania, Faerman et al. (1999) identified TB in a 15-year-old with no bone changes. Conversely, when Mays et al. (2002) analyzed samples of seven individuals with visceral rib lesions from Wharram Percy, England, they found no positive cases of TB.

LEPROSY

Leprosy is a chronic granulomatous infectious disease caused by *Mycobacterium leprae*. The bacillus was first identified by Hansen in 1874 (1875), but recent studies have identified a new strain of bacteria that may also be responsible for diffuse lepromatous leprosy; *Mycobacterium lepromatosis* (Han et al., 2008). This strain may occur instead of or in conjunction with *M. leprae* (Kowalska and Kowalik, 2012). The pathogens enter the body via droplet inhalation from an infected individual or skin-to-skin contact from lesions teeming with bacteria. The respiratory tract is one of the most common portals of entry for leprosy, as bacilli are transmitted via droplets in the breath, or from the highly infectious nasal discharge. Close contact with their parents and other relatives make infants particularly susceptible to this mode of infection (Jopling and McDougall, 1988). Only 10% people will develop clinical signs of the disease, which although highly infectious, has a low pathogenicity meaning most hosts will carry the subclinical form (Barreto et al., 2014). Children aged 3–6 years are particularly susceptible to leprosy, making up to one-third of cases (Newman et al., 1972; Rodriguez, 1926). Nearly 200,000 new cases of leprosy were reported in 105 countries in 2011, with 9% of this figure in children (Butlin and Saunderson, 2014). Today, leprosy is still hyperendemic among the children of Brazil, India, and Indonesia (Barreto et al., 2014; Palit and Inamadar, 2014). As with TB, leprosy in children is indicative of a recent and active infection within the general population (Barreto et al., 2014). Levels of infant and childhood leprosy increase as the disease becomes more endemic, with up to 20% of children infected in hyperendemic areas (Barreto et al., 2014; Noussitou et al., 1976). A survey of 2356 children with leprosy in modern India appeared to show boys were more susceptible to the disease than girls (Palit and Inamadar, 2014). This may reflect the use of hospital records in cultures where boys are brought in for treatment, while lesions in girls tend to be neglected, leading to a greater number of deformities (Sachdeva et al., 2010). In studies of children born within leprosaria, the sex ratio is even, although female cases rise at puberty between 10 and 16 years (Rodriguez, 1926).

While controversial, there is evidence for a congenital form of leprosy resulting from transplacental infection (see below). Infection in utero results in a low feto-placental weight, fetal distress, and spontaneous abortion of the fetus (Duncan, 1980). Once born, children of mothers with lepromatous leprosy are described as small and feeble, and after the first 6 months of life, they grow more slowly than their healthy peers (Duncan, 1985a). Although they suffer from the same ailments as other children, those exposed to leprosy at this early age are particularly susceptible to infantile convulsions, marasmus, skin diseases, gastric, and respiratory problems, and up to 42% of these children may die in infancy (Gomez et al., 1922). Duncan et al. (1981) demonstrated an increase in the transmission of infection to the fetus when mothers descended from the milder tuberculoid to the more severe lepromatous form with pregnancy. This suggests that greater immunological instability and decreased host resistance exposes the child to larger quantities of the bacilli in utero.

Leprosy bacilli have a predilection for cool areas and replicate within skin macrophages, the mucous membrane, and the Schwann cells of the peripheral nerves resulting in damage to the sensory, motor and autonomic nervous systems (Resnick and Kransdorf, 2005). The severity of the disease relies on the immune status of the host, and the spectrum of the disease is often classified using the Jopling–Ridley system (Jopling and Ridley, 1966), spanning tuberculoid leprosy (TT), borderline tuberculosis (BT), borderline (BB), borderline lepromatous (BL), and lepromatous leprosy (LL). A more simple classification describes the disease as paucibacillary or tuberculoid, and multibacillary or lepromatous (Newman et al., 1972). In the tuberculoid form, the host immunity is good and well-contained granulomata with few bacilli are formed; in lepromatous leprosy the immune status of the host is overwhelmed, the granulomata are poorly formed and teaming with bacilli (Waldron, 2009). The skeletal lesions of leprosy result either due to the primary effect of the bacilli on the bone or secondary to neuropathy (Table 7.1). Changes are usually confined to lepromatous or long-term tuberculoid leprosy. In the lepromatous form they invade the skin, peripheral nerves, liver, spleen, bone marrow, kidneys, bladder, ovary, testes, eyes, mucous membranes, and the upper respiratory tract (Newman et al., 1972). The bacilli have a slow multiplication time of around 12–14 days (Duncan, 1980), and while in adults there is an incubation period of 3–5 years, this may be reduced to months in children (Barreto et al., 2014; Sachdeva et al., 2010). In many cases, leprosy heals spontaneously but may reoccur when the child is older.

Infantile Leprosy

New-born children of leprous parents are often as pretty and as healthy in appearance as any… but what an awful infallible certainty, as surely as we inherited it from our fathers do we transmit it to our children.

Thomson (1882, Chapter 43).

TABLE 7.1 Primary and Secondary Lesions Associated With Leprosy in the Skeleton

Area	Primary Bone Lesions	Secondary Bone Lesions
Rhinomaxillary	Localized inflammatory granulomata on the nasal and oral surfaces of the palatine process (Hjørting-Hansen et al., 1965)	Atrophy of the nasal aperture, anterior nasal spine, and alveolar process (Møller-Christensen et al., 1952; Andersen and Manchester, 1992) Diffuse inflammatory pitting of nasal and oral palatine processes (Andersen and Manchester, 1992) Maxillary sinusitis (Barton, 1979; Hauhnar et al., 1992)
Dentition	Leprogenic odontodysplasia (Danielsen, 1968, 1970) (concentric constriction of the roots of the maxillary incisors)	Loss of maxillary incisors as a result of alveolar recession (Andersen and Manchester, 1992; Møller-Christensen, 1961)
Hands and feet	Lepromatous osteomyelitis (Job, 1963) Sensory, motor, and autonomic neuropathy (Jopling and McDougall, 1988) Bone cysts	*Sensory neuropathy:* Pyogenic infections (Andersen et al., 1994) Septic arthritis and ankylosis (Andersen et al., 1992; Singh et al., 1994) Tarsal and carpal disintegration (Kulkarni and Mehta, 1983) Loss of proprioception (Jopling and McDougall, 1988) Fractures, subluxation and dislocation (Andersen et al., 1992; Cooney and Crosby 1944) *Motor neuropathy:* Claw–hand and foot deformities (Andersen and Manchester, 1987; Lewis et al., 1995) Drop-foot and wrist deformities (Andersen et al., 1992; Kulkarni and Mehta, 1983) Navicular squeezing and dorsal barring (Kulkarni and Mehta, 1983; Andersen and Manchester, 1988) Palmer grooves (Andersen and Manchester, 1987) *Autonomic neuropathy:* Concentric remodeling of the phalanges (Møller-Christensen, 1961; Andersen et al., 1992; Cooney and Crosby, 1944) Achroosteolysis (Andersen et al., 1992) Knife-edge remodeling of metatarsals and metacarpals (Møller-Christensen, 1961; Andersen et al., 1992) Osteoporosis (Jopling and McDougall, 1988)
Upper and lower limbs	Lepromatous osteomyelitis (Job, 1963; Andersen et al., 1994)	Diffuse active new bone formation (Andersen et al., 1994) Septic arthritis and ankylosis (Andersen et al., 1992) Ossification of the interosseous membrane (Lewis et al., 1995)

Before the mid-1980s, infantile leprosy was thought to be unlikely due to the slow generation time of *M. leprae* and a long incubation period (Jopling and McDougall, 1988). However in 1985, Brubaker et al. reported 91 cases in children less than 1 year of age and suggested that the infants had become exposed to the infection in utero. Such findings led researchers to argue that favorable conditions, in a highly susceptible host, may reduce the generation time of the bacillus from 13 days to just 26 hours (Brubaker et al., 1985; Girdhar et al., 1989). The placenta is highly vascular and a breach of its integrity may lead to large amounts of the bacilli reaching the fetus (Duncan et al., 1983). In addition, pathogens may be spread through the umbilical vein or through an ingestion of amniotic fluid (Jordan and Spencer, 1949). Congenital leprosy is a controversial issue in the clinical literature but evidence for this form of the disease has been argued since the late 1800s. Navarro (1890) reported two cases of babies born with widespread "leprous spots" with one including a sore on their ear. A similar diffuse rash was later reported in a neonate from India (Ramu, 1959) and considered to be lepromatous. In 1913, Rabinowitsch identified acid-fast bacilli in the heart blood of a fetus during an autopsy of a woman with lepromatous leprosy and argued for a hematogenous spread of the infection. Sugai and Monobe (1913) reportedly isolated leprae bacilli in the 33% of the 12 placenta of leprous mothers and 10 out of 12 of their newborns. Carrying out his own research into this area, Rodriguez (1926, p. 125) stated: "it is evident that the bacilli reach the fetus through placental circulation in a considerable proportion of cases…and is …particularly apt to occur in cases of lepra fever …accompanied by bacteremia." He went on to note that 16% of children with mothers who suffered leprosy-related fevers during pregnancy went on to develop the disease, but that he had not seen any newborns with lesions. Crozier and Cochrane (1929) reported lesions on the heel of a neonate born in a leprosy hospital. The lesion disappeared after treatment with hydnocarpus oil, but some months later an ulcer appeared on the scapula. They considered the possibility of congenital transmission via the infected father's semen as the mother was free from the disease. Since these early discoveries, Melsom et al. (1980) have reported IgA antibodies of *M. leprae* in the cord sera of children with leprous mothers, as IgA itself cannot be passed from the mother to the child across the placenta, the presence of these anti-*M. leprae* antibodies suggests the live passage of bacilli across the placenta and their active proliferation (Melsom et al., 1982).

Some researchers have suggested a gastrointestinal route for infantile infection. In 1778, Schillingii (1980) had stated leprosy could be transmitted from a leprous wet nurse to a suckling infant. In 1967, Pedley first isolated *M. leprae* in the breast milk of a Nepalese woman with lepromatous leprosy; although it is not known if the child ever developed the disease. Further studies revealed bacilli in the breast secretions of a nonlactating woman (Pedley, 1968a), and a leprous male with related gynecomastia (Pedley, 1968b). Girdhar et al. (1981) located bacilli in the breast milk of 8% (n = 1/13) of women with untreated tuberculoid leprosy, 12.5% (n = 1/8) in the borderline group, and 64% (n = 9/14) of women with untreated lepromatous leprosy. It is still not known what the effect of ingesting such vast quantities of infected breast milk has on the child, as exposure to the mother during feeding may also allow transmission through droplet infection and skin-to-skin contact. In addition, the ability of the bacteria to remain viable in the child's gut has yet to be demonstrated.

Pathogenesis in Children

Today, children are mostly diagnosed with the tuberculoid form of the disease, characterized by single nerve involvement and limited deformity (Butlin and Saunderson, 2014; Sundharam, 1990). Lepromatous leprosy in children occurs more often in areas where the disease is hyperendemic (Badger, 1964). Early signs of leprosy in children are usually confined to the skin and peripheral nerves. In a study of 610 children from Burma, the majority of whom were under 15 years of age, Noussitou et al. (1976) noted skin lesions in 79.5% with nerve involvement occurring in around 10% of cases. The most common lesions were hypopigmented patches (or macules), papuloid lesions, nodular lesions, ulcerations and scars (Fig. 7.16), with single lesions on the thighs the most common site and expression. Advanced deformities and bone absorption were rare under 15 years (Noussitou et al., 1976). Lara and Ignatio's (1956) study indicated that only 25% of children exposed to leprosy develop clinical signs of the disease and of those, only 10% are likely to develop full spectrum leprosy in adolescence. Berreman (1984) also reported a high rate of spontaneous healing (75%) in children living in leprosaria but questions the validity of the data arguing that many of these children may never have developed the disease without such high level of exposure. Figures of 12% remission outside the hospital environment have been reported (Berreman, 1984) and may be more representative of the true course of the disease. Given these data, it

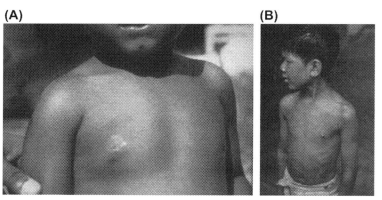

FIGURE 7.16 (A) A child with a single hypopigmented "macule" on the chest and (B) 10-year-old with lepromatous leprosy and diffuse nodular lesions on his nose, cheeks, earlobes, and arms. *From Noussitou, F., Sansarricq, H., Walter, J., 1976. Leprosy in Children, World Health Organisation, Geneva, p. 14.*

is difficult to assess what percentage of children exposed to the disease would go on to produce skeletal manifestations in the past.

Nerve Damage

Neuritis or inflammation of the nerves is the most common feature of leprosy and may be asymptomatic, or extensive with infiltration of the entire nerve and complete loss of muscle function. Symptoms involve pain, tenderness, swelling, loss of sensation, and paralysis. The bacilli enter the nervous system by several routes; direct extension from skin lesions into naked nerve filaments where they travel along the axon; by being engulfed by macrophages where they are protected from the host's immune system; or through the bloodstream entering the nervous system via interneural capillaries where the blood–nerve barrier is compromised (Job, 1989; Scollard, 2000). The most common areas of nerve involvement are the ulnar, median, lateral popliteal, tibial, great auricular, and less commonly, radial nerves (Dayal et al., 1990). In tuberculoid leprosy and the early stage of the disease, nerve damage is often patchy and confined to skin lesions. Loss of sensation may be superficial, or if the nerves of the trunk are involved, there will be a deeper loss of sensation. In the lepromatous form, almost all of the nerves of the body can become involved bilaterally, causing deep loss of sensation and muscle paralysis (Job, 1989). Granulomata form around the nerve, and caseous necrosis and abscesses may be present. The final stage of inflammation involves the formation of fibrous tissue replacing the Schwann cells, axons, and myelin sheaths (Job, 1989), with permanent nerve damage.

Skeletal Manifestations

The diagnosis of leprosy from skeletal remains relies on the quality of bone preservation and the severity of the disease at the time of the individual's death. In isolation, each skeletal lesion of leprosy may represent another condition causing infection or neuropathy. Therefore, a combination of infective and neuropathic lesions in the skeleton is needed before a positive diagnosis can be made.

Rhinomaxillary Syndrome

In 1922, Gomez et al. reported that in children with leprosy, bacilli in the nasal region were rare before the age of 13 years. An accumulation of bacilli in this area is thought to result in facial changes seen in the more advanced cases of lepromatous leprosy, and recognized skeletally as rhinomaxillary syndrome (RMS) (Andersen and Manchester, 1992). Changes within this syndrome are considered pathognomonic of leprosy and include as follows:

1. Inflammatory pitting of the oral palatine surface
2. Inflammatory pitting of the nasal palatine surface
3. Absorption of the anterior nasal spine
4. Absorption of the anterior maxillary alveolus (ceasing at the canines)
5. Absorption of the nasal aperture

Inflammatory pitting is located along the palatine suture, and in advanced cases, results in perforation of the palate. Absorption of the anterior alveolus results in loss of the central and lateral incisors, following the progress of the maxillary nerve, which ceases at the level of the canines (Fig. 7.17). These changes were first described by Møller-Christensen et al. (1952) in the skeletal remains from Naestved, Denmark. The maxillary mucous membrane may be the site of a primary lesion or granuloma (Hjørting-Hansen et al., 1965). Destruction of the nasal cartilage as the result of inflammatory granulomatous destruction causes the collapse of the nose known as "saddle-nose" (Job et al., 1966). Inflammation of the mucous membrane also involves coexistence of a sinus infection (Pinkerton, 1932). Alveolar destruction as the result of osteoclastic stimulation was found to be a slow process and associated most commonly with lepromatous leprosy (Marks and Subramaniam, 1978; Subramaniam et al., 1983). Mirander (1970) suggested that clinical cases of RMS in children were unusual. Previously, Michman and Sagher (1957) noted atrophy of the nasal spine and alveolar process in individuals as young as 14 years after suffering from the disease for 3 years, although changes were more commonly seen after 6 years with the disease. Advanced RMS occurred after 17 years duration. Reichart (1976) found no maxillary changes in 12 patients under 20 years old, who had suffered with the disease for an average of 5 years. In both of these studies, the patients were undergoing chemotherapy. As Subramaniam et al. (1983) report that treatment delays destructive changes to the face, so we might expect earlier and more pronounced changes in children from the archeological record. Although, even in untreated cases facial lesions can take up to 17 years to appear (Reichart, 1976). There are several differential diagnoses for the facial changes seen in leprosy including lupus vulgaris of TB, rhinoscleroma, Binder syndrome, leishmaniasis, yaws, and syphilis.

Dentition

Leprogenic odontodysplasia (LOD) refers to the development of concentrically stunted roots in the developing permanent maxillary incisors, as a direct result of *M. leprae* bacilli, and is thought to be indicative of childhood exposure to the disease. Danielsen (1968) first discussed

168 Paleopathology of Children

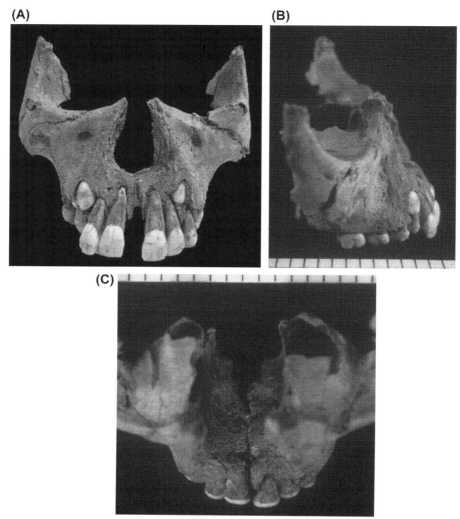

FIGURE 7.17 Rhinomaxillary syndrome in a child from Romano–British Gambier-Parry Lodge showing (A) remodeling of the nasal aperture and reduction of the central alveolar margin, (B) loss of the anterior nasal spine, and (C) diffuse inflammatory pitting on the nasal palatine surface.

these defects in four children with rhinomaxillary changes from Naestved in Denmark aged 8 to 11 years. The most severe case was in an 8- to 9-year-old (Burial 404) with marked dental enamel hypoplasia on the crowns of the maxillary central incisors that terminated in stunted apical buds 2–3 mm in length (Fig. 7.18). It was estimated that the hypoplasia formed at 4 years while the stunted roots occurred around 5 years of age. Danielsen (1970) considered the stunted dental development to be the result of a direct infiltration of leprous bacilli into the pulp cavity during alveolar absorption. Similar changes have been reported from medieval Croatia in a young female (Šilkanjić and Meštrović, 2006), but poor preservation of the maxilla did not allow for an assessment of leprosy, and it was not considered as a potential diagnosis. Matos and Santos (2013) describe a case of RMS and LOD in a 13- to 19-year-old from St Jørgen's hospital in Odense, Denmark, dating to the 13th–17th century. The adolescent had bilateral periosteal new bone formation, acroosteolysis of the proximal foot phalanx, and LOD of the maxillary right central incisor with a constricted tip of the lateral incisor root. Cases of LOD were also identified in four nonadults from the leprosy cemetery at Winchester, England (Tucker pers. comm.).

These dental changes have yet to be reported in the clinical literature of leprosy patients (Roberts, 1986). Some scholars consider hypotrophic roots to be a nonmetric dental trait (Cunha et al., 2006), and they have also been described as symmetrical rhizomicria, a hereditary deformity. These short-rooted teeth usually occur in both central maxillary incisors. Ten percent of Japanese children have this anomaly as do 2% of Swedish children (Schuurs,

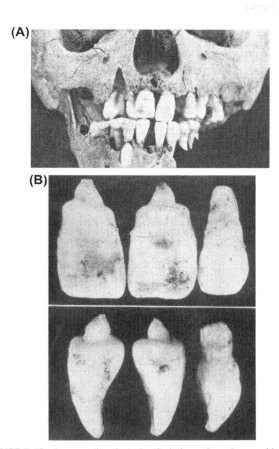

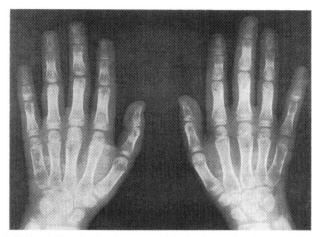

FIGURE 7.18 Leprogenic odontodysplasia in an 8- to 9-year-old from Naestved, Denmark (skeleton 404). (A) There is limited remodeling and inflammatory pitting of the alveolar margin. The left lateral incisor was lost antemortem. (B) The roots of the permanent central incisors and right lateral incisor are severely stunted and concentrically restricted; seen from the front (above) and the side (below). There is a wide banded enamel defect at the base of the crowns. *Used with permission from University Press of Southern Denmark. Møller-Christensen V. 1978. Leprosy Changes of the Skull. Odense: Odense University Press. (B) Danielsen, K., 1970. Odontodysplasia leprosa in Danish medieval skeletons. Tandlaegebladet 74, 7.*

FIGURE 7.19 Hands of a 7-year-old who has suffered leprosy since 2 years old. There is generalized osteopenia of the phalanges, patchy osteoporosis and expansion of the shaft and medullary cavity of the fifth metacarpals. *From Newman, H., Casey, B., Du Bois, J., Gallagher, T., 1972. Roentgen features of leprosy in children. American Journal of Radiology 114 (2), 404.*

2013). Other suggestions are that they represent resorption of previously formed roots due to trauma, occlusal pressure, or exposure to toxins, but the changes seen in leprosy cases are normally asymmetrical and occlusal pressure would be expected to affect all anterior teeth and cause hypercementosis (Cunha et al., 2006). Similar changes may also be seen in Downs and Steven–Johnson syndrome. The direct link between leprosy and short roots is therefore not certain. The presence of the anomaly in cases of childhood leprosy may be the result of exposure to toxins from the bacteria, or it may simply be coincidental appearing in populations with a genetic propensity to demonstrate this trait. The latter argument may be weakened by the more recent identification of LOD outside Scandinavia (i.e., in Winchester England). Until the exact cause of the dental lesions can be ascertained, they should be considered within the possible suite of changes seen in leprosy, rather than pathognomonic of the disease.

Hands and Feet

Children may be subject to peripheral nerve damage, paralysis, anesthesia, and deformity, but would need to survive with permanent changes for such damage to be seen on their skeletons. Newman et al.'s (1972) study of bone changes in the hands and feet of 22 Vietnamese children with leprosy aged 5–15 years identified widespread disuse osteoporosis with cortical thinning of the metacarpals, metatarsals and phalanges due to paralysis of the ulnar nerve in claw–hand deformity. Expansion of the medullary cavity, concentric remodeling, claw–hand deformity, acroosteolysis, enlarged nutrient foramina, and absorptive changes were the most common findings. Enlarged nutrient foramina are thought to a result from infection of the nutrient vessels (Faget and Mayoral, 1944). Bone resorption (concentric remodeling) was found to result from the accelerated activity of osteoclasts and osteolytic osteocytes stimulated by presence of the leprous bacilli, rather than the result of neuropathy alone (Marks, 1979). Newman et al. (1972) described the appearance of metacarpal lesions in a 7-year-old who had suffered from leprosy for 4 years as "an expansion of the shaft, thinned cortices, and loss of normal trabeculae" (Newman et al., 1972, p. 410) an appearance that may mimic dactylitis of TB or syphilis in the absence of new bone formation (Fig. 7.19). The identification of claw–hand in children means that lesions such as grooves on the palmer surface of the proximal

170 Paleopathology of Children

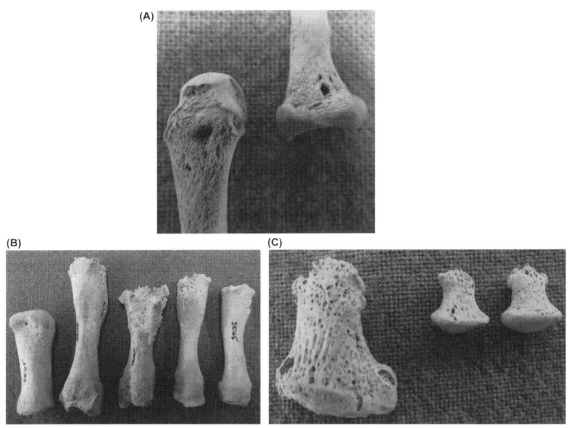

FIGURE 7.20 Changes to the hands and feet in nonadults from the leprosaria site of St Mary Magdalene in Winchester, England. Changes include: (A) enlarged nutrient foramen in the distal metacarpal and proximal phalanx of a 16- to 18-year-old (skeleton 56), (B) inflammatory pitting and lytic destruction of the distal aspects of metacarpals 1–3 in a 13- to 15-year-old (skeleton 45), and (C) acroostolysis of the distal foot phalanges in a 16- to 18-year-old (skeleton 14). *Reproduced with the kind permission of Simon Roffey, University of Winchester.*

phalanges described by Andersen and Manchester (1987) should be visible in the hands of nonadults, due to long standing hyperflexion of the interphalangeal joints and hyperextension of the metacarpophalangeal joints in motor neuropathy.

Foot lesions tend to be less common. For example, Mahajan et al. (1995) examined the level of deformity in 143 leprous Indian children aged 0–14 years but none showed any sign of foot deformity. To date, no examples of dorsal tarsal bars or navicular compression fractures ("squeezing") have been identified in child cases from archeological contexts as the result of flat foot in motor neuropathy (Andersen and Manchester, 1988). Nevertheless, three nonadults from the St Mary Magdalene hospital site in Winchester showed severe foot changes, including osteitis, concentric remodeling, and joint disruption (Fig. 7.20). All were aged between 13 and 16 years (Tucker pers. comm.) and it is likely children need longer walking on a disrupted foot before any changes will occur.

Periostitis and Osteomyelitis

Leprogenic periostitis may occur secondary to neuropathy in the lower legs and extremities. A loss of sensation causes neglected ulcerations that allow toxins from pyogenic bacteria to spread up the muscle planes of the legs, inflaming the periosteum, and resulting in new bone formation on the tibiae and fibulae (Fig. 7.21; Lewis et al., 1995). Ulcerations of the legs and elbows have been reported in clinical cases of childhood leprosy (Noussitou et al., 1976). Skinsnes et al. (1972) examined the skeletal changes of amputated hands and feet from patients in China. They noted more advanced vascular changes in the foot of a 16-year-old compared to a 45-year-old, and secondary arthritis, periostitis and osteitis were not age dependent. Leprosy osteomyelitis as the result of direct infiltration of the bacteria through ulcerated lesions is most common in the hands and feet and may be situated at the joints causing septic arthritis (Job, 1963). Osteomyelitis was found in individuals who had suffered the disease for between 2 and 13 years. Crespo

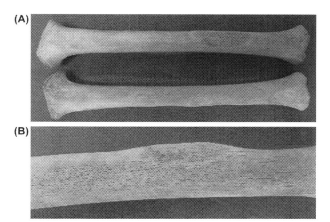

FIGURE 7.21 (A) Active subperiosteal new bone formation and localized osteitis on the left tibia probably as the result of a leg ulcer in a 13- to 16-year-old from St Mary Magdalene, Winchester (B) with close-up. *Reproduced with the kind permission of Simon Roffey, University of Winchester.*

et al. (2017) have suggested that the high prevalence of periostitis in leprosy and other chronic infections may be the result of a stimulated immune system and greater susceptibility to inflammation, rather than to the spread of secondary infections.

Paleopathology

Documentary and artistic evidence suggest childhood leprosy did exist in the past. The portrait of a 13-year-old boy from a Scandinavian leprosy hospital illustrated by Danielsson and Boeck in 1848, clearly shows the nodule expression of lepromatous leprosy. Numerous cases of childhood leprosy have been identified in the archeological record, most commonly from England and Denmark, with the youngest aged between 8 and 9 years (Lewis, 2002). The majority derive from cemeteries associated with leprosy hospitals, which may indicate children entered the institutions with their parents to avoid becoming orphans; as patients with recognizable signs of the disease; or were born in the leprosaria to leprous parents (Lewis, 2002). In England, isolated cases of RMS from lay cemeteries have been reported from Scarborough Castle (Brothwell, 1958), Gambier-Parry Lodge (Lewis, 2002), and Wharram Percy where a 10-year-old with reactive new bone on the nasal palatine surface, a thickened and rounded nasal aperture, and resorption of the anterior nasal spine, tested positive for leprosy aDNA (Taylor et al., 2006). Another potential case of leprosy in a Turkish infant was established on a strongly positive signal for *M. leprae* aDNA (Rubini et al., 2014). The child displayed no skeletal changes other than endocranial lesions, and concerns have been raised about the validity of such strong signals which may indicate modern contamination (Stone et al., 2009). An 11- to 12-year-old from 10th century Sigtuna in Sweden, displayed atrophy of the nasal spine, a rounded nasal aperture, a pitted palatine process, an enlarged incisive fossa, and LOD of central incisors. There was also a lytic lesion on lateral proximal fibula with fine periosteal new bone formation, and concentric atrophy of the first distal phalanx of the foot (Kjellström, 2012).

From leprosaria sites, Møller-Christensen's (1961, 1978) identified leprosy in 16 nonadults (under 14 years) from St. Jørgen's Hospital in Naestved (AD 1250–1550), three (18.7%) with RMS, while 37.5% and 25% had changes to the hands and feet respectively. However, these included isolated nonspecific lesions such as enlarged foramina and osteochondritis dissecans. In the adult group, 68% and 77.5% had hand and foot lesions. None of the children in this age group had periostitis of the legs compared to 85% in the adult group (Møller-Christensen, 1961). Møller-Christensen (1969) reported the greatest prevalence of leprosy in the 14- to 20-year age group, at 83.6%. This demographic profile suggests poor survival of individuals with the disease, and hints at an early age in infection. Anderson (1998) published 11 cases of leprosy in nonadults from Anglo-Saxon St. John de Berstrete Timberhill in Norwich. The children were aged between 12 and 20 years, and five had evidence of RMS with associated postcranial changes. Recent excavations at the later medieval leprosarium of St Mary Magdalene Winchester (AD 1010–1160) have identified possible lepromatous leprosy in nine nonadults aged 7–18 years. (Roffey and Tucker, 2012). By contrast, a review of the skeletons excavated from Sts. James and Mary Magdalene's Hospital in Chichester, England, did not reveal individuals under the age of 17 years with obvious signs of leprosy (Lewis, 2008).

How many children were born of leprous parents in the past is open to some debate. Medieval Scottish law banned women with leprosy from the company of men and threatened the women being buried alive with her child should she become pregnant (Boece, 1535 cited in Duncan, 1985b). Leprosaria practiced the separation of men and women, and in AD 789 Charlemagne forbad the marriage of "lepers". Pope Urban III cited leprosy as the reason to close a betrothal in AD 1186 (Simpson, 1872). If conceived, the weakness of the children and susceptibility to infections may mean they entered the archeological record without chronic skeletal changes. References to the congenital form of leprosy were common in medieval Europe but may have resulted from confusion with congenital syphilis, and a lack of knowledge about how leprosy was transmitted. For example, many considered leprosy to be a venereal disease, perhaps due to the downgrading of some women from less obvious tuberculous pole, to the more evident lepromatous form of the disease during pregnancy (Duncan et al., 1981). The diagnosis of children with leprosy in the past and present is hindered by the subtle nature of the disease in young individuals and its potential to spontaneously heal. Children who develop the disease usually suffer from the indeterminate, borderline or tuberculoid leprosy, which are harder to identify due to the nonspecific nature of the lesions in the skeleton and lack of rhinomaxillary changes. Even if RMS does develop, the rhinomaxilla needs to be complete to identify the earliest changes. Unfortunately, the maxilla is very fragile and is often damaged during burial, excavation, or curation. To identify LOD, the roots of the maxillary permanent incisors need to be fully formed and so defects in individuals under the age of 7 or 8 years can go undetected. In addition, these defects are associated with RMS, but as this condition advances the maxillary incisors are often lost. Without the changes of the skull, we rely on the characteristic lesions of the hands, feet, tibiae, and fibulae. These changes usually only occur in adults and older children. The high susceptibility of children with leprosy to other infections means that they may have died before they became mobile and gross deformities developed. A review of 24 cases of nonadult leprosy (Table 7.2) illustrates how RMS develops at a young age (8–12 years), but postcranial changes mostly occur in the older children (13–16 and 16–19 years), who likely suffered the condition for longer before they died (Fig. 7.22).

The early development of RMS in nonadults not only provides evidence for the route of entry of the disease via the mouth and respiratory tract, but also suggests that cases of leprosy in child skeletal remains can be readily diagnosed. The significance of child cases is that we should expect to see a greater number of cases, and more lepromatous leprosy in areas where the disease was hyperendemic. In both Naestved and Winchester young children were developing the most severe expression of the condition suggesting that in early medieval Europe, leprosy was hyperendemic.

TREPONEMAL DISEASES

Treponemal diseases are four clinically different conditions caused by infection with *Treponema pallidum* a spirochete bacterium. Bejel (endemic syphilis, treponarid), yaws, and pinta have very specific geographical distributions, whereas syphilis and its congenital variant can be found worldwide. Pinta does not affect the skeleton and is not recognized paleopathologically. The skeletal lesions displayed by the other three conditions show considerable overlap often making the exact etiology of the treponematosis impossible to diagnose. Yaws and bejel are childhood conditions normally transmitted through contact with infected skin and mucous membrane, from where they disseminate through the bloodstream. These conditions were originally confined to the dry or tropical zones of Africa and Asia (Mitjà et al., 2013). Grin (1956) states that while these conditions are virtually indistinguishable from one another, the different pattern of lesions is the result of different cultural and environmental factors. Lesions first appear on the legs in yaws as the result of abrasions from vegetation on these uncovered parts of the body, while lesions of the oral area are more common in bejel transmitted through kissing and sharing utensils. In yaws, the mode of transmission allows for a massive amount of bacilli to enter the body, while in bejel the less convenient mode of transmission limits the amount taken in. Both will eventually produce gummatous lesions and ulcerations.

Due to its mode of transmission through sexual contact, syphilis is normally considered an adult condition, with the congenital form occurring in infants and children born to infected mothers. *T. palladium* is readily killed by drying and can only survive outside the body for a few hours (Mitjà et al., 2013). Ortner (2003) discusses the controversy that surrounds the understanding of these diseases as to whether they constitute diseases caused by different strains of a single pathogen, or represent one pathogen with a different expression as the result of individual immune responses and other host factors. The antiquity of venereal syphilis in the Americas and Europe is also a matter of considerable debate. There are two main theories for the spread of the venereal disease. The first theory (Crosby, 1969) is that syphilis was present in the Americas and was brought to the Europe by Columbus and his crew in the 1490s. The reported rapid spread and extreme virulence of the European epidemic seems to attest the introduction of a new disease in a virgin population (Harper et al., 2011). The second popular theory is the "pre-Columbian hypothesis" that purports that syphilis was already in the Europe in the 15th century but was hidden as a low virulent form or reported as venereal "leprosy." Supporters of this theory argue that the epidemic of the 15th century was either the result of the disease's increased virulence, or its greater recognition with the spread of information through the invention of the printing press (Hackett, 1963; Holcomb, 1934; Hudson, 1967). Others theorize that bejel and yaws were also present in Europe before dying out as the result of improved environmental conditions (Grin, 1956; Willcox, 1960). The presence of congenital syphilis is crucial in establishing the endemic nature of venereal form in Europe prior to Columbus (Erdal, 2006; Harper et al., 2011) and contributes to the continuing debate raging between paleopathologists surrounding the origin, evolution, and transmission of treponemal disease (for example, see Baker and Armelagos, 1988; Meyer et al., 2002; Powell and Cook, 2005).

TABLE 7.2 Changes Most Commonly Associated With Leprosy in Nonadult Skeletons From Archeological Contexts

Skeleton	Age (years)	Rhinomaxillary Syndrome					LOD	Periostitis	Postcranial Lesions			References
		PPMN	PPMO	NA	ANS	Alveolar			Hand	Foot	Osteomyelitis	
Gambier-Parry Lodge (?)	8–9	X	X	X	X	X		No postcranium				Lewis (2002)
Naestved (B404)	9			X	X	X	X					Møller-Christensen (1961)
Winchester (B8)	9–10			X			X	X				Tucker (personal communication)
Wharram Percy (B708)	10	X		X				X				Mays (2007)
Naestved (B308)	10						X					Møller-Christensen (1961)
Naestved (B127)	10	X			X	X						Møller-Christensen (1961)
Naestved (B217)	11						X					Møller-Christensen (1961)
Siguna (B3092)	11–12			X	X	X	X	X		X		Kjellström (2010)
Timberhill (B1518)	12–15	X	X					X		X		Anderson (1998)
Winchester (B52)	13–15				X	X	X	X	X			Tucker (personal communication)
Winchester (B54)	13–15		X (p)	X	X		X	X	X	X		Tucker (personal communication)
Scarborough (B4832)	15			X	X	X		No postcranium				Brothwell (1958)
Winchester (B28)	13–16		X	X	X	X	X	X		X		Tucker (personal communication)
Winchester (B41)	13–16	X	X	X				X	X	X		Tucker (personal communication)
Timberhill (B13101)	13–16	X	X					X				Anderson (1998)

Continued

TABLE 7.2 Changes Most Commonly Associated With Leprosy in Nonadult Skeletons From Archeological Contexts—cont'd

Skeleton	Age (years)	Rhinomaxillary Syndrome					Periostitis	Postcranial Lesions			References
		PPMN	PPMO	NA	ANS	Alveolar	LOD		Hand	Foot	Osteomyelitis	
Winchester (B45)	13–17	X			X	X		X	X	X	X	Tucker (personal communication)
Odense (B572)	13–19		X	X	X	X	X	X		X		Matos and Santos (2006)
Timberhill (B11525)	15–18	X	X									Anderson (1998)
Timberhill (B11328)	16	X		X	X			X				Anderson (1998)
Winchester (B46)	16–17		X			X		X		X		Tucker (personal communication)
Winchester (B14)	16–18		X	X					X	X		Tucker (personal communication)
Winchester (B56)	16–18		X			X	X		X		X	Tucker (personal communication)
Winchester (B18)	16–18	X	X		X	X	X	X	X	X	X	Tucker (personal communication)
Winchester (B14)	16–19		X	X					X	X		Tucker (personal communication)

ANS, anterior nasal spine; LOD, leprogenic odontodysplasia; PPMN, inflammatory pitting of the nasal palatine surface; PPMO, inflammatory pitting of the oral palatine surface; NA, nasal aperture.

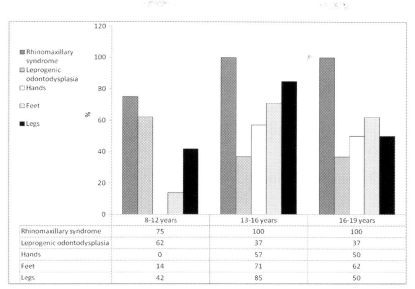

FIGURE 7.22 Percentage prevalence of skeletal changes in nonadults with leprosy from various sites in Scandinavia and England. Lesions on the hands, feet, and legs increase with age.

Yaws

Yaws is a nonvenereal endemic treponemal infection caused by *T. pallidum* subspecies *pertenue*. Yaws is a chronic relapsing disease spread through skin-to-skin contact and causing skeletal and mucosal lesions that can become destructive (Marks et al., 2014). Skeletal involvement is estimated to be between 5% and 15% (Steinbock, 1976). The early skin lesions of yaws are teaming with bacteria and are highly infectious compared to the late yaws lesions (Marks et al., 2014). The existence of congenital yaws is still debated. Today, yaws mainly affects children living in poor densely populated rural areas in warm and humid climates (Marks et al., 2014). Yaws is primarily considered a skin disorder causing lesions of bone and cartilage in the later stages (Mitjà et al., 2013).

Primary yaws starts with a papule (known as the "mother yaw"), at the inoculation site after 21 days, most commonly on the legs and ankles. In up to 15% of patients secondary yaws will develop (Marks et al., 2014), or the disease may become latent reappearing 5–10 years later. Secondary yaws describes the dissemination of infection through the blood and lymphatic system with florid skin and bone lesions appearing between 1 month and 2 years after the spread (Marks et al., 2014). The most commonly involved bones are the tibia, fibula, and femur, with the spine, ribs, and pelvis also affected. Symmetrical spina ventosa of one or multiple fingers and periosteal new bone formation may also be evident. The lesions can heal (Hackett, 1957; Marks et al., 2014). In 10% of untreated cases yaws enters a tertiary stage with ulcerating nodules at the joints and saber tibia. Destruction of the joints including the elbow, phalanges, and interphalangeal joints may be present in child cases. Involvement of the interphalangeal joints may also damage the epiphyses causing shortening of the digits (Fig. 7.23; Ortner, 2003). This destruction of the joints in the hand is not seen in bejel or venereal or congenital syphilis and provides a defining feature of this disease. Before 15 years of age the "boomerang leg" may develop defined as a bowing deformity of the tibia and fibula (Fig. 7.24). Unlike the saber shin of congenital syphilis, this is true bowing where the medullary cavity is abnormally curved (Hackett, 1936). In the cranium there may be gummatous lesions (caries sicca), facial destruction of the nasal cavity and palate (gangosa), and new bone formation and exostoses on the maxilla (goundou).

Based on its early date and location on the Mariana Islands of Australia (AD 850), Stewart and Spoehr (1951) suggested yaws as a diagnosis for the gummatous lesions and caries sicca in a 14-year-old individual and provided images of this rare case. In a wider survey of 23 nonadults under 16 years from a later site in the Pacific Taumako Islands in Melanesia (AD 1530–1700), Buckley and Tayles (2003) suggested yaws as a possible diagnosis for five children aged 1–6 years based on the distribution of lesions on multiple bones, especially the tibia and clavicle. They emphasized the difficulties in providing a diagnosis due to the possible coexistence of scurvy and the lack of caries sicca development in the nonadults. Clinical evidence from the Pacific islands had identified yaws as endemic before European contact with 30% of children infected, many before 3 years of age. In 1980, an outbreak of the infection affected children aged 7 and 13 years (Buckley and Tayles, 2003). While the weight of evidence suggests yaws in these cases, none identified changes to the joints of the hand.

176 Paleopathology of Children

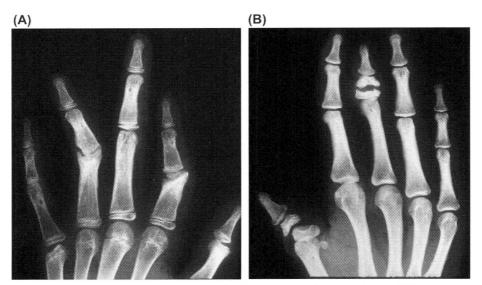

FIGURE 7.23 (A) Joint destruction of the proximal interphalangeal joints in a 12-year-old from Uganda (Case 388), and (B) "opera-glass" fingers due to destruction of the diaphyses of the middle phalanges resulting in shortening of the digits in an 18-year-old male (case 239). These lesions are potentially important in distinguishing tertiary yaws from the other treponemal diseases in children. *From Hackett, C., 1957. An International Nomenclature on Yaws Lesions, World Health Organisation, Geneva.*

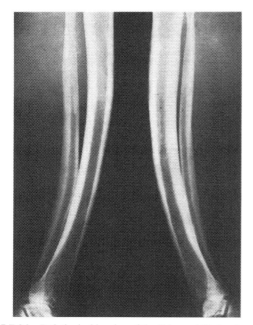

FIGURE 7.24 Pathological bowing of the tibiae and fibulae (boomerang leg) in response to nonsuppurative osteomyelitis in yaws. Note the reduced and bowed medullary cavity. *From musculoskeletakey.com.*

Endemic Syphilis (Bejel, Treponarid)

Caused by *T. pallidum endemicum*, bone lesions are rare in children under 2 years of age in bejel (Ortner, 2003). Bejel is normally confined to drier climates than yaws, such as the Middle East and dry areas of Africa, in poor, overcrowded areas with limited hygiene (Grin, 1956). The bacilli take refuge in moist parts of the body such as the mouth and are spread through kissing and contaminated drinking vessels (Abdolrasouli et al., 2013). Bejel is primarily considered a semimucosal disorder, causing lesions of bone and cartilage in the secondary stages (Mitjà et al., 2013). The primary lesion is small and usually located within the mouth or nose. Later lesions form on the legs and ankles (65%–85%), buttocks, hands, and face (Mitjà et al., 2013), with destruction of the facial bone (gongosa) and ulcerations of the legs a characteristic feature (Abdolrasouli et al., 2013). The potential for new bone and gumma formation on the tibia and ulna of young children make congenital syphilis a potential differential diagnosis (Ortner, 2003).

Congenital Syphilis

Venereal syphilis is the only treponemal disease to have a recognized congenital form. This is thought to be due to its transmission in adulthood. The childhood transmission of yaws and bejel means that they are unlikely to be virulent by the time childbearing age is reached, whereas venereal syphilis is contracted around sexual maturity, and pregnancy can occur shortly after (Grin, 1956). Mothers in the early and secondary stages of infection are most likely to transmit the disease to their child. The longer the mother has the disease the less chance of fetal infection (Fiumara and Lessel, 1970). Hence, congenital syphilis develops in the fetus secondary to active venereal syphilis in the mother (Genç and Ledger, 2000). While it is traditionally reported that *T. pallidum* can be transmitted to the fetus as early as the ninth week of gestation, Fiumara and Lessel (1970) assert that transmission will not occur until after the first 16 weeks of pregnancy. This is because the cylindrical Langerhans cells that make up the early placenta structure provide an effective protective barrier. The pathogen enters the fetal bloodstream and spreads to almost every bone in the body (Steinbock, 1976). In most cases, toxins released from dead microorganisms invoke an allergic response and uterine contractions in the mother, resulting in fetal death and spontaneous abortion in the first half of the pregnancy (Genç and Ledger, 2000). As the body's ability to mount an inflammatory response to infection is not fully developed until the third trimester, these tiny remains, if they survive into the archeological record, will show no signs of disease.

At term, a child may be stillborn due to placentitis, growth retardation, preterm labor, or premature rupture of membranes in utero (Bennett et al., 1997). In some cases a premature or sickly infant will be born alive but infant mortality is around 20% due to hepatitis, respiratory failure, acidosis, and secondary infections (Bennett et al., 1997). In children who initially appear unaffected at birth, 66% will develop symptoms by the time they are 8 weeks old or by 2 years of age (early congenital syphilis) (Hollier and Cox, 1998). Others may not display signs of the infection until they are around 2 years of age or even until puberty (late congenital syphilis) (Ortner, 2003). Harman (1917) reported pregnancies in infected women resulting in spontaneous abortion in 17% of cases and stillbirths in 23%, while 21% of the infants developed congenital syphilis. However, 39% were unaffected at birth. The infection can also be spread to the newborn during their passage through the birth canal or contact with genital lesions, and although not spread through the breast milk, lesions of the breast are a hazard to the sucking child (Genç and Ledger, 2000). In fact, in the 19th century, it was noted that infants taken away from their syphilitic mothers could pass on the infection to the breast of their wet nurse through the sores on their mouths (Lomax, 1979). Genç and Ledger (2000) tabulated the clinical manifestations of congenital syphilis in early and late cases, with skeletal involvement being more common in the early manifestation of the disease, and dental and facial lesions more apparent in late onset congenital syphilis (Table 7.3).

TABLE 7.3 Clinical Manifestations of Congenital Syphilis

Clinical Findings	Percentage
Early Onset	
Abnormal bone X-ray	61
Hepatomegaly	51
Splenomegaly	49
Petechiae	41
Skin lesions	35
Anemia	34
Lymphadenopathy	32
Jaundice	30
Pseudoparalysis	28
Snuffles	23
Late Onset	
Higoumenakis' sign	86
Frontal bossing	30–87
Palatal deformation	76
Dental dystropathies[a]	55
Interstitial keratitis[a]	20–50
Abnormal bone X-ray	30–46
Nasal deformity (saddle nose)[a]	10–30
Eighth nerve deafness	3–4
Neurosyphilis	1–5
Joint disorder	1–3

[a]Hutchinson's triad.
Adapted from Genç, M., Ledger, W., 2000. Syphilis in pregnancy. Sexually Transmitted Infections 76, 75.

Early Onset Congenital Syphilis

Early onset syphilis occurs in infants and children under 2 years of age and is usually characterized by jaundice, pseudoparalysis, convulsions, respiratory tract infections, a diffuse rash on palms and soles of feet, diarrhea, fever, and nasal discharge (Fleming and Bardenstein, 1971). Bone involvement may occur but in 50%–75% of cases lesions heal spontaneously or are asymptomatic (Steinbock, 1976). The first indication of bone involvement is a symmetrical and bilateral widening band of decreased calcification leading to destruction or Wimberger's corner sign. Wimberger's sign is found on the proximal ends of the tibiae on the medial aspect (Steinbock, 1976) and may correspond to defects on the distal femora (Caffey, 1945). These changes are considered pathognomonic of congenital syphilis and are reported in 50% of cases (Steinbock, 1976). Dorfman and Glaser (1990) found these radiological bone changes in children as young as 14-weeks-old in New York where babies with syphilis had been missed and remained untreated. It is important to distinguish Wimberger's sign from Wimberger's ring seen in the osteoporotic epiphyses of scurvy.

The macroscopic lesions of the long bones form a triad of osteochondritis, osteomyelitis, and periostitis (Caffey, 1939). Caffey (1939) asserts that these lesions are more indicative of syphilis when they occur together in the infant skeleton, than when they occur independently. Osteochondritis describes bone and cartilage disruption and has two forms. In the "passive form" the pathogen affects endochondral ossification as it occurs, while in the "active form" syphilitic granulomatous tissue invades already formed bones and joints causing the bone to weaken and fracture, particularly at the growing metaphysis (Ortner, 2003). The bones most affected are the tibia, ulna, and radius followed by the femur, humerus, and fibula. Formation of granular tissue adds to the irregularity of the bone surface as it replaces the normal trabecular bone. Another feature reported by early radiologists is the serration or "sawtooth" appearance of the metaphyseal ends of the long bones (Harris, 1933). These lesions have not been reported in osteological studies so far, and such jagged edges may be lost postmortem, or may be mistaken for the "bristles-of-a-brush" features more typically seen in rickets and scurvy. This sawtooth appearance is caused by focal bone necrosis at the metaphyseal ends, infractions with impaction, and horizontal displacement of fragments (Caffey, 1939). A thick cloak of layered active new bone is characteristic of syphilitic periostitis and is a reactive and reparative response to infection (Steinbock, 1976). The new bone is normally thickest at the midshaft of the long bones (Fig. 7.25). Periostitis is usually accompanied by osteochondritis and osteomyelitis by the fifth month of life (Caffey, 1939). In one study, periostitis was only reported in 7.8% of congenital syphilis cases (Steinbock, 1976), and it has also been described in neonates with trauma, healing rickets and scurvy, anemia, gonorrhea, smallpox, and congenital heart disease (Caffey, 1939). Osteomyelitis normally occurs at or near the metaphyseal ends of the long bones, but similar to the others in the triad, this lesion is not confined to syphilis when it occurs in isolation (Fig. 7.26).

As with TB, the abundance of red bone marrow in the fingers results in dactylitis in the child and the development of a thin bone shell around the shaft. The proximal phalanges are most commonly affected on both hands,

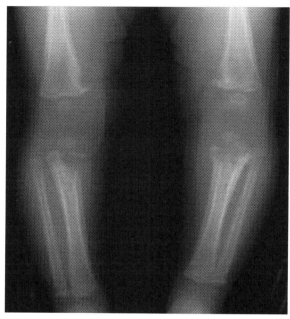

FIGURE 7.25 Classic Wimberger's sign of congenital syphilis with bilateral and symmetrical destruction of the medial metaphyses of the distal femora and proximal tibiae. A cloak of periosteal new bone is also evident on the shafts. *From Palmer, P. and Reeder, M. The Imaging of Tropical Diseases. http://www.isradiology.org/tropical_diseases/tmcr/chapter35/clinical9.htm.*

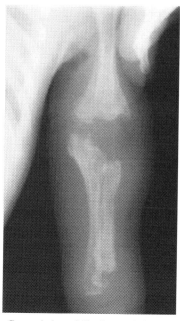

FIGURE 7.26 Congenital syphilis in an infant showing advanced destructive osteochondritis at the distal end of the left humerus, and the proximal left radius and ulna. Florid periosteal reaction gives the diaphyses a "bone within a bone" appearance. *From Palmer, P. and Reeder, M. The Imaging of Tropical Diseases. http://www.isradiology.org/tropical_diseases/tmcr/chapter35/clinical9.htm.*

although the fingers affected may differ (Ortner, 2003). Caffey (1939) did not think these changes could be distinguished from dactylitis seen in TB. Involvement of the skull in early congenital syphilis is not common (5%–10% of clinical cases), but there may be necrosing osteitis affecting both tables of the skull and causing sequestra, or hypertrophic periostitis formation (Steinbock, 1976). One of the other difficulties in diagnosing congenital syphilis in skeletal remains is that it is likely to coexist with nutritional disturbances such as rickets, scurvy, and anemia that will complicate the radiographic signs and contribute to pathological changes at the metaphyses and on the skull. Hence, a series of lesions including the triad is necessary to confirm a diagnosis. Unlike later onset congenital syphilis, there are no dental signatures to aid in a diagnosis, although infants may develop enamel hypoplasia on the central and lateral incisors, and are prone to severe wear and caries (Sarnet and Shaw, 1942). In addition, Hillson (1996) suggested the pitting at the base of the cusps of the deciduous second molars might be associated with this form of congenital syphilis.

Late Onset Congenital Syphilis

Late onset congenital syphilis first manifests after 2 years of age with lesions generally appearing between 5 and 15 years of age (Steinbock, 1976). Around 7% of cases are reported to result in skeletal changes (Steinbock, 1976). Bone lesions in late congenital syphilis are similar to those seen in acquired venereal syphilis in the adult, and comprise mainly of profuse periostitis and gummatous lesions, saddle nose, dental stigmata, Clutton's joints, saber shins, and neuropathy (Steinbock, 1976). Like the early form, the tibia is again the most frequent bone involved (Bennett et al., 1997; Steinbock, 1976). Due to the similarity in the lesions, distinguishing acquired (venereal) syphilis from late onset congenital syphilis in older individuals presents a challenge. However, osteitis at the sternal end of the clavicle or Higoumenakis' sign was a well-recognized feature of late congenital syphilis in the early clinical literature resulting from clogging of the spirochete in the connective tissue in this area (Glickman and Minsky, 1937). First described in 1927, Higoumenakis had recognized the lesion in 86% of his patients aged 15–56 years and it had a right sided prediction (Powell and Cook, 2005). However, Dax and Stewart (1939) also recognized the sign in 5.4% (n = 65) of individuals without syphilis. The "saber shin tibia of Fournier" describes layered bone deposits on the anterior aspect of the tibial midshaft in congenital syphilis. The normally sharp anterior of the tibia becomes rounded and the medullary cavity progressively narrow due to corresponding endosteal bone deposition. There may also be gummatous formation. The bone appears bowed, but unlike saber shin of yaws and the bowing of rickets, the medullary cavity will appear straight when viewed on a radiograph. In some cases, however, bowing may occur if the tibia experiences overgrowth due to the presence of infection, but remains fixed at either end by the attachment of the fibula (Steinbock, 1976). Gummatous lesions, made up of syphilitic granulomatous tissue, are less frequent and more contained than adult forms, and lesions may mimic those seen in TB or metastatic cancer.

Facial changes are more frequent in congenital syphilis than in the acquired form. In their study of adults with congenital syphilis Fiumara and Lessel (1970) reported saddle nose in 73.4% of their patients and considered it an end stage of syphilitic rhinitis occurring early in the neonatal period. The inflamed nasal mucosa destroys the underlying bone and cartilage of the nose, including perforation of the nasal septum resulting in a sunken nose. A respiratory infection develops, known as the "syphilitic snuffles" where "…a profuse discharge of pus, perhaps bloodstained, [is] continually running from the nose, so that the infant cannot suck and is half asphyxiated if it tries to close its mouth" (Still, 1912, p. 776). The base of the skull may be particularly affected causing hydrocephalus and distension of the scalp veins, in addition to spastic paralysis, mental defects, fits, and pituitary disorders (Sheldon, 1943). In the rest of the skull, the palatal arch may appear abnormally high and the mandible and maxilla may be disproportionate in size (Powell and Cook, 2005). On the cranium, the developing gummatous lesions vary from those seen in adult caries sicca outlined by Hackett (1981). Lesions have multiple round lytic foci that do not follow the normal sequence of development (i.e., pitting, destruction, healing). This distinction has yet to be fully explored.

Dentition

The most characteristic changes that will distinguish congenital from acquired syphilis in older children and adolescents are in the dentition. In early studies, Boyle (1932) and De Wilde (1943) indicated the presence of abnormal lacunae in the dentine, and De Wilde (1943) noted a poorly formed root of a lateral incisor in a known case of congenital syphilis. The dental stigmata of the disease are now widely understood and are considered pathognomonic of congenital syphilis (Table 7.4). Known as "Hutchinson's incisors," "Moon's molars," and "mulberry molars," these dental defects occur in the early stages of congenital syphilis, perhaps in the first few months after birth. But they only become apparent with the eruption of the permanent incisors and first molars around the age of 6 years. Dental changes provide the best opportunity to identify congenital syphilis in the archaeological record with between 25% and 45% showing changes in the maxillary incisors and 22%–37% changes in the first molars, compared to 12% that showed skeletal evidence of the disease (Sarnet and Shaw, 1942; Hillson et al., 1998). The incidence of dental stigmata in the mandibular incisors is lower at 5% and in the canines 4.5% (Bradlaw, 1953).

TABLE 7.4 Outline of Dental Lesions Seen in Congenital Syphilis

	Description	Occurrence	References
Hutchinson's incisor	Pumpkin-seed shaped permanent central incisors, caused by a shortened incisal edge and bulging crown and a central notch	10%–63%	Hutchinson (1857, 1858)
Moon's molar	Small, dome-shaped permanent first molars of the upper and lower jaw, with multiple crowded cusps	3%–17%	Moon (1877)
Mulberry (Fournier) molar	Hypoplasia of the occlusal third of the crown with reduced cusps, affecting the permanent upper and lower first molars	3%–37%	Fournier (1884)
"Fanged" canine	Circumferential groove in the occlusal third of the upper and lower permanent canines; wear may result in a notch at the hypoplastic tip of the crown	4.5%	Fournier (1884) and Bradlaw (1953)

Defects of the incisors were first described by Hutchinson (1857, 1858) as being abnormally small, notched, and having dirty gray enamel. The soft nature of the enamel means that the characteristic notches can be worn away with use (Fournier, 1884). The teeth were described as being "peg-shaped" or of a screwdriver appearance or "pumpkin-seed" shaped (Jacobi et al., 1992). Sarnet and Shaw (1942) warned against confusing "true" Hutchinson's incisors of congenital syphilis, with hypoplastic notches on central incisors with a normal morphology that can occur between 3 and 4 months of age. The diagnosis of Hutchinson's incisors in children with an unerupted permanent dentition can be carried out using a radiograph (Putkonen and Paatero, 1961). Moon's or bud molars describe the morphology of the first permanent molars where the tooth is smaller than normal, and narrower at the cusp than the base of the crown (Moon, 1877). Mulberry or Fournier's molars are recognized as first molars with deep hypoplastic defects cutting into the cusps giving a "berry" appearance to the tooth. The second molars can also be affected (Hillson et al., 1998). Although mulberry molars are not specifically diagnostic of congenital syphilis, Hutchinson's incisors and Moon's molars are considered pathognomonic (Figs. 7.27–7.29). In addition to changes in the molars and incisors, Hillson et al. (1998) drew attention to defects in the permanent canines, where deep hypoplasia at the tip of the crown cause it to be broken off to leave a "notch." These were originally described as "fanged" canines (Bradlaw, 1953; Fournier, 1884).

Hutchinson (1848) recognized the difficulties of differentiating between changes to the teeth as the direct result of syphilis and those caused by treatment with mercury. Arsenic and mercury were common remedies for syphilis in the 15th and 16th centuries in Europe and was given to pregnant women and children in the form of arsenic injections and mercury ointments (Coote, 1847). In some cases mercury was also provided in the form of calomel for rubbing on children's gums (Anon, 1919; Sheldon, 1943). While mercury was shown to completely eliminate the signs of syphilis in infancy, it did not completely cure it (Sheldon, 1943). The effect of mercury on the teeth is reflected in severely hypoplastic enamel exposing large areas of dentine and giving the tooth a honeycomb appearance. The deficient enamel leads to the development of "spikes" of dentine protruding through it, with a very abrupt line between the healthy and deficient enamel. Changes are more widespread than in syphilis, affecting pairs of teeth symmetrically, and more often involving the mandibular teeth. While the permanent first molars, incisors and canines are also affected, the premolars, and second and third molars are more likely to be involved, depending on the age of the individual when the treatment was administered (Hutchinson, 1858, p. 56). Hutchinson (1848, p. 54) described mercurial teeth as "rugged, pitted, and dirty" (Fig. 7.30).

Mercury was also used at various times to treat skin lesions in TB and leprosy in adults, although it was seen as a less-effective treatment than in syphilis (Neve, 1889; Wright, 1908). Hence, signs of mercury treatment may be present in the teeth of individuals who did not have congenital syphilis; in individuals where syphilis was present but did not manifest on the teeth or postcranium; or in individuals with additional dental stigmata of congenital syphilis (Ioannou et al., 2015b). The presence of morphologically altered maxillary teeth (small and domed molar; small and pumpkin-shaped incisor) in addition to widespread and severe hypoplastic defects on the mandibular and maxillary permanent dentition would indicate syphilitic-mercurial teeth (Ioannou et al., 2015b). Ioannou et al. (2015b) argue

Infectious Diseases II: Infections of Specific Origin Chapter | 7 **181**

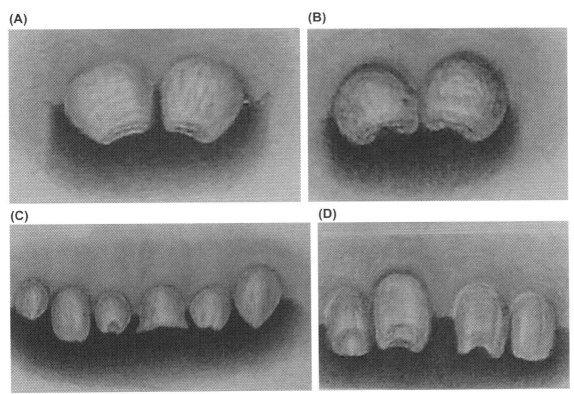

FIGURE 7.27 Variations in the expression of Hutchinson's incisors that all show the unusual morphology of the incisors and characteristic notching. (C) Also features a fanged canine. *From Hutchinson, J., 1848. Illustrations of Clinical Surgery, J&A Churchill, London, p. 10.*

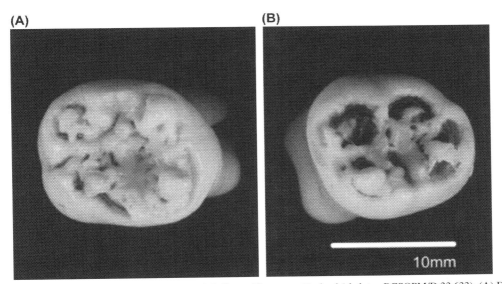

FIGURE 7.28 Mulberry molars in a 9-year-old from the Royal College of Surgeons, England (skeleton RCSOPM/D 33.633). (A) Defects are present in the right maxillary and (B) left mandibular first permanent molars. *From Ioannou, S., Sassani, S., Henneberg, M., Henneberg, R.J., 2015b. Diagnosing congenital syphilis using Hutchinson's method: differentiating between syphilitic, mercurial, and syphilitic-mercurial dental defects. American Journal of Physical Anthropology 159, 13.*

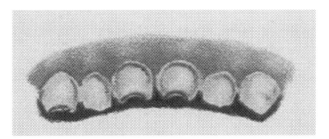

FIGURE 7.29 Fanged canine in congenital syphilis. Note also the notch that has formed on the left canine as the result of exposed dentine wear. *From Hutchinson, J., 1848. Illustrations of Clinical Surgery, J&A Churchill, London, p. 10.*

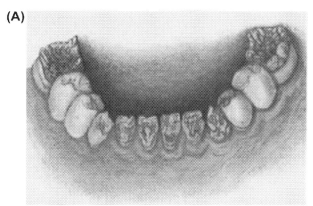

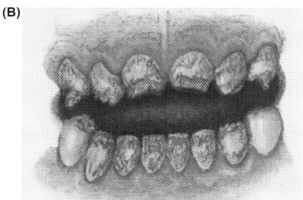

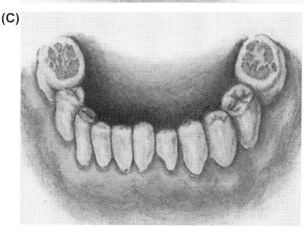

FIGURE 7.30 The effects of mercury on the developing teeth. The defects are more extensive and the enamel has a dirty appearance. *From Hutchinson, J., 1848. Illustrations of Clinical Surgery, J&A Churchill, London, p. 456.*

that as mercury did not form a treatment for any other infant disease besides syphilis, the presence of mercury teeth might be used to identify the disease in the absence of any postcranial changes.

Paleopathology

Numerous cases of probable congenital syphilis have been reported in the literature. The majority come from the New World and three predate Columbus' voyage to those shores (Cook, 1994; Erdal, 2006; Ferencz and Jozsa, 1992; Gaul and Grossschmidt, 2014; Gladykowska-Rzeczycka and Urbanowicz, 1970; Gladykowska-Rzeczycka and Krenz, 1995; Ioannou et al., 2015a; Jacobi et al., 1992; Lauc et al., 2015; Malgosa et al., 1996; Mansilla and Pijoan, 1995; Nystrom, 2011; Pálfi et al., 1992; Piombino-Mascali et al., 2006; Rothschild and Rothschild, 1997; Tomczyk et al., 2015; Blondiaux, 2008; Ortner, 2003, p. 323). Harper et al. (2011) carried out a stringent review of syphilis cases in the Old World, including congenital syphilis, using strict dating and diagnostic criteria. Despite accepting the validity of Erdal (2006) and Blondieux's (2008) pre-Columbian cases of congenital syphilis (see below), they concluded that there was not a single case of treponemal disease in the Old World prior to AD 1493. However, this has been vigorously disputed with new evidence emerging from the United Kingdom (Walker et al., 2014) and possibly Austria (Gaul et al., 2015).

Pálfi et al. (1992) reported on an elderly (c. 50 years) female and associated 7-month fetus recovered from the necropolis of Costebelle, France. The fetus had extensive new bone formation on the long bones, maxilla, ribs and cranial vault, and ankylosis of the hand and foot bones due to calcification of soft tissue. There were also possible destructive lesions on the parietal bones and Wimberger's sign on radiograph. Pálfi et al. (1992) argued that despite her age, the mother had been in the early stages of syphilis, perhaps only 1 year into the infection, where clinical evidence suggests nearly all pregnancies will involve the spread of infection to the developing child. The importance of this diagnosis was that it provided evidence for venereal syphilis in the Mediterranean basin from the 1st century AD, over 1390 years before Columbus returned from the Americas. Mansilla and Pijoan (1995) provided an example of early onset congenital syphilis in a 2-year-old with Hutchinson's incisors still developing within the maxilla, diaphyseal osteomyelitis, and periostitis on the shafts of the long bones (Fig. 7.31). Although less complete, Malgosa et al. (1996) reported on early congenital syphilis in two infants from Huelva in 16th- to 19th-century Spain. The first infant had new bone and a possible lytic lesion on the frontal bone, with sheaths of new bone of the humerus and femur, and the second showed osteochondritis on the distal left humerus. Subsequent aDNA analysis isolated *T. pallidum pallidum* for the first time (Montiel et al., 2012). Previously, Bouwman and Brown (2005) had tested for aDNA in 13 individuals with clear signs

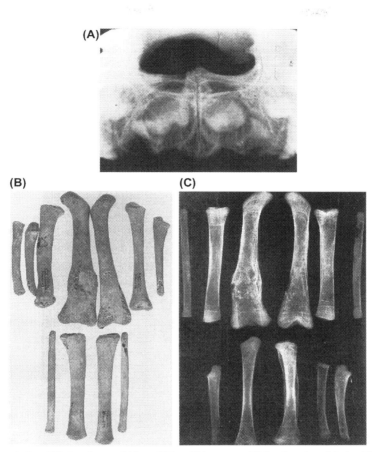

FIGURE 7.31 Early onset congenital syphilis in a 2-year-old from 17th to 18th century AD San Jeronimo, Mexico City (skeleton 43). (A) An X-ray of the maxilla revealed Hutchinson's incisors on the developing central incisors, (B) osteomyelitis was evident on the right femur and tibia diaphysis. (C) Cloaks of periostitis and Harris lines and widened radiolucent bands are evident on X-ray. *From Mansilla, J., Pijoan, C., 1995. Brief communication: a case of congenital syphilis during the colonial period in Mexico city. American Journal of Physical Anthropology 97, 191–193.*

of treponemal disease but were unable to secure a positive result. Montiel et al. (2012) argue that their own success was due to the fact that in neonatal remains abundant numbers of spirochetes invade the system and infiltrate the bone cells making their survival more likely.

Gladykowska-Rzeczycka and Krenz (1995) presented what they considered to be late onset congenital syphilis in a 12- to 15-year-old from medieval Poland. While there were no dental changes, there were gummatous lesions on the distal humerus, clavicle, radius and ulna, and pitting to the skull. Because of the lack of dental stigmata, which only occur in around half of known clinical cases, venereal syphilis or a nonvenereal treponemal disease could not be ruled out. A more definitive case is presented by Erdal (2006) in a 15-year-old from Nicaea in Anatolia, Turkey, dated by artifacts to AD 1222–1254 or pre-Columbian. The adolescent displayed mulberry molars, a Hutchinson's incisor, gummatous lesions of the long bones, saber shin and dactylitis of the hands and feet (Fig. 7.32). Rothschild and Rothschild (1997) highlighted the difficulty in diagnosing the condition in 151 nonadults from Buffalo Site in West Virginia, where clear signs of venereal syphilis were evident in the adults. Only one child had profuse periosteal lesions that may have been indicative of the disease. Periosteal reactions are rare in congenital syphilis compared to yaws and bejel and it may be short lived and remodel quickly, to leave no visible trace on the skeleton (Rothschild and Rothschild, 1995, 1997).

Nystrom (2011) presents a detailed and compelling argument for the use of dental defects alone to diagnose congenital syphilis, describing the deciduous and permanent dentition of a 6-year-old from 19th-entury Newburgh cemetery, New York. Planelike defects of the second deciduous molars were evident in combination with hypoplastic pits and serrated incise edges of the permanent central and lateral maxillary incisors. There were also deep hypoplastic grooves resulting in "waisting" of the mandibular central and lateral incisors. Nystrom (2011) argues that the permanent central incisors represent Hutchinson's incisors in their primary state before eruption and subsequent wear through occlusion. The serrated edges and hypoplastic pits fit Hutchinson's (1857) original description of teeth being originally filled with atrophied "vegetations of dental tissue" and having serrated edges. Once in occlusion, Nystrom (2011) argues the teeth would have developed notches and the pumpkin-seed

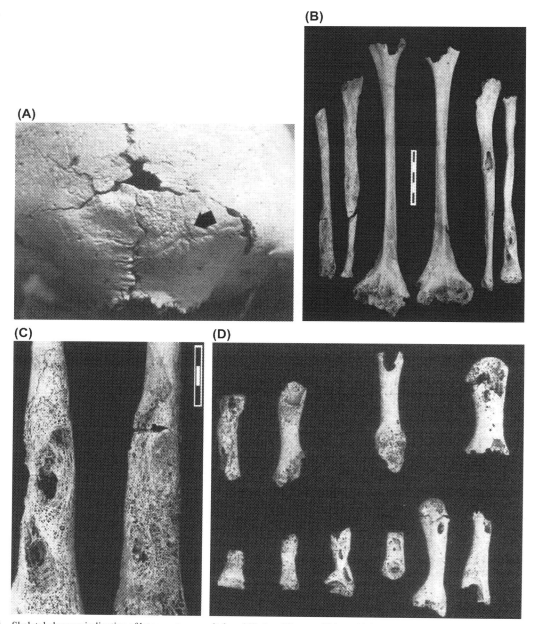

FIGURE 7.32 Skeletal changes indicative of late onset congenital syphilis in a 15-year-old from 13th century Anatolia, Turkey. The skeleton showed (A) a possible radial scar of healed caries sicca on the frontal bone, (B) disuse atrophy of the arm bones with gummatous and nongummatous osteomyelitis (C) viewed close-up, and (D) dactylitis of the hand and foot bones. The individual also displayed a Hutchinson's incisor and mulberry molar. *From Erdal, Y., 2006. A pre-columbian case of congenital syphilis from Anatolia (Nicaea, 13th century AD). International Journal of Osteoarchaeology 16, 20, 23, 25.*

shape of the incisors would have become more pronounced. Another attempt to diagnose congenital syphilis based on dental material alone was made by Gaul and Grossschmidt (2014) on a nonadult from 18th-century Vienna. They demonstrated characteristic changes to the permanent molars and hypoplastic defects of the deciduous teeth but no Hutchinson's incisors. In their study of mercury treatment on the appearance of syphilitic teeth, Ioannou et al. (2015b) reexamined the cases presented by Erdal (2006) and Gaul and Grossschmidt (2014). They argued that the child from pre-Colombian Turkey represented pure syphilitic changes, while the high status child from 18th-century Vienna displayed evidence for treatment with mercury. Taking a different approach, Tomczyk et al. (2015) tested the teeth of a 19th century case of congenital syphilis for mercury and found the levels to be the same as the nonaffected population, suggesting that mercury was not responsible for the hypoplastic defects they identified on the molars. The ability to recognize the presence of mercurial changes on the teeth of children with syphilis represents an exciting prospect in our understanding of how the disease was treated in the past, exploring the social status of those undergoing treatment, and the geographical areas and times at which it was used.

REFERENCES

Abdolrasouli, A., Croucher, A., Hemmati, A., Mabey, D., 2013. A case of endemic syphilis, Iran. Emerging Infectious Diseases 19 (1), 162–163.

Allison, M., Gerszten, E., Munizaga, J., Santoro, C., Mendoza, D., 1981. Tuberculosis in pre-Columbian Andean populations. In: Buikstra, J. (Ed.), Prehistoric Tuberculosis in the Americas. Northwestern University Archeological Program, Illinois, pp. 49–61.

Andersen, J., Manchester, K., 1992. The rhinomaxillary syndrome in leprosy: a clinical, radiological and palaeopathological study. International Journal of Osteoarchaeology 2 (2), 121–129.

Andersen, J.G., Manchester, K., 1987. Grooving of the proximal phalanx in leprosy: a palaeopathological and radiological study. Journal of Archaeological Science 14 (1), 77–82.

Andersen, J.G., Manchester, K., 1988. Dorsal tarsal exostoses in leprosy: a palaeopathological and radiological study. Journal of Archaeological Science 15 (1), 51–56.

Andersen, J.G., Manchester, K., Ali, R.S., 1992. Diaphyseal remodelling in leprosy: a radiological and palaeopathological study. International Journal of Osteoarchaeology 2 (3), 211–219.

Andersen, J.G., Manchester, K., Roberts, C., 1994. Septic bone changes in leprosy: a clinical, radiological and palaeopathological review. International Journal of Osteoarchaeology 4 (1), 21–30.

Anderson, S., 1998. Leprosy in a medieval churchyard in Norwich. In: Current and Recent Research in Osteoarchaeology: Proceedings of the Third Meeting of the Osteoarchaeology Research Group. Oxbow, Oxford, pp. 31–37.

Anon, 1919. The preparation of finely divided calomel. British Medical Journal 1 (3049), 713.

Antunes, J., 1992. Infections of the spine. Acta Neurochirurgica (Wein) 116, 179–186.

Apajalahti, S., Hölttä, P., Turtola, L., Pirinen, S., 2002. Prevalence of short-root anomaly in healthy young adults. Acta Odontologica 60 (1), 56–59.

Arateco, W.M.R., 1998. Mal de Pott en momia de la colección del museo arqueológico Marqués de San Jorge. Maguaré 13, 99–115.

Arriaza, B., Salo, W.L., Aufderheide, A., Holcomb, T., 1995. Pre-Columbian tuberculosis in Northern Chile: molecular and skeletal evidence. American Journal of Physical Anthropology 98, 37–45.

Assis, S., Santos, A.-L., Roberts, C., 2011. Evidence of hypertrophic osteoarthropathy in individuals from the Coimbra skeletal identified collection (Portugal). International Journal of Paleopathology 1, 155–163.

Atkins, P.J., 1992. White poison? The social consequences of milk consumption, 1850-1930. Social History of Medicine 15 (2), 207–226.

Aufderheide, A.C., Rodriguez-Martín, C., 1998. The Cambridge Encyclopedia of Human Paleopathology. Cambridge University Press, Cambridge.

Badger, L., 1964. Epidemiology. In: Cochrane, R., Davey, T. (Eds.), Leprosy in Theory and Practice. Wright, Bristol, pp. 69–97.

Baker, B., Armelagos, G.J., 1988. Origin and antiquity of syphilis: a paleopathological diagnosis and interpretation. Current Anthropology 29 (5), 703–737.

Bancroft, I., 1904. Clinical observations on variola. Journal of Medical Research 11 (1), 322–345.

Barr, J., 1948. Growth and inequality of leg length in poliomyelitis. New England Journal of Medicine 238, 737.

Barreto, J.G., Bisanzio, D., de Souza Guimarães, L., Spencer, J.S., Vazquez-Prokopec, G.M., Kitron, U., Salgado, C.G., 2014. Spatial analysis spotlighting early childhood leprosy transmission in a hyperendemic municipality of the Brazilian Amazon region. PLoS Neglected Tropical Diseases 8 (2), e2665.

Barton, R., 1979. Radiological changes in the paranasal sinuses in lepromatous leprosy. Journal of Laryngology and Otology 93, 597–600.

Baxarias, J., Garcia, A., Gonzalez, J., Perez-Perez, A., Tudo, B., Garcia-Bour, C., Campillo, D., Turbon, E., 1998. A rare case of tuberculosis gonarthropathy from the middle ages in Spain: an ancient DNA confirmation study. Journal of Paleopathology 10 (2), 63–72.

Bennett, M., Lynn, A., Klein, L., Balkowiec, K., 1997. Congenital syphilis: subtle presentation of fulminant disease. Journal of the American Academy of Dermatology 36 (2), 351–354.

Bernard, M., 2002. Tuberculosis in 20th century Britain: a preliminary study of the demographic profile of children admitted to Stannington sanitorium. American Journal of Physical Anthropology 34, 44.

Berreman, J., 1984. Childhood leprosy and social response in South India. Social Science & Medicine 19 (8), 853–865.

Blickman, J., Van Die, C., De Rooy, J., 2004. Current imaging concepts in pediatric osteomyelitis. European Radiology 14 (4), L55–L64.

Blondiaux, J., 2008. La Paléopathologie des tréponématoses. In: Mariaud, O. (Ed.), Ostéo-archaéologie et Techniques Médico-Légales: Tendances et Perspectives. De Boccard, Paris.

Boece, H., 1535. History and Croniklis of Scotland (J. Bellenden, Trans.). Thomas Davidson, Edinburgh.

Bos, K., Harkins, K., Herbig, A., Coscolla, M., Weber, N., Comas, I., 2014. Pre-Columbian mycobacterial genomes reveal seals as a source of New World human tuberculosis. Nature 514 (7523), 494–497.

Bouwman, A., Brown, T., 2005. The limits of biomolecular palaeopathology: ancient DNA cannot be used to study venereal syphilis. Journal of Archaeological Science 32, 703–713.

Boyle, P., 1932. The histopathology of the tooth and gum in congenital syphilis. Journal of Dental Research 12, 425.

Bradlaw, R.V., 1953. The dental stigmata of prenatal syphilis. Medical Oral Pathology 6, 147–158.

Brewerton, D., Sandifer, P., Sweetnam, D., 1963. "Idiopathic" pes cavus. British Medical Journal 2 (5358), 659.

Brothwell, D., 1958. Evidence of leprosy in British archaeological material. Medical History 2, 287–291.

Brubaker, M., Meyers, W., Bourland, J., 1985. Leprosy in children one year of age and under. International Journal of Leprosy 53 (4), 517–523.

Buckley, H., Tayles, N., 2003. Skeletal pathology in a prehistoric Pacific Island sample: issues in lesion recording, quantification, and interpretation. American Journal of Physical Anthropology 122, 303–324.

Buikstra, J., 1976a. Hopewell in the Lower Illinois Valley. Northwestern University Archaeological Program, Evanston.

Buikstra, J., 1976b. The Caribou Eskimo: general and specific disease. American Journal of Physical Anthropology 45, 351–368.

Bukh, N., 1968. Muscle recovery in poliomyelitis. Acta Orthopaedica Scandinavica 39, 579–592.

Butlin, C., Saunderson, P., 2014. Children with leprosy. Leprosy Review 85, 69–73.

Caffey, J., 1939. Syphilis of the skeleton in early infancy. The American Journal of Roentgenology Radium Therapy 42 (5), 637–655.

Caffey, J., 1945. Pediatric X-Ray Diagnosis. Year Book Medical Publishers, Inc., Chicago.

Campbell, J., Hoffman, E., 1995. Tuberculosis of the hip in children. Journal of Bone and Joint Surgery 77-B (2), 319–326.

Cantwell, M., Shehab, Z., Costello, A., Samds, L., Green, W., Ewing, E., CValway, S., Onorato, I., 1994. Brief report: congenital tuberculosis. The New England Journal of Medicine 330 (15), 1051–1054.

Capoor, M.R., Sen, B., Varshney, P., Verghese, M., Shivaprakash, M., Chakrabarti, A., 2014. Coccidioidomycosis masquerading as skeletal tuberculosis: an imported case and review of coccidioidomycosis in India. Tropical Doctor 44 (1), 25–28.

Cappell, D.F., Anderson, J.R., 1971. Muir's Textbook of Pathology. Edward Arnold, London.

Cavanaugh, J.J., Holman, G.H., 1965. Hypertrophic osteoarthropathy in childhood. The Journal of Pediatrics 66 (1), 27–40.

Chiari, H., 1893. Ueber osteomyelitis variolosa. Beitrage Zur Pathologischen Anatomie Und Zur Allgemeinen Pathologie 13, 13–31.

Clough, S., Boyle, A., 2010. Inhumations and disarticulated human bone. In: Booth, P., Simmonds, S., Boyle, A., Clough, S., Cool, H., Poore, D. (Eds.), The Late Roman Cemetery at Lankhills, Winchester Excavations 2000-2005. Oxford Archaeology Ltd., Oxford, pp. 339–403.

Cockshott, P., MacGregor, M., 1959. The natural history of osteomyeltitis variolosa. Journal of the Faculty of Radiologists 10, 57–63.

Cook, D.C., 1994. Dental evidence for congenital syphilis (and its absence) before and after the conquest of the New World. In: Dutour, O., Palfi, G. (Eds.), The Origin of Syphilis in Europe: Before or After 1493? Universite de Provence, France, pp. 169–175.

Cooney, J., Crosby, E., 1944. Absorptive bone changes in leprosy. Radiology 42 (1), 14–19.

Cooper, L., Ziring, P., Ockerse, A., Fedun, B., Kiely, B., Krugman, S., 1969. Rubella: clinical manifestations and management. American Journal of Disease in Childhood 118, 18–29.

Coote, H., 1847. On the administration of mercury in syphilis. Lancet 49 (1234), 437–439.

Crespo, F.A., Klaes, C.K., Switala, A.E., DeWitte, S.N., 2017. Do leprosy and tuberculosis generate a systemic inflammatory shift? Setting the ground for a new dialogue between experimental immunology and bioarchaeology. American Journal of Physical Anthropology 162 (1), 143–156.

Cronjé, G., 1984. Tuberculosis and mortality decline in England and Wales, 1851-1910. In: Woods, R., Woodward, J. (Eds.), Urban Disease and Mortality in Nineteenth-Century England. Batsford Academic and Educational Ltd., London, pp. 79–101.

Crosby, A., 2003. Smallpox. In: Kiple, K. (Ed.), The Cambridge Historical Dictionary of Disease. Cambridge University Press, Cambridge, pp. 300–304.

Crosby, A.W., 1969. The early history of syphilis: a reappraisal. American Anthropologist 71 (2), 218–227.

Crozier, G., Cochrane, R., 1929. Leprosy in an infant. British Medical Journal 1, 501–502.

Crubézy, É.L.B., Poveda, J.-D., Clayton, J., Crouau-Roy, B., Montagnon, D., 1998. Identification of Mycobacterium DNA in an Egyptian Pott's disease of 5400 years old. Correspondance de la Royal Academie des Sciences (Paris) 321, 941–951.

Cruz, A., Starke, J., 2007. Clinical manifestations of tuberculosis in children. Paediatric Respiratory Reviews 8, 107–117.

Cunha, C., Silva, A., Irish, J., Scott, G., Tomé, T., Matquez, J., 2006. Hypotrophic roots of the upper central incisors – a proposed new discrete dental trait. Dental Anthropology 25 (1), 8–14.

Currarino, G., 1966. Premature closure of epiphyses in the metatarsals and knees: a sequel of poliomyelitis 1. Radiology 87 (3), 424–428.

Dabernat, H., Crubézy, E., 2010. Multiple bone tuberculosis in a child from predynastic upper Egypt (3200 BC). International Journal of Osteoarchaeology 20 (6), 719–730.

Danielsen, K., 1968. Leprogenic odontodysplasia. International Journal of Leprosy 36, 552–666.

Danielsen, K., 1970. Odontodysplasia leprosa in Danish medieval skeletons. Tandlaegebladet 74, 603–625.

Danielssen, D., Boeck, W., 1848. Traité de la Spédalskhed og Éléphantiasis des Grecs. Libraire de L'Académie Royale de Médicine, Paris.

Darton, Y., Richard, I., Truc, M.-C., 2013. Osteomyelitis variolosa: a probable medievel case combined with unilateral sacroilitis. International Journal of Paleopathology 3, 288–293.

Davidson, J., Palmer, P., 1963. Osteomyelitis variolosa. The Journal of Bone and Joint Surgery 45B (4), 687–693.

Dax, E.C., Stewart, R., 1939. The sign of the clavicle. British Medical Journal 1 (4084), 771.

Dayal, R., Hashmi, N., Mathur, P., Prasad, R., 1990. Leprosy in childhood. Indian Pediatrics 27 (2), 170–180.

Ddungu, H., Johnson, J.L., Smieja, M., Mayanja-Kizza, H., 2006. Digital clubbing in tuberculosis–relationship to HIV infection, extent of disease and hypoalbuminemia. BMC Infectious Diseases 6 (1), 45.

De Wilde, H., 1943. Stigmata of congenital syphilis in the deciduous dentition. American Journal of Orthodontics and Oral Surgery 29 (7), 368–376.

Derry, D., 1938. Pott's disease in ancient Egypt. The Medical Press and Circular 197, 196–199.

Dorfman, D., Glaser, J., 1990. Congenital syphilis presenting in infants after the newborn period. The New England Journal of Medicine 323 (19), 1299–1302.

Duncan, M., 1980. Babies of mothers with leprosy have small placentae, low birth weights and grow slowly. British Journal of Obstetrics and Gynaecology 87, 471–479.

Duncan, M., 1985a. Leprosy in children – past, present and future. International Journal of Leprosy 53 (3), 468–473.

Duncan, M., 1985b. Leprosy and procreation – a historical review of social and clinical aspects. Leprosy Review 56, 153–162.

Duncan, M., Melsom, R., Pearson, J., Menzel, S., Barnetson, R., 1983. A clinical and immunological study of four babies of mothers with lepromatous leprosy, two of whom developed leprosy in infancy. International Journal of Leprosy 51 (1), 7–17.

Duncan, M., Melsom, R., Pearson, J., Ridley, D., 1981. The association of pregnancy and leprosy. Leprosy Review 52, 245–262.

Duncan, S.R., Scott, S., Duncan, C.J., 1993. The dynamics of smallpox epidemics in Britain, 1550-1800. Demography 30 (3), 405–423.

Erdal, Y., 2006. A pre-columbian case of congenital syphilis from Anatolia (Nicaea, 13th century AD). International Journal of Osteoarchaeology 16, 16–33.

Eyler, W., Monsein, L., Beute, G., Tiley, B., Schultz, L., Schmitt, W., 1996. Rib enlargement in patients with chronic plural disease. American Journal of Radiology 167, 921–926.

Faerman, M., Jankaukas, R., Gorski, A., Bercovier, H., Greenblatt, C., 1999. Detecting mycobacterium tuberculosis in medieval skeletal remains from Lithuania. In: Pálfi, G., Dutour, O., Deák, J., Hutás, I. (Eds.), Tuberculosis: Past and Present. Golden Book Publishers and Tuberculosis Foundation, Budapest, pp. 371–376.

Faget, G.H., Mayoral, A., 1944. Bone changes in leprosy: a clinical and roentgenologic study of 505 cases. Radiology 42 (1), 1–13.

Feldman, F., Auberbach, R., Johnson, A., 1971. Tuberculous dactylitis in the adult. American Journal of Roentgenology 112 (3), 460–479.

Ferencz, M., Jozsa, L., 1992. Congenital syphilis on a medieval skeleton. Anthropologie 30 (1), 95–98.

Fiumara, N., Lessel, S., 1970. Manifestations of late congenital syphilis. Archives of Dermatology 102, 78–83.

Fleming, T.C., Bardenstein, M.B., 1971. Congenital syphilis. Journal of Bone and Joint Surgery 53-A (8), 1648–1651.

Formicola, V., Milanesi, Q., Scarsini, C., 1987. Evidence of spinal tuberculosis at the beginning of the fourth millenium BC from Arene Candide Cave (Liguria, Italy). American Journal of Physical Anthropology 72, 1–6.

Fournier, A., 1884. Syphilitic teeth. Dental Cosmos 26 (12–25), 141–155.

Gaul, J., Grossschmidt, K., 2014. A probable case of congenital syphilis from 18th century Vienna. International Journal of Palaeopathology 6, 34–43.

Gaul, J., Grossschmidt, K., Gusenbauer, C., Kanz, F., 2015. A probable case of congenital syphilis from pre-Columbian Austria. Anthropologischer Anzeiger 72 (4), 451–472.

Genç, M., Ledger, W., 2000. Syphilis in pregnancy. Sexually Transmitted Infections 76, 73–79.

Girdhar, A., Girdhar, B., Ramu, G., Desikan, K., 1981. Discharge of *M. leprae* in milk of leprosy patients. Leprosy in India 53 (3), 390–394.

Girdhar, A., Mishra, B., Lavania, R., Bagga, A., Malaviya, G., Girdhar, B., 1989. Leprosy in infants-a report on two cases. International Journal of Leprosy 57 (2), 472–475.

Gladykowska-Rzeczycka, J.J., Krenz, M., 1995. Extensive change within a subadult skeleton from a medieval cemetery of Slaboszewo, Mogilno district, Poland. Journal of Paleopathology 7 (3), 177–184.

Gladykowska-Rzeczycka, J.J., Urbanowicz, M., 1970. Multiple osseous exostoses of the skeleton from a prehistoric cemetery of a former population of Pruszcz Gdanski. Folia Morphologica 29 (3), 284–296.

Gladykowska-Rzeczycka, J., Smiszkiewicz-Skwarska, A., 1998. Probable poliomyelitis from [a] XVII-XVIII century cemetery in Poland. Journal of Palaeopathology 10 (1), 5–11.

Glickman, L., Minsky, A., 1937. Enlargement of one sternoclavicular articulation: a sign of congenital syphilis. Radiology 28 (1), 85–86.

Gomez, L., Basa, J., Nicolas, C., 1922. Early leprosy and the development and incidence of leprosy in the children of lepers. The Philippine Journal of Science 21 (3), 233–256.

Griffith, J., 1919. The Diseases of Infants and Children. W.B. Saunders and Company, London.

Grin, E.I., 1956. Endemic syphilis and yaws. Bulletin of the World Health Organization 15 (6), 959.

Gupta, M., Singh, M., 2007. Primary tuberculosis of the mandible. Indian Pediatrics 44, 53–54.

Haas, C., Zink, A., Molńar, E., Szeimies, U., Reischl, U., Marcsik, A., Ardagna, Y., Dutour, O., Pálfi, O., Nerlich, A., 2000. Molecular evidence for different stages of tuberculosis in ancient bone samples from Hungary. American Journal of Physical Anthropology 113, 293–304.

Hackett, C., 1957. An International Nomenclature on Yaws Lesions. World Health Organisation, Geneva.

Hackett, C.J., 1936. Boomerang legs and yaws in Australian aborigines. Transactions of the Royal Society of Tropical Medicine and Hygiene 30 (2), 137–143.

Hackett, C.J., 1963. On the origin of the human treponematoses. Bulletin of the World Health Organisation 29, 7–41.

Hackett, C.J., 1981. Development of caries sicca in a dry calvaria. Virchow's Archives A, Pathological Anatomy 391, 53–79.

Han, X.Y., Seo, Y.-H., Sizer, K.C., Schoberle, T., May, G.S., Spencer, J.S., Li, W., Nair, R.G., 2008. A new Mycobacterium species causing diffuse lepromatous leprosy. American Journal of Clinical Pathology 130 (6), 856–864.

Hansen, G., 1875. On the etiology of leprosy. Chirurgie Review 55, 459–489.

Harisinghani, M.G., McLoud, T.C., Shepard, J.-A.O., Ko, J.P., Shroff, M.M., Mueller, P.R., 2000. Tuberculosis from head to toe 1. Radiographics 20 (2), 449–470.

Harman, N., 1917. Staying the Plague. Methuen, London.

Harper, K., Zuckerman, M., Harper, M., Kingston, J., Armelagos, G., 2011. The origin and antiquity of syphilis revisitied: an appraisal of old world pre-Columbian evidence for treponemal infection. Yearbook of Physical Anthropology 54, 99–133.

Harris, H.A., 1933. Bone Growth in Health and Disease. Oxford University Press, London.

Hauhnar, C.Z., Mann, S., Sharma, V.K., Kaur, S., Mehta, S., Radotra, B., 1992. Maxillary antrum involvement in multibacillary leprosy: a radiologic, sinuscopic, and histologic assessment. International Journal of Leprosy and Other Mycobacterial Diseases 60, 390–395.

Hayes, J.T., 1961. Cystic tuberculosis of the proximal tibial metaphysis with associated involvement of the epiphysis and epiphyseal plate. Journal of Bone and Joint Surgery 43-A (4), 560–567.

Hershkovitz, I., Greenwald, C., Latimer, B., Jellema, S.-B., Eshed, V., Dutour, O., Rothschild, B., 2002. Serpens Endocrania Symmetrica (SES): a new term and a possible clue for identifying intrathoracic diseases in skeletal populations. American Journal of Physical Anthropology 118 (3), 201–216.

Hershkovitz, I., Rothschild, B., Dutour, O., Greenwald, C.M., 1998. Clues to recognition of fungal origin of lytic skeletal lesions. American Journal of Physical Anthropology 106, 47–60.

Higoumenakis, G., 1927. A new stigma of hereditary syphilis. Proceedings of the Medical Society of Athens 687–699.

Hillson, S., 1996. Dental Anthropology. Cambridge University Press, Cambridge.

Hillson, S., Grigson, C., Bond, S., 1998. Dental defects of congenital syphilis. American Journal of Physical Anthropology 107 (1), 25–40.

Hjørting-Hansen, E., Kløft, B., Schmidt, H., 1965. Leprotic granuloma in the maxilla. International Journal of Leprosy 33 (1), 83–88.

Hlavenková, L., Teasdale, M., Gábor, O., Nagy, G., Beňuš, R., Marcsik, A., Pinhasi, R., Hajdu, T., 2015. Childhood bone tuberculosis from Roman Pécs, Hungary. HOMO-Journal of Comparative Human Biology 66 (1), 27–37.

Holcomb, R.C., 1934. Christopher Columbus and the American origin of syphilis. US Naval Medical Bulletin 32 (4).

Hollier, L., Cox, S., 1998. Syphilis. Seminars in Perinatology 22 (4), 323–331.

Holloway, K., Henneberg, R., de Barros Lopes, M., Henneberg, M., 2011. Evolution of human tuberculosis: a systematic review and meta-analysis of palaeopathological evidence. HOMO: Journal of Comparative Human Biology 62, 402–458.

Holt, L.E., 1909. Diseases of Infancy And Childhood. D. Appleton and Company, London.

Hudson, E.H., 1967. Christopher Columbus and the history of syphilis. Acta Tropica 25 (1), 1–16.

Hutchinson, J., 1848. Illustrations of Clinical Surgery. J&A Churchill, London.

Hutchinson, J., 1857. On the influence of hereditary syphilis on the teeth. Transactions of the Odontological Society, Great Britain 2, 95–106.

Hutchinson, J., 1858. Report on the effects of infantile syphilis in marring the development of teeth. Transactions of the Pathological Society, London 449–456.

Imamura, M., Kakihara, T., Yamamoto, K., Imai, C., Tanaka, A., Uchiyama, M., 2004. Primary tuberculous osteomyelitis of the mandible. Pediatrics International 46, 736–739.

Ioannou, S., Henneberg, M., Henneberg, R., Anson, T., 2015a. Diagnosis of mercurial teeth in a possible case of congenital syphilis and tuberculosis in a 19th century child skeleton. Journal of Anthropology 2015.

Ioannou, S., Sassani, S., Henneberg, M., Henneberg, R.J., 2015b. Diagnosing congenital syphilis using Hutchinson's method: differentiating between syphilitic, mercurial, and syphilitic-mercurial dental defects. American Journal of Physical Anthropology 159, 617–629.

Jackes, M.K., 1983. Osteological evidence for smallpox: a possible case from seventeenth century Ontario. American Journal of Physical Anthropology 60, 75–81.

Jacobi, K.P., Cook, D.C., Corruccini, R.S., Handler, J.S., 1992. Congenital syphilis in the past: slaves at Newton Plantation, Barbados, West Indies. American Journal of Physical Anthropology 89, 145–158.

James, J., 1956. Paralytic scoliosis. Journal of Bone and Joint Surgery 38B (3), 660–685.

Jankauskas, R., 1999. Tuberculosis in Lithuania: paleopathological and historical correlations. In: Pálfi, G., Dutour, O., Deák, J., Hutás, I. (Eds.), Tuberculosis: Past and Present. Golden Book Publisher Ltd., Tuberculosis Foundation, Szeged, pp. 551–558.

Jankauskas, R., Schultz, M., 1995. Meningeal reactions in a late medieval-early modern child population from Alytus, Lithuania. Journal of Paleopathology 7 (2), 106.

Jensen, C., Jensen, C., Paerregaard, A., 1991. A diagnostic problem in tuberculous dactylitis. The Journal of Hand Surgery 16B, 202–203.

Job, C., 1963. Pathology of leprous osteomyelitis. International Journal of Leprosy 31, 26.

Job, C., Karat, A., Karat, S., 1966. The histopathological appearance of leprous rhinitis and pathogenesis of septal perforation in leprosy. The Journal of Laryngology & Otology 80 (07), 718–732.

Job, C.K., 1989. Nerve damage in leprosy. International Journal of Leprosy and Other Mycobactacterial Diseases 57, 532–539.

Jopling, W., McDougall, A., 1988. Handbook of Leprosy. Heinmann, London.

Jopling, W., Ridley, D., 1966. Classification of leprosy according to immunity. A five-group system. International Journal of Leprosy 34 (3), 255–273.

Jordan, J., Spencer, H., 1949. Congenital tuberculosis. British Medical Journal 1 (4596), 217.

Kant, K.S., Agarwal, A., Suri, T., Gupta, N., Verma, I., Shaharyar, A., 2014. Tuberculosis of knee region in children: a series of eight cases. Tropical Doctor 44 (1), 29–32.

Kelley, M., El-Najjar, M., 1980. Natural variation and differential diagnosis of skeletal changes in tuberculosis. American Journal of Physical Anthropology 52, 153–167.

Kelly, P., Manning, P., Corcoran, P., Clancy, L., 1991. Hypertrophic osteoarthropathy in association with pulmonary tuberculosis. Chest 99 (3), 769–770.

Kjellström, A., 2012. Possible cases of leprosy and tuberculosis in medieval Sigtuna, Sweden. International Journal of Osteoarchaeology 22, 261–283.

Klaus, H., Wilbur, A., Temple, D., Buikstra, J., Stone, A., Fernandez, M., Wester, C., Tam, M., 2010. Tuberculosis on the north coast of Peru: skeletal and molecular palaeopathology of late pre-hispanic and post-contact mycobacterial disease. Journal of Archaeological Science 37, 2587–2597.

Kowalska, M., Kowalik, A., 2012. *Mycobacterium leprae*: pathogenic agent in leprosy. Discovery of new species Mycobacterium lepromatosis. Perspectives in research and diagnosis of leprosy. International Maritime Health 63 (4), 213–218.

Kozłowski, T., Piontek, J., 2000. A case of atrophy of bones of the right lower limb of a skeleton from a medieval (12th–14th centuries) burial ground in Gruczno, Poland. Journal of Paleopatholology 12, 5–16.

Kulkarni, V., Mehta, J., 1983. Tarsal disintegration (T.D.) in leprosy. Leprosy in India 55 (2), 338–370.

Lara, C., Ignatio, J., 1956. Observations on leprosy among children born in the Culion leper colony during the pre-sulphone and the sulphone periods. The Journal of the Philippine Medical Association 32 (4), 189–197.

Lauc, T., Fornai, C., Premužić, Z., Vodanović, M., Weber, G.W., Mašić, B., Šikanjić, P.R., 2015. Dental stigmata and enamel thickness in a probable case of congenital syphilis from XVI century Croatia. Archives of Oral Biology 60 (10), 1554–1564.

Leung, A., Müller, N., Pineda, P., Fitzgerald, J., 1992. Primary tuberculosis in childhood: radiographic manifestations. Radiology 182, 87–91.

Levin, M., Newport, M., 2000. Inherited predisposition to mycobacterial infection: historical considerations. Microbes and Infection 2, 1549–1552.

Lewis, M., 2002. Infant and childhood leprosy: clinical and palaeopathological implications. In: Roberts, C., Lewis, M., Manchester, K. (Eds.), The Past and Present of Leprosy. Archaeopress, Oxford, pp. 163–169.

Lewis, M., 2004. Endocranial lesions in non-adult skeletons: understanding their aetiology. International Journal of Osteoarchaeology 14, 82–97.

Lewis, M., 2007. The Bioarchaeology of Children. Cambridge University Press, Cambridge.

Lewis, M., 2008. The children. In: Magilton, J., Lee, F., Boylston, A. (Eds.), Chichester Excavations 'Lepers Outside the Gate' Excavations at the Cemetery of the Hospital of St. James and St. Mary Magdalene, Chichester, 1986-87 and 1993, vol. 10. Council for British Archaeology, York, pp. 174–186. Research Report, 158.

Lewis, M., 2011. Tuberculosis in the non-adults from Romano-British Poundbury Camp, Dorset, England. International Journal of Paleopathology 1 (1), 12–23.

Lewis, M.E., Roberts, C.A., Manchester, K., 1995. Inflammatory bone changes in leprous skeletons from the medieval hospital of St. James and St. Mary Magdalene, Chichester, England. International Journal of Leprosy and Other Mycobacterial Diseases 63, 77–85.

Lieverse, A., Metcalf, M., Bazaliiskii, V., Weber, A., 2008. Pronounced bilateral asymmetry of the complete upper extremity: a case from the early Neolithic Baikal, Siberia. International Journal of Osteoarchaeology 18 (3), 219–239.

Lind, V., 1972. Short root anomaly. European Journal of Oral Sciences 80 (2), 85–93.

Lomax, E., 1979. Infantile syphilis as an example of nineteenth century belief in the inheritance of acquired characteristics. Journal of the History of Medicine 34, 23–39.

Lorber, J., 1958. Intracranial calcifications following tuberculosis meningitis in children. Acta Radiology 50, 204–210.

Lorin, M.I., 1983. Treatment of tuberculosis in children. Pediatric Clinics of North America 30 (2), 333–348.

Mahajan, P., Jogaikar, D., Mehta, J., 1995. Study of deformities in children with leprosy: an urban experience. Indian Journal of Leprosy 67 (4), 405–409.

Malgosa, A., Aluja, M., Isidro, A., 1996. Pathological evidence in newborn children from the sixteenth century in Huelva (Spain). International Journal of Osteoarchaeology 6, 388–396.

Malhotra, R., Dinda, A., Bhan, S., 1992. Tubercular osteitis of the skull. Indian Pediatrics 30, 1119–1123.

Mansilla, J., Pijoan, C., 1995. Brief communication: a case of congenital syphilis during the colonial period in Mexico city. American Journal of Physical Anthropology 97, 187–195.

Marais, B., Donald, P., Gie, R., Schaaf, H., Beyers, N., 2005. Diversity of disease in childhood pulmonary tuberculosis. Annals of Tropical Paediatrics: International Child Health 25 (2), 79–86.

Marais, B., Gie, R., Schaaf, H., Hesseling, A., Obihara, C., Starke, J., Enarson, D., Donald, P., Beyers, N., 2004. The natural history of childhood intra-thoracic tuberculosis: a critical review of literature from the pre-chemotherapy era. International Journal of Tuberculosis Lung Diseases 8 (4), 392–402.

Marks, M., Lebari, D., Solomon, A.W., Higgins, S.P., 2014. Yaws. International Journal of STD & AIDS 26 (10), 696.

Marks, S., 1979. The cellular basis for extremity bone loss in leprosy. International Journal of Leprosy 47 (1), 26–32.

Marks, S., Subramaniam, K., 1978. The cellular basis for alveolar bone loss in leprosy. Leprosy Review 49, 297–303.

Mathur, N., Bais, A., 1997. Tubercular retropharyngeal abscess in early childhood. Indian Journal of Pediatrics 64 (6), 899–901.

Matos, V., Marques, C., Lopes, C., 2009. Severe vertebral collapse in a juvenile from the graveyard (13th/14th-19th centuries) of the Sao Miguel Church (Castelo Branco, Portugal): differential palaeopathological diagnosis. International Journal of Osteoarchaeology 21, 208–217.

Matos, V., Santos, A.L., 2006. On the trail of pulmonary tuberculosis based on rib lesions: results from the human identified skeletal collection from Museu Bocage (Lisbon, Portugal). American Journal of Physical Anthropology 130 (2), 190–200.

Matos, V.M., Santos, A.L., 2013. Leprogenic odontodysplasia: new evidence from the St. Jørgen's medieval leprosarium cemetery (Odense, Denmark). Anthropological Science 121 (1), 43–47.

Mays, S., 2007. The human remains. In: Mays, S., Harding, C., Heighway, C. (Eds.), Wharram A Study of a Settlement on the Yorkshire Wolds, XI: The Churchyard. York University Archaeological Publications, vol. 13. English Heritage, London, pp. 77–192.

Mays, S., Fysh, E., Taylor, G., 2002. Investigation of the link between visceral surface rib lesions and tuberculosis in a medieval skeletal series from England using ancient DNA. American Journal of Physical Anthropology 119 (1), 27–36.

McKinley, J., 1993. Human Skeletal Report from Baldock, Hertfordshire (Unpublished Report). Wessex Archaeology, Salisbury.

Melsom, R., Duncan, M., Bjune, G., 1980. Immunoglobulin concentrations in mothers with leprosy and in healthy controls and their babies at the time of birth. Leprosy Review 51, 19–28.

Melsom, R., Harboe, M., Duncan, M., 1982. IgA, IgM and IgG anti-*M. leprae* antibodies in babies of leprosy mothers during the first 2 years of life. Clinical and Experimental Immunology 49, 532–542.

Meng, C., 1940. Tuberculosis of the mandible. The Journal of Bone and Joint Surgery 22 (1), 17–27.

Meng, C., Wu, Y., 1942. Tuberculosis of the flat bones of the vault of the skull: a study of 40 cases. Journal of Bone and Joint Surgery 24 (2), 341–353.

Meyer, C., Jung, C., Kohl, T., Poenicke, A., Poppe, A., Alt, K., 2002. Syphilis 2001: a palaeopathological reappraisal. HOMO 53 (1), 39–58.

Michman, J., Sagher, F., 1957. Changes in the anterior nasal spine and the alveolar process of the maxillary bone in leprosy. International Journal of Leprosy 25 (3), 217.

Miles, A., Powers, N., Wroe-Brown, R., Walker, D., 2008. St Marylebone Church and Burial Ground in the 18th-19th Centuries. Excavations at St Marylebone School, 1992 and 2004-6. MOLAS Monograph 46. Museum of London Archaeology Service, London.

Mirander, R., 1970. Efeitos ds lepra na cavidade oral. Publ Cent Estud Lepro 10, 26.

Mitchell, J., 1900. Study of a mummy affected with anterior poliomyelitis. Transactions of the Association of Americn Physicians 15, 134–136.

Mitjà, O., Šmajs, D., Bassat, Q., 2013. Advances in the diagnosis of endemic treponematoses: yaws, bejel, and pinta. PLoS Neglected Tropical Diseases 7 (10), e2283.

Møller-Christensen, V., Bakke, S., Melsom, R., Waaler, E., 1952. Changes in the anterior nasal spine and the alveolar process of the maxillary bone in leprosy. International Journal of Leprosy 20 (3), 335–340.

Møller-Christensen, V., 1961. Bone Changes in Leprosy. Munksgard, Denmark.

Møller-Christensen, V., 1969. Provisional results of the examination of the whole Naestved leprosy hospital churchyard. 1250–1550 AD. Nordisk Medicinhistorik Arsbok 4, 29–36.

Møller-Christensen, V., 1978. Leprosy Changes of the Skull. Odense University Press, Odense.

Montiel, R., Solórzano, E., Díaz, N., Álvarez-Sandoval, B., González-Ruiz, M., Cañadas, M., Simões, N., Isidro, A., Malgosa, A., 2012. Neonate human remains: a window of opportunity to the molecular study of ancient syphilis. PLoS One 7 (5).

Moon, H., 1877. On irregular and defective tooth development. Transactions of the Odontological Society 9 (7), 223–243.

Moon, M.-S., 1997. Tuberculosis of the spine. Controversies and a new challenge. Spine 22 (1), 1791–1797.

Morse, D., 1961. Prehistoric tuberculosis in America. American Review of Respiratory Disease 83, 489–504.

Müller, R., Roberts, C., Brown, T., 2014. Biomolecular identification of ancient *Mycobacterium tuberculosis* complex DNA in human remains from Britain and Continental Europe. American Journal of Physical Anthropology 153 (2), 178–189.

Murphy, E.M., Chistov, Y., Rutland, P., Taylor, G., 2009. Tuberculosis among Iron Age individuals from Tyva, South Siberia: palaeopathological and biomolecular findings. Journal of Archaeological Science 36, 2029–2038.

Musgrave, W., Sison, A., Crovvel, B., 1913. The bone lesions of smallpox. Philippine Journal of Tropical Medicine 8, 67.

Naeye, R., Blanc, W., 1965. Pathogenesis of congenital rubella. Journal of the American Medical Association 194 (12), 1277–1283.

Navarro, R., 1890. Congenital leprosy. British Medical Journal 2, 766.

Neve, E., 1889. Leprosy in Kashmir: its distribution and etiology. Lancet 134 (3455), 999–1000.

Newman, H., Casey, B., Du Bois, J., Gallagher, T., 1972. Roentgen features of leprosy in children. American Journal of Radiology 114 (2), 402–410.

Nicklisch, N., Maixner, F., Ganslmeier, R., Friederich, S., Dresely, V., Meller, H., Zink, A., Alt, K.W., 2012. Rib lesions in skeletons from early Neolithic sites in Central Germany: on the trail of tuberculosis at the onset of agriculture. American Journal of Physical Anthropology 149 (3), 391–404.

Norris, C., Landis, H., 1918. Pregnancy and pulmonary tuberculosis: with a report on one hundred and three cases. Journal of the American Medical Association 70, 362–365.

Noussitou, F., Sansarricq, H., Walter, J., 1976. Leprosy in Children. World Health Organisation, Geneva.

Novak, M., Čavka, M., Šlaus, M., 2014. Two cases of neurogenic paralysis in medieval skeletal samples from Croatia. International Journal of Paleopathology 7, 25–32.

Nystrom, K., 2011. Dental evidence of congenital syphilis in a 19th century cemetery from the mid-Husdon Valley. International Journal of Osteoarchaeology 21 (3), 371–378.

Ortner, D., 1979. Disease and mortality in early Bronze age people of Bab edh-Dhra, Jordan. American Journal of Physical Anthropology 51, 589–598.

Ortner, D., 2003. Identification of Pathological Conditions in Human Skeletal Remains. Academic Press, New York.

Ortner, D.J., Bush, H., 1993. Destructive lesions of the spine in a 17th century child's skeleton from Abingdon, Oxfordshire. Journal of Paleopathology 5 (3), 143–152.

Pálfi, G., Ardagna, Y., Maczel, Y., Berato, J., Aycard, P., Panuel, M., Zink, A., Nerlich, A., Dutour, O., 2000. Traces des infections osseuses dans la série anthropologique de la Celle (var, France): Résultats preliminaries. In: Paper Presented at the Colloque 2000 du Groupe des Palaeopathologistes des Langue Francaise, February 11–13. Toulon.

Pálfi, G., Dutour, O., Borreani, M., Brun, J.-P., Berato, J., 1992. Pre-Columbian congenital syphilis from the late antiquity in France. International Journal of Osteoarchaeology 2, 245–261.

Palit, A., Inamadar, A., 2014. Childhood leprosy in India over the past two decades. Leprosy Review 85, 93–99.

Pedley, J., 1967. The presence of *M. leprae* in human milk. Leprosy Review 38 (4), 239–242.

Pedley, J., 1968a. The presence of *M. leprae* in the breast secretion of a non-lactating woman with lepromatous leprosy. Leprosy Review 39 (3), 111.

Pedley, J., 1968b. Presence of *M. leprae* in the nipple secretion and lumina of the hypertrophied mammary gland. In a case of gynaecomastia associated with active and untreated lepromatous leprosy. Leprosy Review 39 (2), 67–70.

Pfeiffer, E., 1984. Paleopathology in an Iroquoian Ossuary, with special reference to tuberculosis. American Journal of Physical Anthropology 65, 181–189.

Pinkerton, F., 1932. Leprosy of the ear, nose and throat. Archives of Otolaryngology 16 (4), 467–487.

Piombino-Mascali, D., Lippi, B., Mallegni, F., D'Anastasio, R., Capasso, L., 2006. A possible case of congenital syphilis from Sienna (Central Italy). In: Paper Presented at the 16th Paleopathology Association European Meeting Santorini Island.

Powell, M., Cook, D. (Eds.), 2005. The Myth of Syphillis. University of Florida, Gainesville.

Putkonen, T., Paatero, Y.V., 1961. X-ray photography of unerupted permanent teeth in congenital syphilis. British Journal of Venereal Diseases 37 (3), 190.

Puzzilli, F., Salvati, M., Ruggeri, A., Raco, A., Bristot, R., Bastianello, S., Lundari, P., 1977. Intracranial actinomycosis in juvenile patients. Case report and review of the literature. Child's Nervous System 14 (9), 463–466.

Rabinowitsch, M., 1913. Leprabacillen im kreisenden blute der lepra-kranken und im herzblute eines leprafötus. Berliner Klinisch Wochenscrift 50 (6), 252–253.

Rajeshwari, K., Sharma, A., 1994. Multifocal skeletal tuberculosis presenting as osteitis skull and atlantoaxial dislocation. Indian Pediatrics 32, 1214–1219.

Ramu, G., 1959. Adult type lepromatous leprosy in a child of 6 months. Indian Journal of Child Health 8, 313–314.

Rankin, K., Tuli, S., 2009. Skeletal tuberculosis. Children's Orthopaedics and Fractures 3 (4), 161–178.

Rasool, M., Givender, S., Naidoo, K., 1994. Cystic tuberculosis of bone in children. The Journal of Bone and Joint Surgery 76-B (1), 113–117.

Ratliff, A., 1959. The short leg in poliomyelitis. The Journal of Bone and Joint Surgery 41B (1), 56–69.

Reed, G., 1969. Rubella bone lesions. The Journal of Pediatrics 74 (2), 208–213.

Regan, J., 1918. The hydrocephalus of poliomyelitis. American Journal of Diseases in Children 15, 259–270.

Reichart, P., 1976. Facial and oral manifestations in leprosy: an evaluation of seventy cases. Oral Surgery, Oral Medicine, Oral Pathology 41 (3), 385–399.

Resnick, D. (Ed.), 1995. Diagnosis of Bone and Joint Disorders, third ed. W.B. Saunders Company, Philadelphia.

Resnick, D., Kransdorf, M., 2005. Bone and Joint Imaging, third ed. Elsevier Saunders, Philadelphia.

Rida, A., 1962. A dissertation from the early eighteenth century, probably the first description of poliomyelitis. Journal of Bone and Joint Surgery 44B (3), 735–740.

Roberts, C., 1986. Leprogenic odontodysplasia. In: Cruwys, E., Foley, R. (Eds.), Teeth and Anthropology. Archaeopress, Oxford, pp. 46–59.

Roberts, C., Buikstra, J., 2003. The bioarchaeology of tuberculosis. A global view on a reemerging disease. University Press Florida, Gainsville.

Roberts, C., Cox, M., 2003. Health and Disease in Britain. Sutton Publishing Ltd., Gloucestershire.

Roberts, C., Knusel, C., Race, L., 2004. A foot deformity from a Romano-British cemetery at Gloucester, England, and the current evidence for Talipes in palaeopathology. International Journal of Osteoarchaeology 14, 389–403.

Roberts, C., Lucy, D., Manchester, K., 1994. Inflammatory lesions of ribs: an analysis of the Terry collection. American Journal of Physical Anthropology 95 (2), 169–182.

Rodriguez, J., 1926. Studies on early leprosy in children of lepers. The Philippine Journal of Science 31 (2), 115–148.

Roffey, S., Tucker, K., 2012. A contextual study of the medieval hospital and cemetery of St Mary Magdalen, Winchester, England. International Journal of Paleopathology 2, 170–180.

Rohnbogner, A., 2015. Dying Young: A Palaeopathological Analysis of Child Health in Roman Britain (Ph.D. thesis). University of Reading, England.

Rothschild, B., Naples, V., Barbian, L., 2006. Bone manifestations of actinomycosis. Annals of Diagnostic Pathology 10, 24–27.

Rothschild, B.M., Rothschild, C., 1995. Treponemal disease revisited: skeletal discriminators for yaws, bejel and venereal syphilis. Clinical Infectious Diseases 20, 1402–1408.

Rothschild, B.M., Rothschild, C., 1997. Congenital syphilis in the archaeological record: diagnostic insensitivity of osseous lesions. International Journal of Osteoarchaeology 7, 39–42.

Rubini, M., Erdal, Y., Spigalman, M., Zaio, P., Donogue, H., 2014. Paleopathological and molecular study on two cases of ancient childhood leprosy from the Roman and Byzantine empires. International Journal of Osteoarchaeology 24 (5), 570–582.

Rudolf, A., Singleton, E., Rosenberg, H., Singer, D., Phillips, C., 1965. Osseous manifestations of the congenital rubella syndrome. American Journal of Disease in Childhood 110, 428–433.

Sachdeva, S., Zulfia, K.S.A., Pranav, K.S., 2010. Childhood leprosy: a retrospective study. Journal of Public Health and Epidemiology 2 (9), 267–271.

Santos, A., 2015. Archives and skeletons: an interdisciplinary approach to the study of paleopathology of tuberculosis. Tuberculosis 95, S109–S111.

Santos, A.L., Roberts, C., 2006. Anatomy of a serial killer: differential diagnosis of tuberculosis based on rib lesions of adult individuals from the Coimbra identified skeletal collection, Portugal. American Journal of Physical Anthropology 130 (1), 38–49.

Santos, A.L., Roberts, C.A., 2001. A picture of tuberculosis in young Portuguese people in the early 20th century: a multidisciplinary study of the skeletal and historical evidence. American Journal of Physical Anthropology 115 (1), 38–49.

Sarnet, B., Shaw, N., 1942. Dental development in congenital syphilis. American Journal of Diseases of Children 64 (5), 771–788.

Schillingii, G., 1778. De Lepra Commentationes. Lugduni Batavorum.

Schuurs, A., 2013. Pathology of the Hard Dental Tissues. Wiley-Blackwell, West Sussex.

Scollard, D., 2000. Endothelial cells and the pathogenesis of lepromatous neuritis: insights from the armadillo model. Microbes and Infection 2, 1835–1843.

Sekeles, E., Ornoy, A., 1974. Osseous manifestations of gestational rubella in young human fetuses. American Journal of Obstetrics and Gynecology 122 (3), 307–312.

Shapiro, F., 2001. Pediatric Orthopedic Deformities: Basic Science, Diagnosis and Treatment. Academic Press, New York.

Sharma, M., Bhatia, V., 2004. Abdominal tuberculosis. Indian Journal of Medical Research 120, 305–315.

Sharrard, W., 1955. Muscle recovery in poliomyelitis. Journal of Bone Joint and Surgery 37B (1), 63–79.

Sharrard, W., 1967. Paralytic deformity in the lower limb. Journal of Bone and Joint Surgery 49B (4), 731–747.

Sheldon, W., 1943. Diseases of Infancy and Childhood. J. & A. Churchill Ltd., London.

Shingadia, D., Novelli, V., 2003. Diagnosis and treatment of tuberculosis in children. The Lancet: Infectious Diseases 3, 624–632.

Siegal, M., Greenberg, M., 1956. Poliomyelitis in pregnancy: effects on fetus and newborn infant. Journal of Pediatrics 49 (3), 280–288.

Šilkanjić, P., Meštrović, S., 2006. A case of short-root anomaly in a female from medieval Ostria. International Journal of Osteoarchaeology 16, 177–180.

Silverman, F., 1976. Virus diseases of bone: do they exist? American Journal of Roentgenology 126 (4), 677–703.

Simpson, J.Y., 1872. Archaeological Essays: On Leprosy and Leper Hospitals in Scotland and England. Edmonston and Douglas.

Singh, I., Kaur, S., Khandelwal, N., Kaur, I., Deodar, S., 1994. Arthritis in leprosy: clinical, laboratory, and radiological assessments. International Journal of Leprosy 62 (3), 428–433.

Singh, A., Chatterjee, P., Pai, M., Chacko, T., 2009. Tuberculous osteomyelitis of the scapula masquerading as metastasis. Radiology Case Reports 3 (1), 27–31.

Singh, R., Monga, A.K., Bais, S., 2013. Polio: a review. International Journal of Pharmeceutical Sciences and Research 4, 1714–1724.

Skinsnes, O., Sakurai, I., Aquino, T., 1972. Pathogenesis of extremity deformity in leprosy. International Journal of Leprosy 40, 375–388.

Sorrel, E., Sorrel-Dejerine, M., 1932. Tuberculose Osseuse et Osteoarticulaire. Masson et Cie, Paris.

Spiro, H., 1995. Protean manifestation of gastrointestinal tuberculosis: report on 130 patients. Journal of Clinical Gastroenterology 20 (3), 181–268.

Steinbock, R.T., 1976. Paleopathological diagnosis and interpretation: bone diseases in ancient human populations. Charles C Thomas, Illinois.

Stewart, T.D., Spoehr, A., 1951. Evidence on the paleopathology of yaws. Bulletin of the History of Medicine 26 (6), 538–553.

Steyn, M., Meiring, J.-H., Nienaber, W., Loots, M., 2002. Large fontanelles in an early 20th century rural population from South Africa. International Journal of Osteoarchaeology 12, 291–296.

Still, G., 1912. Common Disorders and Diseases of Childhood. Froude, London.

Stone, A., Wilbur, A., Buikstra, J., Roberts, C., 2009. Tuberculosis and leprosy in perspective. Yearbook of Physical Anthropology 52, 66–94.

Subramaniam, K., Marks Jr., S.C., 1978. Alveolar bone loss in leprosy–a clinical and radiological study. Leprosy Review 49 (4), 287.

Subramaniam, K., Marks, S., Seang, H.N., 1983. The rate of loss of maxillary anterior alveolar bone height in patients with leprosy. Leprosy Review 54 (2), 119.

Sugai, T., Monobe, K., 1913. Hematological studies in newborn babies and leprosy bacilli in the blood. Sei-i-Kwai Medical Journal 32, 102–103.

Sugarman, J., Calvin, C., Moran, A., Oxlade, O., 2014. Tuberculosis in pregnancy: an estimate of the global burden of disease. Lancet 2, 710–716.

Sundharam, J., 1990. Leprosy in childhood. Indian Pediatrics 27, 1126–1128.

Tata, H., 1978. Tuberculosis osteomyelitis of the skull. Indian Journal of Tuberculosis 25 (4), 208–209.

Taylor, G., Watson, C., Bouwman, A., Lockwood, D., Mays, S., 2006. Variable nucleotide tandem repeat (VNTR) typing of two palaeopathological cases of lepromatous leprosy from medieval England. Journal of Archaeological Science 33, 1569–1579.

Teklali, Y., El Alami, Z., El Madhi, T., Gourinda, H., Miri, A., 2003. Peripheral osteoarticular tuberculosis in children: 106 case-reports. Joint Bone Spine 70, 282–286.

Teo, H., Peh, W., 2004. Skeletal tuberculosis in children. Pediatric Radiology 34 (11), 853–860.

Teschler-Nicola, M., Gerold, F., Prodinger, W., 1998. Endocranial features in tuberculosis. In: Twelfth European Meeting of the Paleopathology Association, p. 92 Prague.

Thompson, A., 2014. Differential diagnosis of limb length discrepenancy in a nineteenth century burial from Southwest Mississippi. International Journal of Osteoarchaeology 24 (4), 517–530.

Thomson, W., 1882. The Land and the Book. Nelson, London.

Tomczyk, J., Mańkowska-Pliszka, H., Palczewski, P., Olczak-Kowalczyk, D., 2015. Congenital syphilis in the skeleton of a child from Poland (Radom, 18th–19th century AD). Anthropological Review 78 (1), 79–90.

Veiby, G., Daltveit, A., Gilhus, N., 2007. Pregnancy, delivery and perinatal outcome in female survivors of polio. Journal of Neurological Sciences 258, 27–32.

Waldron, T., 2009. Palaeopathology. Cambridge University Press, Cambridge.

Walker, D., Powers, N., Connell, B., Redfern, R., 2014. Evidence of skeletal treponematosis from the medieval burial ground of St. Mary Spital, London, and implications for the origins of the disease in Europe. American Journal of Physical Anthropology 156 (1), 90–101.

Wallgren, A., 1948. The time-table of tuberculosis. Tubercle 29, 245–251.

Walls, T., Shingadia, D., 2004. Global epidemiology of pediatric tuberculosis. Journal of Infection 48, 13–22.

Wells, C., 1982. The human burials. In: McWhirr, A., Viner, L., Wells, C. (Eds.), Romano-British Cemeteries at Cirencester. Corinium Museum, Cirencester, pp. 135–202.

Wilbur, A., Bouwman, A., Stone, A., Roberts, C., Pfister, L.-A., Buikstra, J., Brown, T., 2009. Deficiencies and challenges in the study of ancient tuberculosis DNA. Journal of Archaeological Science 36, 1990–1997.

Willcox, R., 1960. Evolutionary cycle of the treponematoses. British Journal of Venereal Diseases 36, 78–91.

Willows, M., 2015. Palaeopathology of the Isle of May. In: Gerdau-Radonić, K., McSweeney, K. (Eds.), Trends in Biological Anthropology. Oxbow Books, Oxford, pp. 42–53.

Winkler, E.-M., Grosschmidt, K., 1987. A case of poliomyelitis from an early medieval cemetery at Georgenberg/Upper Austria. OSSA 13, 217–231.

Wright, B.L., 1908. The treatment of tuberculosis by the administration of mercury at the United States hospital, New Fort Lyon, Colo. Journal of the American Medical Association 51 (22), 1854–1856.

Wyatt, H., 2003. Poliomyelitis. In: Kiple, K. (Ed.), The Cambridge Historical Dictionary of Disease. Cambridge University Press, Cambridge, pp. 258–261.

Chapter 8

Hemopoietic and Metabolic Disorders

Chapter Outline

Hemopoietic Disorders	193	Thalassemia	200
Cribra Orbitalia, Porotic Hyperostosis, and the "Cribrous Syndrome"	194	Sickle Cell Anemia	203
		Leukemia	206
Dietary Iron-Deficiency Anemia	197	Hemophilia A and B	207
Malaria	198	**Metabolic Disorders**	209
Other Parasitic Infections	199	Rickets and Osteomalacia (Vitamin D Deficiency)	209
Folate Deficiency	199	Infantile Scurvy (Vitamin C Deficiency)	213
Vitamin B_{12} Deficiency	199	Comorbidity and Cooccurrence in Rickets and Scurvy	218
Lead Poisoning	199	**References**	218

HEMOPOIETIC DISORDERS

Hemopoietic or blood-borne disorders are those that result from abnormalities of the red blood cells (erythrocytes). They are characterized by marrow hyperplasia, vascular occlusion, and anemia, which affect the blood's capacity to transport oxygen around the body (Resnick and Kransdorf, 2005). Anemia is a symptom of preexisting conditions, rather than a diagnosis in itself, and understanding its skeletal manifestation and cause in archeological groups has been the subject of much controversy. This section will discuss the issues surrounding the interpretation of the most common lesions associated with anemia in the past, cribra orbitalia and porotic hyperostosis, as well as the more specific conditions of hemolytic anemia and leukemia.

The protein molecule hemoglobin is formed by four polypeptide chains with each molecule (HbA) containing two alpha and two beta chains. Each chain contains heme, a compound with an embedded iron atom that is responsible for the transportation of oxygen and carbon dioxide around the body. During development different polypeptide chains are present, reflecting the specialized transportation of oxygen in utero (Simpson, 1991). In the fetus, HbF replaces embryonic hemoglobins from 6 weeks gestation until birth. After birth, HbF is replaced by HbA (and smaller amounts of HbA_2) as the lungs expand and tissue uptake of oxygen becomes a priority. At birth all of the bodily iron is of maternal origin reducing to 70% during infancy and 30% by 2 years of age (Simpson, 1991). In the fetus blood cell formation, or hemopoiesis, occurs at numerous sites including the bone marrow, liver, spleen, and lymph nodes, but by birth bone marrow is almost entirely responsible for this process.

Postnatal skeletal development is characterized by the conversion of the majority of hematopoietic red bone marrow into fatty yellow bone marrow. This process begins at the terminal phalanges of the hands and feet from birth and occurs at different rates in different bones. Conversion starts from the distal to the proximal aspect of each bone. It is complete in the feet by 1 year of age and by 7 years the long bones start their conversion, first at the distal epiphyses and by 12–14 years at the midshaft (Figs. 8.1 and 8.2). By 25 years red bone marrow has migrated from all of the long bones with the exception of the proximal humerus and femur, pelvis, sternum and margins of the scapula (Kricun, 1985). At any stage, conversion from red to yellow bone marrow may be halted or reversed. This occurs in the presence of marrow infiltrating disorders such as leukemia and hemolytic anemia (sickle cell and thalassemia) causing abnormal expansion of the remaining red bone marrow (Kricun, 1985). As children have more reactive bone marrow than adults they present more severe skeletal changes with relatively smaller stimuli (Bolton-Maggs and Thomas, 2008). In anemia, the body responds to the decreased oxygen in the blood by stimulating the kidneys to secrete erythropoietin to stimulate erythropoiesis in bone marrow (Kwong et al., 2004). Red bone marrow is able to increase erythrocyte production (erythropoiesis) beyond 120 days by six- to eightfold without failing, and so mild anemia will not produce any visible change on the skeleton (Bolton-Maggs and Thomas, 2008).

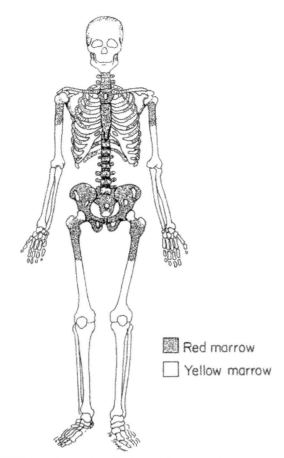

FIGURE 8.1 Conversion of red (*shaded*) to yellow bone marrow in the long bones from birth to 25 years. At birth the epiphyses (i.e., distal femur, proximal humerus) do not contain any marrow. *From Kricun, M., 1985. Red-yellow marrow conversion: its effect on the location of some solitary bone lesions. Skeletal Radiology 14, 11.*

Cribra Orbitalia, Porotic Hyperostosis, and the "Cribrous Syndrome"

Anemia manifests on the skeleton primarily in the form of marrow expansion. Cribra orbitalia (usura orbitae, hyperostosis spongiosa orbitae) refers to porous lesions on the orbital roof thought to be associated with similar lesions on the cranial vault known as porotic hyperostosis (Figs. 8.3 and 8.4). Cribra orbitalia was a term first used by Welcker in 1885. Similar porotic changes to the frontal endocranial and ectocranial surfaces were termed "cribra cranii" by Henschen (1961). However, these names are rarely used by clinicians (Campillo, 2006) who prefer the term porotic hyperostosis. Porotic hyperostosis describes the changes to the cranial vault (including the orbital roofs) as a result of overreacting red marrow in anemia. In severe cases of anemia, hyperplastic marrow widens the diploë and thins the outer table, which may be totally obliterated. There is trabecular destruction and thickening of residual trabeculae as the marrow proliferates under the periosteum, and new bony spicules are laid down perpendicular to the inner

table in a "hair-on-end" pattern (Hollar, 2001; Ponec and Resnick, 1984). Hair-on-end trabeculae have been identified in numerous hemopoietic disorders (Moseley, 1965, 1974; Steinbock, 1976), including sickle cell disease, thalassemia major, and spherocytosis, as well as several metabolic conditions that may coexist with anemia (Table 8.1).

In the absence of anemia, conversion from red to yellow marrow in the frontal bone, and hence the orbits, is reported to occur around the age of 10 years in boys and girls, and the parietals at around 11.5 years (Simonson and Kao, 1992). The location of lesions associated with red marrow is dependent on the age of the individual and the site of red marrow at the time of the pathology, so we should not expect porotic changes in the skull and orbits to occur in response to new episodes of anemia after 10–11 years of age. There is debate about whether these lesions will heal after the anemia has resolved (Moseley, 1974; Sebes and Diggs, 1979). In paleopathology, cribra orbitalia and porotic hyperostosis should serve as descriptive terms only, and while thalassemia, sickle cell anemia, and rickets have discernible postcranial features that may help in diagnosis, they need to be taken into consideration when attempting to identify iron-deficiency anemia. An illustration that cribrotic lesions may have other etiologies is highlighted by a histological study of adolescent and adult individuals from Missiminia in northern Sudan. In the 333 individuals with cribra orbitalia, Wapler et al. (2004) only found 56.5% with microscopic signs of anemia.

Porous lesions of the femoral and humeral neck (cribra femoralis and cribra humeralis) were included in studies of anemia in Spain when Miquel-Feucht et al. (1999a,b) noted that the porous lesions at the metaphyseal ends of nonadult long bones were morphologically identical to those seen in the orbit (Fig. 8.5). Through histological analysis they described expansion of bone marrow, thinning of the cortex and substitution by trabeculae bone in the proximal aspects of the humerus and femur. In combination with cribra orbitalia, they termed these changes the "cribrous syndrome." The lesions occurred symmetrically in hyperplatycnemic and platycnemic femora and were often associated with changes in the humerus and orbits in the same individual (Miquel-Feucht et al., 1999a,b). In a further study in which they induced iron and magnesium deficiency in rats, Polo-Cerdá et al. (2001) asserted that the resulting cribra orbitalia was part of a cribrous syndrome seen in the rest of the skeleton, although they did not demonstrate any evidence of porotic lesions on the cranial vault, humerus, or femur. Since that time, a handful of researchers have published femoral and humeral lesions in association with anemia (Baxarias, 2002; Djuric et al., 2008; Mendiela et al., 2014; Paredes et al., 2015). Djuric et al. (2008) reported a prevalence of 83.2% and 58.5% for femoral and humeral cribra, respectively, in nonadults from later medieval Serbia. While they had lower rates of cribra orbitalia at 46.1%, 33.3% of individuals had both orbital and postcranial lesions. This association

Hemopoietic and Metabolic Disorders **Chapter | 8** 195

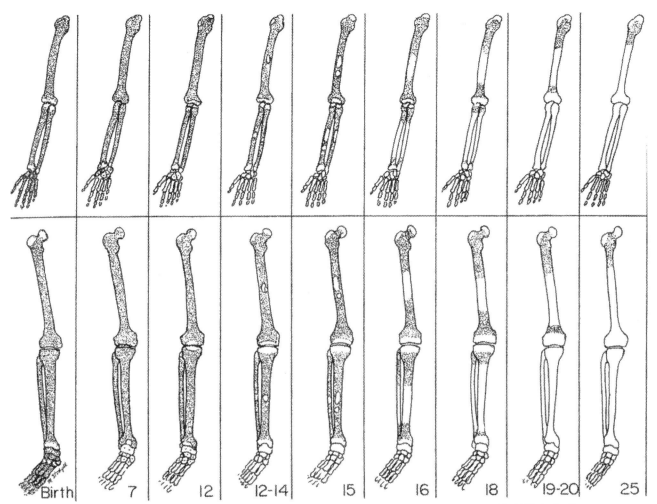

FIGURE 8.2 Distribution of red bone marrow in the upper and lower limbs from birth to 25 years. *From Kricun, M., 1985. Red-yellow marrow conversion: its effect on the location of some solitary bone lesions. Skeletal Radiology 14, 12.*

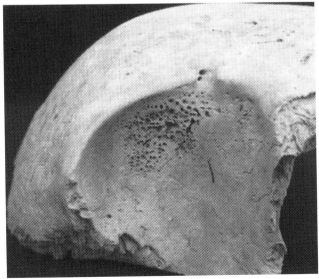

FIGURE 8.3 Cribra orbitalia on the orbital roof of a 1.5-year-old from Kültepe, Turkey (Kültepe Excavation Archive skeleton 07M90B2). *Photographs reproduced with the kind permission of Handan Üstündağ, University of Anadolu, Turkey.*

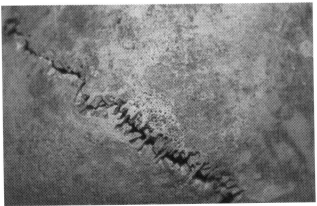

FIGURE 8.4 Mild porotic hyperostosis on the right parietal bone of a 5-6-year-old from St Oswald's Priory in Gloucester, England (skeleton 398).

TABLE 8.1 List of Conditions Associated With Hyperblastic Changes to the Cranium

Thalassemia major

Thalassemia intermedia

Thalassemia minor

Sickle-cell disease

Hereditary elliptocytosis

Glucose-6-phosphate dehydrogenase (G6PD) deficiency

Microangiopathic hemolytic anemia

Pyruvate kinase (PK) deficiency

Hereditary spherocytosis

Iron-deficiency anemia

Rickets

Scurvy

After Moseley, J.E., 1974. Skeletal changes in the anemias. Seminars in Roentgenology 9 (3), 169–184 and Steinbock, R.T., 1976. Paleopathological Diagnosis and Interpretation: Bone Diseases in Ancient Human Populations, Charles C Thomas, Illinois.

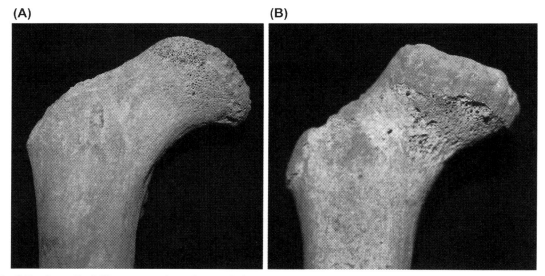

FIGURE 8.5 Cribra femoralis. Different expressions of porous lesions at the proximal metaphyses of the femur from (A) fine porosity to (B) a large circumscribed area of pitting, more commonly interpreted as a nonmetric trait (Allen's fossa) in adults.

was not statistically significant. Mendiela et al. (2014) also recorded a high prevalence of femoral cribra at 80.9% in Copper Age nonadults from Spain. Paredes et al. (2015) recorded humeral and femoral lesions in 52.0% and 45.5% of nonadults from later medieval Faro in Portugal, with 40% of individuals displaying cribra orbitalia. The retention of red bone marrow at the metaphyses of growing children and the thin cortex in these areas could cause visible hyperplastic changes in a pathological condition. However, unlike the cranial lesions, these changes require further investigation and have yet to be demonstrated in the clinical literature in association with anemia or any other deficiency. In addition we need to be able to differentiate any lesions caused by anemia from other features in these areas, such as the cutback zone, or in the proximal femur, Allen's fossa, a nonmetric trait.

Cribra orbitalia and porotic hyperostosis are often graded according to the scheme described by Stuart-Macadam (1991, p. 109) who provided photographs and a written description of the different appearances. But other grading schemes exist (Knip, 1971; Nathan and Haas, 1966; Robledo et al., 1995; Schultz, 1988; Buikstra and

Ubelaker, 1994). Further details should be added using Mensforth et al.'s (1978) description of active (sharp-edged) and remodeled (smooth-edged, filled-in) lesions. Orbital lesions are often seen in isolation, particularly in European samples, making it important to make a distinction between orbital and cranial lesions as this may provide some indication as to the cause or severity (Blom et al., 2005). Prevalence rates of cribra orbitalia vary considerably in the literature and are often based on low sample sizes. A review of cribra orbitalia prevalence rates from sites across the world with over 40 nonadults who had orbits to observe revealed crude prevalence rates that vary considerably from just 4% in 75 early medieval children from Gloucestershire, England (Boyle et al., 1995), to 78% in 41 Iron Age/early Roman children from Alvastra, Sweden (Liebe-Harkort, 2012). Some researchers omit Stuart-Macadam's Grades 1 (capillary-like impressions) and 2 (i.e., small isolated pits) from their analyses as these mild lesions can be ambiguous (Lewis, 2007). However, not all researchers are specific about the grades they include, and the impact on reported prevalence rates can be dramatic. For example, Novak and Šlaus (2010) recorded a prevalence rate of 50% cribra orbitalia in nonadults from Roman Period Zadar in Croatia, providing high rates compared to many other child samples in Europe. When only their moderate to severe forms (Grades 3–5) were taken into account, the prevalence was 15.6% producing rates lower than those of similar grades reported for the same period in England. If grades are not reported, valid comparisons between sites are impossible.

The earliest reported case of porotic hyperostosis in a child is in a 2-year-old hominin from Olduvai Gorge, Tanzania, with porotic lesions on both parietals (Dominguez-Rodrigo et al., 2012). Studies into the likely causes of cribra orbitalia have included orbital hemangioma or chronic eye infections in leprous individuals (Duggan and Wells, 1964; Møller-Christensen and Sandison, 1963), optic nerve entrapment (Naveed et al., 2012), and iron-deficiency anemia due to a dependency on maize (Cohen and Armelagos, 1984; El-Najjar et al., 1979; Gilbert and Mielke, 1985; Palkovich, 1987), parasitic infection (Blom et al., 2005; Reinhard, 1992; Trinkaus, 1977), weaning diarrhea (Walker, 1986), or an immune response to an increased pathogen load (Brown and Holden, 2002; Weinberg, 1974, 1992). Fairgrieve and Molto (2000) argued that early weaning onto goat's milk led to cribra orbitalia at 6 months in the infants from the Dakhleh Oasis, and that their iron-deficiency anemia was exacerbated by the use of honey during weaning, exposing the children to botulism. While the precise etiology of cribra orbitalia and porotic hyperostosis remains controversial (Walker et al., 2009), at present orbital lesions are considered the result of severe anemia acquired due to deficiencies in folic acid and vitamin B_{12}, available in fresh meat and leafy vegetables, or a deficiency in dietary iron. Porotic hyperostosis is considered to have an acquired and inherited etiology (Oxenham and Cavill, 2010). Anemia as the result of chronic infections, toxicosis, and congenital anomalies (for example, Fanconi's anemia, Diamond–Blackfans anemia, transient erythroblastopenia) is aplastic in that it suppresses erythropoietic activity and is unlikely to result in marrow expansion (Simpson, 1991). The most often cited causes for iron-deficiency anemia in archeological contexts are discussed below.

Dietary Iron-Deficiency Anemia

Iron is necessary for the healthy development of the brain and normal red blood cell production (Bolton-Maggs and Thomas, 2008). Iron-deficiency anemia is a common condition affecting as much as 80% of the world's population (Kwong et al., 2004). The combined effect of deficiencies in iron, vitamin A, and zinc is linked to high child mortality, poor mental health, retarded motor skills, impaired growth, and limited resistance to infection (Ryan, 1997). The clinical symptoms of anemia in the child include pallor, tiredness, breathlessness on minor exertion, and a poor appetite (Simpson, 1991). They are also prone to pica (eating mouthfuls of earth, stones, and sand). To grow, the young child relies on the iron derived from maternal stores being gradually replaced by iron-rich weaning foods. Hence, iron deficiency anemia is most common after 6 months of age (Kwong et al., 2004; Saarinen, 1978). Preterm and low for birth weight infants may become deficient at 3 months due to lower maternal stores gathered in utero and an increased need for iron due to catch-up growth (Schulman, 1959). Similar to infants, adolescents have different nutritional requirements to the rest of the population due to their rapid growth during the growth spurt. Their iron requirement rises from ~1.0 to 2.5 mg/day in boys, due to an increased blood volume and rise in hemoglobin concentration. At peak growth, females require ~1.5 mg/day iron that finally decreases to 1.3 mg/day reflecting the need to supplement menstrual loss throughout adulthood (Brabin and Brabin, 1992).

The most common cause of iron-deficiency anemia is an inappropriate diet. Dietary iron is produced in two forms: heme and nonheme. Heme iron is available in red meat, fish, and poultry and is readily absorbed by the body. Nonheme iron is less bioavailable. It is present in beans, pulses, fruit, and green leafy vegetables. Absorption is enhanced by vitamin C and proteins but inhibited by legumes, eggs, and phytates of unrefined cereals (Bolton-Maggs and Thomas, 2008). In children iron deficiency may be accentuated by the use of cow's milk for weaning before the age of 1 year, which can cause intestinal bleeding from an irritation of the immature digestive system (Jelliffe and Blackman, 1962). This would be further exacerbated by the use of cereal based pap and low amounts of vitamin C. Interestingly, McCullough et al. (2015) have suggested that hemochromatosis, caused by a recessive gene disorder (allele C282Y), was an adaptation to high diary and low iron diets during the transition to agriculture in the Neolithic. They identified high levels of the gene mutation, coupled with cribra orbitalia and porotic hyperostosis in Northwestern European skeletons in areas where dairying was widely adopted. Although individuals with the severest form of hemochromatosis will die due to toxic levels of iron being stored in the liver and kidneys, heterozygotes may have been actively selected for their ability to absorb higher levels of iron from their diets.

Specific cranial lesions associated with iron deficiency include frontal bossing and the absence of the lamina dura outlining the tooth socket (Lanzkowsky, 1968, 1977). It is essential to differentiate between true cases of iron-deficiency anemia, where gracile trabeculae are orientated in a perpendicular hair-on-end pattern extending from the diploë, from porotic lesions caused by remodeled appositional new bone as the result of hemorrhage due to trauma or scurvy, tumors, poorly mineralized osteoid in rickets, or inflammation (Fig. 8.6; Schultz, 1997, 2001). While cranial changes get the most focus in paleopathology, iron-deficiency anemia may also produce postcranial changes, commonly at the elbow (Steinbock, 1976), with osteoporosis and coarse trabecular striations at the distal humerus and proximal radius and ulna. While the hands and feet may be mildly affected, changes are not as extensive as in thalassemia, and the condition lacks the vertebral changes and thrombosis of sickle cell. Due to malnutrition, it is likely that iron-deficiency anemia and the skeletal changes associated with it will coexist with other changes due to rickets, scurvy, or other missing nutrients.

Malaria

Malaria is carried by a parasite of the *Plasmodium* species and transmitted to humans by mosquito bites. There are several strains of malaria; *Plasmodium malariae*, *P. vivax*, *P. ovale*, and *P. falciparum*, with the latter considered the most virulent (Sallares and Gomzi, 2001). In high endemic areas children younger than 5 years are at the most risk of infection, whereas in low endemic areas all age groups can be affected (Miller et al., 1994). The parasites (sporozoites) enter the bloodstream after multiplying in the liver and invading the red blood cells. Premature rupture (hemolysis) of the red blood cells in 3- to 4-day cycles releases the sporozoites that then invade other cells. Capillaries become clogged with subsequent kidney and spleen disorders causing anorexia, nausea, and headaches followed by vomiting, fevers, and anemia. In severe cases, renal failure and noncardiac pulmonary edema may develop. The pattern of disease in African children is slightly different as they are not infected by *P. vivax* and do not develop renal or cardiac symptoms (Miller et al., 1994). The disease is exacerbated by pregnancy and may result in death of the fetus and blood poisoning in the mother (Miller et al., 1994). While the acute form of infection caused by *P. falciparum* may leave little trace of the skeleton, low grade recurring infections caused by *P. vivax* may be present in the form of cribra orbitalia or porotic hyperostosis (Setzer, 2014), and today severe anemia is only identified in highly endemic areas (Miller et al., 1994). Setzer (2014) argues for the use of more multidisciplinary techniques such as immunology and red blood cells preservation to help study malaria in future paleopathological investigations.

Malaria is considered an ancient disease that may have been transmitted to humans from other primates during the Holocene. *P. vivax* and *P. malariae* appear to have been present in Greece during the 4th to 5th century BC, due to the low grade fever described in texts (Sallares and Gomzi, 2001). The more malignant form, *P. falciparum* seems to have evolved out of Africa, and was well known in Greece by the 5th century BC appearing in Italy by the 1st century AD (Sallares and Gomzi, 2001). Malaria (known as ague) is then thought to have been brought to the British Isles during the Roman conquest. Ague was a common condition in marshy areas in the 16th–17th century (Dobson, 1989; Reiter, 2000). One of the first studies to consider malaria as a cause of high infant mortality in archeological material was Soren et al. (1995) while excavating Poggio Gramignano, in Teverina, Italy. This cemetery sample comprised 87%

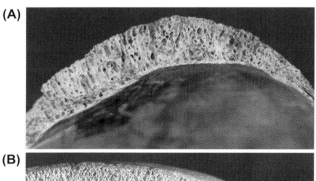
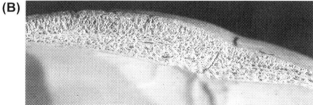

FIGURE 8.6 Differences in the cross-sectional appearance of porous cranial lesions. (A) Anemia in a 1- to 2-year-old from Pueblo Bonito, New Mexico, with complete obliteration of the outer table of the cranium (Skeleton NMNH 327,072; AD 950–1250). (B) Rickets in a child from 19th century Vienna. The skull displays porous periosteal new bone on the outer surface, and on cross section a layer of fine cancellous bone is evident both internally and externally to the original cortex (skeleton FPAM 5051). *From Ortner, D., 2003. Identification of Pathological Conditions in Human Skeletal Remains, Academic Press, New York, p. 374 and 395.*

perinates and 13% infants. It was located in an area known for malaria outbreaks, which may cause spontaneous abortions (Miller et al., 1994; Soren et al., 1995). Offerings of mutilated puppies and other votives suggest the unusual nature of the site. Charred honeysuckle seeds, used to treat diseases of the spleen, and a toad used to ward off fevers, adds weight to the argument that the burials occurred as the result of a malaria epidemic (Soren et al., 1995). While this original assertion has proved controversial, later aDNA analysis of the oldest child proved to be positive for *P. falciparum* malaria (Fig. 8.7). Interestingly this child appeared to have been "held down in death" using a tile and pebbles on their hands and feet (Soren, 2003). The plasmodium parasite does not preserve well in bones and the fact that the child from Lugnano was positive for malaria suggests a high-grade infection that may have caused his or her death (Sallares and Gomzi, 2001).

P. falciparum was also later isolated in a muscle sample from a 15- to 18-month-old mummy from Gebelein, Egypt (2820–2630 BC) (Bianucci et al., 2008). The earliest possible evidence for malaria (*P. vivax*) in England was provided by Gowland and Western (2012) who plotted the prevalence rates of cribra orbitalia in nonmarshy and marshy areas. They showed a positive correlation between elevated levels of cribra orbitalia and areas with favorable conditions for the presence of the *Anopheles atroparvus* mosquito. Cribra orbitalia as the result of both malaria and its comorbidities was considered a likely explanation for the distribution, particularly as enamel hypoplasia, that might be expected in a more generally sick and malnourished population, did not follow the same pattern.

Other Parasitic Infections

Clinical studies have suggested parasitic infections are likely to exacerbate anemia in malnourished people, rather than being the primary cause of anemia (Oguntibeju, 2003). Several forms of parasite have been linked to the development of anemia in humans; *Ascaris lumbricoides* (roundworm), *Necator americanus* (hookworm), *Trichuris trichiura* (whipworm), and *Entamoeba histolytica* resulting in amoebiasis, causing multiple deficiencies in iron, folic acid, and protein. Heavy burdens of hookworms and *T. trichiura* in particular cause chronic bleeding in the gut (Oguntibeju, 2003). Bathurst (2005) identified *A. lumbricoides* in multiperiod shell middens from British Colombia, Canada. Given the availability of iron-rich marine foods and the absence of genetic anemia prior to European contact, she suggested parasitic load may have been a contributing factor to cribra orbitalia and porotic hyperostosis seen in the skeletons. This parasite has been found in numerous contexts throughout America, with the oldest sample of *Ascaris* recovered dating to 3700–3490 BC (Bathurst, 2005).

Folate Deficiency

Megaloblastic anemia, a form where unusually large, structurally abnormal, immature red blood cells are formed is rare in childhood, but may be caused by a deficiency in folic acid. Maternal stores of folate last for 3–4 months, and absorption is rapid and efficient, but levels are in constant need of replenishment as they are required for nucleic acid synthesis in growing tissues. Rapid growth, fever, infection, diarrhea, and hemolysis all increase folate requirements. Mothers with low folate stores will pass this deficiency on to their children, and preterm children with lower maternal stores may develop megaloblastic anemia by 8 weeks. Severe cases of maternal deficiency result in neural tube defects such as spina bifida, anencephaly, and Down syndrome (Bolton-Maggs and Thomas, 2008). The best source of folate is from breast milk, but folate is also found in cow's milk, liver, green vegetables, and nuts. Goat's milk is a poor source of folate, and it can be easily destroyed by heating (Simpson, 1991).

Vitamin B_{12} Deficiency

This is very rare in children today and is usually only seen in those whose mothers are vegetarian or in children who have undergone gastric bypass surgery to combat obesity (Bolton-Maggs and Thomas, 2008). B_{12} is transported preferentially to the fetus and can stay within the system for 3–4 years, meaning deficient infants have enough B_{12} stores for 2–3 years (Simpson, 1991). B_{12} is found in all animal by-products.

Lead Poisoning

Lead poisoning has been associated with anemia since it was first described by Laennec in 1831. A shortened life span of red blood cells below 40 days, results in newly formed hypochromic cells and mild anemia (Rubino et al., 1962; Waldron, 1966), although severe lead

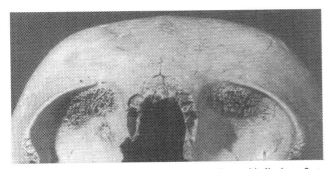

FIGURE 8.7 Malaria. Active "air-on-end" cribra orbitalia in a 2- to 3-year-old from 5th century AD Lugnano, Italy (skeleton IB36). This skeleton tested positive for aDNA *Plasmodium falciparum* malaria. *From Soren, D., Fenton, T., Birkby, W., 1995. The late Roman infant cemetery near Lugnano in Teverina, Italy: some implications. Journal of Paleopathology 7 (1), 25.*

toxicity can occur without anemia, or the anemia may be coincidental (Bolton-Maggs and Thomas, 2008). Some research has indicated an increased susceptibility to lead poisoning in cases of iron deficiency, while high iron intake may reduce lead absorption in children (Wright et al., 2003). When iron deficiency and lead poisoning occur in combination, the resulting anemia is much more severe, particularly in infants and children (Kwong et al., 2004). Lead poisoning is associated with impaired neurobehavioral development, lower intelligence, reduced birth weight, and slower nerve conduction velocity. While iron-deficiency anemia stimulates erythropoiesis, lead poisoning inhibits the production of erythropoietin, perhaps due to the effects of lead toxicity on renal cells (Kwong et al., 2004). Hence, it is unlikely anemia as the result of lead toxicity would be evident in the skeleton in the form of expanded bone marrow, and it may also reduce the appearance of iron-deficiency anemia in the skull.

Thalassemia

Thalassemia is one of a group of conditions caused by a failure or depression in the synthesis of one or two of the polypeptide chains of hemoglobin (alpha or beta) as the result of genetic mutations (Steinbock, 1976). Hemoglobin is substituted by amino acids, leading to the formation of red blood cells with reduced hemoglobin content (Aufderheide and Rodriguez-Martín, 1998) and, hence, a reduced ability to transport oxygen around the body. These abnormal red blood cells increase in response to low hemoglobin and are destroyed within the marrow from where they are recycled into new red blood cells (ineffective erythropoiesis) causing unusually high quantities of marrow (Aufderheide and Rodriguez-Martín, 1998). Classification of the condition is based on the globin chain that is affected: α-thalassemia occurs as the result of gene deletions, whereas β-thalassemia is caused by gene mutations of or near the β-globin (beta) genes. Alterations to the red blood cells provide protection against invasion from the malaria parasite, and hence mutations originally evolved in areas where malaria was endemic (Hedrick, 2011). The classic and most common form of thalassemia is beta-thalassemia, which affects groups from the central and eastern Mediterranean (i.e., Italians, Greeks, and North Africans). Both beta and alpha thalassemia may be found in other areas of the world including India, Thailand, Malaysia, and China (Ortner and Putschar, 1985). There are three types of genetic transmission: heterogeneous, homozygous, or compound heterogeneous. The terms major, minor, or intermedia thalassemia refer to the degree of clinical expression. β-thalassemia major (T-major) is the most serious form and results from the inheritance of two β-thalassemia alles (homozygote), one from each parent. Children need blood transfusions to survive, and if left untreated bones become thin and brittle, and the heart, liver, and spleen become greatly enlarged. Death usually occurs as the result of heart failure and stroke (Resnick, 1995) that may occur due to an uncontrolled iron build up in the body (Olivieri, 1999). It is unlikely that children born with T-major would survive beyond infancy in the past, and specific changes would be difficult to identify in the archeological record. β-thalassemia minor (T-minor) is less serious in its clinical expression than T-major. It is caused by one affected gene (heterozygote). The condition is usually asymptomatic, with no skeletal changes, and only mild clinical symptoms. It is most common in 1% of Black Americans and in the Mediterranean (Ortner, 2003). β-thalassemia intermedia is more severe than T-minor and is characterized by mild hemolytic anemia. Symptoms usually manifest by 2 years of age, when children become pale, fatigued, develop jaundice, and have growth deficiencies and facial deformities. This form of the condition does not usually require blood transfusions (Parano et al., 1999) but may manifest as extensive marrow proliferation and skeletal abnormalities. As sufferers can survive for years without a blood transfusion they should be visible in older children in antiquity (Lagia et al., 2006).

In the skull, changes affect the vault and the facial bones and can manifest in children as young as 18 months (Cooley et al., 1927). The cranial changes are particularly severe in T-major with the frontal bone affected first as the enlarged marrow is forced between two curved plates of the inner and outer tables. The plates expand vertically and the outer table becomes thinned (Resnick, 1995). The occipital bone is usually spared (Steinbock, 1976). In a study of 60 Thai thalassemia patients aged 11–16 years by Wisetsin (1989), only 8.3% (n=5) developed hair-on-end changes, but this figure may be higher without treatment. Lawson et al. (1984) suggest that endocranial vascular impressions that result from skull enlargement were most evident in individuals without blood transfusions. In infancy and later childhood, marrow enlargement also affects the face, and the maxillary and frontal sinuses fail to develop, resulting in a characteristic "rodent" face (Cooley and Lee, 1925; Resnick, 1995). The lack of sinus development is thought to be linked to the failure of red bone marrow to convert to yellow marrow during the normal conversion period (Simonson and Kao, 1992). Facial changes occur because the maxilla, zygomatic bones, and other facial bones are comprised mainly of cancellous bone. The facial appearance is characterized by high and bulging cheek bones, retraction of the upper lip, protrusion of the anterior teeth, wide dental spacing, and abnormal dental occlusion (Kaplan et al., 1964). Resnick (1995) reports that postcranial changes occur in the axial and appendicular skeleton before puberty and only in the axial skeleton after puberty. There is fanlike trabeculae organization of the pelvis, cortical thinning and porosity of the long bones, and thinning and enlargement of the phalanges (Ortner, 2003).

Skeletal manifestations in treated patients includes metaphyseal flask-shaped deformities, premature epiphyseal fusion most commonly of the proximal humerus and distal femur (Lawson et al., 1983), dwarfism, osteoporosis, and honeycomb hand and foot bones (osteopenia). There may also be metaphyseal flaring as the result of accompanying conditions such as rickets (Moseley, 1974; Resnick, 1995). Pathological fractures may occur in the femur, vertebrae, and forearms, healing slowly. There may also be rheumatoid arthritis, ischemic necrosis, osteomyelitis, and enlarged foramen of the phalanges (motheaten phalanges). Osseous changes increase with age and are manifest in varying degrees throughout the skeleton (Aksoy et al., 1973). In modern cases, sustained regular blood transfusions prevent the development of extramedullary hematopoiesis and severe bone changes. While such information is useful, the effect of treatment on skeletal expression should always be considered when using recent cases to inform the type and distribution of lesions we might expect to see in children with thalassemia intermedia in the past. Perhaps less well known in the diagnosis of skeletal thalassemia are the changes to the thorax. Lawson et al. (1981a) describe widening of the entire rib, which was more pronounced posteriorly with localized lucent areas evident within the medulla. The radiographic appearance is that of a "rib-within-a-rib," depicted by a band of radioopaque bone. In addition to this change, bulbous expansion of the ribs has been noted (Lawson et al., 1981b). These are described as costal osteomas caused by prolific hypermarrow within a bony shell sitting on top of the original cortex, with localized erosions. Caffey (1957) was the first to describe these masses in the ribs of a 3-year-old. On autopsy the osteoma was a large shell of bone, containing red bone marrow with the periosteum of the mass continuous with the cortex of the rib (Aksoy et al., 1973). In a wider survey, Singcharoen et al. (1988) examined rib changes in 33 children with β-thalassemia, aged between 6 months and 14 years. 26 (9%) had widening of the anterior rib surfaces, with 13 also exhibiting widening of the posterior rib surfaces. They noted cortical erosions (70%), subcortical radiolucency (61%), and localized radiolucency (36%), as well as the "rib-within-a-rib" appearance in 42% of cases, they also found soft tissue masses related to rib expansion and erosion in three cases (9%). Rib lesions were highlighted in the clinical case of Lagia et al. (2006) (Fig. 8.8) and by Moseley (1974), who considered them pathognomonic of thalassemia. These changes are particularly useful for the paleopathologists, they are more common in people who have not received blood transfusions (Pfeiffer et al., 1995).

Today, migration has resulted in a spread of the condition, and thalassemia now encompasses regions such as the Mediterranean basin, the Middle East, West Africa, Saudi Arabia, Southeast Asia, the Indian subcontinent, and China (Aufderheide and Rodriguez-Martín, 1998). In these areas, the presence of genetic anemia has been suggested in archeological groups on the basis of porotic hyperostosis and/or cribra orbitalia. These lesions vary in their severity and appear to be much milder in places such as Greece, where thalassemia and sickle cell diseases are prevalent among the modern population (Whipple and Bradford, 1936). Despite the lack of conclusive evidence for genetic anemia, several studies have highlighted possible cases. In 1964, Angel described 11 children from Lerna, Corinth, and Cyprus with porotic hyperostosis, but also thickening of the sphenoid, maxilla, and ribs, which could suggest thalassemia. But Angel's attention was on the parietal bone changes, and the postcranial lesions were not fully described. Mutations in the β-globin gene for thalassemia have been identified in children from 16th century Achziv, Israel (Filon et al., 1995), Roman period Isola Sacra in Italy (Yang, 1997) and three Egyptian mummies from Marro (c. 3200 BC) held at the museum in Turin (Massa, 1977). Genetic anemia was suggested as a possible diagnosis for thickened zygomatic bones in infants from prehistoric Thailand by Tayles (1996). Here, there were also enlarged foramen on the phalanges, but the form of genetic anemia (i.e., thalassemia or sickle cell disease) was not specified. The authors used an assessment of the thickness of the cortical vault (i.e., the ratio of cortex to diploë), to aid in their diagnosis. Baggieri and Mallegni (2001) describe the skeleton of an 8-year-old from Piazza dei Miracoli of Pisa, Italy, with porotic hyperostosis of the occipital–parietal region, porous cortex on the long bones, exaggerated sulci on the tibiae and femora that were interpreted as newly formed small blood vessels, and hypertrophic metacarpals and phalanges. The location of the site near marsh land suggested the presence of malaria and added weight to their assertion that the child was suffering from thalassemia. A similar connection was made for the infants recovered at the unusual villa site of Poggio Gramignano, in Teverina, Italy (Soren et al., 1995). Five of the older infants (4–6 months) and one child (2–3 years) in the sample of 47 displayed porotic hyperostosis and/or cribra orbitalia, with profuse new bone formation creating a "bone-within-a-bone" appearance to the long bones on radiograph, which they determined could have been caused by thalassemia, as malaria was endemic in the region. In 1991, Hershkovitz and Edelson (1991) identified premature epiphyseal fusion in the proximal humerus of a 16- to 17-year-old male from Neolithic (6000 BCE) Atlit-Yam, Israel. As the proximal humerus is the growth plate most often affected in thalassemia (Lawson et al., 1983), the authors considered the finding pathognomonic of genetic anemia. No other changes were described and a differential diagnosis of trauma, or the form of the disease that allowed the individual to live to such an age without treatment was not explored.

Lagia et al. (2006) provide the first in-depth study of dry bone changes of thalassemia in a modern case in a 14-year-old girl from Athens. They describe hair-on-end

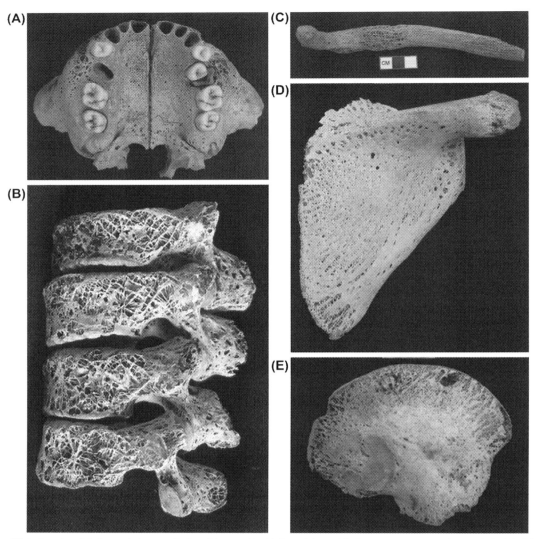

FIGURE 8.8 Clinical study of thalassemia intermedia in a 14-year-old girl from Athens. The bones are porous and expanded with diffuse large and small pits. Images show changes on the (A) maxilla, (B) vertebrae, (C) rib, (D) scapula, and (E) ilium. *From Lagia, A., Eliopoulos, C., Manolis, S., 2006. Thalassemia: macroscopic and radiological study of a case. International Journal of Osteoarchaeology 17 (3), p. 276, 277, and 279.*

porotic hyperostosis, obliteration of the cranial sutures, and expanded maxilla, widened intraorbital space, protrusion of the upper incisors, dental retardation, and bony masses on the ribs. The postcranial bones have changes associated with widespread osteopenia, and there are fanlike thickened trabeculae on the ilia. The child was treated with blood transfusions and so it is difficult to predict the natural progression of the disease on the skeleton without treatment. The other most commonly cited skeletal example of thalassemia is an 8-year-old from modern Thailand, who exhibits extensive porosity and cortical thinning of the long bones (Ortner, 2003, p. 366; Aufderheide and Rodriguez-Martín, 1998, p. 347). In England one site, late Roman Poundbury Camp in Dorset, revealed high levels of both porotic hyperostosis (75%) and cribra orbitalia (31%), which was uncharacteristic of similar dated sites from the British Isles (Stuart-Macadam, 1991). Reexamination of 364 Poundbury nonadults revealed children with general "wasting" of the bones and three young children who demonstrated a variety of severe lesions (e.g., zygomatic bone and rib hypertrophy, porotic hyperostosis, rib calluses, osteopenia, and pitted diaphyseal shafts) consistent with a diagnosis of genetic anemia. Two of these children displayed rib lesions typical of those seen in modern cases of thalassemia intermedia (Fig. 8.9). The children of Poundbury Camp represent the first cases of genetic anemia identified in a British archeological population (Fig. 8.10), and this is the first study to clearly demonstrate the pathognomonic rib changes. High infant mortality and children demonstrating severe osteopenia indicating a wasting condition that may also point to

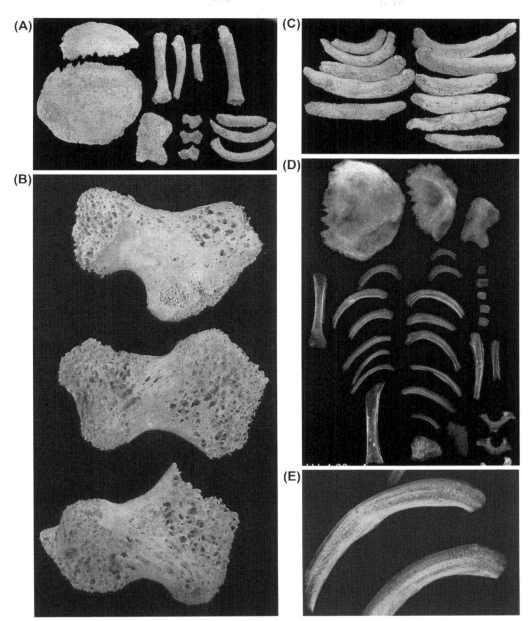

FIGURE 8.9 Thalassemia intermedia in an infant from late Roman Poundbury Camp in Dorset, England (skeleton 525). (A) The surviving bones show diffuse expansion and porosity, (B) with the fragile nature of the bones particularly evident on the vertebral neural arches. (C) The ribs are thickened with accentuated pitting along the costal margin and what appear to be fracture calluses on the central aspects of the shafts. (D) On X-ray thick layers of subperiosteal new bone are evident on the long bone shafts and the ribs have a "rib-within-a-rib" appearance. (E) On the ribs, costal osteomas caused by prolific hypermarrow within a bony shell sit on top of the original cortex, mimicking fracture calluses macroscopically. *Photographs taken with the kind permission of the Natural History Museum, London.*

the presence of T-major at the site (Lewis, 2010). As thalassemia is a condition strongly linked to the Mediterranean, the presence of this condition suggests the children were born to wealthy immigrant parents living in this small Roman settlement (Lewis, 2011). Rohnbogner (2015) identified a further probable case of β-thalassemia in a 1-year-old from Romano–British Colchester, England. She also highlighted the difficulty in distinguishing this condition from nonspecific respiratory infections, rickets, and trauma in cases where the remains are poorly preserved.

Sickle Cell Anemia

Sickle cell is a homogenous genetic anemia caused when an abnormal gene (hemoglobin S or HbS) causes the substitution of the amino acid valine, for another, glutamic

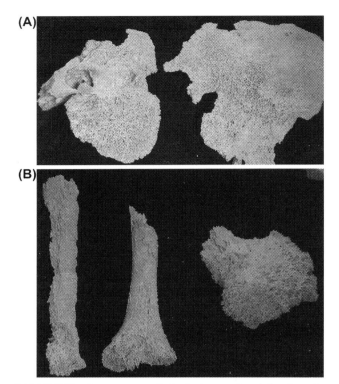

FIGURE 8.10 Severe osteopenia in the bones of an infant from late Roman Poundbury Camp in Dorset, England (skeleton 915) (A) with porosity and thinning of the cranial bones and (B) thickened and sparse trabecular bone on the long bones and ilium. These changes are suggestive of a severe metabolic disorder and potentially β-thalassemia major. *Photographs taken with the kind permission of the Natural History Museum, London.*

acid (Amundsen et al., 1984). The sickle gene protects heterogeneous carriers (HbC) from *P. falciparum* in malaria endemic areas, but migration has disseminated the gene more widely (Stuart and Nagel, 2004). Individuals may carry the sickle cell trait without producing any symptoms. Sickle cell disease occurs where HbS makes up more than 50% of the hemoglobin (Bolton-Maggs and Thomas, 2008). Hemoglobin S crystallizes causing the red blood cells to take on a "sickle" or "C" shape and limiting their capacity to transport oxygen around the body. In addition, they cause the blood to thicken and the deformed cells block the blood vessels preventing adequate oxygen reaching the body's systems, causing necrosis of tissues (Moseley, 1974). The gene for hemoglobin S is almost exclusively limited to people of African descent, where the trait may be as high as 50%, although some adjacent Mediterranean populations may be slightly affected, such as Southern Italy, Greece, and Armenia (Ortner, 2003). Despite the high number of Africans that may carry the trait, the disease may only manifest in around 2% of the carriers (Ortner, 2003). In general, sickle cell disease follows the same geographical distribution as malaria, leading to the theory that like thalassemia, the condition evolved to provide protection against this disease in the crucial childhood years (Serjeant, 2005).

Although the genetic abnormality is present at birth, infants are protected from sickling red blood cells for around 6 months, but as HbF levels fall, HbS levels dominate (Simpson, 1991). Without treatment most individuals will die in infancy or certainly before the age of 10 years (Steinbock, 1976, p. 255). So in the past it is a condition that would only be present in nonadult skeletal remains. Today, around 200,000–250,000 children are born with sickle cell disease with a high infant mortality rate (Sylvester et al., 2003). Sufferers are at risk from a sickling crisis, that includes severe pain caused by bone infarctions, which are susceptible to secondary infections such as osteomyelitis. They may also experience a series of related conditions including spleen disruption resulting in septicemia; pneumonia, pulmonary vasoocclusion, and chest infections (i.e., acute chest syndrome). With stokes usually occurring between the ages of 2 and 8 years in modern-treated cases (Almeida and Roberts, 2005; Quinn et al., 2004). Despite low hemoglobin levels, many children lead active lives as their bodies become used to the reduced oxygen levels. In addition, as HbS has a low affinity for oxygen it readily releases it into the tissues (Simpson, 1991). Bone changes occur due to two processes: marrow hyperplasia caused by the need to produce more red blood cells, and blood clots (thrombosis) most often in the long bones. Blood clots prevent nutrients reaching the bones and other tissues causing necrosis (Steinbock, 1976). The skeletal elements most commonly affected are the skull, vertebrae, tibia, and fibula, but the extent and severity of the skeletal manifestations are not considered to be related to the severity of the disease (Ortner, 2003). The changes seen in sickle cell disease, in comparison to thalassemia and iron-deficiency anemia are outlined in Table 8.2.

In the skull, changes are less pronounced than in thalassemia. The outer table of the skull thins as the diploë is enlarged. This enlargement is bilateral, and usually limited to the parietals, although enlargement may extend to the zygomatic bones and orbital roof. Of the 194 individuals with sickle cell disease examined by Sebes and Diggs (1979) aged from 4 months to 55 years, only 5% (n = 10) showed hair-on-end changes, although these individuals would have been undergoing treatment. Punched-out lesions, similar to multiple myeloma may result due to thrombosis and are estimated to occur in 7.3% cases (Steinbock, 1976). In all the affected bones, thickened coarse trabecular are a common feature, but the collapse and squaring of the vertebral bodies seen in adults with sickle cell is not evident in children. In the tibia and fibula new bone formation, osteomyelitis and thickening of the cortex results in the reduction of the medullary cavity (Burnett et al., 1998; Moseley, 1974). This is in contrast

TABLE 8.2 Features Associated With the Most Common Anemic Conditions

Feature	Iron-Deficiency Anemia	Thalassemia	Sickle-Cell Anemia
Cranial bossing	Yes	Yes	Yes
Osteomyelitis	No	No	Yes
Hair-on-end changes	Yes	Severe	Rarely
Facial bones	No	Yes	Yes
Femoral head necrosis	No	No	Yes
Retarded sinus formation	No	Yes	No
Hand and foot bones	Rarely	Yes	No
Necrosis	No	No	Yes
Vertebral compression	No	Yes	Yes
Vertebral osteoporosis	No	Yes	Yes

to the cortical thinning seen in thalassemia. Due to the sickling and blocking of the blood vessels, epiphyses may become necrotic, and on radiograph, the bone will have a patchwork of radiolucent areas next to radiodense areas. One of the most prominent features of the disease is necrosis of the femoral head, present in between 20% and 60% of all patients (Ortner, 2003). In addition, children with the disease have impaired growth, delayed puberty, and poor nutritional status (Barden et al., 2002). In the postcranium, marrow hyperplasia may be limited to the vertebrae and pelvis (30% cases). Central zone vertebral collapse causes the space between the vertebrae to have a gaping or "fishmouth" appearance on lateral radiographs with a flat base of dense bone apparent due to circulatory stasis. These lesions may be indistinguishable from Schmorl's nodes and are less likely to occur in younger individuals (Hershkovitz et al., 1997). Salmonella osteomyelitis, due to an increased risk of salmonella in gut thrombosis is frequently associated with sickle cell (Steinbock, 1976). Marrow infarction at the epiphyses may cause secondary septic arthritis. Children younger than 3 years may develop dactylitis with subperiosteal new bone formation, which can lead to premature epiphyseal fusion and digit shortening (Fig. 8.11; Stuart and Nagel, 2004). Infarcts can occur in any bone but are most common in the tibia and fibula, femur, radius, ulna, and humerus (Almeida and Roberts, 2005). Hershkovitz et al. (1997) provide a comprehensive table of the expected skeletal changes in sickle cell, as distinguished from thalassemia or leukemia, cautioning that not all changes will occur in every case, and that the most characteristic features may not be evident before the age of 9 years.

Few cases of sickle cell have been identified in the archeological literature and this is likely due to high mortality that would have prevented sufferers reaching beyond

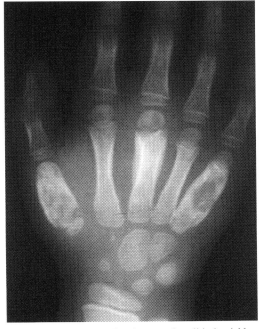

FIGURE 8.11 Clinical example of severe dactylitis in sickle-cell disease. Osteitis is evident on the first and fifth metacarpals and sheaths of new bone cover the expanded third metacarpal. *Image taken from http://img.medscapestatic.com/pi/meds/ckb/52/22352.jpg.*

the age of 10 years in the past. Bohrer and Connah (1971) described bone infarcts in a series of nonadult tibiae from Benin City in Midwest Nigeria dating from c. AD 1180–1310. They believed sickle cell anemia to be the cause of the lesions. Maat (1991) provided remarkable evidence for preserved sickled cells in skeletons from the Persian Gulf (330–150 BC) and this was followed by Massa (1977) who isolated sickled cells in histological slides in the Benin City collection and described well-preserved red blood cells in a mummy that demonstrated ipocromacy and hair-on-end porotic hyperostosis. One clinical case of a 6-year-old boy from Mexico was reported by Hershkovitz et al. (1997), demonstrating limited changes to the spine, long bone and calcanei, but clear signs of porotic hyperostosis on the parietals. Faerman et al. (2000) successfully isolated β-globin gene sequences for sickle cell anemia in a male from Midwestern Africa, thought to be a descendent of Africans brought to Jamaica during the Trans-Atlantic African slave trade. A further possible case of genetic anemia was recovered from the Liberated African cemetery in Rupert's Valley, St Helena. The child was aged 7- to 12-years-old and had bilateral premature fusion of the proximal humeral epiphyses and flattening and elongation of the distal ends of the bone, which may have been the result of necrosis (Fig. 8.12). Although trauma and rickets could not be ruled out, premature epiphyseal fusion and subsequent shortening is a common signature of sickle cell disease (Witkin, 2011).

Leukemia

The leukemias are a group of neoplasms that frequently affect the myeloid and lymphoid hematopoietic stem cells of the bone marrow (Ortner, 2003; Waldron, 2009). There blood-borne pathogenesis is the reason for their inclusion here. Today, leukemia is the most common form of cancer seen in children and accounts for 1 in every 3 cases. It may be inherited or spontaneous with close links to both radiation exposure and to chromosomal abnormalities such as Down syndrome (Cappell and Anderson, 1971). There are four main types of leukemia: acute lymphoblastic leukemia, acute myeloid leukemia, chronic lymphocytic leukemia, and chronic myeloid leukemia. Acute lymphoblastic leukemia is the most common form in children, with a peak between the ages of 2 and 5 years (Isler and Turcotte, 2003; Rothschild et al., 1997), followed by acute myeloid leukemia. Chronic conditions are rare in children. Acute leukemia appears abruptly with weakness, fever, pallor, bleeding of the gums, and bruising (Kobayashi et al., 2005) and children may develop a limp due to bone and joint pain in the hips, knees, or ankles (Kobayashi et al., 2005; Tuten et al., 1998). The whole course of the condition from onset to death may only take a few weeks if infection sets in (Cappell and Anderson, 1971), potentially limiting the number of cases we may be able to identify in the past. Nevertheless, children are more likely to demonstrate skeletal changes as normal bone marrow cells are gradually replaced by tumor cells during the growth process (Rothschild et al., 1997; Willson, 1959). Hence lesions tend to occur in rapidly growing areas such as the knee and wrist. When they do occur, lytic lesions and periosteal new bone formation is widespread along the bones and ribs, and sclerotic changes are unusual (Isler and Turcotte, 2003; Sinigaglia et al., 2008). In Kobayashi et al.'s (2005) survey of 16 modern children diagnosed with

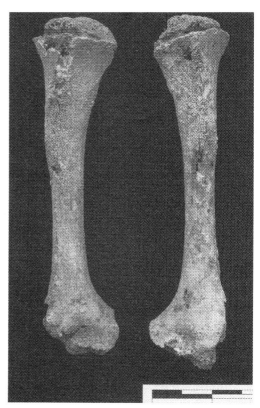

FIGURE 8.12 Possible sickle-cell disease in a 7- to 12-year-old from Rupert's Valley, St Helena (skeleton 438). Premature fusion of the proximal humeral epiphyses has resulted in stunted growth. The disruption to the distal ends of the bones may be related to necrosis. The skeleton also had rickets and overall growth was retarded in comparison to others in the same age group. *From Witkin, A., 2011. The human skeletal remains. In: Pearson, A., Jeffs, B., Witkin, A., MacQuarrie (Eds.), Infernal Traffic: Excavations of a Liberated African Graveyard in Rupert's Valley, St Helena. Council for British Archaeology, Oxford, p. 80.*

leukemia, 31.2% had periosteal reactions. The metaphysis may become severely vascular and grooved as tumor cells emerge through the foramina (Ortner, 2003). Collapse of the spine due to lytic lesions may be misdiagnosed as tuberculosis, and a small number of children may develop bilateral transverse fractures of the lower limbs due to diffuse osteopenia.

A critical feature of leukemia is the early occurrence of a highly characteristic transverse radiolucent metaphyseal band (Isler and Turcotte, 2003; Kobayashi et al., 2005). This thick line of radiolucency occurs immediately below the metaphyseal surface, which itself appears as a thinner radioopaque band (Fig. 8.13). These bands have been shown to be present in 10%–89% of leukemia patients, in areas of rapid growth (Bolton-Maggs and Thomas, 2008). They measure between 1 and 15 mm in thickness and occur more commonly in leukemia than other condition that display similar bands, such as scurvy, healing rickets, syphilis, and juvenile rheumatoid arthritis (Willson, 1959). In Willson's

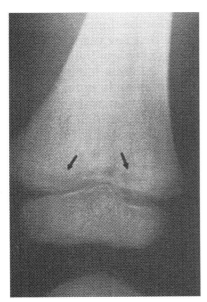

FIGURE 8.13 Willson's metaphyseal (radiolucent) band in leukemia. *Arrows* indicate the thick radiolucent band above a thin and radioopaque metaphyseal edge. *From Resnick, D., Kransdorf, M., 2005. Bone and Joint Imaging, third ed. Elsevier Saunders, Philadelphia, p. 686.*

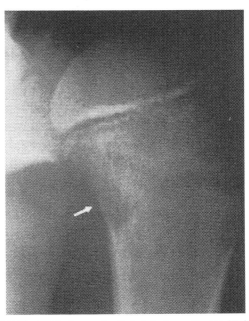

FIGURE 8.14 Clinical example of a lytic lesion on the proximal metaphysis of the humerus in leukemia. *From Resnick, D., Kransdorf, M., 2005. Bone and Joint Imaging, third ed. Elsevier Saunders, Philadelphia, p. 686.*

(1959) study of 740 individuals with radiolucent lines, 32 (4.3%) had leukemia, but after 2 years, only four individuals with radiolucent bands did not have leukemia. Kobayashi et al. (2005) reported that only two out of the 16 children in their study (12.5%) had metaphyseal bands leading them to suggest that this is a less reliable diagnostic sign than previously thought, although the sample was much smaller. Nevertheless, these bands may prove to be a crucial factor in distinguishing leukemia from other metastatic cancers in children (Rothschild et al., 1997).

The next most common feature Willson (1959) noted was osteolytic lesions within the long bones (present in 38% cases), which extended further down the shaft as the disease progressed (Fig. 8.14). He noted both multiple lytic lesions and large single discreet lesions that were often symmetrical. Rothschild et al. (1997) explored the nature of lytic lesions in a 3-year-old black girl whose skeleton is housed within the Hamann–Todd collection, Cleveland, USA. They explored whether it was possible to distinguish between acute lymphocytic leukemia and acute myelogenous leukemia based on the distribution and nature of the skeletal lesions. In the facial bones there were isolated or coalescing superficial pits that rarely perforated the cortex, and a small foramen was often present at the base of the pits. There was minimal periosteal reaction on the ectocranium, with more widespread changes endocranially. Some pitting and new bone formation was noted on the facial bones and mandible. The pits on the scapulae and upper limb were larger than on the skull but spared the humeral epiphyses. There were also areas of endosteal and intracortical bone resorption on radiograph, as well as the presence of 2 mm wide radiolucent bands. In the lower limbs, the epiphyses were only affected by mild periostitis with the largest pits located at the metaphyses. In the fibula these pits were in the form of linear oval defects. The vertebrae, ribs, and pelvis were all affected by lytic lesions that did not extend to the joints. There was also the probable appearance of gout in the child with large lytic lesions on the tibial tarsal joint. Gout is a known complication of hyperplastic diseases such as leukemia (Rothschild et al., 1997). They concluded that lytic lesions were more widely distributed in lymphocytic leukemia and periosteal reactions more extensive on the skull, while rib and vertebra involvement was rare in myelocytic leukemia, probably due to the limited distribution of red bone marrow in older individuals with this condition.

The first archeological case of leukemia was proposed by Klaus (2016) in a child from Lambayeque Valley, Peru. Accentuated porosity on the clavicles, scapulae, neural arches, and long bones, in addition to areas of finely deposited new bone suggested a blood-borne condition, with leukemia considered the most likely diagnosis (Fig. 8.15). The femora were not preserved, and as no radiographs were presented the presence of lytic lesions or radiolucent bands seen in clinical cases could not be assessed.

Hemophilia A and B

Hemophilia is a group of disorders that affect the body's ability to control blood clotting. Inherited bleeding disorders occur in 1:10,000 births today with 80% the result of

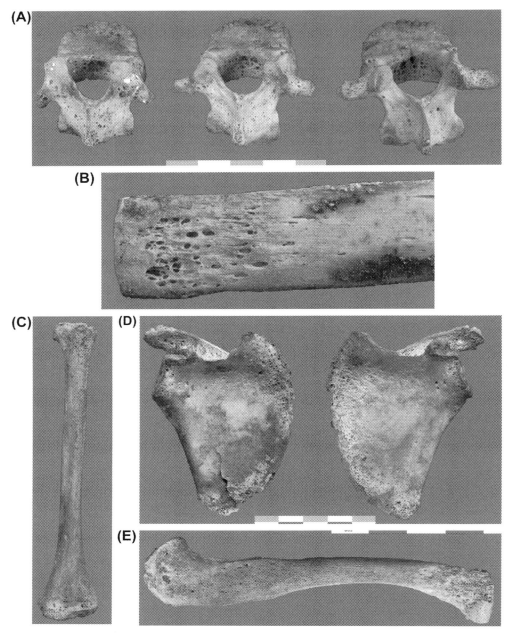

FIGURE 8.15 Possible leukemia in a 5- to 6-year-old from Santa María de Magdalena de Eten Lambayeque Valley, Peru (skeleton U3-1 S1). Abnormal metaphyseal porosity is evident on the areas overlying red bone marrow in the (A) neural arches, (B) ribs, (C) humerus, and (D) scapulae (E) with fine reactive new bone also present on the clavicles. *From Klaus, H., 2016. A probable case of acute childhood leukemia: skeletal involvement, differential diagnosis, and the bioarchaeology of cancer in South America. International Journal of Osteoarchaeology 26 (2), 350–354.*

hemophilia A (Simpson, 1991). Hemophilia B (Christmas disease) is five time less common. Both hemophilia A and B are disorders of the X-chromosome seen almost entirely in males. Hemophilia produces mild, moderate, or severe symptoms depending on the degree of deficiency of the plasma coagulation factors, VIII or IX. In severe cases, boys present with joint bleeds when they start to walk around 12–18 months, or have bleeding in their mouths. The blood oozes slowly allowing a friable clot to form that is easily dislodged causing the bleeding to start again. Children with moderate forms may not show symptoms before 5 years of age with untreated severe hemophilia causing recurrent bleeding into the joints and muscles, progressive joint deformity, destructive arthropathy, and eventually ankylosis (Bolton-Maggs and Thomas, 2008). The most commonly affected joints are the weight bearing joints of the knees and ankles, followed by the elbow. The condition rarely affects the hands and feet (Simpson, 1991).

Minor trauma can lead to life-threatening amounts of bleeding, or for example, biting the tongue can lead to prolonged bleeding and subsequent anemia (Bolton-Maggs and Thomas, 2008). In 2009, Rogaev et al. identified hemophilia B as the condition suffered by Alexis Romanov passed down through the Royal family line of Queen Victoria. Without medical support it is unlikely hemophiliacs would have survived long beyond childhood, but the condition should be considered a possibility in archeological cases with widespread new bone formation and lytic joint lesions.

METABOLIC DISORDERS

Metabolic disorders are problems associated with the way the body extracts nutrients from the diet. They result from malnutrition due to a diet deficient in certain nutrients, undernutrition where the diet fails to meet the body's energy requirements, or are secondary to congenital disorders and chronic conditions. Nutrition and infection are intrinsically linked, and there is growing awareness that the nutritional status of a mother and her child play a role in the genesis of adult chronic diseases (Langley-Evans, 2015). Children have different energy requirements to adults. Their diet has to supply sufficient energy to compensate for what is normally expended during the day, and the additional energy required for growth. Rapidly growing infants expend 35% of their energy intake on growth compared to around 2% in childhood and adolescence (Golden and Reilly, 2008). Metabolic disorders cause a reduction in bone mass due to one of three mechanisms that may occur independently or together: inadequate osteoid production, inadequate osteoid mineralization, or excessive deossification of normal bone. A detailed account of metabolic disorders and how they are identified in archeological skeletal material is provided by Brickley and Ives (2008). This section will concentrate on two conditions most commonly identified in nonadult skeletal material; rickets and scurvy.

Rickets and Osteomalacia (Vitamin D Deficiency)

Rickets and osteomalacia result from inadequate osteoid mineralization due to a deficiency in vitamin D_2 and D_3. Vitamin D is required to promote the absorption and mobilization of calcium and phosphorus from previously formed bone, as well as for the maturation and mineralization of the organic matrix (Pitt, 1988). Small amounts of vitamin D are present in foodstuffs such as fish oil and egg yolks (Fraser, 1995) and stored in the liver as ergocalciferol (vitamin D_2). Vitamin D status is primarily maintained by exposure to sunlight (cholecalciferol or vitamin D_3) and is produced internally by the interaction of ultraviolet light with 7-dehydrocholesterol in the deep layers of the skin (Levene, 1991a). Vitamin D is hydroxylated into an active form (1,25-dihydroxyvitamin D or 1,25$(OH)_2D_3$) in the liver and kidneys, the latter under the influence of the parathyroid hormone (Axon, 1991). In utero there is active transfer of calcium between mother and child, with fetal blood calcium levels 10% higher than the mother. This hypercalcemic state is corrected within 4–5 days after birth with the release of the parathyroid hormone (McKintosh and Stenson, 2008). Skeletal growth, and hence the requirement for calcium and other minerals, begins from midgestation and reaches its height during the third trimester. This requirement declines at birth and again after the first few months after birth (Prentice, 2003). At birth, the skeleton comprises c.20–30g calcium, making up to 98%–99% of the total body mineral of the infant (Prentice, 2003).

As vitamin D is normally passed to the fetus in utero, maternal vitamin D deficiency can result in neonatal rickets, where babies are born with broadened metaphyses and cupping of the epiphyses (Levene, 1991a), which may also be delayed in their appearance (Prentice, 2003). However, children can maintain high calcium levels despite hypocalcemia in the mother (Kovacs, 2003). Most cases of nutritional rickets occur between 6 months and 2 years of age and are related to the gradual depletion of the maternal calcium store coupled with a deficiency in the infant diet (Foote and Marriott, 2003). Premature babies miss out on the last 2 months of fetal life when the storage of calcium salts occurs (Arneil, 1973), making them more susceptible to hypocalcemia, loss of bone mass, and reduced growth in later childhood (Bishop and Fewtrell, 2003). In addition, low birth weight and twinned babies are at risk of neonatal rickets due to their greater need of calcium and phosphorus as the result of "catch-up" growth after birth. These babies require up to 1000 units of vitamin D per day. Breastfed infants are also at risk if they are fed indoors, covered-up, kept away from the sunlight, or if their mothers are vitamin D deficient, as the milk is low in both vitamin D and phosphorus (Golden and Reilly, 2008; Levene, 1991a).

Some cases of rickets are the result of defects in the individual's metabolism rather than access to vitamin D, and therefore are not indicative of a poor diet or environmental circumstances. These include chronic glomerular deficiency due to kidney malformation and low calcium, and raised phosphate levels due to hyperparathyroidism (Levene, 1991b). Late rickets is defined as occurring between the ages of 6 and 15 years and today is usually associated with kidney disorders Steinbock, 1976). Vitamin D-resistant rickets is an X-linked genetic disorder causing renal tubular acidosis due to bicarbonate loss, presenting at 1–2 years of age. The resulting severe dehydration may result in a coma (Levene, 1991b) and in the past, death of the child. Today, the increasing prevalence of rickets in countries with high levels of sunlight and "Asian rickets" in British immigrants has highlighted the influence of full body clothing, low calcium diets, and darker skin in limiting exposure to UV light (Narchi et al., 2001). The incidence of modern rickets has also raised new questions about the synergistic effects of lead, zinc, and calcium metabolism in the etiology of the condition (Thacher et al., 1999).

Skeletal abnormities occur due to defective mineralization of newly formed bone (Table 8.3). Children suffer from the dual effects of reduced osteoid mineralization on both endochondral growth (rickets) and intramembranous modeling and remodeling (osteomalacia) (Pettifor, 2003). When vitamin D is lacking, parathyroid hormone is secreted to maintain normal plasma calcium levels. It does this by stimulating bone absorption and releasing greater quantities of stored calcium and phosphorus into the bloodstream. In cases of chronic deficiency, this exacerbates the condition by weakening the normal bone tissue (Shapiro, 2001; Steinbock, 1976) and causes secondary hyperparathyroidism, which again increases bone resorption.

TABLE 8.3 Skeletal Lesions Associated With Rickets and Osteomalacia in Nonadults

Location	Macroscopic Features	Radiographic Features
Cranium	Delayed fontanel closure	Generalized osteopenia
	Craniotabes, or flattening, normally of the occipital bone	
	Frontal and parietal bossing	
Mandible and dentition	Dental hypoplasia	
	Caries	
	Deformed mandibular ramus	
	Delayed dental eruption of deciduous and permanent dentition	
Ribs and sternum	Rachitic rosary enlargement (beading) and cupping of the costochondral junction	
	Abnormal curvature/flattening	
	Fractures	
Pelvis	Curvature of iliac crest	
	Small, plump ilia	
Long bones	Widening, cupping, and fraying of metaphyses of long bones (esp. radius and ulna in early stages)	"Fuzzy" or undefined metaphyseal margin
	Windswept deformity of femur and tibia (varus of one leg, valgus of the other)	Coarsening of remaining trabeculae
	Anterior bowing of tibia	
	Anteroposterior flattening of fibula	
	Coxa vara of femoral neck	
	"Knock-knees" (genu valgum) and bowleg (genu varum) at knees	
	Metaphyseal fractures	Looser's zones (pseudofractures)
	Cortical thinning	

List compiled from Mankin, H.J., 1974. Rickets, osteomalacia, and renal osteodystrophy. Journal of Bone and Joint Surgery 56-A (1–2), 101–128 and 352–386; Sheldon, W., 1943. Diseases of Infancy and Childhood, J. & A. Churchill Ltd., London; Holt, L.E., 1909. Diseases of Infancy and Childhood, D. Appleton and Company, London; Caffey, J., 1945. Pediatric X-Ray Diagnosis, Year Book Medical Publishers, Inc., Chicago; Stuart-Macadam, P.L., 1989. Nutritional deficiency diseases: a survey of scurvy, rickets and iron-deficiency anemia. In: Iscan, M.Y., Kennedy, K.A.R. (Eds.), Reconstruction of Life from the Skeleton. Alan R. Liss, Inc., New York, pp. 201–222; Resnick, D., Niwayama, D. (Eds.), 1988. Diagnosis of Bone and Joint Disorders. W.B. Saunders Company, Philadelphia; Pettifor, J., 2003. Nutritional rickets. In: Glorieux, F., Pettifor, J., Jüppner, M. (Eds.), Pediatric Bone: Biology and Diseases. Academic Press, New York, pp. 541–565; Ortner, D., 2003. Identification of Pathological Conditions in Human Skeletal Remains, Academic Press, New York; Schamall, D., Teschler-Nicola, M., Kainberger, F., Tangl, S., Brandstätter, F., Patzak, B., Muhsil, J., Plenk, H., 2003. Changes in trabecular bone structure in rickets and osteomalacia: the potential of a medico-historical collection. International Journal of Osteoarchaeology 13, 283–288; Harris, H.A., 1933. Bone Growth in Health and Disease, Oxford University Press, London; Adams, J.E., 1997. Radiology of rickets and osteomalacia. In: Feldman, D., Glorieux, F., Pike, J. (Eds.), Vitamin D. Academic Press, New York, pp. 619–642; Brickley, M., Ives, R., 2008. The Bioarchaeology of Metabolic Bone Disease. Academic Press, Oxford; Brickley, M., Moffat, T., Watamaniuk, L., 2014. Biocultural perspectives of vitamin D deficiency in the past. Journal of Anthropological Archaeology 36, 48–59.

In normal physeal development, five processes work in equilibrium to provide growth: cell multiplication, cell growth, calcification of the matrix, cartilage removal, and bone mineralization. In nutritional rickets the earliest lesions are observed at the metaphyses of the long bones. Cartilage removal and bone mineralization are disrupted as uncalcified and poorly mineralized cartilage cells buildup at the growth plate causing crushing and flattening of the cell columns and expansion of the metaphyses (or "trumpeting"). Cupping occurs because the cells at the periphery are more affected than the centrally placed cells, altering the physical shape of the growth plate (Shapiro, 2001). The characteristic smooth epiphyseal surface of the metaphysis is lost, and the metaphyses develop frayed edges, resembling "bristles of a brush" (Fig. 8.16; Caffey, 1945). The wrist is usually the first area where changes to the growth plate are noticed on radiograph. Thacher et al. (2000) published a radiographic scoring method for rating the severity of metaphyseal changes in the wrist and knee, which may prove useful in assessment and comparison of rickets severity in archeological samples (Fig. 8.17).

In the youngest children, the cranium is thinned and the posterior aspects of the parietal bones and superior aspect of the occipital bone become flattened (craniotabes) on the side the infant habitually lays (Mankin, 1974). Cranial thinning is also usually unilateral and may cover an area of 2–4 cm (Steinbock, 1976). Once rapid growth has ceased after around 9 months, these changes may disappear (Steinbock, 1976). Around the ages of 2 or 3 years, the cranium can become abnormally thick as new bone and osteoid are deposited on the outer surface of the skull this thickening is more pronounced on the frontal and parietal bones. If all four bosses are affected, the skull takes on a "squared" appearance (Steinbock, 1976). These cranial lesions may appear pitted on the surface and hence mimic porotic hyperostosis of anemia. In addition, the anterior fontanel may remain open until the third year and the sutures appear wider than normal (Shapiro, 2001). Seow et al. (1984) found enamel hypoplasia in 80% (n = 13/15) of neonates with rickets, with dental opacities evident in the remaining two children. The defects occurred mostly in the deciduous incisors along the incisal edge or labial surface. Dental development may be delayed (Holt, 1909; Sheldon, 1943), and this delay varies in its extent between individuals and between teeth,

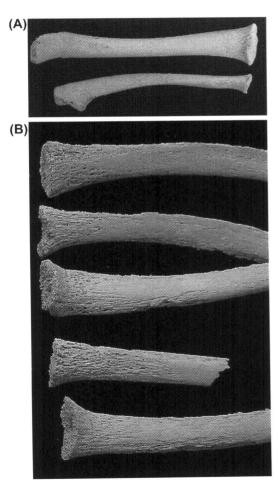

FIGURE 8.16 Infantile rickets. (A) Frayed metaphysis of the distal tibia and ulna (skeleton 484) and (B) abnormal pitting and frayed margins at the sternal ends of the ribs (skeleton 882) in two infants from Poundbury Camp, Dorset. *Photographs taken with the kind permission of the Natural History Museum, London.*

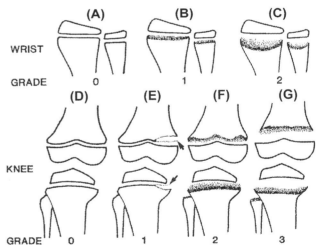

FIGURE 8.17 Radiographic scoring method for the assessment of rickets severity. (A) Normal wrist; (B) irregularity and widening at the growth plate, without cupping; (C) metaphyseal cupping and frayed margins. (D) Normal knee; (E) medial portions of the femoral and tibial metaphyses are affected. There is partial lucency of the metaphyses, but the margins are clearly visible (*arrow*); (F) partial lucency of the metaphyses, but the margins are not sharply defined. Zones of provisional calcification are not completely lucent and display some calcification; (G) complete lucency of the zone of provisional calcification. The epiphyses appear widely separated from the distal metaphyses. *From Thacher, T.D., Fischer, P., Pettifor, J., Lawson, J., Manaster, B., Reading, J., 2000. Radiographic scoring method for the assessment of the severity of nutritional rickets. Journal of Tropical Pediatrics 46, 133.*

which is a matter of concern when trying to estimate the age of an affected child (Liversidge and Molleson, 2001).

The manifestation of nutritional rickets and osteomalacia on the postcranial nonadult skeleton is related to the extent of malnutrition, the age at which the condition occurs, their rate of growth, and their mobility (Harris, 1931). In the undernourished rachitic child, the cortices are thinned, trabeculae become sparse, and marrow spaces enlarged with general atrophy, and other conditions, such as scurvy, may be present. In a well-nourished child, the hypertrophic form of rickets is seen, and children are described as having "plump bones" where the cortex becomes thickened and the medullary cavity is reduced (Steinbock, 1976). The long bones, ilia and scapulae thicken under the periosteum, with "several layers of friable, spongy vascular tissue, [and] large vascular spaces" (Griffith, 1919, p. 588). Well-nourished vitamin D deficient children are also more likely to maintain good muscle tone and remain mobile leading to the development of more severe bowing, cupping, and flaring deformities. By contrast, their poorly nourished peers are generally weaker and tend to remain stationary (Stuart-Macadam, 1988). Throughout the skeleton, bowing deformities are secondary to increasingly softening bone that deforms under normal mechanical strain, cortical thinning, and generalized osteopenia. In the infant, bowing of the arms, where the humeral head is bent medially and inferiorly, suggests the child was crawling at the time of onset. Abnormal anterior-lateral concavity of the femoral shaft, a bowed tibia, and anteroposterior flattening of the fibula may indicate that the child had begun to walk (Fig. 8.18; Stuart-Macadam, 1988). However, anterior bowing of the tibia may occur in severe cases if the child lies with one leg on top of the other (Pettifor, 2003). In fact, children with rickets have a habit of sitting cross-legged whilst rocking to and fro, exacerbating the deformities (Holt, 1909). Older children develop "knock-knee" deformities ("genu valgum") and severe cases may develop "windswept" deformity, where one leg is bent toward the midline ("varus") and the other away from it ("valgus"). There

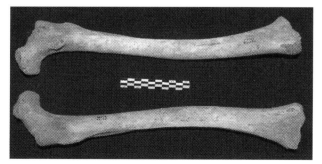

FIGURE 8.18 Bilateral bowing deformities of rickets in the femora of a 17-year-old from St Mary Spital, London (AD 1200–1250, skeleton 33,220). *Photograph by F. Shapland with the kind permission of the Museum of London.*

may also be coxa vara of the femoral neck (Pettifor, 2003). Subperiosteal new bone may form on the concave surface, stemming from abnormal osteoid deposition and accentuated by healing calluses from stress fractures in osteopenic bone. In particular, new bone formation has been noted on the anterior aspect of the ribs, posterior surface of the femur, and medial and posterior aspects of the tibia (Ortner, 2003). The combination of an unmineralized growth plate and softened bone can result in severe deformities of the rib cage. Cupping deformities present on the costal ends of the ribs from an abnormal accumulation of osteoid result in beading known as the "rachitic rosary" (Resnick and Kransdorf, 2005). Pressure of the arms and strain on the diaphragm during breathing results in a constricted "pigeon chest," where the costochondral junctions are inwardly displaced (Caffey, 1945). Affected children have difficulty in breathing, and it is for this reason that they are believed to be particularly susceptible to respiratory infections such as pneumonia (Pettifor, 2003). In infants, rib fractures due to general osteopenia may be the first clinical sign of this disease (Pettifor and Daniels, 1997). In the spine, thickened and irregularly arranged trabeculae, with enlarged cavities in the center of the vertebral bodies causes partial collapse and reduced height of the bodies (Schamall et al., 2003). While vitamin D deficiency is more easily identified on nonadult skeletons due to their rapid growth and the amount of uncalcified material put down, signs of the disease can disappear just as quickly. Within 2–3 days of treatment, a zone of dense calcification appears at the end of the bone (Fig. 8.19). The radiolucent rachitic metaphysis is remodeled and becomes normal in appearance as the calcification band is gradually incorporated into the diaphysis (Caffey, 1945). The gross enlargements at the joint ends become "trimmed" and there is a period of intense remodeling, similar to catch-up growth. All signs of the disease may have disappeared within 3–4 months (Harris, 1931). Bowing due to faulty fetal positioning can persist for up to 2 years after birth, and trauma in the child may result in plastic bowing (Borden, 1974; Caffey, 1945). Both should be considered as a differential diagnosis for the bowed limbs caused by rickets, although plastic bowing due to trauma is normally unilateral (Verlinden and Lewis, 2015).

The clinical changes of rickets were first described in Germany by Whistler in 1645, while Mellanby (1919) and McCollum et al. (1922) finally isolated the cause of the condition. Prior to the Industrial Revolution in Europe, rickets was a disease of affluence, where wealthy children were kept fully clothed and remained indoors (Pettifor and Daniels, 1997). Later, urban overcrowding and air pollution created a rickets epidemic, which was so rampant in Britain that it was termed the "English Disease" (Mankin, 1974). In 1889, a collective investigation committee of the British Medical Association found that the further individuals lived from industrial and mining areas, the lower the frequency of

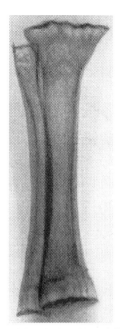

FIGURE 8.19 Healing rickets in the tibia and fibula of a child 14 days after treatment with cod-liver oil. The radiopaque band follows a wide radiolucent area and indicates a zone of dense calcification during the healing process. *From Harris, H.A., 1933. Bone Growth in Health and Disease, Oxford University Press, London, p. 99.*

rickets, cementing its reputation as a disease of industrialization. Similarly, in 1900 Morse reported rickets in 79.5% of 400 infants living in Boston and in Germany, 89% of Dresden infants aged between 2 and 4 years had the disease. Rickets was closely associated with whooping cough and measles in the 19th century, and this contributed to the high mortality rates from the disease (Hardy, 1992). Studies on postmedieval skeletal material reflect the documentary sources and indicate rickets was a widespread disease affecting children from all social classes. Environmental pollution in addition to cultural practices such as prolonged breastfeeding, prolonged swaddling, keeping children indoors, and heavy clothing were determining factors, illustrating the complexity of the social and cultural factors that contribute to the disease (Brickley et al., 2014). Archeologically, Pêterstone et al. (2013) reported rickets in 7.1% (n=2/28) of their high status children from 17th to 18th century Germany, this is similar to the 7.5% (n=14/186) reported from Christ Church Spitalfields, London (Lewis, 2002). Much higher levels were found from the 19th century burial vault in Spring Street, New York, where 34% (n = 30/86) of children showed evidence for rickets (Ellis, 2010). Ellis (2010) suggests that the possible presence of children of African descent may have contributed to this high occurrence due to the inhibiting effects of melanin in their skin, in addition to the effects of air pollution, cultural swaddling, and dietary regimes. Among the most privileged, rickets was a major cause of morbidity.

Examination of the nine Medici children from 16th to 17th century Italy revealed that all had some signs that they were suffering from rickets. In the lower classes, such as those from St Martin's Church in Birmingham, England, rates of 13% have been reported (Brickley and Ives, 2006). Even in rural areas rickets remained high with 9.5% of under fifteens, and 30.4% of 2- to 3-year-olds in 17th century Beemster, The Netherlands, showing signs of the condition (Veselka et al., 2015). Ortner and Mays (1998) had previously reported a prevalence of 2% rickets in 327 nonadults from later medieval Wharram Percy in rural Yorkshire, UK. Here it was suggested that the condition was exacerbated by mothers keeping their sickly children indoors. The presence of rickets (in addition to scurvy) in 11.2% of children from Romano–British Dorset, indicates that urbanization and its devastating effects were also a factor during the Roman occupation (Lewis, 2010). Littleton (1998) argued that the cultural practice of avoiding sunlight through prolonged swaddling was the cause of rickets in 10 of the 663 (1.5%) children from Bahrain in the Middle East (1000 BC–AD 250). The impact of swaddling on the development of childhood rickets is a commonly cited cause. Swaddling has been shown to calm the child and regulate their temperature and today at least, it is practiced for short periods of time during infancy. But despite its reputation, even in constant swaddling cases, modern studies have not shown any association between swaddling and rickets (Van Sleuwen et al., 2007). In the past, swaddling in combination with high levels of air pollution, extended breastfeeding or a deficient weaning diet may have predisposed to rickets. Brickley et al. (2014) call for a bicultural approach to further understand the complex development of rickets in past populations, including an assessment of socioeconomic status, place of residence, migration, house structure, clothing, infant diet and care, and climate.

Infantile Scurvy (Vitamin C Deficiency)

Vitamin C (ascorbic acid) is necessary for the synthesis of osteoid through the hydroxylation of the amino acid proline to hydroxyproline within collagen. Type 1 collagen forms the basis of all connective tissues for the skin, blood vessels, cartilage, and bone. Vitamin C also protects and regulates the biological processes of other enzymes (Steinbock, 1976; Stuart-Macadam, 1989). Vitamin C deficiency results in scurvy, which is characterized by the primary effect of ascorbic acid deficiency on the collagen matrix and the secondary effects of trauma to weakened bone and vessels. Unlike other mammals, humans and other primates cannot synthesize this vitamin internally and it must be ingested (Brickley and Ives, 2008). Vitamin C is available in fruit and uncooked vegetables, milk, and fish, with smaller amounts gained from potatoes. Cereals are totally lacking in vitamin C, and meat contains very little of the vitamin. However, consumption of the liver and glandular tissue of animals will provide adequate amounts of vitamin C (Steinbock, 1976). Breast milk contains high levels of vitamin C providing protection for breast-fed babies (Axon, 1991), whereas children fed on cow's milk will receive much lower levels (Brickley and Ives, 2008). Hence, scurvy is unlikely to develop in children of well-nourished mothers in societies where artificial feeding has not been adopted (Brickley and Ives, 2008).

The disease is clinically recognizable when the vitamin has been deficient for 4–10 months, or in infants once the birth stores have been depleted. Hence like rickets, scurvy is most common between 6 months and 2 years of age or earlier in premature births, low birth weight babies, and twins (Griffith, 1919). Cases of scurvy have been identified in children as young as 5 days old leading to speculation of a neonatal or congenital form of the disease caused by malnourished mothers (Hirsch et al., 1976; Jackson and Park, 1935). However, differentiating periosteal lesions that may be associated with neonatal scurvy from birth trauma or congenital syphilis is problematic. Scorbutic infants are highly susceptible to secondary infections that can prove fatal (Jackson and Park, 1935). Excessive internal bleeding may lead to shock and heart failure. Anemia, causing growth retardation, results not just from bleeding but also from the body's inability to produce normal erythroblastic areas, as the marrow produced is gray and gelatinous rather than red bone marrow. This effect is more severe in individuals with both scurvy and rickets (Harris, 1933).

Hemorrhage of the defective connective membranes is the most significant sign of scurvy, with minor trauma resulting in bleeding into neighboring tissues and calcified hematomas, which appear as irregular subperiosteal new bone in the skeleton. Hematomas are particularly marked in children due to a loose periosteum that accommodates normal transverse growth. Harris (1933) surveyed lesions in scorbutic children under 3 years of age and found that hemorrhage into the skeletal system occurred in 93% of cases and 37% of cases had bilateral or unilateral orbital lesions. If the hematomas are absorbed rather than calcified, increased osteoclastic activity causes weakening of the cancellous bone. Osteopenia further develops, particularly in the metaphyses, as the result of defects in osteoid synthesis, the virtual cessation of new bone formation (Brickley and Ives, 2008), and disuse atrophy (Steinbock, 1976). Osteopenia is recognized as areas of thinned cortex with sparse trabeculae that may appear thickened. Early radiographic signs of the disease have been reported most commonly at the distal tibia, and distal radius and ulna, with the formation of a "cleft" under a torn periosteum, a rounded, bulging margin ("bagging"), and a thinned cortex (Park et al., 1935). Steinbock (1976, p. 256) describes the beading at the costochondral junction of the ribs in scurvy as more angular and less "knobbly" than that caused by rickets, and notes that it may be accompanied by new bone formation along the shaft of the ribs. Harris (1933, p. 104) tabulated the most common sites for bleeding in children compared to adults, with bleeding into bone most common in children up to 2 years of age (93%), followed by the intestinal tract (60%), gums (43%), eyelids (37%), and nasal and oral palatine surfaces (3%). In contrast, the gums made up the main site of bleeding for adults at 94%–97% followed by the periosteum in 5%–18% of his selected adult sample.

Historically, scurvy was not recognized as a childhood disease until the rise of urbanization. Initially described as Möller–Barlow disease (Barlow, 1883; Möller, 1862), rickets and scurvy were considered part of the same disease process. This may have been due to their similar age of onset, and the fact that the skeletal lesions of scurvy only appear in advanced cases and can be masked by the lesions of rickets (Barlow, 1935; Follis and Park, 1952). In the 1980s, cases of scurvy were also rarely reported in the archeological record. Ortner (1984) had described lesions of the skull in a child from Alaska, which he suspected as being indicative of scurvy. This was followed by a case in a young Iron Age child from Beckford, Worcestershire, displaying new bone formation around a deciduous maxillary molar, the mandible, tibia, and in the orbits (Roberts, 1987). Using histological techniques to distinguish hemorrhage from anemia and inflammation, Schultz (1989) diagnosed scurvy in 13.8% of infants from Bronze Age Europe. In the late 1990s, Ortner set out to tackle the problems behind the diagnosis of scurvy in past populations, carrying out a series of studies on the skulls of nonadults from Peru and North America (Ortner et al., 1999, 2001; Ortner and Ericksen, 1997). The "Ortner Criteria" is now considered diagnostic of childhood scurvy in the skull and scapulae, and includes bilateral porosity and new bone formation, most commonly on the orbital roof, maxilla, and the greater wing of the sphenoid, due to hemorrhaging of the anterior deep temporal artery underlying the temporalis muscle (Fig. 8.20; Ortner et al., 1999). New bone formation around the foramina rotunda of the sphenoid was found to be present in 27% of nonadults from the Kilkenny Workhouse in Ireland who suffered from scurvy, similar to the changes seen in the infraorbital foramina noted by Ortner (Geber and Murphy, 2012). Ossifying hematomas ("Parrot's swellings") may develop on the parietal, occipital, and frontal bones mimicking porotic hyperostosis (Fig. 8.21; Melikian and Waldron, 2003). This remains a controversial feature of scurvy and need to be distinguished from changes due to congenital syphilis, rickets and anemia (Brickley and Ives, 2008). Due to the weakened vascular structure, slight movement of the eyes causes bleeding resulting in new bone formation on the orbital roof. It is possible that in some cases, endocranial lesions may result from slow hemorrhage of the dura mater as a result of scurvy (Lewis, 2004), and

Hemopoietic and Metabolic Disorders Chapter | 8 215

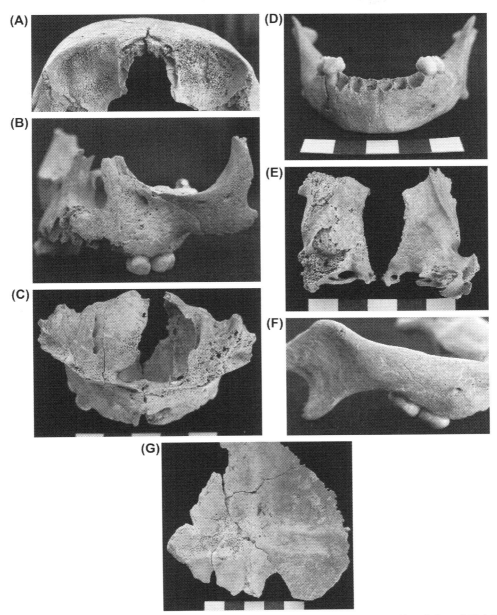

FIGURE 8.20 Scurvy in a 2.5-year-old child of Roman date from Kültepe in Turkey (Kültepe Excavation Archive, skeleton 7-51a). There is (A) profuse new bone formation on the orbits with abnormal pitting on the (B) maxilla and zygomatic bones, (C) orbital floor, (D) anterior mandible, and (E) wings of the sphenoid, with a fine layer of reactive new bone formation on the (F) inferior mandibular ramus and (G) endocranial surfaces. *Photographs reproduced with the kind permission of Handan Üstündağ, University of Anadolu, Turkey.*

Klaus (2013) highlighted the association of vascular ectocranial lesions and scurvy in his nonadult from Lambayeque Valley in Peru. A study of 557 North American nonadult skeletons showed that cranial lesions were most frequently in children aged between 3 and 7 years, perhaps as a result of their rapid growth at this age (Ortner et al., 2001).

Postcranial lesions have received much less attention and in many cases, the more subtle lesions associated with scurvy may be masked or indistinguishable from the lesions caused by accompanying rickets (Schattmann et al., 2016). Ortner et al. (2001) suggest that porous lesions that extend 10 mm past the growing metaphyseal end of the diaphyses are indicative of scurvy. Normally, these vascular channels would be filled in by osteoblasts during bone development. Subperiosteal hemorrhage and subsequent new bone formation is most frequently seen at the ends of the femur, tibia, and humerus but may be present on the entire length of the diaphysis. However, such ossification can only occur in cases where vitamin C has been ingested and osteoid formation has been reinitiated

216 Paleopathology of Children

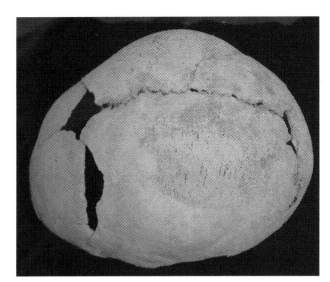

FIGURE 8.21 Parrot swelling of scurvy in the parietal bones of a 1- to 2-year-old from late Roman Poundbury Camp in Dorset, England (skeleton 1096). *Photographs taken with the kind permission of the Natural History Museum, London.*

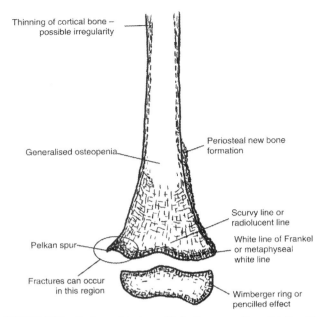

FIGURE 8.22 Radiographic signs of infantile scurvy. *From Brickley, M., Ives, R., 2008. The Bioarchaeology of Metabolic Bone Disease, Academic Press, Oxford, p. 63.*

(Brickley and Ives, 2008). The new bone formed as a result of hemorrhage remodels resulting in a slight thickening of the affected bones (Caffey, 1945). A similar process is seen in the flat bones of the scapulae and ilia (Ortner, 2003).

Radiographs can aid in the diagnosis of scurvy, particularly when the condition has healed, as lesions are often still present some years after the other signs of the condition have been remodeled (Caffey, 1945). At the metaphyses, cartilage cells become reduced in size and number and are thickened by continuous layers of osteoid (Caffey, 1945). This heavily calcified band, known as the "white line of Frankel" is weak and made up of irregular trabeculae, which are susceptible to fracture. Directly preceding this white line is an area of thinned trabeculae, appearing as a radiolucent band or "scurvy line" on radiographs (Caffey, 1945), also known as the Trümmerfeld zone (Fig. 8.22). Once healing begins, this radiolucent scurvy line will disappear rapidly leaving a band of dense calcification, recognized only as a Harris line. In the epiphyses, a shell of heavily calcified bone, known as "Wimberger's ring" surrounds a radiolucent ossification center. Healing microfractures may leave bony projections known as the Pelkan spurs on the lateral edge or corner of the metaphysis (Brickley and Ives, 2008). Stark (2014) emphasizes three phases of scorbutic lesion development, from the initial radiological indicators that will be macroscopically invisible (phase 1), radiological and macroscopically visible skeletal lesions (phase 2), and predominant skeletal lesions with "remnant" radiological features (phase 3). Hence, many cases of scurvy may go unnoticed in the archeological record, especially if it is not possible to carry out large scale radiographic or histological analysis. A list of the macroscopic and radiological features of scurvy in the skull and postcranium is provided in Table 8.4.

Difficulties in distinguishing the macroscopic porous lesions caused by iron-deficiency anemia from those as the result of scurvy in the cranium remain, with some attempts to make a distinction using cranial vault thickness (Zuckerman et al., 2014). Stark (2014, p. 23) suggests a stepwise approach to aid in the macroscopic diagnosis of scurvy in nonadults stating that:

if clinical radiological indicators, periosteal new bone and abnormal porosity in long bones…co-occur with cranial lesions…a stronger argument can be made to support cranial porous lesions being the result of scurvy…[while] periosteal new bone formation and abnormal porosity in long bones occurring in conjunction with porous cranial lesions, but in the absence of clinical radiological indicators, can be taken as indicative of subadult scurvy.

Differential diagnoses for the pitting and new bone formation seen in scurvy should include rickets, isolated hematomas as the result of trauma and other factors, infantile cortical hyperostosis, tuberculosis, leukemia, thalassemia, congenital syphilis, and normal growth particularly in infants. The likely existence of other deficiency disease, such as anemia or comorbidly with rickets should also be considered (Armelagos et al., 2014; Crandall and Klaus, 2014). To advance our understanding of this important condition, Crandall and Klaus (2014) reflect the arguments made for rickets by calling for a contextualized approach

TABLE 8.4 Macroscopic and Radiological Features Associated With Nonadult Scurvy

Location	Macroscopic Appearance	Radiographic Appearance
Cranium (specifically vault, greater wing of sphenoid, orbital roof, temporal bone, zygomatic bone, maxillary alveolus)	Abnormal regions of porosity over 1 mm Pores penetrate the surface New bone formation on orbits, cranial bosses (Parrot's swellings), infraorbital foramen, foramina rotunda of the sphenoid and palatine process Ectocranial vascular impressions, endocranial new bone formation	–
Mandible and maxilla	New bone formation on coronoid process, ramus, alveolus and sockets, antemortem tooth loss	–
Scapula	New bone formation on the supra and infraspinous fossa, abnormal porosity	
Ribs	Fractures or enlargement adjacent to costochondral junction (scorbutic rosary)	White line of Frankel Trümmerfeld zone
Vertebrae	–	Microfractures due to osteopenia causing "ground glass appearance"
Long bone diaphyses	New bone formation particularly at metaphyses Abnormal porosity >5–10 mm superior to metaphysis, possible thickening of shaft	White line of Frankel Trümmerfeld zone Cortical thinning Corner sign (clefting along zone of calcification) Pelkan spurs Metaphyseal cupping/mushrooming
Long bone epiphyses	–	Wimberger's ring Invagination/ball-in-socket appearance (with premature fusion)
Ilium	Porosity on external and internal surface, possible thickening of bone	Microfractures due to osteopenia causing "ground glass appearance"

List compiled from Brickley, M., Ives, R., 2008. The Bioarchaeology of Metabolic Bone Disease, Academic Press, Oxford; Stark, R.J., 2014. A proposed framework for the study of paleopathological cases of subadult scurvy. International Journal of Paleopathology 5, 18–26; Klaus, H., 2013. Subadult scurvy in Andean South America: evidence for vitamin C deficiency in the late pre-Hispanic and Colonial Lambayeque Valley, Peru. International Journal of Paleopathology 5, 34–45.

to our understanding of the disease, considering ecological, social, and historical aspects of the sample under study.

Since the refinement of the criteria, cases of nonadult scurvy are now commonly reported in the paleopathological literature. Initially represented by isolated cases (Mays, 2008; Ferreira, 2002; Brown and Ortner, 2011), more large scale studies have demonstrated its existence across a wide geographical area dating from the prehistoric to postmedieval periods. In nonadult samples current prevalence rates for scurvy range widely from 0.8% to 68% (Bourbou, 2014; Buckley, 2014; Geber and Murphy, 2012; Klaus, 2013; Krenz–Niedbała, 2016; Lewis, 2010; Lovasz et al., 2013; Mahoney-Swales and Nystrom, 2009; Pêterstone et al., 2013). The highest rates come from children buried at the Kilkenny Workhouse in Ireland during the Irish potato famine, there 68% (n = 371/545) of the nonadults showed characteristic lesions, with 28% neonates and 32% in infant skeletons affected, indicating scurvy in their mothers (Geber and Murphy, 2012). In the samples studied above, it is likely that the prevalence rates represent an underestimate of the cases of scurvy that actually existed in the child population as early radiological signs are invisible. Reasons for the occurrence of scurvy in such diverse areas include seasonal availability of fresh foods, and food shortages as the result of earthquakes and their consequences (Buckley, 2000), potato famine (Geber and Murphy, 2012), cultural practices related to weaning (Bourbou, 2014; Lewis, 2010), economic strategies (Wrobel, 2014), subsistence transition (Buckley, 2014), social control, and marginalization (Crandall, 2014). Nondiet factors include genetic susceptibility (Halcrow and Tayles, 2011) and the coexistence of absorption inhibiting conditions such as cancer and gastrointestinal diseases

(Halcrow et al., 2014). Other factors that may increase an individual's requirement for vitamin C, such as burns, major trauma, and malaria have been outlined by Halcrow et al. (2014) and have the potential to provide a new dimension to our interpretation of scurvy in the past.

Comorbidity and Cooccurrence in Rickets and Scurvy

As it is unlikely a malnourished child will be deficient in just one nutrient, the presence of more than one condition in the skeleton is highly likely (Armelagos et al., 2014; Crandall and Klaus, 2014). The identification of comorbidity, where several conditions are active at once, or cooccurrence where one disease may manifest after another has been resolved is highly complex. For example, if a child is suffering from marasmus (severe protein-calorie deficiency) and has retarded growth, the signs and symptoms of rickets will not appear unless the marasmus is cured (Griffith, 1919). Hence, in the past, children suffering from a suite of malnutrition diseases may not show any visible signs of the disease on the skeleton. Geber and Murphy's (2012) study of the Kilkenny workhouse in Ireland identified three cases of scurvy with active TB and 14 probable cases of rickets and scurvy. Lewis (2011) suggested comorbidity of rickets and scurvy in 11.2% of the Roman sample from Poundbury in Dorset, while Pêterstone et al. (2013) found new bone formation in the orbits of their two individuals diagnosed with rickets based on bowed femora and flared sternal rib ends. While the coexistence of rickets, scurvy, and anemia has been suggested, few studies have examined this in detail. Klaus (2013) suggested the new bone formation in the cranium in rickets is much finer than that produced in scurvy. It is also not clear which of the conditions, rickets or scurvy, will dominate in cases of comorbidity, with some studies showing scurvy signs can inhibit or eliminate traces of rickets (Bromer and Harvey, 1948), and others that rickets will be the dominant manifestation (Schattmann et al., 2016). While subperiosteal new bone formation should be hindered in rickets due to poor mineralization, it has been shown that small traces of vitamin C will allow it to occur, and the calcification of hematomas of scurvy are not affected by the presence of rickets (Schattmann et al., 2016).

REFERENCES

Aksoy, M., Camli, N., Dincol, K., Erdem, S., Dincol, G., 1973. On the problem of 'rib-within-a-rib' appearance in thalassemia intermedia. Radiological Clinical Biology 42, 126–133.

Almeida, A., Roberts, I., 2005. Bone involvement in sickle cell disease. British Journal of Haematology 129 (4), 482–490.

Amundsen, T., Siegal, M., Siegal, B., 1984. Osteomyelitis and infarction in sickle cell hemoglobinopathies: differentiation by combined Technetium and Gallium scintigraphy. Radiology 153 (3), 807–812.

Angel, L., 1964. Osteoporosis; thalassemia? American Journal of Physical Anthropology 22, 369–374.

Armelagos, G.J., Sirak, K., Werkema, T., Turner, B.L., 2014. Analysis of nutritional disease in prehistory: the search for scurvy in antiquity and today. International Journal of Paleopathology 5, 9–17.

Arneil, G., 1973. Rickets in Glasgow today. The Practitioner 210 (1257), 331–339.

CICotBM Association, 1889. Report of the collective investigation committee of the BMA. British Medical Journal 1, 113–116.

Aufderheide, A.C., Rodriguez-Martín, C., 1998. The Cambridge Encyclopedia of Human Paleopathology. Cambridge University Press, Cambridge.

Axon, J., 1991. Paediatrics in developing countries. In: Levene, M. (Ed.), Jolly's Diseases of Children. Blackwell Scientific Publications, London, pp. 529–575.

Baggieri, G., Mallegni, F., 2001. Morphopathology of some osseous alterations of thalassic nature. Paleopathology Newsletter 116, 10–16.

Barden, E., Kawchak, D., Ohene-Frempong, K., Stallings, V., Zemel, B., 2002. Body composition in children with sickle cell disease. American Journal of Clinical Nutrition 76, 218–225.

Barlow, T., 1883. On cases described as 'acute rickets' which are probably a combination of scurvy and rickets, the scurvy being an essential, and the rickets a variable element. Medico-chirurical Transactions 66, 159–219.

Barlow, T., 1935. On cases described as 'acute rickets' which are probably a combination of scurvy and rickets. Archives of Diseases in Children 10, 223–252.

Bathurst, R., 2005. Archaeological evidence of intestinal parasites from coastal shell middens. Journal of Archaeological Science 32 (1), 115–123.

Baxarias, J., 2002. La Enfermedad en la Hispania Romana: estudio de una necrópolis tarraconense. Libros Pórtico, Zaragoza.

Bianucci, R., Mattutino, G., Lallo, R., Charlier, P., Jouin-Spriet, H., Peluso, A., Higham, T., Torre, C., Massa, E., 2008. Immunological evidence of Plasmodium falciparum infection in an Egyptian child mummy from the Early Dynastic period. Journal of Archaeological Science 35, 1880–1885.

Bishop, N., Fewtrell, M., 2003. Metabolic bone diseases of prematurity. In: Glorieux, F., Pettifor, J., Jüppner, M. (Eds.), Pediatric Bone: Biology and Diseases. Academic Press, New York, pp. 567–581.

Blom, D., Buikstra, J., Keng, L., Tomczak, P., Shoreman, E., Stevens-Tuttle, D., 2005. Anemia and childhood mortality: latitudinal patterning along the coast of pre-Columbian Peru. American Journal of Physical Anthropology 127, 152–169.

Bohrer, S., Connah, G., 1971. Pathology in 700-year-old Nigerian bones. Diagnostic Radiology 98, 581–584.

Bolton-Maggs, P., Thomas, A., 2008. Disorders of the blood and bone marrow. In: McIntosh, N., Helms, P., Smyth, R., Logan, S. (Eds.), Forfar and Arneil's Textbook of Pediatrics. Churchill Livingstone, London, pp. 959–990.

Borden, S., 1974. Traumatic bowing of the forearm in children. Journal of Bone and Joint Surgery 56-A (3), 611–616.

Bourbou, C., 2014. Evidence of childhood scurvy in a middle Byzantine Greek population from Ctere, Greece (11th-12th centuries A.D.). International Journal of Paleopathology 5, 86–94.

Boyle, A., Dodd, A., Miles, D., Mudd, A., 1995. Two Oxfordshire Anglo-Saxon Cemeteries: Berinsfield and Didcot. Oxford Archaeological Unit, Oxford.

Brabin, L., Brabin, B.J., 1992. The cost of successful adolescent growth and development in girls in relation to iron and vitamin A status. The American Journal of Clinical Nutrition 55 (5), 955–958.

Brickley, M., Ives, R., 2006. Skeletal manifestations of infantile scurvy. American Journal of Physical Anthropology 129, 163–172.

Brickley, M., Ives, R., 2008. The Bioarchaeology of Metabolic Bone Disease. Academic Press, Oxford.

Brickley, M., Moffat, T., Watamaniuk, L., 2014. Biocultural perspectives of vitamin D deficiency in the past. Journal of Anthropological Archaeology 36, 48–59.

Bromer, R.S., Harvey, R.M., 1948. The roentgen diagnosis of rickets associated with other skeletal diseases of infants and children. Radiology 51 (1), 1–10.

Brown, J., Holden, D., 2002. Iron acquisition by gram-positive bacterial pathogens. Microbes and Infection 4, 1149–1156.

Brown, M., Ortner, D.J., 2011. Childhood scurvy in a medieval burial from Macvanska Mitrovica, Serbia. International Journal of Osteoarchaeology 21 (2), 197–207.

Buckley, H., 2000. Subadult health and disease in prehistoric Tonga, Polynesia. American Journal of Physical Anthropology 113, 481–505.

Buckley, H., 2014. Scurvy in a tropical paradise? Evaluating the possibility of infant and adult vitamin C deficiency in the Lapita skeletal sample of Teouma, Vanuatu, Pacific Islands. International Journal of Paleopathology 5, 72–85.

Burnett, M., Bass, J., Cook, B., 1998. Etiology of osteomyelitis complicating sickle cell disease. Pediatrics 101 (2), 296–297.

Buikstra, J.E., Ubelaker, D. (Eds.), 1994. Standards for Data Collection from Human Skeletal Remains. Arkansas Archeological Survey, Fayetteville.

Caffey, J., 1957. Cooley's anaemia: a review of the roentgenographic findings in the skeleton. The American Journal of Roentgenology 78 (3), 381–391.

Caffey, J., 1945. Pediatric X-Ray Diagnosis. Year Book Medical Publishers, Inc., Chicago.

Campillo, D., 2006. Paleoradiology VI. Metabolic osteopathies. Journal of Paleopathology 18 (3), 117–133.

Cappell, D.F., Anderson, J.R., 1971. Muir's Textbook of Pathology. Edward Arnold, London.

Cohen, M.N., Armelagos, G.J. (Eds.), 1984. Paleopathology at the Origins of Agriculture. Academic Press, Inc, New York.

Cooley, T., Lee, P., 1925. A series of cases of splenomegaly in children with anemia and peculiar bone changes. Transactions of the American Pediatric Society 37, 29–30.

Cooley, T., Witwer, E., Lee, P., 1927. Anemia in children. American Journal of Diseases of Children 34, 347–363.

Crandall, J.J., 2014. Scurvy in the Greater American Southwest: modeling micronutrition and biosocial processes in contexts of resource stress. International Journal of Paleopathology 5, 46–54.

Crandall, J.J., Klaus, H.D., 2014. Advancements, challenges, and prospects in the paleopathology of scurvy: current perspectives on vitamin C deficiency in human skeletal remains. International Journal of Paleopathology 5, 1–8.

Djuric, M., Milovanovic, P., Janovic, A., Draskovic, M., Djukic, K., Milenkovic, P., 2008. Porotic lesions in immature skeletons from Stara Torina, late medieval Serbia. International Journal of Osteoarchaeology 18, 458–475.

Dobson, M., 1989. History of malaria in England. Journal of the Royal Society of Medicine 82 (17), 3.

Dominguez-Rodrigo, M., Pickering, T., Diez-Martin, F., Mabulla, A., Musiba, C., et al., 2012. Earliest porotic hyperostosis on a 1.5-million-year-old hominin, Olduvai Gorge, Tanzania. PLoS One 7 (10).

Duggan, A., Wells, C., 1964. Four cases of archaic disease of the orbit. Eye, Ear, Nose and Throat Digest 26, 63–68.

El-Najjar, M., Ryan, D., Turner II, C., Lozoff, B., 1979. The etiology of porotic hyperostosis among the prehistoric and historic Anasazi Indians of southwestern United States. American Journal of Physical Anthropology 44, 477–488.

Ellis, M.A., 2010. The children of Spring Street: rickets in an early nineteenth-century urban congregation. Northeast Historical Archaeology 39, 120–133.

Faerman, M., Nebel, A., Fion, D., Thomas, M., Bradman, N., Ragsdale, B., Schultz, M., Oppenheim, A., 2000. From a dry bone to a genetic portrait: a case study of sickle cell anaemia. American Journal of Physical Anthropology 111 (2), 153–163.

Fairgrieve, S.I., Molto, J., 2000. Cribra orbitalia in two temporally disjunct population samples from the Dakhleh Oasis, Egypt. American Journal of Physical Anthropology 111, 319–331.

Ferreira, M.T., 2002. A scurvy case in an infant from Monte da Cegonha (Vidigueira-Portugal). Anthropologia Portuguesa 19, 57–63.

Filon, D., Faerman, M., Smith, P., Oppenheim, A., 1995. Sequence analysis reveals a B-thalassaemia mutation in the DNA of skeletal remains from the archeological site of Akhziv, Israel. Nature Genetics 9, 365–368.

Follis, R.H., Park, E.A., 1952. Some observations on bone growth, with particular respect to zones of increased density in the metaphysis. The American Journal of Roentgenology 68 (5), 709–724.

Foote, K., Marriott, L., 2003. Weaning of infants. Archives of Diseases in Childhood 88, 488–492.

Fraser, D.R., 1995. Vitamin D. The Lancet 345 (8942), 104–105.

Geber, J., Murphy, E., 2012. Scurvy in the Great Irish Famine: evidence of vitamin C deficiency from a mid-19th century skeletal population. American Journal of Physical Anthropology 148 (4), 512–524.

Gilbert, R.I., Mielke, J.M. (Eds.), 1985. The Analysis of Prehistoric Diets. Academic Press, Inc, Florida.

Golden, B., Reilly, J., 2008. Nutrition. In: McIntosh, N., Helms, P., Smyth, R., Logan, S. (Eds.), Forfar and Arneil's Textbook of Pediatrics. Churchill Livingstone, London, pp. 513–529.

Gowland, R., Western, A., 2012. Morbidity in the marshes: using spatial epidemiology to investigate skeletal evidence for malaria in Anglo-Saxon England (AD 410–1050). American Journal of Physical Anthropology 147 (2), 301–311.

Griffith, J., 1919. The Diseases of Infants and Children. W.B. Saunders and Company, London.

Halcrow, S., Harris, N., NBeavan, N., Buckley, H., 2014. First bioarchaeological evidence of probable scurvy in Southeast Asia: multifactoral etiologies of vitamin C deficiency in a tropical environment. International Journal of Paleopathology 5, 63–71.

Halcrow, S., Tayles, N., 2011. The bioarchaeological investigation of children and childhood. In: Agarwal, S., Glencross, S. (Eds.), Social Bioarchaeology. Wiley-Blackwell, Chichester, pp. 333–360.

Hardy, A., 1992. Rickets and the rest: child-care, diet and the infectious children's diseases, 1850-1914. Social History of Medicine 5 (3), 389–412.

Harris, H.A., 1931. Lines of arrested growth in the long bones in childhood. British Journal of Radiology 18, 622–640.

Harris, H.A., 1933. Bone Growth in Health and Disease. Oxford University Press, London.

Hedrick, P.W., 2011. Population genetics of malaria resistance in humans. Heredity 107 (4), 283–304.

Henschen, F., 1961. Cribra cranii, a skull condition said to be of racial or geographical nature. Pathological Microbiology 24, 724–729.

Hershkovitz, I., Edelson, G., 1991. The first case of thalassaemia? Human Evolution 6 (1), 49–54.

Hershkovitz, I., Rothschild, B.M., Latimer, B., Dutour, O., Leonetti, G., Greenwald, C.M., Rothschild, C., Jellema, L.M., 1997. Recognition of sickle cell anemia in skeletal remains of children. American Journal of Physical Anthropology 104 (2), 213–226.

Hirsch, M., Mogle, P., Barkli, Y., 1976. Neonatal scurvy. Report of a case. Pediatric Radiology 4, 251–253.

Hollar, M., 2001. The hair-on-end sign. Radiology 221, 347–348.

Holt, L.E., 1909. Diseases of Infancy and Childhood. D. Appleton and Company, London.

Isler, M., Turcotte, R., 2003. Bone tumors in children. In: Glorieux, F., Pettifor, J., Jüppner, M. (Eds.), Pediatric Bone: Biology and Diseases. Academic Press, New York, pp. 703–743.

Jackson, D., Park, E.A., 1935. Congenital scurvy: a case report. The Journal of Pediatrics 7 (6), 741–753.

Jelliffe, D.B., Blackman, V., 1962. Bahima disease: possible 'milk anemia' in late childhood. Tropical Pediatrics 61, 774–779.

Kaplan, R., Werther, R., Castano, F., 1964. Dental and oral findings in Cooley's anemia: a study of fifty cases. Annals of the New York Academy of Sciences 119, 664–666.

Klaus, H., 2013. Subadult scurvy in Andean South America: evidence for vitamin C deficiency in the late pre-Hispanic and Colonial Lambayeque Valley, Peru. International Journal of Paleopathology 5, 34–45.

Klaus, H., 2016. A probable case of acute childhood leukemia: skeletal involvement, differential diagnosis, and the bioarchaeology of cancer in South America. International Journal of Osteoarchaeology 26 (2), 348–358.

Knip, A., 1971. Frequencies of non-metrical varients in Tellem and Nokara skulls from Mali Republic. Proceedings of the Koninklijke Nederlandse Akademie van Wetenschappen 74 (5), 422–443.

Kobayashi, D., Satsuma, S., Kamegaya, M., Haga, N., Shimomura, S., Fujii, T., Yoshiya, S., 2005. Musculoskeletal conditions of acute leukemia and malignant lymphoma in children. Journal of Pediatric Orthopaedics B 14, 156–161.

Kovacs, C., 2003. Fetal mineral homeostasis. In: Glorieux, F., Pettifor, J., Jüppner, M. (Eds.), Pediatric Bone: Biology and Diseases. Academic Press, New York, pp. 271–302.

Krenz-Niedbała, M., 2016. Did children in medieval and post-medieval Poland suffer from scurvy? Examination of the skeletal evidence. International Journal of Osteoarchaeology 26, 633–647.

Kricun, M., 1985. Red-yellow marrow conversion: its effect on the location of some solitary bone lesions. Skeletal Radiology 14, 10–19.

Kwong, W., Friello, P., Semba, R., 2004. Interactions between iron deficiency and lead poisoning: epidemiology and pathogenesis. Science of the Total Environment 330, 21–37.

Laennec, R., 1831. Traité de L'auscultaticn Médiate. Chaudé, Paris.

Lagia, A., Eliopoulos, C., Manolis, S., 2006. Thalassemia: macroscopic and radiological study of a case. International Journal of Osteoarchaeology 17 (3), 269–285.

Langley-Evans, S., 2015. Nutrition in early life and the programming of adult disease: a review. Journal of Human Nutrition and Dietetics 28 (s1), 1–14.

Lanzkowsky, P., 1968. Radiological features of iron-deficiency anemia. American Journal of Diseases in Children 116, 16–29.

Lanzkowsky, P., 1977. Osseous changes in iron deficiency anemia – implications for paleopathology. In: Cockburn, E. (Ed.), Porotic Hyperostosis: An Enquiry. Paleopathology Association, Detroit, pp. 23–34.

Lawson, J., Ablow, R., Pearson, H., 1981a. The ribs in thalassemia I: the relationship to therapy. Pediatric Radiology 140, 663–672.

Lawson, J., Ablow, R., Pearson, H., 1981b. The ribs in thalassemia II: the pathogenesis of the changes. Pediatric Radiology 140, 673–679.

Lawson, J., Ablow, R., Pearson, H., 1983. Premature fusion of the proximal humeral epiphyses in thalassemia. American Journal of Radiology 140, 239–244.

Lawson, J., Ablow, R., Pearson, H., 1984. Calvarial and phalangeal vascular impressions in thalassemia. American Journal of Roentgenology 143, 641–645.

Levene, M., 1991a. Special care of the sick newborn infant. In: Levene, M. (Ed.), Jolly's Diseases of Children, sixth ed. Blackwell Scientific Publications, London, pp. 77–115.

Levene, M., 1991b. Metabolic disorders. In: Levene, M. (Ed.), Jolly's Diseases of Children, sixth ed. Blackwell Scientific Publications, London, pp. 370–381.

Lewis, M., 2002. The impact of industrialisation: comparative study of child health in four sites from medieval and post-medieval England (AD 850-1859). American Journal of Physical Anthropology 119 (3), 211–223.

Lewis, M., 2004. Endocranial lesions in non-adult skeletons: understanding their aetiology. International Journal of Osteoarchaeology 14, 82–97.

Lewis, M., 2007. The Bioarchaeology of Children. Cambridge University Press, Cambridge.

Lewis, M., 2010. Life and death in a civitas capital: metabolic disease and trauma in the children from late Roman Dorchester, Dorset. American Journal of Physical Anthropology 142, 405–416.

Lewis, M., 2011. Thalassaemia: its diagnosis and interpretation in past skeletal populations. International Journal of Osteoarchaeology 21 (2), 685–693.

Liebe-Harkort, C., 2012. Cribra orbitalia, sinusitis and linear enamel hypoplasia in Swedish Roman Iron Age adults and subadults. International Journal of Osteoarchaeology 22, 387–397.

Littleton, J., 1998. A Middle Eastern paradox: rickets in skeletons from Bahrain. Journal of Palaeopathology 10 (1), 13–30.

Liversidge, H., Molleson, T., 2001. Variation in deciduous tooth formation in humans. American Journal of Physical Anthropology 33, 98.

Lovasz, G., Schultz, M., Goedde, J., Bereczki, Z., PÁLFI, G., Marcsik, A., Molnar, E., 2013. Skeletal manifestations of infantile scurvy in a late medieval anthropological series from Hungary. Anthropological Science 121 (3), 173–185.

Maat, G., 1991. Ultrastructure of normal and pathological red blood cells compared with pseudo-pathological biological structures. International Journal of Osteoarchaeology 1, 209–214.

Mahoney-Swales, D., Nystrom, P., 2009. Skeletal manifestation of non-adult scurvy from early medieval Northumbria: the Black Gate cemetery, Newcastle-upon-Tyne. In: Lewis, M., Clegg, M. (Eds.), Proceedings of the Ninth Annual Conference of the British Association for Biological Anthropology and Osteoarchaeology. BAR International Series 1981, Archaeopress, Oxford, pp. 31–41.

Mankin, H.J., 1974. Rickets, osteomalacia, and renal osteodystrophy. Journal of Bone and Joint Surgery 56-A (1–2)) 101–128 and 352–386.

Massa, E., 1977. Presence of thalassaemia in Egyptian mummies. Journal of Human Evolution 6 (3), 225.

Mays, S., 2008. A likely case of scurvy from early Bronze Age Britain. International Journal of Osteoarchaeology 18, 178–187.

McCollum, E., Simmonds, N., Becker, J., Shipley, P., 1922. An experimental demonstration of the existence of a vitamin which promotes calcium deposition. Journal of Biological Chemistry 53, 293–298.

McCullough, J.M., Heath, K.M., Smith, A.M., 2015. Hemochromatosis: Niche construction and the genetic domino effect in the European neolithic. Human Biology 87 (1), 39–58.

McKintosh, N., Stenson, B., 2008. The newborn. In: McIntosh, N., Helms, P., Smyth, R., Logan, S. (Eds.), Forfar and Arneil's Textbook of Pediatrics. Churchill Livingstone, London, pp. 191–366.

Melikian, M., Waldron, T., 2003. An examination of skulls from two British sites for possible evidence of scurvy. International Journal of Osteoarchaeology 13, 207–212.

Mellanby, E., 1919. An experimental investigation on rickets. Lancet 1, 407–412.

Mendiela, S., Rissech, C., Haber, M., Pujol-Bayona, A., Lomba, J., Turbón, D., 2014. Childhood growth and health in Camino del Molino (Caravaca de la Cruz, Murcia, Spain) a collective burial of the III Millennium cal. BC. A preliminary approach. In: Adés, Ao (Ed.), Estudis D'evolució Etologia, pp. 101–106 Barcelona.

Mensforth, R.P., Lovejoy, O.C., Lallo, J.W., Armelagos, G.J., 1978. The role of constitutional factors, diet and infectious disease in the etiology of porotic hyperostosis and periosteal reactions in prehistoric infants and children. Medical Anthropology 2 (1), 1–59.

Miller, L.H., Good, M.F., Milon, G., 1994. Malaria pathogenesis. Science 264 (5167), 1878–1883.

Miquel-Feucht, M., Polo-Cerdá, M., Villalaín-Blanco, J., 1999a. Anthropological and paleopathological studies of a mass execution during the War of Independence in Valencia, Spain (1808-1812). Journal of Paleopathology 11 (3), 15–23.

Miquel-Feucht, M., Polo-Cerdá, M., Villalaín-Blanco, J., 1999b. El síndrome cribroso: cribra femoral vs cribra orbitalia. In: Sánchez, J. (Ed.), Sistematización metodológica en Paleopathología Actas del V Congreso Nacional de Paleopatología. Asociación Española de Paleopatología, Alcalá la Real, Spain, pp. 221–237.

Møller-Christensen, V., Sandison, A.T., 1963. Usura orbitae (cribra orbitalia) in the collection of crania in the Anatomy Department of the University of Glasgow. Pathological Microbiology 26, 175–183.

Möller, V., 1862. Zwei von acuter rachitis. Königsberger Medicinische Jahrbüker 3, 136–149.

Morse, J., 1900. The frequency of rickets in infancy in Boston and vicinity. Journal of the American Medical Association 34 (12), 724–726.

Moseley, J.E., 1965. The paleopathologic riddle of 'symmetrical osteoporosis'. American Journal of Roentgenology 95 (1), 135–142.

Moseley, J.E., 1974. Skeletal changes in the anemias. Seminars in Roentgenology 9 (3), 169–184.

Narchi, H., El Jamil, M, Kulaylat, N., 2001. Symptomatic rickets in adolescence. Archives of Disease in Childhood 84 (6), 501–503.

Nathan, H., Haas, N., 1966. On the presence of cribra orbitalia in apes and monkeys. American Journal of Physical Anthropology 24, 351–360.

Naveed, H., Abed, S.F., Davagnanam, I., Uddin, J.M., Adds, P.J., 2012. Lessons from the past: cribra orbitalia, an orbital roof pathology. Orbit 31 (6), 394–399.

Novak, M., Šlaus, M., 2010. Health and disease in a Roman walled city: an example of Colonia Iulia Iader. Journal of Anthropological Sciences 88, 189–206.

Oguntibeju, O., 2003. Parasitic infestation and anaemia: the prevalence in a rural hospital setting. Journal of the Indian Academy of Clinical Medicine 4, 210–212.

Olivieri, N., 1999. The B-Thalassaemias. The New England Journal of Medicine 341 (2), 99–109.

Ortner, D., 2003. Identification of Pathological Conditions in Human Skeletal Remains. Academic Press, New York.

Ortner, D., Kimmerle, E., Diez, M., 1999. Probable evidence of scurvy in subadults from archaeological sites in Peru. American Journal of Physical Anthropology 108, 321–331.

Ortner, D., 1984. Bone lesions in a probable case of scurvy from Metlatavik, Alaska. MASCA Journal 3, 79–81.

Ortner, D., Butler, W., Cafarella, J., Milligan, L., 2001. Evidence of probable scurvy in subadults from archaeological sites in North America. American Journal of Physical Anthropology 114 (4), 343–351.

Ortner, D., Ericksen, M.F., 1997. Bone changes in the human skull probably resulting from scurvy in infancy and childhood. International Journal of Osteoarchaeology 7, 212–220.

Ortner, D., Mays, S., 1998. Dry-bone manifestations of rickets in infancy and early childhood. International Journal of Osteoarchaeology 8, 45–55.

Ortner, D., Putschar, W.G.J., 1985. Identification of Pathological Conditions in Human Skeletal Remains. Smithsonian Institution Press, Washington.

Oxenham, M., Cavill, I., 2010. Porotic hyperostosis and cribra orbitalia: the erythropoietic response to iron-deficiency anaemia. Anthropological Science 118 (3), 199–200.

Palkovich, A.M., 1987. Endemic disease patterns in palaeopathology: porotic hyperostosis. American Journal of Physical Anthropology 74, 527–537.

Parano, E., Pavone, V., Di Gregorio, F., Trifiletti, R., 1999. Extraordinary itrathecal bone reaction in B-thalassaemia intermedia. Lancet 354, 922.

Paredes, J., Ferreira, M.T., Wasterlain, S.N., 2015. Growth problems in a skeletal sample of children abandoned at Santa Casa da Misericórdia, Faro, Portugal (16th–19th centuries). Anthropological Science 123, 49–59.

Park, E., Guild, H., Jackson, D., Bond, M., 1935. The recognition of scurvy with especial reference to the early x-ray changes. Archives of Diseases in Childhood 10 (58), 265–294.

Pêterstone, E., Gerhards, G., Jakob, T., 2013. Nutrition-related health problems in a wealthy 17-18th century German community in Jelgava, Latvia. International Journal of Paleopathology 3, 30–38.

Pettifor, J., 2003. Nutritional rickets. In: Glorieux, F., Pettifor, J., Jüppner, M. (Eds.), Pediatric Bone: Biology and Diseases. Academic Press, New York, pp. 541–565.

Pettifor, J., Daniels, E., 1997. Vitamin D deficiency and nutritional rickets in children. In: Feldman, D., Glorieux, F., Pike, J. (Eds.), Vitamin D. Academic Press, New York, pp. 663–678.

Pfeiffer, E., Coppage, L., Conway, W., 1995. General case of the day. Radiographics 15, 235–238.

Pitt, M., 1988. Rickets and osteomalacia. In: Resnick, D., Niwayama, G. (Eds.), Diagnosis of Bone and Joint Disorders. W.B.Saunders Company, Philadelphia, pp. 2087–2126.

Polo-Cerdá, M., Miquel-Feucht, M., Villalaín-Blanco, J., 2001. Experimental cribra orbitalia in Wistar rats: an etiopathogenic model of porotic hyperostosis and other porotic phenomena. In: La Verghetta, M., Capasso, L. (Eds.), Proceedings of the XIIIth European Meeting of the Paleopathology Association. Chieti, Italy: Journal of Paleopathology, pp. 253–259.

Ponec, D.J., Resnick, D., 1984. On the etiology and pathogenesis of porotic hyperostosis of the skull. Investigative Radiology 19 (4), 313–317.

Prentice, A., 2003. Pregnancy and lactation. In: Glorieux, F., Pettifor, J., Jüppner, M. (Eds.), Pediatric Bone: Biology and Diseases. Academic Press, New York, pp. 249–269.

Quinn, C., Rogers, Z., Buchanan, G., 2004. Survival of children with sickle cell disease. Blood 103 (11), 4023–4027.

Reinhard, K.J., 1992. Patterns of diet, parasitism and anemia in prehistoric West North America. In: Stuart-Macadam, P., Kent, S. (Eds.), Diet, Demography and Disease: Changing Patterns of Anemia. Aldine de Gruyter, New York, pp. 219–260.

Reiter, P., 2000. From Shakespeare to Defoe: malaria in England in the little ice age. Emerging Infectious Diseases 6 (1), 1–11.

Resnick, D. (Ed.), 1995. Diagnosis of Bone and Joint Disorders, third ed. W.B. Saunders Company, Philadelphia.

Resnick, D., Kransdorf, M., 2005. Bone and Joint Imaging, third ed. Elsevier Saunders, Philadelphia.

Roberts, C., 1987. Case report No. 9. Paleopathology Newsletter 57, 14–15.

Robledo, B., Trancho, G., Brothwell, D., 1995. Cribra orbitalia: health indicator in the late Roman population of Cannington (Somerset, Great Britain). Journal of Paleopathology 3, 185–193.

Rogaev, E.I., Grigorenko, A.P., Faskhutdinova, G., Kittler, E.L., Moliaka, Y.K., 2009. Genotype analysis identifies the cause of the "royal disease". Science 326 (5954), 817.

Rohnbogner, A., 2015. Dying Young: A Palaeopathological Analysis of Child Health in Roman Britain (Ph.D. thesis). University of Reading, England.

Rothschild, B., Hershkovitz, I., Dutour, O., Latimer, B., Rothschild, C., Jellema, L., 1997. Recognition of leukemia in skeletal remains: report and comparison of two cases. American Journal of Physical Anthropology 102, 481–496.

Rubino, G., Rasetti, L., Giarrusso, P., 1962. Effect of glycine administration on gamma-aminolaevulic acid and porphobilinogen excretion in lead poisoning. Panminerva Medica 4, 340–388.

Ryan, A.S., 1997. Iron-deficiency anemia in infant development: implications for growth, cognitive development, resistance to infection, and iron supplementation. Yearbook of Physical Anthropology 40 (25), 25–62.

Saarinen, U.M., 1978. Need for iron supplementation in infants on prolonged breast feeding. The Journal of Pediatrics 93 (2), 177–180.

Sallares, R., Gomzi, S., 2001. Biomolecular archaeology of malaria. Ancient Biomolecules 3 (3), 195–213.

Schamall, D., Teschler-Nicola, M., Kainberger, F., Tangl, S., Brandstätter, F., Patzak, B., Muhsil, J., Plenk, H., 2003. Changes in trabecular bone structure in rickets and osteomalacia: the potential of a medicohistorical collection. International Journal of Osteoarchaeology 13, 283–288.

Schattmann, A., Bertrand, B., Vatteoni, S., Brickley, M., 2016. Approaches to co-occurrence: scurvy and rickets in infants and young children of 16–18th century Douai, France. International Journal of Paleopathology 12, 63–75.

Schulman, I., 1959. The anemia of prematurity. Journal of Pediatrics 54, 663–672.

Schultz, M., 1988. Palaopathologische diagnostik. In: Knussmann, R. (Ed.), Anthropologie: Handbuch der Vergleichenden Biologie des Menschen Wesen und Methoden der Anthropologie. Fischer Verlag, Stuttgart and New York, pp. 480–496.

Schultz, M., 1989. Causes and frequency of diseases during early childhood in Bronze Age populations. In: Capasso, L. (Ed.), Advances in Palaeopathology. Marino Solfanelli Editore, Chieti, pp. 175–179.

Schultz, M., 1997. Porotic hyperostosis in Spanish Florida: nature and etiology of a frequently observed phenomenon. American Journal of Physical Anthropology (Suppl. 24), 206.

Schultz, M., 2001. Palaeohistopathology of bone: a new approach to the study of ancient diseases. Yearbook of Physical Anthropology 44, 106–147.

Sebes, J., Diggs, L., 1979. Radiographic changes to the skull in sickle cell anemia. American Journal of Roentgenology 132, 373–377.

Seow, W., Brown, J., Tudehope, D., O'Callaghan, M., 1984. Dental defects in the deciduous dentition of premature infants with low birth weight and neonatal rickets. Pediatric Dentistry 6 (2), 88–92.

Serjeant, G., 2005. Mortality from sickle cell disease in Africa. British Medical Journal 330, 432–433.

Setzer, T.J., 2014. Malaria detection in the field of paleopathology: a meta-analysis of the state of the art. Acta Tropica 140, 97–104.

Shapiro, F., 2001. Epiphyseal Involvement with Metabolic, Inflammatory, Neroplastic, Infectious and Hematologic Disorders. Pediatric Orthopedic Deformities: Basic Science, Diagnosis and Treatment. Academic Press, New York, pp. 872–905.

Sheldon, W., 1943. Diseases of Infancy and Childhood. J. & A. Churchill Ltd., London.

Simonson, T., Kao, S., 1992. Normal childhood developmental patterns in skull bone marrow by MR imaging. Pediatric Radiology 22, 556–559.

Simpson, E., 1991. Hematological disorders. In: Levene, M. (Ed.), Jolly's Diseases of Children, sixth ed. Blackwell Scientific Publications, London, pp. 423–441.

Singcharoen, T., Piyachon, C., Kulapongs, P., 1988. Radiographic abnormalities of ribs in β-thalassaemia children. Birth Defects 23 (5A), 417–420.

Sinigaglia, R., Gigante, C., Bisinella, G., Varotto, S., Zanesco, L., Turra, S., 2008. Musculoskeletal manifestations in pediatric acute leukemia. Journal of Pediatric Orthopedics 28, 20–28.

Soren, D., 2003. Can archaeologists excavate evidence of malaria? World Archaeology 35 (2), 193–209.

Soren, D., Fenton, T., Birkby, W., 1995. The late Roman infant cemetery near Lugnano in Teverina, Italy: some implications. Journal of Paleopathology 7 (1), 13–42.

Stark, R.J., 2014. A proposed framework for the study of paleopathological cases of subadult scurvy. International Journal of Paleopathology 5, 18–26.

Steinbock, R.T., 1976. Paleopathological Diagnosis and Interpretation: Bone Diseases in Ancient Human Populations. Charles C Thomas, Illinois.

Stuart-Macadam, P.L., 1988. Rickets as an interpretative tool. Journal of Paleopathology 2 (1), 33–42.

Stuart-Macadam, P.L., 1989. Nutritional deficiency diseases: a survey of scurvy, rickets and iron-deficiency anemia. In: Iscan, M.Y., Kennedy, K.A.R. (Eds.), Reconstruction of Life from the Skeleton. Alan R. Liss, Inc., New York, pp. 201–222.

Stuart-Macadam, P.L., 1991. Anemia in Roman Britain: Poundbury Camp. In: Bush, H., Zvelebil, M. (Eds.), Health in Past Societies: Biocultural Interpretations of Human Skeletal Remains in Archaeological Contexts. British Archaeological Research International Series, Oxford, pp. 101–113.

Stuart, M.J., Nagel, R.L., 2004. Sickle-cell disease. Lancet 364 (9442), 1343–1360.

Sylvester, K., Patey, R., Milligan, P., Dick, M., Rafferty, G., Rees, D., Thein, S., Greenough, A., 2003. Pulmonary function abnormalities in children with sickle cell disease. Thorax 59, 67–70.

Tayles, N., 1996. Anemia, genetic diseases, and malaria in prehistoric mainland Southeast Asia. American Journal of Physical Anthropology 101 (1), 11–27.

Thacher, T.D., Fischer, P., Pettifor, J., Lawson, J., Manaster, B., Reading, J., 2000. Radiographic scoring method for the assessment of the severity of nutritional rickets. Journal of Tropical Pediatrics 46, 132–139.

Thacher, T.D., Fischer, P.R., Pettifor, J.M., Lawson, J.O., Isichei, C.O., 1999. A comparison of calcium, vitamin D, or both for nutritional rickets in Nigerian children. The New England Journal of Medicine 341 (8), 563–568.

Trinkaus, E., 1977. The Alto Salaverry child: a case of anemia from the Peruvian preceramic. American Journal of Physical Anthropology 46, 25–28.

Tuten, H., Gabos, P., Kumar, S., Harter, G., 1998. The limping child: a manifestation of acute leukemia. Journal of Pediatric Orthopedics 18, 625–629.

Van Sleuwen, B.E., Engelberts, A.C., Boere-Boonekamp, M.M., Kuis, W., Schulpen, T.W., L'Hoir, M.P., 2007. Swaddling: a systematic review. Pediatrics 120 (4), e1097–e1106.

Verlinden, P., Lewis, M., 2015. Childhood trauma: methods for the identification of physeal fractures in nonadult skeletal remains. American Journal of Physical Anthropology 157 (3), 411–420.

Veselka, B., Hoogland, M., Waters-Rist, A., 2015. Rural rickets: vitamin D deficiency in a post-medieval farming community from The Netherlands. International Journal of Osteoarchaeology 25 (5), 665–675.

Waldron, H., 1966. The anaemia of lead poisoning: a review. British Journal of Industrial Medicine 23, 83–100.

Waldron, T., 2009. Palaeopathology. Cambridge University Press, Cambridge.

Walker, P., Bathurst, R., Richman, R., Gjerdrum, T., Andrushko, V., 2009. The causes of porotic hyperostosis and cribra orbitalia: a reappraisal of the iron-deficiency anemia hypothesis. American Journal of Physical Anthropology 139, 109–125.

Walker, P.L., 1986. Porotic hyperostosis in a marine-dependent California Indian population. American Journal of Physical Anthropology 69, 345–354.

Wapler, U.Crubézy, E., Schultz, M., 2004. Is cribra orbitalia synonymous with anemia? Analysis and interpretation of cranial pathology in Sudan. American Journal of Physical Anthropology 123, 333–339.

Weinberg, E.D., 1974. Iron susceptibility to infectious disease. Science 184, 952–956.

Weinberg, E.D., 1992. Iron withholding in prevention of disease. In: Stuart-Macadam, P., Kent, S. (Eds.), Diet, Demography and Disease: Changing Perspectives on Anemia. Aldine de Gruyer, New York, pp. 105–150.

Welcker, H., 1885. Die Abstammung der Bevölkerung von Socotra (the origin of the people of Socotra). Deutsch Geographentag, Hamburg.

Whipple, G., Bradford, W., 1936. Mediterranean disease – thalassemia (erythroblastic anemia of Cooley). The Journal of Pediatrics 9 (3), 279–311.

Whistler, D., 1645. De Morbo Puerli Anglorum, Quem Patrio Ideiomate Indigenae Vocant "The Rickets". Lugduni, Batavorum.

Willson, J.K., 1959. The bone lesions of leukemia: a survey of 140 cases. Radiology 72 (5), 672–681.

Wisetsin, S., 1989. Cephalography in thalassemic patients. The Journal of the Dental Association of Thailand 40 (6), 260–268.

Witkin, A., 2011. The human skeletal remains. In: Pearson, A., Jeffs, B., Witkin, A., MacQuarrie (Eds.), Infernal Traffic: Excavations of a Libertated African Graveyard in Rupert's Valley. Council for British Archaeology, St Helena. Oxford, pp. 57–98.

Wright, R.O., Tsaih, S.-W., Schwartz, J., Wright, R.J., Hu, H., 2003. Association between iron deficiency and blood lead level in a longitudinal analysis of children followed in an urban primary care clinic. The Journal of Pediatrics 142 (1), 9–14.

Wrobel, G., 2014. Brief communication: a likely case of scurvy in a rural early classic Maya burial from Actun Uayazba Kab, Belize. American Journal of Physical Anthropology 155 (3), 476–481.

Yang, D., 1997. DNA Diagnosis of Thalassemia from Ancient Italian Skeletons (Ph.D. thesis). McMaster University, Canada.

Zuckerman, M., Garofalo, E., Frolich, B., Ortner, D., 2014. Anemia or scurvy: a pilot study on differential diagnosis of porous and hyperostotic lesions using differential cranial vault thickness in subadult humans. International Journal of Paleopathology 5, 27–33.

Chapter 9

Neoplastic Disease, Tumors, and Tumor-Like Lesions

Chapter Outline

Introduction	225	Osteofibrous Dysplasia	235
Classification of Lesions and Terminology	226	**Bone Cysts**	**236**
Recognition of Tumors	226	Unicameral (Solitary) Bone Cyst	236
Benign Primary Tumors	**230**	Aneurismal Bone Cyst	236
Osteoid Osteoma	230	**Langerhans Cell Histiocytosis**	**236**
Osteoblastoma (Codman's Tumor)	230	Eosinophilic Granuloma	238
Giant-Cell Tumor (Osteoclastoma)	231	Hand–Schüller–Christian Disease	238
Osteochondroma	231	Letterer–Siwe Disease	239
Hereditary Multiple Osteochondromas	232	**Malignant Primary Tumors**	**240**
Chondromas and Ollier's Disease	232	Osteosarcoma (Osteogenic Sarcoma)	240
Chondroblastoma	234	Ewing's Sarcoma	240
Chondromyxoid Fibroma	234	Chordoma	241
Desmoid Fibroma (Desmoplastic Fibroma)	234	**Non-Hodgkin's Lymphoma**	**242**
Fibrous Cortical Defects	234	**References**	**242**
Nonossifying Fibroma	235		

INTRODUCTION

Today, cancer is the second biggest killer of children between the ages of 1 and 14 years in the developed world, second only to deaths due to accidents. Cancers affect 186.6 per million children and in the United States contribute to 11.9 million deaths (Ward et al., 2014). The majority of cases (75%–90%) are of unknown origin making childhood cancer one of the most poorly understood branches of medicine (Buka, 2009). Children have the potential to develop the disease after long periods of latency and tend to have a longer life expectancy than affected adults (Buka, 2009). Today, exposure to UV light, radiation, tobacco, and other air pollutants are the main environmental carcinogens, while viral infections are the primary biological agents. As children are growing they are more likely to develop cancer after carcinogen exposure than adults. There is a recognized peak in malignant bone cancers in adolescence that may be related to the hormonal changes at puberty. There are also variations in susceptibility due to sex, with, for example, females suffering more commonly from malignant myeloma than males (Buka, 2009). Glass and Fraumeni (1970) surveyed the death records of 1532 children dying from primary malignant bone tumors in the United States between 1960 and 1966. They found the incidence of tumors was more related to ancestry, age and sex, and genetic factors rather than the presence of environmental carcinogens.

As the incidence of neoplastic disease increases with age, it is considered rare in nonadult skeletal remains. Similar to congenital disease, the significance of tumors and neoplasms in the past relates to how much we can determine about the causes of the disease. As cancers can occur spontaneously or have a genetic origin, they may tell us little about past environmental conditions. Nevertheless, numerous carcinogens would have been present in the past, including those that occur naturally such as radon gas and ultraviolet light, and viruses can stimulate gene mutations that give rise to tumors (Aufderheide and Rodriguez-Martín, 1998; Cappell and Anderson, 1971). Today, cancers of the brain and nervous system are the most common in children under 14 years, followed by acute lymphoblastic leukemia, neuroblastoma, and non-Hodgkin's lymphoma. In adolescence, thyroid carcinomas and testicular germ cell tumors make an appearance (Ward et al., 2014). Osteosarcomas are the most prevalent malignant primary tumors, while giant-cell tumors make up the most common benign primary tumors in children. By contrast, in archeological contexts by far the most commonly diagnosed "cancer" in children is Langerhans cell histiocytosis (LCH), although this condition is not strictly neoplastic, it will be discussed here.

Classification of Lesions and Terminology

Various conditions are listed under the broader heading of neoplasms in the paleopathological and clinical literature, with researchers choosing to further define them into "tumors and tumor-like diseases" to highlight complications in their classification. For example, hereditary multiple osteochondromas (HMO), while characterized by tumors that may become malignant, is primarily a congenital condition. While leukemia is a cancer as it arises from the bone marrow, it is mainly a hemopoietic disorder (and is discussed in Chapter 8), and LCH is no longer classified as a cancer, but rather a disorder of the reticuloendothelial or immune system. Cancer is an umbrella term for diseases that are characterized by uncontrolled cell growth. The word "tumor" simply means a swelling of tissues. Tumors have a reduced power of repair and a low resistance to infection, and many external soft tissue tumors are prone to ulceration (Cappell and Anderson, 1971). Bone cysts may exhibit uncontrolled growth, and in some cases uncontrolled function (i.e., they produce hormones or enzymes), but they are not considered neoplastic (Cappell and Anderson, 1971). Neoplasms (or new growths) are masses of abnormal tissue that exceed normal growth in an uncoordinated manner and continue to increase once the stimulus has been removed. A neoplasm can arise in any tissue or organ of the body regardless of an individual's age, sex, ethnicity, or social group, although certain neoplasms have a higher incidence in some of these groups (Roberts and Manchester, 2007). Neoplasms may arise as a mass of "differentiated" cells that resemble the original tissue from which they arise (e.g., breast or lung cells) or may be "undifferentiated" (anaplastic), not resembling any organ or cell within the body (Roberts and Manchester, 2007; Cappell and Anderson, 1971). In the main, benign neoplasms are well differentiated and grow slowly, remaining within the area they arose, causing localized effects due to compression of the surrounding tissue, and restricting joint movement. However, some benign tumors may transform into malignant tumors (Steinbock, 1976). Malignant neoplasms are poorly differentiated and grow rapidly (Cappell and Anderson, 1971). They are characterized by an uncontrolled spread from the primary area of growth into the surrounding tissues and distant organs of the body. This is achieved through the bloodstream and lymphatic system, or by direct implantation of cells into surrounding areas (Roberts and Manchester, 2007). These secondary deposits are known as metastases. The uncontrolled growth and spread of both the primary neoplasm and metastases ultimately leads to the death of the individual as the invaded organs fail.

Tumors that affect the skeleton can arise directly from bone, or originate in cartilage, fibrous tissue, and blood vessels (Ortner, 2003). Broders (1925) established a system that classifies tumors according to the tissue from which they originate, whereas the International Classification of Childhood Cancer uses codes that relate to the morphology, topography, and behavior of the neoplasms (Ward et al., 2014). Others choose to list tumors according to the location of the bone in which they most commonly appear (Khurana and Unni, 2003). Table 9.1 draws together these various systems to outline the most common neoplasms in children, their age of occurrence, and usual location. According to Broders' (1925) system, tumors originating in bone have the prefix "osteo," while the suffix "oma" identifies a tumor according to the tissue of origin, for example, chondro-, osteo-, fibro- (Aufderheide and Rodriguez-Martín, 1998). Adenoma suggests the neoplasm forms in a gland, and tumors named after people are usually of unknown cell origin (Aufderheide and Rodriguez-Martín, 1998). Chondrogenic tumors (e.g., endochondroma) originate in cartilage, angiomas arise in vessels, and fibromas occur in fibrous tissue. Malignant tumors are classified as either sarcomas or carcinomas. Sarcomas develop in tissue or their mesodermal layer (e.g., bone, muscle). Carcinomas arise in the epithelial tissue that is associated with many organs of the body (Steinbock, 1976). According to Steinbock (1976), most malignant neoplasms metastasize into bone, usually the pelvis and spine, and this may be as high as 85% for neoplasms of the prostate, breast, kidney, lung, or thyroid.

Recognition of Tumors

Strouhal (1994) carried out a review of neoplastic disease and listed 37 cases of tumors and metastatic carcinomas in archeological contexts. He argued that the discovery of malignant tumors is hindered by a low mean life expectancy in the past, with many tumors occurring only in people who live to over 60 years of age. In addition, there were fewer carcinogens in ancient environments, and many cancers are missed as bone histology is rarely employed to look for them, and finally, fragile tumor shells often fail to survive the burial environment. Strouhal (1994, p. 1) also asserted that the "geographical distribution of ancient malignant tumors often reflects the research activities of an individual paleopathologist, rather than the actual prevalence of tumors." This lack of systematic research means that our attempt to understand the true extent of cancer in the past is currently limited, and given their earlier age at death the situation is likely to be worse for children.

Diagnosing neoplastic diseases in archeological remains is certainly difficult and depends on the identification of distinct macroscopic and radiographic changes. Narrowing down the most likely neoplasm relies on an understanding of the individual's age, sex, and the specific bones that are affected, as well as the nature of the lesions themselves. For example, Roberts and Manchester (2007) cite the osteoid osteoma; a benign tumor that is twice as common in males as females, has a 50% occurrence in 11- to 20-year-olds,

TABLE 9.1 Classification, Age, Location, and Characteristics of Tumors That Commonly Affect Children

	Age of Presentation (Years)	Tissue Formation Type	Location	Bones Most Commonly Affected (in Order of Prevalence)	Specific Feature
Benign					
Osteoid osteoma	5–20	Bone	Diaphysis	Femur, tibia, fibula	Up to 1.5 cm
Osteoblastoma	15–30	Bone	Diaphysis	Spine, sacrum, hands and feet	Over 1.5 cm
Giant-Cell tumor (osteoclastoma)	Older child to adolescent	Bone	Epiphysis, metaphysis	Femur, tibia, humerus, radius	
Osteochondroma	0–20	Cartilage	Metaphysis	Knee, humerus, fibula, ilium, hands and feet	
Chondroma	10–30	Cartilage	Metaphysis, diaphysis	Hands and feet, pelvis, sternum, skull	
Chondroblastoma	5–25	Cartilage	Epiphysis	Proximal humerus, proximal femur, knee	
Chondromyxoid fibroma	10–30	Cartilage	Metaphysis	Knee, foot, pelvis	
Desmoid fibroma	10–30	Fibrous	Diaphysis	Ilium, mandible	
Fibrous cortical defect	4–8	Fibrous	Metaphysis	Distal femur, distal tibia, proximal tibia and fibula	
Nonossifying fibroma	Older child to adolescent	Fibrous	Metaphysis	Distal femur, distal tibia, proximal tibia and fibula	
Unicameral (solitary) bone cyst	0–20	–	Metaphysis	Proximal humerus, femur	
Aneurismal bone cyst	5–25	–	Metaphysis, diaphysis	Humerus, femur, tibia, ilium, spine	
Osteofibrous dysplasia	0–5	Fibrous	Diaphysis	Tibia	
Langerhans cell histiocytosis	5–10		Metaphysis, diaphysis	Frontal bone, mandible, ribs, femur	Not strictly neoplastic Single and multiple lesions
Malignant					
Osteosarcoma	10–25	Bone, fibrous, cartilage	Metaphysis (epiphysis rare)	Knee, humerus	Metastatic, onion-peel periostitis
Ewing's sarcoma	10–20	–	Diaphysis	Femur, tibia, humerus	Metastatic
Chordoma	0–20	–		Skull (clivus), spine	
Non-Hodgkin's lymphoma	Any age			Spine, pelvis, skull, ribs, facial bones	Metastatic, "moth-eaten" lytic lesions

and affects the femur and tibia equally. It is rare that a complete radiographical survey of a skeletal collection can be undertaken meaning that many early cancers still forming within the bone will go unnoticed, although the increase in available digital radiographic equipment in archeological departments is making such skeletal surveys more possible.

Accurate differential diagnosis relies on good preservation of the entire skeleton and bone surface, in fact Waldron (2009) warns against making any diagnosis of cancer without the aid of a radiologist or medical pathologist. It may be that often, defining a lesion as a benign or malignant tumour is the only diagnosis we will be able to achieve.

In clinical practice, tumors are diagnosed on the basis of fresh tissue pathology, usually as a method to determine if a lesion is benign or malignant. Understanding which tumors arise from which area of the bone is also crucial (Fig. 9.1). Benign tumors are recognized by their lamellar tissue architecture and the lack of osteolytic activity, whereas malignant tumors will display both osteolytic and osteoblastic activity in abundance. Their invasive quality is demonstrated by numerous Howship's lacunae, while new bone is deposited in a patchwork manner (De Boer et al., 2013). In dry bone cases, De Boer et al. (2013) argue that histology is rarely conclusive, and the morphology of the tumor, and the age and sex of the individual usually provides the best basis for a diagnosis. While histology is not always accessible or useful to the researcher, radiography is essential for tumor recognition. New bone formation within the bone in response to a tumor can often be distinguished from the response to an infection or trauma by its radiographic features. Neoplastic new bone appears either as a nest or nests of ivory-like dense bone, or as multiple flecks. These nests are normally the result of an osteosarcoma or osteoblastoma, whereas dense flecks are considered indicative of a cartilage origin, and due to a chondrosarcoma, chondroblastoma, and chondroma. These are the only tumors that produce new bone, allowing diagnosis to be narrowed down (Edeiken et al., 1966). Ragsdale (1993) argues that the presence of a sclerotic margin around a lesion on radiograph normally suggests a benign disorder, where slow growth allows time for an accumulation of bone around the lesion. This appearance is characteristic of unicameral cysts, nonossifying fibromas, fibrous dysplasias, enchondromas, and chondroblastomas. Malignant tumors such as a chondrosarcoma can also elicit this response (Ragsdale, 1993). Rapidly expanding malignant tumors often have no such margins visible on the radiograph. The amount of periosteal reaction is proportionate to the intensity, aggressiveness, and duration of the lesion, and is more prominent on the long bones, and in younger individuals (Ragsdale, 1993). Within 10–21 days after the initial stimulus the osteoid mineralizes sufficiently to be seen on radiograph. The ridged shell ("soap bubble") of some tumors signals a relatively slow process, and a thin uniform, lobulated shell is caused by ridges on the endosteal surface that form where bone deposition has lagged behind bone removal. These shells represent newly deposited bone rather than an expanded cortex, and become thicker and therefore more likely to preserve archeologically, the longer

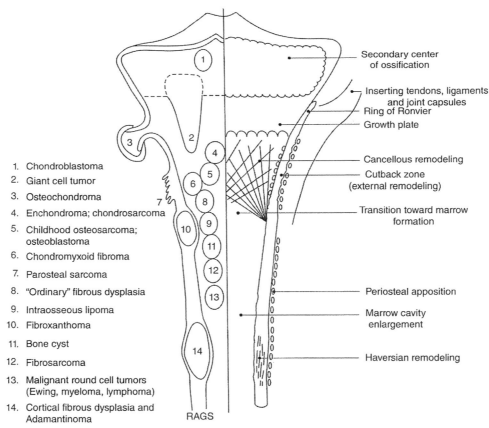

FIGURE 9.1 Typical locations of bone tumors (numbered list on the left) in relation to anatomical landmarks of growth and development (right). *From Ragsdale, B., Lehmer, L., 2012. A knowledge of bone at the cellular (histological) level is essential to paleopathology. In: Grauer, A. (Ed.), A Companion to Paleopathology. Wiley Blackwell, Chichester, p. 237.*

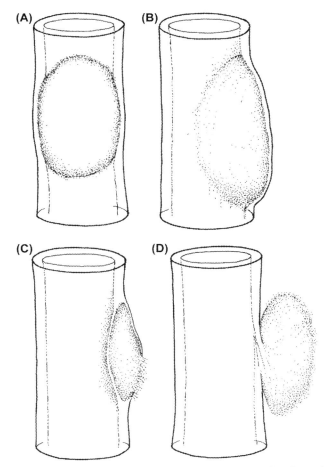

FIGURE 9.2 Position of lesions: (A) central, (B) eccentric, (C) cortical, and (D) juxtacortical. The lesions in (B) and (C) have produced bony shells around the lesion. Lesions extend from the medullary cavity (A, B) or within the cortex (C). *From Resnick, D., Kransdorf, M., 2005. Bone and Joint Imaging. Elsevier Saunders, Philadelphia, p. 1117.*

the lesion is present (Ragsdale, 1993). Tumors that form in the medullary cavity may be much more difficult to recognize, as a nonaggressive cortical lesion will show a sharp interface between the surrounding bone on radiograph, whereas a medullary lesion may not (Fig. 9.2; Resnick et al., 2005).

Where a dense sclerotic margin around the tumor characterizes a benign lesion, malignancy is suggested by permeative destruction with a gradual zone of transition away from the normal bone structure. The reaction of the periosteum is also helpful in a diagnosis (Fig. 9.3). If the periosteum has time to lay down mature bone, it is benign and slow growing, if there are sequential layers in an "onion-skin" pattern this suggests a rapidly evolving process that is usually malignant in nature. The "Codman's triangle" describes an area at the corner of rapid periosteal elevation that is usually the sign of an active malignant process, as are "sunburst" lesions on the cortex, although Codman's triangle signifies a raised

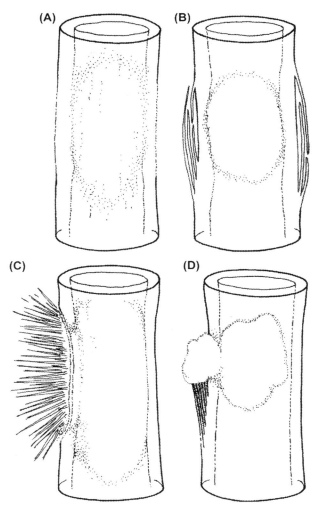

FIGURE 9.3 Examples of the appearance of tumors on radiograph. (A) Permeative bone destruction with poorly defined margins; (B) "onion-peel" pattern with multiple concentric periosteal layers surrounding the lesion; (C) "sunburst" pattern with radiating spicules of periosteal new bone; and (D) Codman's triangle: triangular elevation of the periosteum above an aggressive cortex-invading lesion. *Adapted from Resnick, D., Kransdorf, M., 2005. Bone and Joint Imaging. Elsevier Saunders, Philadelphia, pp. 1111–1116.*

periosteum that can also occur in infections (Edeiken et al., 1966). If the tumor destroys bone, then the type will be defined by the calcification and ossification of the lesion (Isler and Turcotte, 2003), and the metaphyseal or diaphyseal location of the lesion may also aid in the differential diagnosis. Hence, to aid in the diagnosis of a primary bone tumor, the following should be considered:

1. Appearance on radiograph (evidence of sclerotic margin)
2. Periosteal reaction (lamellar bone, onion skin, sunburst)
3. Nature of bone destruction (evidence of ossification)
4. Location (metaphyseal, diaphyseal, epiphyseal involvement).

BENIGN PRIMARY TUMORS

Osteoid Osteoma

An osteoid osteoma is a relatively rare, benign, and solitary tumor presenting as an oval nidus composed of osteoid with the trabeculae of newly formed bone deposited within the periosteum (Steinbock, 1976). The majority of osteoid osteomas occur before 30 years of age but most common between the ages of 5 and 20 years (Isler and Turcotte, 2003; Khurana and Unni, 2003), and they are three times more likely to occur in males than females (Isler and Turcotte, 2003). Individuals experience severe unremitting pain, especially at night, and if the tumor is left untreated it may cause spinal scoliosis or joint flexion (Khurana and Unni, 2003). Jaffe (1958) reported that these tumors were most common in the femur (25%) and tibia (25%) but also present in the fibula, humerus, vertebrae, and feet. Osteoid osteomas have a very distinctive radiographic appearance with a well-defined radiolucent core representing an area once occupied by osteoid (the nidus) (Fig. 9.4). The area of sclerotic reactive bone surrounding the lesion is out of proportion to the size of the lesion itself (Ortner, 2003; Steinbock, 1976) and may cause it to be confused with osteomyelitis, an osteosarcoma, or an osteoblastoma. However, osteoblastomas are almost always larger than 1.5 cm, whereas osteoid osteomas are almost always below 1.5 cm in length (Khurana and Unni, 2003; Steinbock, 1976). Some lesions are very small and may be easily missed in archeological material. Despite the epidemiology of this tumor, no cases have been identified in nonadult individuals and this may reflect the fact that the tumor is both rare and nonfatal.

Osteoblastoma (Codman's Tumor)

Osteoblastomas occur in adolescents and young adults below the age of 30 years, with males reported to be more affected than females. This rare benign tumor is one of the most common lesions affecting the spine in children (Isler and Turcotte, 2003). Although similar radiographically to the osteoid osteoma, osteoblastomas can reach a greater size (i.e., between 2 and 10 cm) and occur in the posterior elements of the spine (Khurana and Unni, 2003; Ortner, 2003) and sacrum (Isler and Turcotte, 2003), with 10% of tumors located in the bones of hands and feet (Resnick and Kransdorf, 2005, p. 1126). Osteoblastomas are difficult to diagnose on dry bone as, while some of these tumors are heavily mineralized with sclerosis and extensive periosteal reactions, others remain merely as osteoid seams (Ortner, 2003). However, their more circumscribed appearance makes them distinguishable from osteosarcomas (Fig. 9.5; Khurana and Unni, 2003).

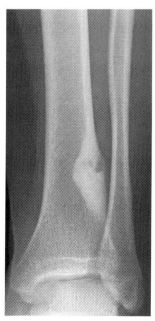

FIGURE 9.4 Classic presentation of an osteoid osteoma on the distal tibia. Note the central radiolucent oval lesion (nidus) surrounded by extensive sclerotic bone and cortical thickening. *From http://img.medscapestatic.com/pi/meds/ckb/50/7650.jpg.*

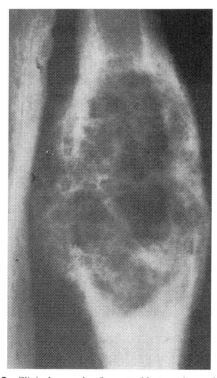

FIGURE 9.5 Clinical example of an osteoblastoma in an ulna. There is irregular osteolysis and sclerosis with cortical thickening and bone enlargement. *From Resnick, D., Kransdorf, M., 2005. Bone and Joint Imaging. Elsevier Saunders, Philadelphia, p. 1128.*

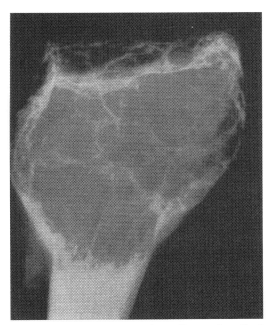

FIGURE 9.6 Clinical example of a giant-cell tumor in a distal radius. Note the fine trabecular bone distributed through and surrounding the expansive lesion. *From Resnick, D., Kransdorf, M., 2005. Bone and Joint Imaging. Elsevier Saunders, Philadelphia, p. 1112.*

Giant-Cell Tumor (Osteoclastoma)

The osteoclastoma is one of the most common primary bone tumors in children, and is made up of stromal cells and multinucleated giant cells similar to osteoclasts. Tumors arise in metaepiphyseal areas of newly fused long bones, particularly the femur, tibia, humerus, and radius (Isler and Turcotte, 2003). For this reason giant-cell tumors occur in older children and adolescents. They also have preponderance for females around 17 years of age (Isler and Turcotte, 2003). These tumors are painful and aggressive and may break through the cortex resulting in a hard tissue mass contained within a thin cortical shell. Its presence may result in muscular atrophy. Although they may be located near articular surfaces, they do not normally penetrate the joint (Ortner, 2003). On radiograph these tumors show lytic destruction of the epiphysis extending into the metaphysis and subchondral bone (Fig. 9.6). The fragile cortical shell displays internal reinforcing ridges giving it the appearance of a "soap bubble" on radiograph (Resnick et al., 2005). Differential diagnosis should consider a nonossifying fibroma, chondroblastoma, osteoblastoma, and osteosarcoma (Isler and Turcotte, 2003). A possible case of a giant-cell tumor was reported in a child from Roman Age Corinth (AD 43–450), but the location of the tumor on the tibia makes this diagnosis uncertain (Fox, 2004) and the large expansion of the lesion and central location on the tibia means that osteofibrous dysplasia or a desmoid fibroma cannot be ruled out (Fig. 9.7). The layers of periosteal new

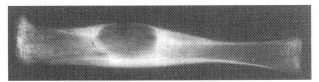

FIGURE 9.7 Possible giant-cell tumor in a child from ancient Corinth, Greece (skeleton 61–10). *From Fox, S.C., 2004. The case studies of Paphos, Cyprus and Corinth, Greece. In: King, H. (Ed.), Health in Antiquity, Routledge, London, p. 74.*

bone producing a Codman's triangle, as well as the ill-defined margins are also more suggestive of a malignant tumor such as an intramedullary osteosarcoma.

Osteochondroma

While being one of the most commonly cited neoplasms, an osteochondroma is not strictly neoplastic as it is not caused by cell proliferation, but rather an aberration of development caused by faulty ossification of the growth plate. It causes a localized swelling on the bone that remains in the position it arose after the growth plate has moved on. Osteochondromas may be present at birth (and hence potentially recognized in an infant's remains) but do not usually become clinically significant until later in life (Steinbock, 1976). The tumor consists of bone marrow and trabeculae capped with a thick layer of cartilage. If the cartilage cap is very thick (c. 1.5 cm), it may give rise to the more malignant chondrosarcoma (Khurana and Unni, 2003). On radiograph there is a continuation of cancellous bone into the defect (Steinbock, 1976). Growth of the tumor ceases with the end of the growing period. As these lesions develop out of the growth plate, the closer the lesion is to the end of the fused bone, the later in life the tumor arose. Osteochondromas are classified as either sessile (broad and bulbous) or pedunculated (spurlike). Pedunculated osteochondromas arise on a "stalk" directly from the cortex and at right angles from the affected long bone, leaning toward the diaphysis and away from the epiphysis (Steinbock, 1976). Single osteochondromas may also appear on the ilium and small bones of the hands and feet (Steinbock, 1976). Osteochondromas are usually solitary tumors, but where there are multiple appearances they are classed as hereditary multiple osteochondromas (HMO, below).

Eight possible cases of ostechondroma have been identified in the paleopathological literature (Antikas and Graeaekos, 2010; Walker, 2012a,b; WORD database, 2011). Walker (2012a,b) identified two cases of a single osteochondroma in nonadults from London, the first a 10-year-old from the Roman period and the second a 1.6-year-old from postmedieval London. Both lesions were situated on the medial aspect of the proximal tibia (one right, one left) in the form of an inferiorly pointing spur (Fig. 9.8). An additional case was identified on the fibula of a 16-year-old from St Mary Spital, London (Shapland pers. comm.). A

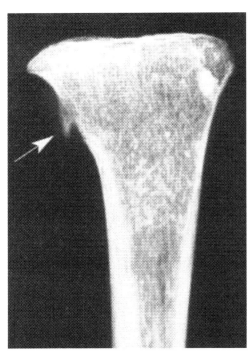

FIGURE 9.8 Pedunculated osteochondroma in a 1.5-year-old from St Mary and St Michael, London (AD 1843–1854, skeleton 349). The radiograph shows a spur of bone at the medial edge of the metaphysis that is continuous with the medullary cavity and is directed towards the diaphysis. *From Walker, D., 2012a. Disease in London, 1st-19th Centuries, Museum of London Archaeology, London, p. 218.*

possible case of sessile osteochondroma is evident on the humerus of a child from later medieval St. Helen-on-the-Walls in York, England (Fig. 9.9). Nerlich and Zink (1995) reported on a possible osteochondroma in the spine of an adolescent from Thebes, Egypt (1500–1000 BC), which had resulted in scoliosis, and Antikas and Graeaekos (2010) identified a raised blastic lesion as an osteochondroma on the scapula of a 9-year-old from Berio, Greece.

Hereditary Multiple Osteochondromas

This condition is also known by a series of other names including: multiple exostoses, diaphyseal aclasis, Bessel-Hagen disease, and osteochondromatosis, but HMO is the favored clinical term. HMO is an autosomal dominant condition caused by a mutation of the exostosis in the genes on chromosome 8 (EXT_1) and chromosome 11 (EXT_2) (Waldron, 2009) and 19 (EXT_3) (Vanhoenacker et al., 2001). It has an incidence of 1 in 50,000 and in 62% of cases is inherited, usually passing from the father to the child (Bovée, 2008). The condition may be present in several generations (Caffey, 1945) but in 10% of cases HMO occurs spontaneously (Patil et al., 2012). Errors in the regulation of chondrocyte proliferation and maturation produce a wide spectrum of skeletal expressions. Individuals may have a shorter stature than their peers, display discrepancies in limb length, suffer wrist subluxation and coxa vara of the femoral neck, have widened distal metaphyses, display short and bowed ulnae, and more rarely, show changes to the small bones of the hands and feet (Clement et al., 2012; Patil et al., 2012; Waldron, 2009). As the name suggests, the most characteristic feature of HMO is the formation of multiple osteochondromas, and it is diagnosed when at least two exostoses are present near the epiphyseal area (Bovée, 2008). These osteochondromas are usually bilateral, symmetrical, and directed away from the nearest joint. They are most common, numerous, and largest at the knee (70%), followed by the humerus (50%) and fibula (30%) (Patil et al., 2012; Vanhoenacker et al., 2001; Waldron, 2009). The skull is not affected (Bovée, 2008). The mean number of osteochondromas can be between 15 and 18 (Bovée, 2008) and exostoses may be asymptomatic, or cause the individual pain (Clement et al., 2012). In rare cases, a pelvic obstruction will cause difficulty in childbirth. Sometimes two sides of the same epiphyseal growth plate will grow unequally causing oblique joint and shortening of the bone (Caffey, 1945). There may also be restricted joint movement and fractures of the bony projections (Bovée, 2008; Patil et al., 2012). Formation of exostoses stops at around 12 years of age with the closing of the growth plates but just like the solitary form, they are potentially malignant (Bovée, 2008; Caffey, 1945). Today the risk of sarcoma is 1%–2%, or up to 8.3% where the condition is familial (Waldron, 2009).

Several cases have reported in the nonadult paleopathological literature. Sjøvold et al. (1974) identified HMO in a full-term fetus from Visby in Gotland found within the abdominal area of a female with the same condition. A 4-year-old from early medieval Winchester, England, has also been identified (Fig. 9.10; Ortner, 2003, p. 519), as have adolescents from Jericho (Lyall and Mann, 1993) and Poland (Gladykowska-Rzeczycka and Urbanowicz, 1970).

Chondromas and Ollier's Disease

Chondromas are tumors of the mature hyaline cartilage that today account for 25% of all benign bone tumors. Chondromas arise endochondrally (an enchondroma) or less frequently, in the periosteum (a juxtacortical chondroma) and usually appear at the metaphyseal zone of the hands and feet. In rare cases they have been reported on the pelvis, sternum, or skull (Khurana and Unni, 2003). Ortner (2003) suggests rickets may have been a predisposing factor in the past, as tumors can occur in fragments of growth cartilage that become detached from the growth plate. The tumor spares the joint surfaces and has a limited external appearance in long bones, but a thin cortical shell may form in the hands and feet that may be perforated. The juxtacortical chondroma can occur on any long bone

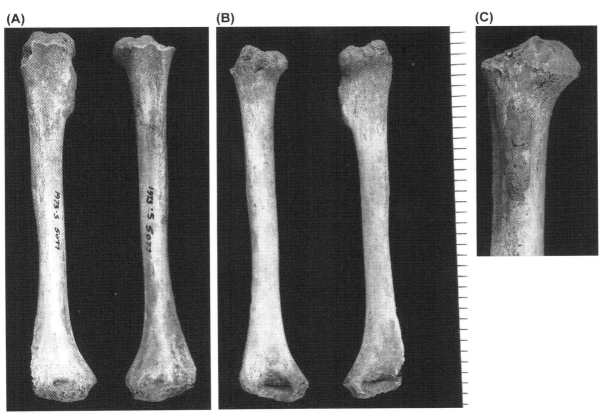

FIGURE 9.9 Sessile osteochondroma in a 5- to 6-year-old from later medieval St Helen-on-the-Walls, York, England (skeleton 5077). The lesion is continuous with the cortical surface and sits below the proximal metaphysis of the right humerus. Viewed from the (A) anterior, (B) posterior, and (C) medial aspects.

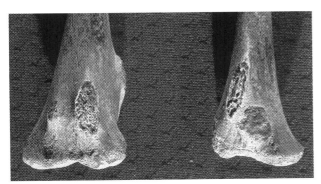

FIGURE 9.10 Possible hereditary multiple osteochondromas in a 3-year-old from Cathedral Green in Winchester, England (Anglo-Saxon, skeleton 932). Exostoses were evident on the anterior and medial aspects of the distal femora (shown), the proximal right femur, and the left ilium. *From Ortner, D., 2003. Identification of Pathological Conditions in Human Skeletal Remains, Academic Press, New York, p. 519.*

at the metaphyseal–diaphyseal border. As they arise from the periosteum they are located on top of the original cortex potentially causing cupping of the area beneath (Ortner, 2003). Enchondromas may cause thinning of the cortex and fractures, particularly of the hands and feet (Khurana and Unni, 2003). Bone cysts, nonossifying fibromas, chondroblastomas, and chondrosarcomas should all be considered among the differential diagnoses.

The development of numerous chondromas (enchondromatosis) in childhood is known as Ollier's disease and normally occurs after the age of 10 years (Khurana and Unni, 2003; Ortner, 2003; Isler and Turcotte, 2003). Lesions form in multiple sites along one side of the skeleton, with the affected bones becoming shortened and deformed (Resnick et al., 2005). Ollier's disease is considered to result from a congenital defect in osseous development, rather than being a true neoplasm (Isler and Turcotte, 2003). In the hands and feet, tumors appear within the bone as unilateral ballooned lesions with a thin cortical shell. Unlike the solitary form, chondromas occur both endochondrally and as numerous smaller chondromas within the periosteum. Large cartilage masses disrupt growth causing uneven elongation and bowing deformities, widened metaphyses, and delayed or incomplete remodeling (Ortner, 2003). The lower extremities are more often affected than upper extremities, and the cranial base and facial skeleton are usually spared. An estimated 25% of people with Ollier's disease will develop malignancy (chondrosarcoma) by the age of 40 years (Isler and Turcotte, 2003).

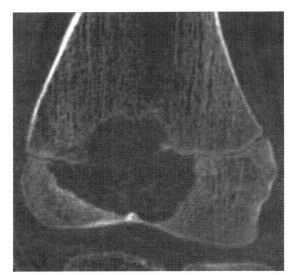

FIGURE 9.11 Clinical case of a chondroblastoma in the distal femur of an adolescent. The lesion penetrates both the epiphysis and metaphysis. *Case courtesy of Dr Angela Byrne, Radiopaedia.org, rID: 8112.*

Chondroblastoma

These epiphyseal tumors represent 5% of all benign bone tumors with 90% occurring in individuals aged 5–25 years old (Resnick et al., 2005). The proximal humerus appears to be the most common area affected, followed by the proximal and distal ends of the femur and proximal tibia (Resnick et al., 2005). Lesions may be latent, active, or aggressive. Latent lesions remain within the bone, whereas active lesions may penetrate the cortex with a surrounding rim of periosteal reaction, and aggressive lesions are fast growing, poorly defined with minimal periosteal reaction (Isler and Turcotte, 2003). On radiograph, the chondroblastoma presents as a radiolucent lesion with a sclerotic border that may extend to the metaphysis (Fig. 9.11).

Chondromyxoid Fibroma

This is a rare benign bone tumor, occurring between the ages of 10 and 30 years, and is twice as common in males as females (Fig. 9.12). The tumor arises in the metaphyseal area of the bone, most commonly in the knee, foot, and pelvis (Isler and Turcotte, 2003). Ten percent of cases present with a pathological fracture at the site. In the foot, chondromyxoid fibromas appear more aggressive and affect the whole of bone, while larger tumors are noted in the pelvis. The tumor presents as a sharp circumscribed lesion, with marginal sclerosis and a thinned cortex, and there may be periosteal reaction. Spicules (coarse and thick trabeculae) forming inside the lesion are a common sign on radiograph (Resnick et al., 2005). The diameter of the lesion is usually 1–10 cm making smaller lesions difficult to distinguish from a chondroblastoma, but other tumors such as a nonossifying fibroma, aneurismal bone cyst, and endochondroma should also be considered (Isler and Turcotte, 2003).

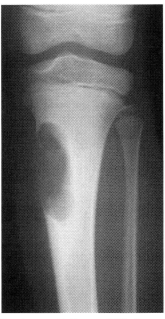

FIGURE 9.12 Chondromyxoid fibroma. Well-circumscribed lytic defect with scalloped, sclerotic margins similar to a metaphyseal fibrous defect. *From chondromyxoid fibroma http://pathologyoutlines.com/wick/chondromyxoid%20fibroma%20tibia%20xray.jpg. Courtesy of Pathology Outlines.com.*

Desmoid Fibroma (Desmoplastic Fibroma)

Desmoid fibromas are rare and slowly progressive soft tissue tumors seen in children and adolescents, with 75% of cases occurring before 30 years (Resnick et al., 2005). Males and females are equally affected. Tumors occur most commonly on the ilium and mandible as an expanding mass arising from the bone. The tumors may result in a pathological fracture although they are generally asymptomatic (Isler and Turcotte, 2003). The tumor is mainly well demarcated and osteolytic with a bubbly pattern and thinned cortex, and coarse thick trabeculae on radiograph (Resnick and Kransdorf, 2005). If the tumor does occur in the long bones it is centrally located and causes large expansion of bone.

Fibrous Cortical Defects

Today up to 35% of all children are said to have a metaphyseal fibrous cortical defect (Khurana and Unni, 2003). They are most common in children aged between 4 and 8 years and are seen predominantly in males (Ortner, 2003). Lesions do not appear before a child can walk and their appearance may be related to the strain exerted on muscles during walking (Waldron, 2009). The majority of lesions are asymptomatic, measure less than 0.5 cm in size, and usually persist for 2 years before healing spontaneously.

The most commonly affected sites are close to the growth plate of the distal femur, followed by the distal tibia, and proximal tibia and fibula (Khurana and Unni, 2003). The defects are always longer than they are wide, symmetrical and multiple, and move away from the metaphyseal area as the bone increases in length (Ortner, 2003).

Anderson (2002) reported metaphyseal fibrous defects in two nonadults from medieval St Faith's Lane in Norwich, England, affecting the distal femur and proximal tibia, respectively. The children were aged between 12–15 and 15–17 years. In the 12- to 15-year-old, there was smooth cystic lesion at the proximal metaphysis of the left femur, about 4 cm above the metaphyseal edge, and 20 mm in length. No swelling or bone reaction was evident although sclerosis was noted on the radiograph. In the 15- to 17-year-old there was an oval smooth-edged lesion on the lateral aspect of the proximal tibia. Again sclerosis was evident on radiograph and the base of the lesion was lobulated suggesting a slow benign process (Fig. 9.13). The size, depth, and base appearance of this lesion may be suggestive of a nonossifying fibroma (see the following section). Anderson (2002) argued that the lack of swelling ruled out cysts, but that it was rare to find two cases of this condition in same site (prevalence of 4.65%). Anderson (2001) also noted one case in the 587 nonadults from St Gregory's Priory, Canterbury (0.17%). Waldron (2007) later suggested a fibrous cortical defect as a likely diagnosis for a 20×10 cm lytic lesion with sclerotic margins in the fibula of an infant from Barton-upon-Humber, England. Djukić et al. (2010) identified a fibrous cortical defect in the distal left femur of a 15- to 17-year-old from Serbia, and there are several other mentions of these lesions in nonadult skeletons within various skeletal reports, although they are rarely illustrated and generally remain unpublished.

Nonossifying Fibroma

In some cases a fibrous cortical defect will give rise to a nonossifying fibroma, an aggressive expanding neoplasm. The lesion is normally unilateral and occurs in older children and adolescents. The lesion will penetrate the medullary cavity but will be separated from it by a scalloped bony shell. Tumors may reach up to 10 cm in length and can result in pathological fractures, although they are normally asymptomatic (Ortner, 2003). The trabeculae within and around the tumor are lobulated described as a "soap-bubble" appearance (Resnick et al., 2005) and on radiograph, the defects appear as "streaklike." Lesions will migrate away from the metaphyseal area as the child grows (Fig. 9.14).

Osteofibrous Dysplasia

Osteofibrous dysplasia is a rare congenital neoplasm that almost exclusively affects a single tibia at the midshaft but may expand to involve the fibula (Hindman et al., 1996). Osteofibrous dysplasia is usually diagnosed in children around 5 years of age. However, Hindman et al. (1996) describe two cases in neonates, one in a 4-week-old and

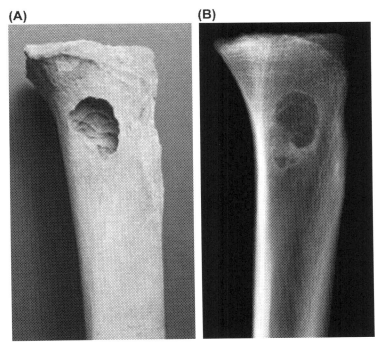

FIGURE 9.13 (A) Lobulated appearance of the cortical defect in the proximal tibia of a 15- to 17-year-old from medieval St Faith's Lane, Norwich (skeleton 98). The radiograph (B) shows a sclerotic margin to the lesion suggestive of a benign tumor. The scalloped base of the lesion may indicate the tumor transformed into a nonossiying fibroma. *From Anderson, T., 2002. Metaphyseal fibrous defects in juveniles from medieval Norwich. International Journal of Osteoarchaeology 12, 146.*

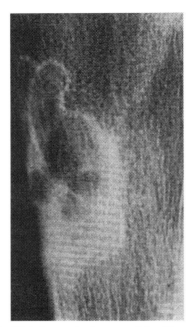

FIGURE 9.14 Clinical example of a nonossifying fibroma in a proximal tibia. *From Resnick, D., Kransdorf, M., 2005. Bone and Joint Imaging. Elsevier Saunders, Philadelphia, p. 1112.*

one in a 17-day-old newborn, both were boys and one case also involved the fibula. The lesion comprises fibrous and osseous tissue and its progressive growth results in intracortical bone destruction, expansion of the outer cortical surface, and subsequent bowing of the diaphysis. The tumor may result in a pathological fracture. On radiograph, there is a hazy "ground-glass" appearance to the lesion, and a "bubble" within a sclerotic margin is evident. The medullary canal may be obliterated (Isler and Turcotte, 2003). Macroscopically, a patch of woven bone is surrounded by a band of lamellar bone (Isler and Turcotte, 2003). An adamantinoma should be considered as a differential diagnosis as it can occur in teenagers and affects the tibia, but it is much rarer (Isler and Turcotte, 2003). The lesion can be confused with a monostotic fibrous dysplasia, but the young age of the individual should aid in differentiation.

BONE CYSTS

Unicameral (Solitary) Bone Cyst

Some describe solitary bone cysts as developmental anomalies rather than of neoplastic origin (Isler and Turcotte, 2003); however, they may give rise to a primary bone tumor (Khurana and Unni, 2003). These are common lesions in children and in individuals under 20 years of age (Khurana and Unni, 2003). The majority of lesions (80%) arise in the metaphyses of the proximal humerus or distal and proximal femur, in close proximity to the growth plate (Isler and Turcotte, 2003; Khurana and Unni, 2003). The epiphysis is always spared. Similar to a fibrous cortical defect, during growth the cyst migrates toward the diaphysis. In life the cyst is filled with a clear or straw-colored fluid (Khurana and Unni, 2003) and presents with pain and stiffness. Enlargement of the cyst causes smooth tapering of the overlying cortex that is gradually replaced by a new shell of cortical bone that may have reinforcing ridges in the inner surface. Pathological fractures that heal well are common (Ortner, 2003).

Lagier et al. (1987) published a possible case of a unicameral bone cyst in the proximal right femur of a 6- to 8-year-old from Vaud, Switzerland. There was a thinned and expanded cortex, with a central cavity and a clear delineation of the original cortex and the lesion (Fig. 9.15).

Aneurismal Bone Cyst

These are less common than unicameral cysts but again can give rise to a primary bone tumor (Khurana and Unni, 2003). These blood-filled bone cysts run in families and occur in individuals between the ages of 5 and 25 years (Khurana and Unni, 2003; Waldron, 2009). Pain and visible swelling is evident at the site. Any bone can be affected but they are most common in the humerus, femur, tibia, or ilium. Again lesions will spare the epiphysis (Ortner, 2003). In the vertebrae, multiple sites can be involved, usually in the posterior arch and spinous process (Khurana and Unni, 2003) of the lumbar, thoracic, and sacral vertebrae (Isler and Turcotte, 2003). In the skull, lesions generally affect the frontal bone (Darsaut et al., 2001). Initially, the aneurismal bone cyst presents as a small lytic lesion that does not expand the bone, however, as it progresses the cyst becomes a "balloon" of thin cortical bone (Khurana and Unni, 2003) that would be susceptible to postmortem damage in archeological contexts. On radiograph, there may be a sclerotic margin to the radiolucent area (Waldron, 2009) but delicate trabeculae are horizontally orientated within and around the lesion (Fig. 9.16; Resnick et al., 2005). In the healing phase, progressive ossification results in a bony mass (Khurana and Unni, 2003). Differentiating this form of lesion, at least in its early stages, from a solitary bone cyst may be challenging, although it tends to occur in many more locations. The delicate nature of the shell means that lytic lesions on the cortex may be the only remnants of the cyst evident postmortem.

LANGERHANS CELL HISTIOCYTOSIS

LCH is one of the most commonly cited conditions in nonadult archeological material. Although it has not been considered a true neoplastic disease since the 1980s, it behaves in a similar way to cancer and children are usually referred to cancer clinics (Broadbent et al., 1994). LCH is a benign condition that occurs when the body produces too many

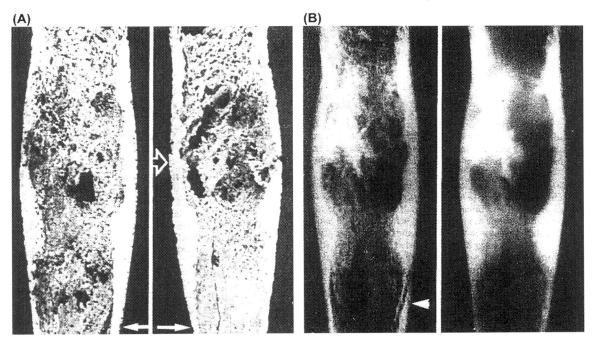

FIGURE 9.15 Possible solitary unicameral bone cyst in the femur of a 6- to 8-year-old from Nyon Clementy, Vaud in Switzerland (5th–7th century, skeleton 38). Seen in transverse section (A) the macroscopic view shows a space occupying lesion in the medullary cavity with an expanded cortex (*black arrow*). On radiograph (B) a clear delineation between the lesion and the original cortex can also be seen (*white arrows*). *From Lagier, R., Kramar, C., Baud, C.A., 1987. Femoral unicameral bone cyst in a medieval child: radiological and pathological study. Pediatric Radiology 17, 498.*

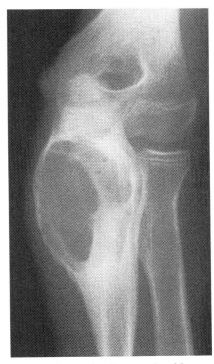

FIGURE 9.16 Clinical example of an aneurismal bone cyst in a proximal ulna. There is expansion of the cortical bone with an intact cortical shell and reactive subperiosteal new bone formation. *From Resnick, D., Kransdorf, M., 2005. Bone and Joint Imaging. Elsevier Saunders, Philadelphia, p. 1113.*

histiocytes known as Langerhans cells. These white blood cells normally help fight infection, but they buildup in the body causing granulomatous destruction of bone and organ damage (Resnick and Kransdorf, 2005; Steinbock, 1976). LCH was originally described as three separate conditions: eosinophilic granuloma, Hand–Schüller–Christian disease, and Letterer–Siwe disease, but when it was recognized that they were all variations in the severity of a single disease, they were joined under the single term "histiocytosis X" (Lichtenstein, 1953). Final recognition of abnormal histiocytes as Langerhans cells led to a change in the name (Broadbent et al., 1994). In the older paleopathological literature, eosinophilic granuloma and histiocytosis X are common terms used to describe the condition.

LCH can occur between the ages of 1 and 60 years but has a peak between 5 and 10 years (Isler and Turcotte, 2003) and has an incidence of 3–4 per 1,000,000 (Broadbent et al., 1994). Males are affected twice as commonly as females. As the three original classifications suggest, the disease has a wide spectrum of presentation. In the very young, LCH causes multiple organ failure and is fatal (Broadbent et al., 1994). In other cases there may be serious involvement of the brain, pituitary system, lungs or heart, or there may be spontaneous resolution (Resnick and Kransdorf, 2005). The majority of deaths result from pulmonary disease (Sims, 1977), while involvement of the pituitary system can lead to severely retarded growth. Mastoiditis and otitis media

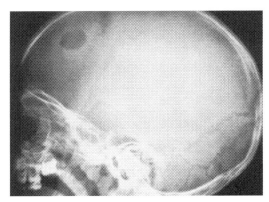

FIGURE 9.17 Clinical radiograph of the cranium of a 2.5-year-old with Langerhans cell histiocytosis. There is a lytic lesion in the frontal bone with sharply outlined borders and a "punched-out" appearance. Uneven involvement of the inner and outer tables results in a beveled lesion. *From http://radiologykey.com/round-cell-lesions/.*

can be present resulting in deafness and damage to the ear ossicles (Broadbent et al., 1994). LCH is known as the "great imitator" of bone tumors (Isler and Turcotte, 2003, p. 739), especially in children under 12 years of age who have large punched-out lesions in the skull (Fig. 9.17; Isler and Turcotte, 2003). If the cortex of the long bone is destroyed by a lesion within the medullary cavity, secondary periosteal new bone may occur leading to confusion with Ewing's sarcoma or osteomyelitis (Steinbock, 1976). Other differential diagnoses should include leukemia, and when there is spinal involvement, Pott's disease of tuberculosis. In skeletal remains, it may be possible to differentiate between the three forms (severities) of the condition.

Eosinophilic Granuloma

This is the most common form of LCH occurring in 70% of all cases with death rare after early childhood. It is characterized by a solitary and purely lytic lesion usually located in cranial vault (Isler and Turcotte, 2003). The lesion has a beveled edge and unequal destruction of the inner and outer tables, causing a "hole within a hole" appearance of the lesion on flat bones (Fig. 9.18; Resnick and Kransdorf, 2005, pp. 674–675). In the long bones, epiphyseal lesions can occur and cross the open physeal plate. When the mandible is involved, a radiolucent area may make the teeth appear to be "floating" on radiograph. In Sims' (1977) study of 29 children with solitary lesions, the majority affected the frontal bone, followed by the lumbar spine and the humerus, although solitary lesions have been described in almost every bone of the skeleton (Fowles and Bobechko, 1970). When the vertebrae are affected, lesions are focused on the vertebral body and may cause collapse. Asymmetrical collapse creates a wedge-shaped vertebra, whereas anterior collapse will cause local kyphosis, without fusion (Robert et al., 1987). The lesion may be located only in the posterior

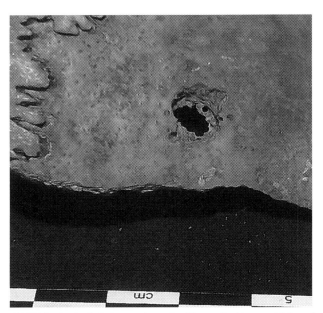

FIGURE 9.18 Lytic lesion on the parietal bone of a 10-year-old from St Mary Spital, London (AD 1200–1250, skeleton 31,254). The lesion is beveled with a wider ectocranial margin. This type of lesion is consistent with cranial lesions associated with an eosinophilic granuloma in Langerhans cell histiocytosis. *Photograph taken by F. Shapland, with the kind permission of the Museum of London.*

arch, especially in the cervical spine, and simultaneous involvement of the arch and body is rare. If collapse occurs in younger children, initial kyphosis may become corrected if the child survives (Robert et al., 1987). In their study of 28 children displaying vertebral lesions from France during 1970 to 1985, Robert et al. (1987) observed the thoracic vertebrae were affected in the majority of cases (51.1%), followed by the lumbar (26.5%), and the cervical vertebrae (22.4%). In the long bones the lesion begins in the medullary cavity of the diaphysis, it usually has an ill-defined edge and the cortex is eroded and expanded with some lamination and new bone formation. In the femur, the lesion will spread distally to a considerable degree but will not affect the femoral neck (Fowles and Bobechko, 1970). Children who initially present with solitary lesions consistent with eosinophilic granuloma may develop the more widespread lesions of Hand–Schüller–Christian disease 1–2 years later (Sims, 1977).

Hand–Schüller–Christian Disease

This form of the disease is characterized by large multiple confluent lesions in the skull, spine, and long bones that are purely lytic and that occur sequentially over several years. It is a chronic disease with periodic bouts of illness affecting the bone, the middle ear and the skin causing diabetes, mastoiditis, and dermatitis. Today, this form of the disease is fatal in 10%–30% of cases, while in others it will slowly regress (Resnick and Kransdorf,

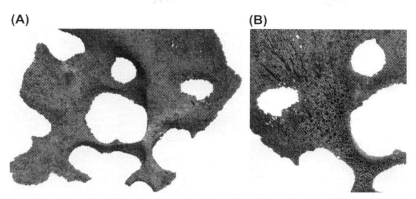

FIGURE 9.19 Possible Letterer–Siwe disease in a 36-week-old perinate from Cross Bones, London (AD c. 1850, Skeleton 125). Large lytic lesions with defined margins are evident on the (A) endocranial and (B) ectocranial surfaces of all surviving cranial bones. *From Walker, D., 2012a. Disease in London, 1st-19th Centuries, Museum of London Archaeology, London, p. 262.*

2005). It affects children between ages of 3 and 12 years (Isler and Turcotte, 2003) but is most common in those under 5 years.

Letterer–Siwe Disease

Making up around 10% of all cases, this is the most serious manifestation of the disease, in which granulomatous lesions are widely disseminated in the hard and soft tissues (Steinbock, 1976). There are multiple skull lesions, involving the sphenoid and facial bones, but hands and feet are usually spared. Seen primarily in children less than 3 years of age it is fatal with most individuals dying within 1–2 years (Resnick and Kransdorf, 2005). Walker (2012a,b) identified a probable case of LCH in the skull of a 36-week-old from postmedieval Cross Bones in London (Fig. 9.19). The young age of this child makes the fatal Letterer–Siwe form most likely. Only the skull survives, displaying large lytic lesions with some reactive new bone formation, perhaps as the result of secondary hemorrhaging.

At least 16 cases of LCH have been identified in nonadult skeletons (Steinbock, 1976; Campillo, 1977; Morse, 1978; Strouhal, 1976–1977; Gregg et al., 1982; Williams, 1993; Hargreaves and MacLeod, 1994; Nerlich and Zink, 1995; Barnes and Ortner, 1997; Mays and Nerlich, 1997; Oxenham et al., 2005; Spiegelman et al., 2006; Einwögerer and Teschler-Nicola, 2008; Vidal, 2010; Walker, 2012a,b; Colombo et al., 2015). Steinbock (1976) reinterprets a case first presented by Williams et al. (1941) as a multiple myeloma, in a 10-year-old dating from 13th-century Rochester, New York. The child displayed "punched-out" lesions of 3–10 mm in diameter on the cranial vault, mandible, ribs, vertebrae, pelvis, and scapula. Barnes and Ortner (1997) present a case in a 12- to 14-year-old from medieval Corinth, Greece. The adolescent had multifocal coalescing lesions, 1–2 cm in size and limited to skull. They also noted a healing trepanation on the right parietal that may have been carried out to treat the individual. The long

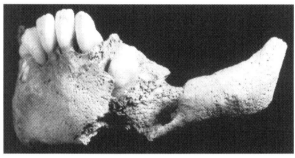

FIGURE 9.20 Possible Langerhans cell histiocytosis. Lytic lesion in the left mandibular body of an 8-year-old from Wharram Percy, England (skeleton NA135). The destruction of the supporting alveolar structure has left the developing canine "floating" in the jaw. *From Mays, S., Nerlich, A., 1997. A possible case of Langerhans' cell histiocytosis in a medieval child from an English cemetery. Journal of Palaeopathology 9 (2), 75.*

slender bones of the adolescent suggests they had associated paralysis. Williams (1993) reported on a younger possible case from Wilson Mounds, Minnesota, on the basis of an infant cranium with multiple round and elliptical lytic lesions that in some cases involved both skull plates. Mays and Nerlich (1997) published a possible case in an 8-year-old from Wharram Percy, England. Here the mandible showed large remodeled lytic lesions (Fig. 9.20). On radiograph the lesions were sharply defined and lacked sclerosis. While the histology was inconclusive, the authors ruled out tuberculosis osteomyelitis due to a lack of reactive new bone formation. The difficulty in distinguishing this condition from infections such as tuberculosis was also highlighted in the skeleton of a young child from Vác, Hungary. Punched out lytic lesions were found throughout the skeleton, but the child also tested positive for aDNA tuberculosis. Although miliary tuberculosis may have been responsible for the lesions, the authors attributed them to LCH based on their radiographic appearance. They conclude that the depressed immune system characteristic of the disease may have predisposed the child to TB (Spiegelman et al., 2006).

MALIGNANT PRIMARY TUMORS

Malignant primary tumors in children are rare (Isler and Turcotte, 2003). Waldron (2009, p. 185) suggests primary metastatic tumors can arise in the ovaries as early as 6 years, the uterus from 8 years, the colon and rectum between 6 and 11 years, the bladder at 13 years, the mouth by 14 years, and the stomach between 2 and 18 years. However, these tumors rarely metastasis to bone and so are unlikely to be identified in the archeological record. Children with neuroblastoma have a 70% chance of presenting with metastatic skeletal disease with spinal involvement causing destructive lesions and periosteal reaction (Isler and Turcotte, 2003). Rhabdomyosarcoma is a common soft tissue malignancy in children that will cause spinal involvement in 40% of cases, and may result in collapse of the spine.

Osteosarcoma (Osteogenic Sarcoma)

An osteosarcoma is the most common malignant form of neoplasm in people between the ages of 10 and 25 years (Steinbock, 1976) and is characterized as the abnormal production of osteoid by malignant cells (Resnick et al., 2005). Osteosarcomas can occur secondary to osteogenesis imperfecta, Paget's disease, a bone infarct, chronic osteomyelitis, fibrous dysplasia, a giant-cell tumor, bilateral retinoblastomas, or an osteoblastoma, and there is some suggestion that they may also arise from traumatic calluses or hematomas (Khurana and Unni, 2003). In individuals under 25 years, 80% of all lesions occur in the long bones, especially the knee (50%–70%), femur (40%), proximal humerus (15%), or tibia (16%) (Resnick et al., 2005). Glass and Fraumeni (1970) noted that children who developed sarcomas were taller than their peers, and that as very actively growing bones are prone to lesions, they argued this explained the common predilection for the femur in adolescent tumors. Osteosarcomas of the mandible and flat bones of the skull and pelvis occur at an older age than at other locations (Khurana and Unni, 2003). The precise location of the tumor may be medullary (or central), cortical, surface, periosteal, or parosteal (at the outer layer of the periosteum). Tumors may be single or multifocal, and despite their name may also be chondroblastic or fibroblastic among others (Resnick et al., 2005).

The primary site for the tumor is the metaphysis, with the epiphysis having only rare secondary involvement. Lesions metastasize into other bones via ligament attachments (Khurana and Unni, 2003; Steinbock, 1976; Isler and Turcotte, 2003). The appearance of these tumors varies widely. They may be completely lytic or mostly sclerotic but are usually both lytic and blastic. The tumor destroys the trabeculae and cortex as it quickly spreads leaving as indistinct margin. In life, the tumor contains large amounts of osteoid and may stimulate secondary periosteal new bone as it elevates the periosteum. This periosteal reaction is usually in the form of several layers resulting in an "onion-peel" appearance (Steinbock, 1976). If new bone occurs along the vascular channels that remain attached to the cortex and periosteum, a "sunburst" pattern can occur (Steinbock, 1976). In archeological material, these fast growing tumors may be very large, measuring up to 20 cm, as they will have run their natural course uninhibited by radiation therapy, chemotherapy, or amputation (Steinbock, 1976). The osteosarcoma is distinctive and other tumors that may mimic its appearance, such as a chondrosarcoma or fibrosarcoma, are less common in children. A solitary fibrous dysplasia may also been confused with an osteosarcoma, but the lesions are smaller and much better defined. By contrast, Ewing's sarcoma has both the sunburst and onion-peel appearance of the osteosarcoma and occurs in a similar age group so should always be considered as a differential diagnosis (Steinbock, 1976).

Alt et al. (2002) described a case of an osteosarcoma in the right proximal femoral metaphysis of an 8- to 10-year-old from medieval Germany. On radiograph, the tumor is isolated from the original cortex and has affected an area below the osseous mass. Codman's triangles are present on the diaphysis suggesting the cortex had been breached. The "chessboard-like" appearance of the tumor histologically suggested the presence of osteoid, bone, and cartilage within the mass, confirming a diagnosis of osteosarcoma (Fig. 9.21). The presence of osteoid differentiated it from a chondrosarcoma. Alt et al. (2002) suggest possible exposure to lead from the lead–silver mine may have caused the cancer, with lead lines found on radiographs of other nonadult bones. Uhlig (cited in Alt et al., 1982) had diagnosed an osteosarcoma in a 16- to 18-year-old "warrior" from early medieval Germany located at the distal metaphysis of the femur. Czarnetzki and Pusch (2000) also report the case of an osteosarcoma in a 12- to 14-year-old from Minden, Germany, affecting the distal right humerus and proximal ulna. A pear-shaped tumor is evident arising from the diaphysis of the humerus. On radiograph, the tumor was isolated from the original cortex, but there was no Codman's triangle. The authors suggest the tumor arose in the humerus and extended to the ulna via the periosteum which then sustained a pathological fracture. The left mandibular ramus had new bone formation and there was a possible lytic lesion on the base of the ramus and on the mandibular fossa. Czarnetzki and Pusch (2000) argue that the presence of spiculation and the older age of the individual negate a Ewing's sarcoma or chondrosarcoma.

Ewing's Sarcoma

This small, round-cell tumor is another common and aggressive tumor in children (Isler and Turcotte, 2003).

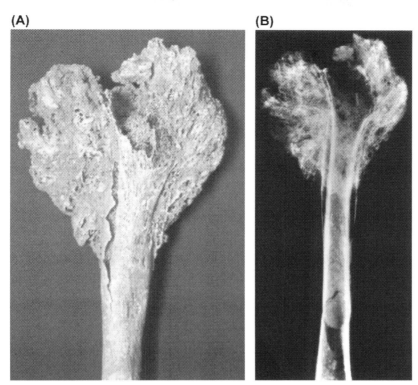

FIGURE 9.21 Osteosarcoma on the proximal right femur of an 8-year-old from Sulzberg, Germany (12th-century AD, skeleton 71). (A) A large tumor has formed at the proximal metaphysis and would have extended into the soft tissue. (B) On radiograph the predominantly blastic tumor is superimposed onto the original cortex. The location of the tumor at the femoral metaphysis and age of the child make osteosarcoma the most likely diagnosis. *From Alt, K., Alder, C., Buitrago-Tellez, C., Lohrke, B., 2002. Infant osteosarcoma. International Journal of Osteoarchaeology 12, 443–444.*

It has a peak prevalence at 10–20 years (Steinbock, 1976), with 90% of those affected being between the ages of 5 and 30 years (Resnick et al., 2005). It affects males twice as commonly as females and is rare in black and Asian populations (Isler and Turcotte, 2003; Glass and Fraumeni, 1970). Ewing's sarcomas arise in the nonhematopoietic elements of the medullary cavity from immature mesenchymal round cells (Isler and Turcotte, 2003; Ortner, 2003; Steinbock, 1976). Tumors can appear in any bone, but lesions in the pelvis, femur, humerus, and ribs are most common, especially in children where the bones are predominantly occupied by red bone marrow. The epiphyses are rarely affected. Metastasis from the original site is estimated to occur in 30% of cases (Isler and Turcotte, 2003) and results in "punched-out" lesions, particularly in the flat bones of the skull and pelvis. At the diaphyseal midshaft the tumor is usually centrally located, while its position varies in the metaphysis (Steinbock, 1976). On radiograph there may be a mottled appearance to the cortex and medullary cavity as the tumor causes ischemia of the affected bone, until it occupies the space. As the tumor extends, the periosteum is elevated causing lesions similar sunburst and onion-skin lesions of the osteosarcoma. The absence of massive destruction and involvement of the long axis should raise suspicions of a Ewing's sarcoma (Ortner, 2003). Osteomyelitis should be considered as a differential diagnosis.

No clear cases of Ewing's sarcoma have been identified in the archeological record, although Waldron (2007) describes a possible round-cell tumor in the left tibia of a 13- to 15-year-old from Barton-on-Humber, England. There was a thick layer of woven bone interrupted by an active lytic lesion passing through the new cortical layer penetrating the original surface.

Chordoma

These rare low grade malignant tumors arise from the embryonic notochord along the axial skeleton where they expand and destroy bone. They occur most commonly in adults but are recognized in children between 8 and 12 years, with a peak at 10 years, and have been described in infants (Habrand et al., 2016). Chordomas follow a more aggressive course in childhood (Coffin et al., 1993). They have a particular predilection for the extremities of the spine, and the clivus at the base of the cranium (Khurana and Unni, 2003). These tumors may form part of a differential diagnosis for tuberculosis in children.

NON-HODGKIN'S LYMPHOMA

Lymphomas are a series of neoplasms grouped into two main categories: Hodgkin's lymphoma and malignant lymphoma. Today, non-Hodgkin's lymphoma is one of the most common forms of metastatic cancer in children (Ward et al., 2014). Tumors arise in the lymph nodes, spleen and gut, with abdominal masses, fever, night sweats, and weight loss common symptoms (Resnick and Kransdorf, 2005). Non-Hodgkin's lymphoma affects the skeleton in 20%–30% of child cases depending on its grade of severity (Resnick and Kransdorf, 2005). The axial skeleton is most commonly affected, with lesions occurring in the spine, pelvis, ribs, and facial bones, with the long bones involved through hematogenous spread or via the lymph nodes. Lesions may be single or multiple and have a moth-eaten appearance, with some sclerosis and periosteal reaction (Waldron, 2009). Non-Hodgkin's lymphoma is similar to Ewing's sarcoma in that it displays permeative lytic changes but may be identified through an atypical location for Ewing's. Differential diagnoses should also include LCH and leukemia (Isler and Turcotte, 2003).

REFERENCES

Alt, K., Alder, C., Buitrago-Tellez, C., Lohrke, B., 2002. Infant osteosarcoma. International Journal of Osteoarchaeology 12, 442–448.

Anderson, T., 2001. The human remains. In: Hicks, M., Hicks, A. (Eds.), St Gregory's Priory, Northgate, Canterbury Excavations 1988-1991. Canterbury Archaeological Trust, Canterbury, pp. 338–370.

Anderson, T., 2002. Metaphyseal fibrous defects in juveniles from medieval Norwich. International Journal of Osteoarchaeology 12, 144–148.

Antikas, T., Graeaekos, I., 2010. Scapular lesions in a juvenile of the 3rd c. CE from Northern Greece. Paleopathology Newletter 149, 19–20.

Aufderheide, A.C., Rodriguez-Martín, C., 1998. The Cambridge Encyclopedia of Human Paleopathology. Cambridge University Press, Cambridge.

Barnes, E., Ortner, D., 1997. Multifocal eosinophilic granuloma with a possible trepanation in a fourteenth century Greek young individual. International Journal of Osteoarchaeology 7, 542–547.

Bovée, J., 2008. Multiple osteochondromas. Orphanet Journal of Rare Diseases 3 (3), 1–7.

Broadbent, V., Egeler, R., Nesbit Jr., M., 1994. Langerhans cell histiocytosis–clinical and epidemiological aspects. The British Journal of Cancer Supplement 23, S11.

Broders, A.C., 1925. The grading of carcinoma. Minnosota Medicine 8, 726–730.

Buka, I., 2009. Children and cancer. In: Organization W.H. (Ed.), WHO Training Package for the Health Sector.

Caffey, J., 1945. Pediatric X-Ray Diagnosis. Year Book Medical Publishers, Inc., Chicago.

Campillo, D., 1977. Paleopatología del cráneo en Cataluña, Levante y Baleares. Montbanc-Martín, Barcelona.

Cappell, D.F., Anderson, J.R., 1971. Muir's Textbook of Pathology. Edward Arnold, London.

Clement, N., Duckworth, A., Baker, A., Porter, D., 2012. Skeletal growth patterns in hereditary multiple exostoses: a natural history. Journal of Pediatric Orthopaedics B 21 (2), 150–154.

Coffin, C., Swanson, P.E., Wick, M., Dehner, L., 1993. Chordoma in childhood and adolescence. A clinicopathologic analysis of 12 cases. Archives of Pathology & Laboratory Medicine 117 (9), 927–933.

Colombo, A., Saint-Pierre, C., Naji, S., Panuel, M., Coqueugniot, H., Dutour, O., 2015. Langerhans cell histiocytosis or tuberculosis in a medieval child (Oppidum de la Granède, Millau, France 10th–11th centuries AD). Tuberculosis 95, S42–S50.

Czarnetzki, A., Pusch, C., 2000. Identification of sarcomas in two burials of the 9th century in Western Germany. Journal of Paleopathology 12 (3), 47–62.

Darsaut, T., Lanzino, G., Lopes, M., Newman, S., 2001. An introductory overview of orbital tumours. Neurosurgical Focus 10, 1–9.

De Boer, H., Van der Merwe, A., Maat, G., 2013. The diagnostic value of microscopy in dry bone palaeopathology: a review. International Journal of Paleopathology 3 (2), 113–121.

Djukić, M., Janović, A., Milnovanović, P., Djukić, K., Milenković, P., Drašković, M., Roksandic, M., 2010. Adolescent health in medieval Serbia: signs of infectious diseases and risk of trauma. HOMO-Journal of Comparative Human Biology 61, 130–149.

Edeiken, J., Hodes, P.J., Caplan, L.H., 1966. New bone production and periosteal reaction. American Journal of Roentgenology 97 (3), 708–718.

Einwögerer, T., Teschler-Nicola, M., 2008. Barred from the common? A case of Langerhans cell histiocytosis among early Bronze Age storage pit burial in Ziersdorf, lower Austria. In: 7th European Meeting of the Paleopathology Association, Copenhagen, Denmark, pp. 25–27.

Fowles, J., Bobechko, W., 1970. Solitary eosinophilic granuloma in bone. The Journal of Bone and Joint Surgery 52B (2), 238–243.

Fox, S.C., 2004. The case studies of Paphos, Cyprus and Corinth, Greece. In: King, H. (Ed.), Health in Antiquity. Routledge, London, pp. 59–82.

Gladykowska-Rzeczycka, J.J., Urbanowicz, M., 1970. Multiple osseous exostoses of the skeleton from a prehistoric cemetery of a former population of Pruszcz Gdanski. Folia Morphologica 29 (3), 284–296.

Glass, A., Fraumeni, J., 1970. Epidemiology of bone cancer in children. Journal of the National Cancer Institute 44 (1), 187–199.

Gregg, J., Steele, J., Bass, W., 1982. Unusual osteolytic defects in ancient South Dakota skulls. American Journal of Physical Anthropology 58, 243–254.

Habrand, J.-L., Datchary, J., Bolle, S., Beaudré, A., de Marzi, L., Beccaria, K., Stefan, D., Grill, J., Dendale, R., 2016. Chordoma in children: case-report and review of literature. Reports of Practical Oncology & Radiotherapy 21 (1), 1–7.

Hargreaves, A., MacLeod, R., 1994. Did Edward V suffer from histiocytosis X? Journal of the Royal Society of Medicine 87, 98–101.

Hindman, B., Bell, S., Russo, T., Zuppan, C., 1996. Neonatal osteofibrous dysplasia: report of two cases. Pediatric Radiology 26, 303–306.

Isler, M., Turcotte, R., 2003. Bone tumors in children. In: Glorieux, F., Pettifor, J., Jüppner, M. (Eds.), Pediatric Bone: Biology and Diseases. Academic Press, New York, pp. 703–743.

Jaffe, H., 1958. Tumors and Tumorous Conditions of the Bones and Joints. Lea & Fibiger, Philadelphia, pp. 298–303.

Khurana, J., Unni, K., 2003. Pathological diagnosis of common tumours of bone and cartilage. In: Yuehuei, H., Martin, K. (Eds.), Handbook of Histology Methods for Bone and Cartilage. Humana Press, New Jersey, pp. 447–494.

Lagier, R., Kramar, C., Baud, C.A., 1987. Femoral unicameral bone cyst in a medieval child: radiological and pathological study. Pediatric Radiology 17, 498–500.

Lichtenstein, L., 1953. Histiocytosis X. Integration of eosinophilic granuloma of bone, "Letterer-Siwe disease" and "Schuller-Christian disease" as related manifestations of a single nosologic entity. AMA Archives of Pathology 56, 84–102.

Lyall, H., Mann, G., 1993. Diaphyseal aclasis in citizens of ancient Jericho. International Journal of Osteoarchaeology 3, 233–240.

Mays, S., Nerlich, A., 1997. A possible case of Langerhans' cell histiocytosis in a medieval child from an English cemetery. Journal of Palaeopathology 9 (2), 73–81.

Morse, D., 1978. Ancient Disease in the Midwest. Illinois State Museum, Springfield.

Nerlich, A., Zink, A., 1995. Evidence of Langerhans cell histiocytosis in an infant of a late Roman cemetery. Journal of Paleopathology 7 (2), 119.

Ortner, D., 2003. Identification of Pathological Conditions in Human Skeletal Remains. Academic Press, New York.

Oxenham, M., Kim Thuy, N., Lan Cuong, N., 2005. Skeletal evidence for the emergence of infectious disease in Bronze and Iron Age northern Vietnam. American Journal of Physical Anthropology 126 (4), 359–377.

Patil, K., Patil, M., Khemka, A., 2012. Osteochondromatosis: a rare clinical condition. Journal of the Scientific Society 39 (1), 40–41.

Ragsdale, B., 1993. Polymorphic fibro-osseous lesions of bone: an almost site-specific diagnostic problem of the proximal femur. Human Pathology 24 (5), 505–512.

Resnick, D., Kransdorf, M., 2005. Bone and Joint Imaging. Elsevier Saunders, Philadelphia.

Resnick, D., Kyriakos, M., Greenway, G., 2005. Bone and joint imaging. In: Resnick, D., Kransdorf, M. (Eds.), Bone and Joint Imaging. Elsevier Saunders, Philadelphia, pp. 1120–1198.

Robert, H., Dubousset, J., Miladi, L., 1987. Histiocytosis X in the juvenile spine. Spine 12 (2), 167–172.

Roberts, C.A., Manchester, K., 2007. The Archaeology of Disease. Cornell: Cornell University Press.

Sims, D., 1977. Histiocytosis X. Follow-up of 43 cases. Archives of Diseases in Childhood 52, 433–440.

Sjøvold, T., Swedborg, I., Diener, L., 1974. A pregnant woman from the Middle Ages with exostosis multiplex. Ossa 1, 3–23.

Spiegelman, M., Pap, I., Donogue, H., 2006. A death from Langerhans cell histiocytosis and tuberculosis in 18th century Hungary – what palaeopathology can tell us today. Leukemia 20, 740–742.

Steinbock, R.T., 1976. Paleopathological Diagnosis and Interpretation: bone diseases in ancient human populations. Charles C Thomas, Illinois.

Strouhal, E., 1976–1977. Two cases of polytopic osteolytic lesions in the pyramid age Egyptians. OSSA 3/4, 11–52.

Strouhal, E., 1994. Malignant tumours in the Old World. Paleopathology Newsletter No. 85 (Suppl.), 1–2.

Uhlig, C., 1982. Zur palaopathologischen Differentialdiagnose von Tumoren an Skeletteilen. Reichert, Stuttgart.

Vanhoenacker, F., Van Hul, W., Wuyts, W., Willems, P., De Schepper, A., 2001. Hereditary multiple exostoses: from genetics to clinical syndrome and complications. European Journal of Radiology 40, 208–217.

Vidal, P., 2010. About a medieval case of Langerhans cell histiocytosis. XVIII European Meeting of the Paleopathology Association, Copenhagen, Denmark, p. 133.

Waldron, T., 2007. St Peter's, Barton-upon-Humber, Lincolnshire, Vol 2. The Human Remains. Oxbow Books, Oxford.

Waldron, T., 2009. Palaeopathology. Cambridge University Press, Cambridge.

Walker, D., 2012a. Disease in London, 1st-19th Centuries. Museum of London Archaeology, London.

Walker, D., 2012b. St Mary Spital in context. In: Connell, B., Gray Jones, A., Redfern, R., Walker, R. (Eds.), A Bioarchaeological Study of Medieval Burials on the Site of St Mary Spital. Museum of London Archaeology, London, pp. 149–194.

Ward, E., DeSantis, C., Robbins, A., Kohler, B., Jemal, A., 2014. Childhood and adolescent cancer statistics, 2014. CA: A Cancer Journal for Clinicians 64 (2), 83–103.

Williams, J., 1993. Possible histiocytosis X in a plains Woodland burial. American Journal of Physical Anthropology Supplement 16, 208–209.

Williams, G., Ritchie, W., Titterington, P., 1941. Multiple bony lesions suggesting myeloma in a Pre-Columbian Indian aged ten years. American Journal of Roentgenology 46, 351–355.

WORD database, 2011. Wellcome Osteological Research Database (WORD). Museum of London, London.

Chapter 10

Juvenile Arthropathies, Circulatory, and Endocrine Disorders

Chapter Outline

Juvenile Idiopathic Arthritis	245
Systemic Arthritis	247
Seronegative Idiopathic Arthritis	248
Juvenile-Onset Adult-Type Rheumatoid Arthritis	249
Juvenile-Onset Ankylosing Spondylitis	250
Juvenile Psoriatic Arthritis	250
Hemophilic Arthritis	252
Schmorl's Nodes	252
Circulatory Disorders	252
Osteochondroses	252
Osgood-Schlatter Disease	254
Blount's Disease (Tibia Vara)	255
Legg–Calvé–Perthes' Disease	255
Scheuermann's Disease (Juvenile kyphosis, Spinal Osteochondrosis)	256
Endocrine Disturbances	258
Hypopituitarism (Pituitary Dwarfism)	259
Hyperpituitarism (Pituitary Gigantism, Acromegaly)	259
Hypothyroidism (Myxedema)	260
Hyperthyroidism (Thyrotoxicosis)	261
Cushing's Disease	261
Hypogonadism	261
Hypergonadism	262
Hypoparathyroidism	262
Hyperparathyroidism	262
References	263

JUVENILE IDIOPATHIC ARTHRITIS

Juvenile idiopathic arthritis (JIA) is a broad term encompassing a clinically heterogeneous group of chronic arthropathies that occur before 16 years of age and may become asymptomatic in adulthood. This group includes systemic arthritis, seronegative idiopathic arthritis, seropositive juvenile-onset adult-type rheumatoid arthritis (JORA), juvenile-onset ankylosing spondylitis (JOAS), and psoriatic arthritis. JORA should be distinguished from juvenile rheumatoid arthritis (JRA), a term that was used to encompass all of the above before JIA was adopted (Ortner, 2003; Resnick and Kransdorf, 2005). Today, the prevalence of JIA is high and reported in 16–150 per 100,000 individuals, although this is probably an underestimate (Ravelli and Martini, 2007). While girls are considered to be more susceptible than boys (Berntson et al., 2003), much of the epidemiological work has been carried out in Nordic countries and data for other populations are limited. JIA is classified in the clinical literature as inflammation of the joints causing pain, tenderness and limited movement that persists for more than 6 weeks (Ravelli and Martini, 2007). Still (1896) was the first to recognize JIA as a condition that had unique characteristics and a different progression to adult forms of arthritis. The childhood form includes additional clinical features such as spleen and lymph enlargement, a fever and a rash, symptoms that together are termed "Still's disease." Not all individuals with Still's disease will develop arthritis, but all children with persistent joint lesions are recognized as suffering from Still's disease, no matter what the form of arthritis is (Rothschild et al., 1997). Children with JIA demonstrate immune system involvement with a characteristic inflammatory response. Regulating these are cytokines or polypeptide mediators. Interleukins are the cytokines responsible for cell growth, and in JIA activation of these interleukins is both proinflammatory and antiinflammatory causing persistent inflammation. JIA has both autoimmune and inflammatory responses and is thought to be caused by a complex interaction of multiple genetic and environmental factors (Woo, 1998; Cobb et al., 2014).

Juvenile idiopathic arthropathies appear in early childhood with a second peak shortly before puberty. The severity of the disease relies on several parameters including sex and the age of onset, with onset before 5 years potentially life-threatening. As well as being more commonly affected, females suffer the most debilitating forms of the disease (Ravelli and Martini, 2007). Skeletal lesions are similar to those seen in the adult condition, but a third of cases involve the cervical spine, which is higher than in adults. These changes include fusion of the articular facets and vertebral bodies, hypoplasia, and possible fusion of the atlas with the axis that can mimic Klippel–Feil syndrome. Scoliosis may also occur. Joint erosions and loss of articular space (on clinical radiograph) are later manifestations in children; instead they display metaphyseal radiolucency, subperiosteal new bone formation, bony ankylosis, compression fractures of the epiphyses, subluxation and dislocation of the joints, and growth disturbances (Resnick and Kransdorf, 2005). Although any joint can be affected, involvement of the hand, wrist, foot, knee, hip, neck, mandible, and temporomandibular joint (TMJ) are most common (Resnick and Kransdorf, 2005, p. 256). If the child is young when the disease develops, chronic inflammation causes hyperemia and increased vascularization resulting in overgrowth of the affected bone in comparison to the unaffected side. If the child is nearing the end of the maturity, then the epiphyses may fuse prematurely causing the affected bone to be shorter (Bernstein et al., 1977). In addition to limb length discrepancy, persistence of the disease for more than 5 years can result in disuse atrophy and ankylosis of the carpals and tarsals (Resnick and Kransdorf, 2005). JIA has also been shown to cause delayed puberty (Umlawska and Prusek-Dudkiewicz, 2010), and this may be as the result of the prolonged presence of proinflammatory interleukins causing inhibition of the pituitary growth hormone (Tsatsoulis et al., 1999).

The involvement of the TMJ occurs in 11% of clinical cases. Lesions include joint surface erosion, decreased bone density, and collapse of the condyle (flattening). These changes may be bilateral or unilateral. TMJ lesions may be established by 8 years of age; and as changes are seen in the absence of modern corticosteroid treatment (Pearson and Rönning, 1996), they would be expected in archeological cases of the disease. Involvement may cause micrognathia due to flattened TMJ and shortened rami. In advanced cases, the TMJ may fuse (Guyuron, 1988) causing disuse atrophy and a receding chin, known as "bird-face" deformity. There may also be exaggerated antegonial notching (the concavity on the inferior mandibular body adjacent to the gonial angle), forward sloping of the mandibular symphysis, and reduced height of the maxilla. Retrognathism of the mandible is reported to be more pronounced in females, with ramus height and mandibular body measurements consistently shorter in females (Sidiropoulou-Chatzigianni et al., 2014).

Paleopathology has the potential to extend our knowledge of the antiquity of juvenile arthropathies. JIA was only recognized as a clinical condition in 1810, although Thomas Phaer writing in 1545 refers to "stiffness of the lymes" after exposure to the cold in his *The Boke of Chyldren* that may be a reference to the disease (cited in Schaller, 2005). The earliest artistic example is Botticelli's 1483 "Portrait of a Youth," although arguments revolve around whether such portraits are true representations of pathology or mere artistic convention (Yeap, 2009). Art historians point to several other paintings that may illustrate that JIA has a long history, including Caravaggio's painting of 1608, *Il Amore Dormiente* ("the sleeping cupid"), showing ulna deviation and swelling of the left hand, micrognathia, puffiness of the face, and a protruded abdomen suggestive of Still's disease. While these interpretations are controversial, the lack of similar characteristics in these artists' other paintings suggest they were at pains to emphasize these deformities in their models (Fig. 10.1; Yeap, 2009). Given the high occurrence of JIA in more recent populations, we may expect a number of cases in the archeological record; however, these are limited, and diagnosis relies on a complex pattern of lesions that may not be present in every case (Table 10.1). Ortner (2003, p. 568) cautions that given the complexity of the lesions, and issues of poor preservation, it may only be possible to describe the lesions of JIA by nature of their distribution, i.e., as polyarticular or monoarticular, rather than identifying a specific subtype.

Ortner and Utermohle (1981), Ortner (2003, pp. 566–568), Hawkey (1998), and Walker (2012, pp. 174–175) suggest JIA for the lesions seen in adult individuals from Kodiak Island, Alaska (AD 1200); Puye and Gran Quivira, New Mexico (AD 1550–1672), and London (AD 1200–1250) respectively, based on the severity of changes in these young adults, and the concentration of lesions in the major and minor joints.

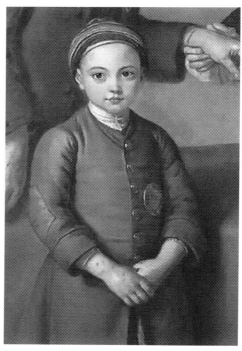

FIGURE 10.1 Detail of a child with a rash and swollen hands considered to be an example of juvenile arthropathy. From William Hoare's (AD 1707–92) "Dr Oliver and Mr Pierce, the First Physician and Surgeon Examining Patients Afflicted with Paralysis, Rheumatism and Leprosy." This painting hangs in the Royal National Hospital for Rheumatic Diseases, London. Royal United Hospital NHS Foundation.

The skeletons from New Mexico show the most extreme changes including ballooning of the metaphyses in the Puye individual (Ortner, 2003, pp. 568–570), which may suggest hemophilia (see below). In nonadults, the first and earliest case of JIA was reported by Buikstra et al. (1990) who describe lesions in a 12- to 15-year-old from Peru in South America (AD 900–1050). The child was found buried in the traditional way for the region, in a seated and flexed position within an unlined cylindrical tomb. Examination of the bones suggested the child was possibly female. She displayed bilateral degeneration of her joints and had a small face and teeth, dental enamel hypoplasia, and porotic hyperostosis. The joints affected included the TMJ, shoulder, elbow, and wrists, with degeneration of the atlanto–occipital and C1–C2 joints, and underdevelopment of the vertebral bodies. The femoral heads were flattened and eburnated, and the carpals distorted. Long bone lengths were short and similar to that of a 7- to 9-year-old. There were signs of disuse atrophy of the legs and feet, with the left thigh appearing to have been habitually flexed and rotated medially, leaving the child in a permanently seated position (Fig. 10.2).

Garralda and Herrerín (2003) described a case of probable JIA in a 16- to 17 year-old female from Soria, Spain, buried between the 17th and 18th century. The individual displayed subchondral cysts, erosions of the radial head, cervical vertebrae and sacrum, premature epiphyseal fusion and smooth ankylosis of the elbow joint bilaterally, fusion of the right shoulder, congenital dislocation of the right acetabulum, deformation of the radial and femoral heads, and generalized osteopenia. They concluded that the right leg and left arm would have been immobile. The absence of the mandible, hand, and foot bones prevented a distinction between JIA and JORA being made, the latter more commonly affecting the hands. The authors suggest that the extensive disability suffered by the adolescent may explain their burial in the poorer section of the cemetery.

Systemic Arthritis

This form is unlikely to be identified in the archeological record as joint lesions are rare (Resnick and Kransdorf, 2005, p. 256). It has its onset in children under 5 years of age, and death occurs in 5%–8% of cases due to macrophage activation syndrome causing sustained fever, hemorrhage, liver, and renal failure (amyloidosis) (Ravelli and Martini, 2007).

TABLE 10.1 Skeletal Lesions Associated With Juvenile Idiopathic Arthritis

Location	Abnormality
Mandible	Underdevelopment of the jaw (bird face), shortening of the body and ascending rami, widened mandibular notch, flattened condyles, joint erosion.
Cervical spine	Most commonly affected area of the spine. Fusion of the atlas and axis, vertebral body ankylosis, erosion of the odontoid process, ankylosis of apophyseal joints, and/or spinous processes of C2–C3, decreased vertebral height.
Thoracic and lumbar spine	Direct involvement rare. May be compression fractures as the result of osteopenia and scoliosis due to limb length discrepancy.
Arm	Degenerative changes of the shoulder, short ulna relative to radius, ulnar deviation, bowed radius, enlarged radial head.
Hand, foot, wrist, and ankle	Short and broad MCs, MTs, and phalanges (brachydactyly); ankylosis of MCP, MTP, or IP joints; severe flexion deformities, erosion, or ankylosis of carpals and tarsals; periostitis (especially in seronegative form), osteoporosis, tilting of the distal tibial epiphysis. Hands more commonly affected in JORA.
Hip	Impaired iliac bone development, coxa valga, premature fusion of the femoral head, osseous erosions, protruding acetabulum, osteophytosis.
Knee	Ballooned distal femoral and proximal tibia epiphyses, squaring of the patella, flattened femoral condyles, wide intercondylar notch.
Joints	Symmetrical involvement of more than four joints (polyarticular). Joint erosion more common in JORA form.
Long bones	Translucent metaphyseal bands (active) or Harris lines (healed).

IP, interphalangeal; *JORA*, juvenile-onset adult-type rheumatoid arthritis; *MCP*, metacarpophalangeal; *MCs*, metacarpals; *MTP*, metatarsophalangeal; *MTs*, metatarsals. Compiled from Rothschild, B., Hershkovitz, I., Bedford, L., Latimer, B., Dutour, O., Rothschild, C., Jellema, L., 1997. Identification of childhood arthritis in archaeological material: juvenile rheumatoid arthritis versus juvenile spondyloarthropathy. Amerian Journal of Physical Anthropology 102, 249–264 and Resnick, D., Kransdorf, M., 2005. Bone and Joint Imaging. Elsevier Saunders, Philadelphia.

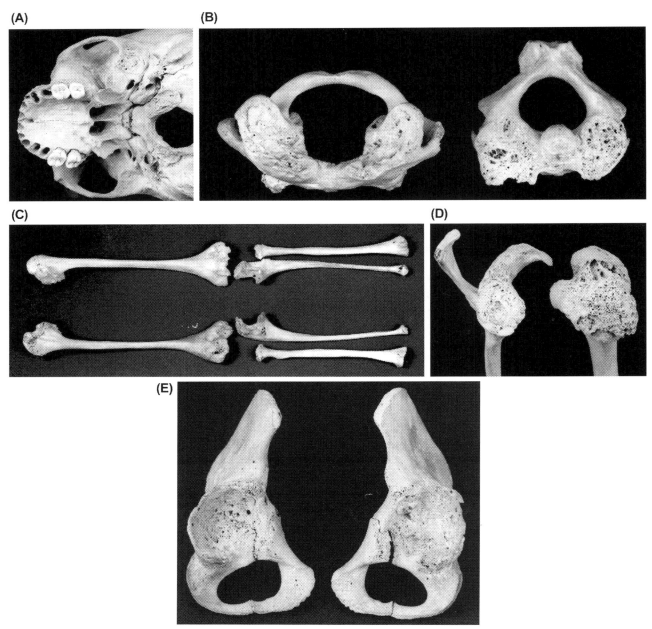

FIGURE 10.2 Juvenile idiopathic arthritis in a 12- to 15-year-old from Peru (AD 900–1050, skeleton omo M11-2030). Detail of arthritic lesions in the (A) temporomandibular and atlanto–occipital joints; (B) atlas and axis; (C) elbows; (D) shoulders; and (E) hips. *From Buikstra, J., Poznanski, A., Cerna, M., Goldstein, P., Hioshower, L. 1990. A case of juvenile rheumatoid arthritis from pre-Colombian Peru. In: Buikstra, J. (Ed.), A Life Science Papers in Honor of J Lawrence Angel. United States, Central American Archaeology, pp. 99–137. Courtesy of the Center for American Archeology, Kampsville.*

Seronegative Idiopathic Arthritis

Seronegative idiopathic arthritis is the most common form of JIA (70% cases) and has three variants depending on the number of joints affected and age of onset: monoarticular (affecting one joint), oligoarticular (2–3 joints), and polyarticular (4+ joints). Arthritis of fewer than four joints is the most common pattern, making up 30%–70% of the seronegative cases. Monoarticular involvement may develop into the polyarticular form after 2 years, and a diagnosis of tuberculosis, trauma, brucellosis, and syphilis should be considered before JIA, when only one joint is affected (Bywaters and Ansell, 1965; Al-Matar et al., 2002). Oligoarthritis is divided into two types. Type I occurs in children under 7 years of age and is more common in girls, often leading to severe visual impairment as the result of eye inflammation (iridocyclitis) (Ravelli and Martini, 2007). Type II is more common in boys over the age of 5 years and usually affects the knees, ankles, and in some cases, the sacroiliac joint (Resnick and Kransdorf, 2005, p. 258). In 20% of cases, seronegative idiopathic arthritis occurs in polyarticular form. This affects males and females of all ages.

The extent and severity of changes seen in a child with seronegative idiopathic arthritis is related to the variant they develop. Cervical spine involvement is an early manifestation and is characteristically the only part of the spine affected. In the hands and feet there is symmetrical involvement with flexing deformities of the fingers at the proximal interphalangeal (IP) joints and periostitis. There may be malformation and ankylosis of the carpals and shortening of the ulna in comparison with the radius, resulting in ulnar deviation of the hand. Changes to the foot and ankle are similar to the hands, with other deformities including hammertoe, pes cavus, hindfoot varus, or valgus (Resnick and Kransdorf, 2005, p. 256). Due to accelerated epiphyseal maturation, phalanges of the hand and foot may be shorter and broader than normal (Resnick and Kransdorf, 2005). Reduced long bone length as the result of premature epiphyseal fusion may also occur, with ballooned or enlarged epiphyses in relation to the diaphysis. In the knee, there is enlargement of the epiphyses, osteoporosis, flattening of the femoral condyles, widening of the intercondylar notch, as well as squaring of the patella due to flattening of the inferior aspect. In 35%–45% of patients the hip is involved, with premature fusion of the femoral head, coxa valga, hypoplasia of the iliac bones, and a protruding acetabulum (where the socket protrudes into the pelvis) common in older children. Juxta-articular and diffuse osteoporosis may be evident at the knee and hip joints, although this will take time to develop with 41% of untreated children showing low bone mass after 11 years. Those who develop the condition closer to complete maturity are less likely to develop osteopenia (Lien et al., 2003). Osteoporosis may lead to secondary compression fractures of the epiphyseal, diaphyseal, or metaphyseal regions of tubular bones or vertebral compression fractures (Resnick and Kransdorf, 2005, p. 258). Translucent metaphyseal bands, similar to those seen in leukemia may be present and will eventually heal to mimic Harris lines. Unlike rheumatoid arthritis, joint erosions are not common in seronegative idiopathic arthritis or are a later manifestation. Whereas periostitis is common in the seronegative form of arthritis it is less common in JORA. Similar to the adult form of the disease, there may be calcification of the joint capsule beyond the margin of the joint in JIA.

Juvenile-Onset Adult-Type Rheumatoid Arthritis

In adults, rheumatoid arthritis typically develops between 25 and 55 years of age (Ortner, 2003). However, this seropositive form of JIA, or JORA, makes up 10% of modern clinical juvenile cases. It is more common in girls than in boys with a ratio of 3:1 and usually occurs after the age of 10 years. JORA is usually divided into two forms: polyarticular (4+ joints) and oligoarticular (fewer than 4 joints), with polyarticular involvement more common in the first decade of life. Around 50% of children with the oligoarticular expression progress to polyarticular involvement after 6 months (Al-Matar et al., 2002). The disease is characterized by synovial hyperplasia and cartilage destruction, with the small bones of the hands and feet more commonly affected than in the adult form (Fig. 10.3). Hand and foot involvement is interphalangeal and metacarpophalangeal or metatarsophalangeal. The knees, wrists, ankles, and cervical vertebrae are also affected (Rothschild et al., 1997) with subcutaneous cysts present at the elbow in 10%–20% cases (Resnick and Kransdorf, 2005). Osteoporosis, premature epiphyseal fusion, and in advanced stages, joint erosions are also evident. Extensive subperiosteal new bone formation may occur on the hands and feet but is more common in seronegative JIA.

Oligoarticular arthritis may indicate the presence of psoriatic arthritis, while polyarticular changes may occur prior to the development of chronic bowel disease or Lyme's disease in children (Resnick and Kransdorf, 2005). When considering a diagnosis, Reiter's syndrome, which may also affect children, should be considered. In addition, periarticular osteoporosis, apparent overgrowth of the epiphyses, premature epiphyseal closure, and bone atrophy are all features found in neuromuscular disorders such as cerebral palsy, poliomyelitis and muscular dystrophy, and in hemophilia. Therefore, the need to identify joint erosions in the diagnosis of JORA is essential (Richardson et al., 1984).

The first clinical description of rheumatoid arthritis was made in 1800 by Landré-Beauvais (Snorrason, 1952). Since then debate has surrounded the evolution and antiquity of the disease. The identification of clear paleopathological cases is central to this debate (Leden et al., 1988). Hawkey's (1998) description of likely JORA in an adult skeleton from New Mexico provides a detailed hypothetical progression of the disease from late childhood until their death aged 30–40 years. A similar case is described by Campillo (1990) in an adult female from 3rd to 5th century, Tarragona, Spain. Child cases are rare. Rothschild et al. (1997) described extensive changes in a 7-year-old girl from the Hamann–Todd collection in the United States, diagnosed during the 1930s with JORA. The child demonstrates enlarged ankle, hip and knee joints, and a permanently flexed left leg with severe atrophy. The child was of short stature with diaphyseal lengths suggesting an age of 4 years. The ilia were atrophied with subperiosteal new bone formation. Premature epiphyseal fusion of both elbows and wrists resulted in shortened arms, and the humeral and femoral heads were flattened and eroded. The most severe spinal lesions were of the cervical vertebrae, which exhibited erosive destruction of the facets and fusion of the spinous processes of C2–C3 and C7–T1. Erosive lesions were also evident on the

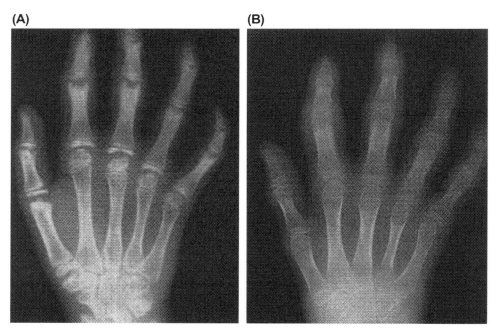

FIGURE 10.3 Clinical example of rheumatoid arthritis in the hand; (A) with epiphyseal compression fractures and lytic lesions at the metacarpophalangeal and proximal interphalangeal joints as the result of osteoporotic bone. (B) Still's disease showing osteoporosis at the metacarpophalangeal and interphalangeal joints and periosteal new bone formation on the phalanges. *From Resnick, D., Kransdorf, M., 2005. Bone and Joint Imaging. Elsevier Saunders, Philadelphia, p. 261.*

carpus, which had fused, and the TMJ. Dental development was normal (Fig. 10.4). Based on this case, Rothschild et al. (1997) set out the following diagnostic criteria for JORA:

- Peripheral articular marginal subchondral erosions
- Apophyseal and sacroiliac erosions
- Fusion of cervical apophyseal joints or peripheral joints
- Premature epiphyseal fusion
- Shortened long bones
- Short mandibular rami
- Osteopenia

Distinguishing JORA from other forms of inflammatory rheumatic diseases such as ankylosing spondylitis is challenging, although a lack of involvement of the hands and feet in that latter may aid diagnosis (Rothschild et al., 1997).

Juvenile-Onset Ankylosing Spondylitis

Ankylosing spondylitis is a form of enthesis-related arthritis causing spondyloarthropathy and is among a group of inflammatory rheumatic disease. It occurs five times more often in boys than girls (Ansell, 1978; Ravelli and Martini, 2007). JOAS may occur in the presence of the human leukocyte antigen (HLA-B27) a histocompatibility antigen. The mean age of onset is 10–12 years, although the range includes 3–15 years (Ansell, 1978). In the spine there is ankylosis and sclerosis of the vertebral corners and squaring of the vertebral anterior surface, with syndesmophytes (bony outgrowths arising within ligaments) and apophyseal joint fusion. Atlantoaxial subluxation has also been reported (Resnick and Kransdorf, 2005). The spinal lesions appear to spread symmetrically as syndesmophytes extending from the sacroiliac joint through to the lumbar, thoracic, and cervical spine. However, making a diagnosis in younger individuals may be problematic as these characteristic spinal changes are usually delayed until the early 20s, and sacroiliitis can take up to 5 years to develop (Ansell, 1978). To date, no nonadult cases of JOAS have been identified.

Juvenile Psoriatic Arthritis

In living individuals, the presence of psoriatic skin lesions and pitted nails aids in the diagnosis of psoriatic arthritis. It is rare in children but can occur between 9 and 10 years of age (Ansell, 1978). The clinical mechanisms behind the juvenile form of this disease are still not understood (Ravelli and Martini, 2007). Asymmetry of joint involvement is characteristic, and the condition is prone to remission and exacerbation. Dactylitis and involvement of both small and large joints is characteristic, as is the risk of iridocyclitis (Ravelli and Martini, 2007) causing light phobia and decreased vision. Distinguishing this disease from other forms of JIA in the skeleton is challenging.

Juvenile Arthropathies, Circulatory, and Endocrine Disorders Chapter | 10 251

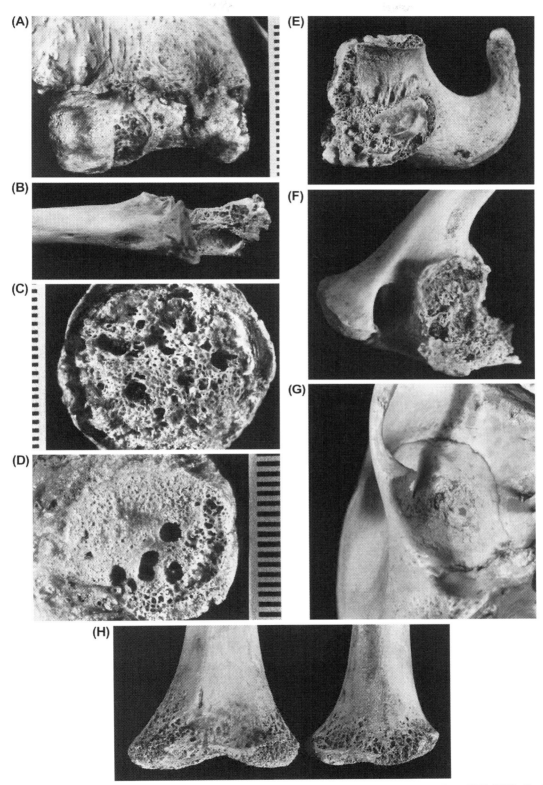

FIGURE 10.4 Juvenile-onset rheumatoid arthritis in a 7-year-old from the Hamann–Todd collection (AD 1930; skeleton HTC, 2039). Erosive lesions are evident on the (A) distal humerus; (B) ulna; (C) proximal femur; (D) patella; (E) acetabulum; (F) cervical vertebra facets; and (G) the temporomandibular joint. Premature epiphyseal fusion resulted in shortened arms and legs, and (H) the left femur was atrophied. The femoral metaphyseal aspects were also abnormally porous. *From Rothschild, B., Hershkovitz, I., Bedford, L., Latimer, B., Dutour, O., Rothschild, C., Jellema, L., 1997. Identification of childhood arthritis in archaeological material: juvenile rheumatoid arthritis versus juvenile spondyloarthropathy. Amerian Journal of Physical Anthropology 102, 253–260.*

Hemophilic Arthritis

Hemophilia is an X-linked recessive congenital disorder characterized by suppressed blood coagulation. The disease affects males almost exclusively but is carried by the mother (Jaganathan et al., 2011). The main characteristic of the disease is repeated bleeding into the joint capsule. This is a more frequent complication in children than adults, probably due to their greater activity levels and subsequent trauma to the joints. Bleeding into the soft tissues and under the periosteum is less common (Jaganathan et al., 2011). Chronic hemoarthrosis causes lesions similar to JIA including osteopenia, overgrowth, epiphyseal enlargement, premature epiphyseal fusion, subluxation, and periostitis (Rodriguez-Merchan, 1996). It affects the knees, ankles, elbows, shoulders, and hips, in that order. Unlike other forms of JIA, changes are rare in the hands and feet, and it does not tend to affect the spine. Similar to the seronegative juvenile arthropathies subchondral cysts and bone erosions appear only in the later stages (Jaganathan et al., 2011). In chronic hemoarthrosis, 1%–2% individuals will develop well-defined large expensive lytic lesions adjacent to the joint, particularly in the femur, ilium, tibia, and small bones of the hand. These hemophilic pseudotumors can mimic neoplasms (Resnick and Kransdorf, 2005, p. 703; Jaganathan et al., 2011). Thickened trabeculae may extend across the lytic lesion, and there may be endosteal scalloping, cortical thinning, and subperiosteal new bone formation as the lesion expands as the result of continued bleeding into the area (Jaganathan et al., 2011). Pseudotumors may be multiple causing severe deformation of the bone and leaving it vulnerable to pathological fractures and secondary infections. Hemophilia is not fatal, provided steps are taken to stem any bleeding, and so there is potential for cases to have existed in the past. Hence, hemophilia should be considered as a possible cause of arthritis, especially in the presence of cysts within the bone or as a differential diagnosis for a giant-cell tumor in the presence of arthropathy.

Lewis (1998) described a possible case of JIA, suggested to be the result of Lyme's disease, in an adolescent from precontact Louisiana (Fig. 10.5). The skeleton was extremely gracile, with underdeveloped muscle attachments, and widened fused joints in comparison to thinned diaphyses, eburnation of the radius, and flexion of the knee, which was suggested by a deep groove in the corresponding patella. Erosive lesions were minimal and changes to the hands, feet, and mandible were not described. A radiograph revealed a well-defined lytic lesion within the shaft of the humerus with a clear sclerotic margin, attributed to osteomyelitis by the author (Fig. 10.5E). This lesion is similar to the pseudotumor of hemoarthritis, suggesting hemophilia as an alternative diagnosis.

Schmorl's Nodes

Schmorl's nodes are common, often asymptomatic depressions caused by herniation of the nucleus pulposus on the superior and inferior surfaces of the vertebral bodies (Mattei and Rehman, 2014). The prevalence of Schmorl's nodes is reported as being from 5% to 76% in archeological samples (Waldron, 2009). Their etiology is complex, and there is a likely hereditary component, although spinal trauma caused by vigorous activity, and flexion and extension of the spine is most often associated with their formation (Kyere et al., 2012). While most commonly associated with degenerative disc disease, the age of their occurrence is not clear, and clinically they generally appear before the age of 18 years (Resnick, 1995). Some studies have also suggested a link between the early appearance of these lesions and Scheuermann's disease (juvenile kyphosis) (Mattei and Rehman, 2014). Plomp et al. (2012) argue that males are more susceptible to these lesions due to the size and shape of their vertebrae. The pathophysiology of a node's development suggests a relationship with abnormal vertebral vessel development, perhaps due to the persistence of fetal blood vessels that feed the endplate in utero, which when they finally disappear result in an avascular intervertebral disc (Mattei and Rehman, 2014). The persistence of these vessels weakens the endplate resulting in herniation of the nucleus pulposus. Others suggest a circulatory disorder as an etiological factor (Resnick, 1995).

Given the potential for a hereditary or developmental etiology of these lesions, the presence of Schmorl's nodes should be recorded in a nonadult sample. Although not the focus of any paleopathological study so far, Lewis (2016) reported Schmorl's nodes in 1.1% (n = 8/732) of English medieval urban children aged 10–13 years, rising to 7.8% (n = 58/736) in both urban and rural children by 14–16 years (Fig. 10.6).

CIRCULATORY DISORDERS

Osteochondroses

All conditions described under the heading of osteochondroses share a common theme: (1) they all affect young individuals in the first decade of life; (2) they normally affect males; (3) they involve fragmentation and sclerosis of the epiphyseal or apophyseal center; and (4) they often involve reossification. The most commonly reported osteochondroses in nonadult paleopathology discussed here, are Osgood–Schlatter and Blount's disease of the tibia, Legg–Calvé–Perthes disease of the femoral head, and Scheuermann's disease of the spine. Many of these conditions have been found to have a traumatic origin and may cause bone necrosis (death) (Resnick and Kransdorf, 2005, p. 1089), where a reduction or loss of the blood supply causes irreversible damage to the

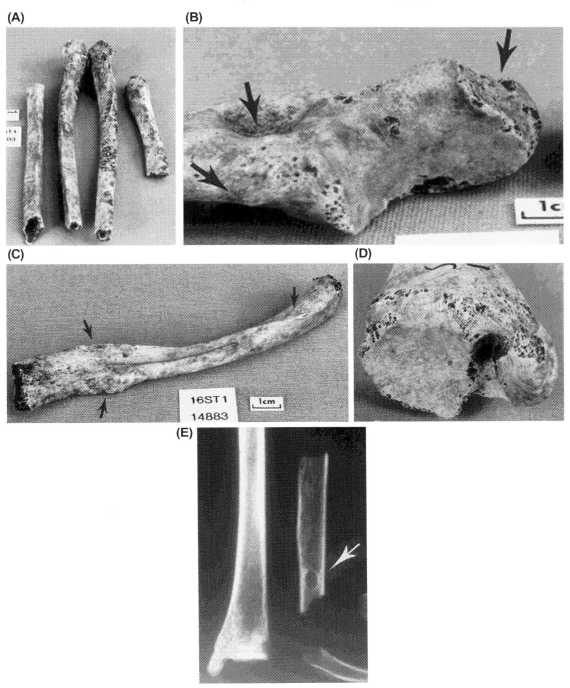

FIGURE 10.5 Possible juvenile idiopathic arthritis in an 18-year-old from the Tchefuncte group in Louisiana, USA (2000 BP, skeleton 16ST1-14,883b). There is (A) a diminished interosseous margin and bowing of the left and right radius and ulna; (B) a reduced attachment for musculus triceps brachii on the olecranon process of the ulna and a cavitation at the usual location of the supinator crest; (C) the clavicle is gracile with reduced attachments for the deltoid; and the (D) distal right radius has a cavitation adjacent to the medial malleolus. (E) A sharply delineated cyst with a sclerotic margin is evident on the radiograph of the humerus (*arrow*). *From Lewis, B., 1998. Prehistoric juvenile rheumatoid arthritis in a Precontact Louisiana Native population reconsidered. American Journal of Physical Anthropology 106, 231–235.*

254 Paleopathology of Children

FIGURE 10.6 Schmorl's nodes. (A) Smooth-based, shallow Schmorl's nodes in a 14-year-old from Romano–British Poundbury Camp in Dorset, England (Skeleton 1168) compared to (B) deeper impressions on the thoracic vertebrae of a 17-year-old from St Mary Spital in London (AD 1250–1400, Skeleton 31,404). *Photographed with the kind permission of (A) the Natural History Museum, London, and (B) the Museum of London.*

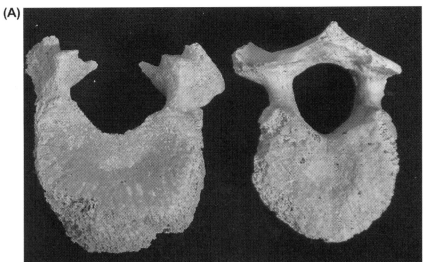

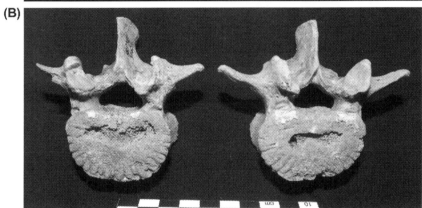

bone cells. A complete loss of oxygen will then cause necrosis in 12–28 hours (Sweet and Madewell, 1995). In clinical practice, "ischemic necrosis" usually refers to circulatory disruption to the epiphysis and subchondral bone, while an "infarct" refers to loss of circulation to the metaphysis or diaphysis (Sweet and Madewell, 1995).

Osgood-Schlatter Disease

Osgood-Schlatter (OS) lesions are defined as avulsions of the unfused tibial tuberosity (or apophysis) where fragments of bone are torn away from the anterior surface of the proximal tibia. It was first described by Paget and Goodhart (1885), and then it was defined independently by Osgood (1903) and Schlatter (1903). Originally classified as a circulatory disorder, the blood supply of the tibia is now considered normal, and the etiology is thought to be the result of multiple small avulsion fractures caused by repetitive strain at the attachment for the quadriceps (Maher and Ilgen, 2013). This muscle acts to extend the knee. There may also be lesions on the apex of the patella suggesting additional trauma to the patellar ligament (Resnick and Kransdorf, 2005, p. 1099). Pain is gradual but can persist for around 2 years and is aggravated by running, jumping, kneeling, squatting, and climbing. The patient presents with a localized swelling at the insertion of the patella ligament (Sponseller and Stanitski, 2001). Today, 25%–30% of these lesions are bilateral (Resnick and Kransdorf, 2005, p. 1098; Gholve et al., 2007).

The lesion usually occurs in boys between the ages of 11 and 15 years and between 8 and 12 years of age. This pattern is directly related to strenuous activity that coincides with the development of the tibial tuberosity (Gholve et al., 2007). The tibial tuberosity is both part of, and distinct from, the ossification center of the proximal tibial epiphysis. The tubercle initially forms as a separate epiphysis on the anterior aspect of the shaft (known as the "apophyseal stage"), and it is at this point that it is most vulnerable to avulsion. The proximal epiphysis and tuberosity finally unite around 14 years in girls and 16.5 years in boys (Scheuer and Black, 2000, p. 408). Later in the development of the epiphysis, OS lesions may still occur, but they are rare. After avulsion the bone fragments will continue to ossify and enlarge merging together to either become a "separate persistent ossicle" or reunite with the underlying tibia and evident only as mild enlargement (Gholve et al., 2007; Resnick and Kransdorf, 2005, p. 1099). These lesions should be differentiated from acute fractures of the tibial tuberosity as unlike acute trauma, OS lesions are not associated with a specific incident, and sufferers are still able to stand and walk after injury (Sponseller and Stanitski, 2001). In OS, there is no separation of the growth plate from the metaphysis. However, preexisting OS lesions have been associated with later physeal fractures that cause separation of the entire tubercle (Ogden, 2006). Individuals with cerebral palsy are also vulnerable to developing the lesion (Sponseller and Stanitski, 2001).

The only published cases of OS from archeological contexts are in adults (Wells, 1968; DiGangi et al., 2010), although they do provide indirect evidence for trauma during adolescence. In theory, the separate ossicle should be recoverable archeologically, although no such discovery has ever been published; and in dry bone, OS is normally identified as a rough rectangular depression at the site of the tuberosity (Wells, 1968). If the fragment reunites, changes may be more subtle with the tubercle on the affected side more prominent when compared to the normal opposite side (Sponseller and Stanitski, 2001). In nonadult remains we are unlikely to be able to determine whether the separate epiphysis that makes up the tubercle is missing as the result of OS or because this unfused fragment was not excavated. After 14–16 years, an intact proximal tibial epiphysis with an undeveloped tubercle extension should be discernible.

Blount's Disease (Tibia Vara)

Resulting from aseptic necrosis of the medial tibial condyle, Blount's disease can develop in infancy and adolescence. Infantile Blount's disease is usually bilateral (50%–75%) (Caffey, 1945). It occurs five times more frequently than the adolescent type, between the ages of 1 and 3 years and can heal spontaneously (Resnick and Kransdorf, 2005). There may be prominent bowing deformity or a slightly shortened leg. The infantile type is likely to lead to the greatest deformity (Resnick and Kransdorf, 2005). In the adolescent form (8–15 years), the tibia is affected unilaterally. Necrosis results in a depression of the medial aspect of the epiphysis causing the joint surface to become sloped (at 10–20 degrees) as the direction of medial growth changes its orientation. There is subsequent lateral bowing of the shaft (Fig. 10.7; Caffey, 1945). The deformed medial condyle that has a "beaklike" extension and there is medial wedging of the tibial epiphysis (Resnick and Kransdorf, 2005).

Lagier et al. (1991) suggested Blount's disease as a diagnosis for the severe shortening of the tibia and sloping of the proximal articular surface in a 17-year-old male from early medieval Switzerland (Fig. 10.8). To date, no other nonadult cases have been identified in the published literature.

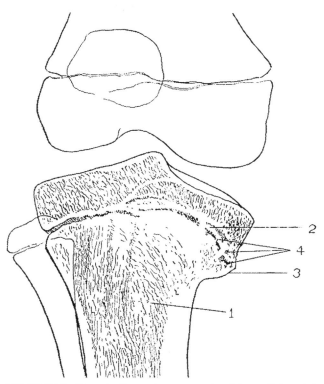

FIGURE 10.7 Blount's disease due to necrosis of the medial condyle of the tibia; (1) the shaft is bowed laterally; (2) the medial aspect of the epiphyses is depressed; (3) a "beaklike" medial projection of the condyle is formed; and (4) radiolucent areas evident on radiograph indicate necrotic bone and islands of growth plate. *From Caffey, J., 1945. Pediatric X-Ray Diagnosis, Year Book Medical Publishers, Inc., Chicago, p. 658.*

Legg–Calvé–Perthes' Disease

Caused by idiopathic avascular necrosis of the femoral neck and proximal epiphysis, Legg-Calvé-Perthes' disease usually appears between the ages of 4 and 8 years. Boys are four times more likely to be affected than girls. It has a modern occurrence of 1 in 1200 children (Waldron, 2009). The condition is usually unilateral but may be bilateral in 10%–20% of cases and a family history is noted in 6% of cases (Resnick and Kransdorf, 2005).

There are four progressive stages to the condition (Caffey, 1945):

1. Onset of avascular necrosis
2. Fragmentation of the femoral head
3. Revascularization and regeneration
4. Healing

Necrosis begins at the neck extending into the head, with the dome of the head the last location to be affected. This destruction phase persists for around 18 months, with the cycle of necrosis and regeneration occurring over 4 years (Caffey, 1945). While some cases may heal without deformity, in other cases there may be lateral displacement of the epiphysis and a fractured fragment; shortening and widening of the

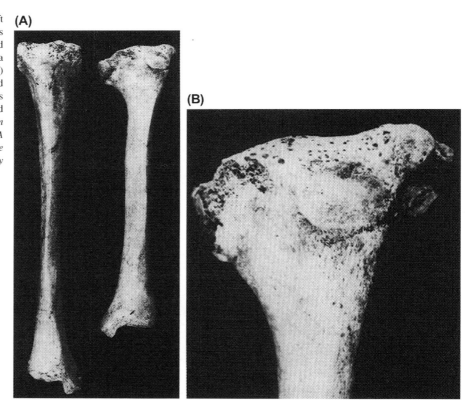

FIGURE 10.8 Blount's disease of the left tibia in a 16- to 17-year-old from the Clos d'Aubonne Necropolis in Vaud, Switzerland (5th to 9th century AD). (A) The left tibia is 5.5 cm shorter than the right, and the (B) proximal articular surface is severely sloped toward the medial aspect with an osseous projection. The left fibula was also affected measuring 3.8 cm shorter than the right. *From Lagier, R., Baud, C.-A., Kramar, C., 1991. A case of tibia vara (Blount's Disease) from the early Middle Ages. Journal of Paleopathology 4 (1), 26–27.*

femoral neck (coxa magna) with varus deformity; flattening and enlargement of the femoral head with or without mushroom deformity; and a shallow acetabulum, shortening of the limb, and secondary arthritis (Waldron, 2009). Flattening of the femoral head occurs both due to compression fractures and a lack of endochondral growth (Ortner, 2003). The short thickened neck may aid in distinguishing Perthes' from the later changes associated with a slipped femoral epiphysis (Waldron, 2009), although both may develop metaphyseal cysts (Resnick and Kransdorf, 2005). The clinical presentation of the disease is limping, pain, and limited movement. Osteochondritis dissecans is present in 2%–4% of cases, particularly in males (Resnick and Kransdorf, 2005).

Burwell et al. (1978) suggest that individuals with Perthes' disease have underlying problems with growth and development that predisposes them to avascular necrosis of the hip, and that this growth deficiency may be genetic due to the presence of other congenital anomalies in affected individuals (Hall et al., 1979). Burwell (1988) also noted different body proportions in those affected with Perthes' disease in particular, a shorter radius and ulna relative to the humerus, and a delay and variability in development of the wrist. In some cases, development of the carpal bones halted with bones failing to form (Burwell, 1988). This feature would be impossible to identify in skeletonized remains where carpal bones are often lost postmortem. Where evidence of necrosis is absent in a flattened and enlarged femoral head, a "cretin hip" in hypothyroidism should be considered as a differential diagnosis (see below). Resnick and Kransdorf (2005) also advise consideration of other conditions in bilateral cases, such as sickle cell anemia and epiphyseal dysplasia.

Published cases of Perthes' disease in nonadult material are not uncommon, with two reported in individuals around 6 years of age, the first from medieval Jarrow, England, and the second at the Crow Creek massacre site in Arizona (Anderson et al., 2006; Loveland et al., 1985). A further four cases have been identified in older individuals. Hinkes (1983) identified a possible case in an adolescent male from Grasshopper Pueblo; Walker (2012) identified a case of a prematurely fused and mushroom-shaped left femoral head epiphysis, with a thickened neck in a 12-year-old from St Mary Spital in London; and another possible case comes from Roman Queensmill, Oxfordshire, in a 10-year-old (Rohnbogner, 2015). The most recent published case comes from Argentina, where Ponce and Novellino (2014) report a 14- to 16-year-old with expanded right femoral head, thickened femoral neck, and shallow acetabulum (Fig. 10.9) from 16th- to 17th-century Cápiz Alto.

Scheuermann's Disease (Juvenile kyphosis, Spinal Osteochondrosis)

Scheuermann's disease results from protrusion of the vertebral endplate into the vertebral body. This causes anterior narrowing of the disc space, retarded growth of the cartilage endplate, anterior wedging of the bodies, and sclerosis of the adjoining

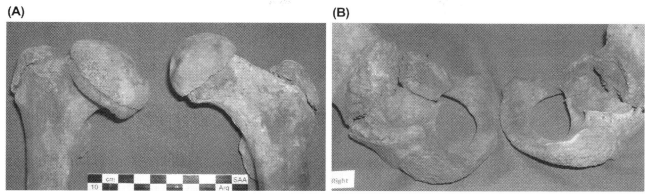

FIGURE 10.9 Legg–Calvé–Perthes' disease in a 14- to 16-year-old from Cápiz Alto, Argentina (16th to 17th century AD, skeleton 12). (A) The right femoral epiphysis is widened with a central necrotic area visible on radiograph; the neck is also thicker and shorter in comparison to the left side. (B) The acetabulae are still unfused but the right acetabulum is clearly broad and shallow in comparison to the normal left side. *From Ponce, P., Novellino, P., 2014. A palaeopathological example of Legg-Calvé-Perthes disease from Argentina. International Journal of Palaeopathology 6, 32.*

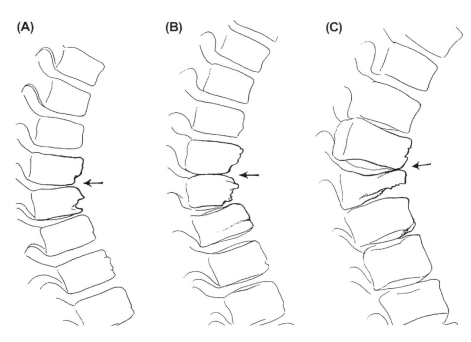

FIGURE 10.10 Progressive changes of Scheuermann's disease in a child aged between 11 and 15 years of age; (A) at age 11 notched deformities are present on the anterior aspect of T6 and T7, and kyphosis is evident; (B) shows progression of the deformity after 2 years; and (C) demonstrates anterior collapse of T7 with elongation (Edgren's sign) of T6 in the child aged 15 years. *From Caffey, J., 1945. Pediatric X-Ray Diagnosis, Year Book Medical Publishers, Inc., Chicago, p. 805.*

vertebrae (Aufdermaur and Spycher, 1986). Changes may be confined to the intervertebral disc (primary) or affect the vertebrae themselves (secondary) (Ortner, 2003). The condition is characterized by anterior collapse and wedging of the thoracic spine resulting in increased curvature (kyphosis). There may also be flattening of the whole vertebral body, rather than just the anterior section, with lengthening of the adjacent vertebrae as compensation (Edgren's sign) (Fig. 10.10; Palazzo et al., 2014), but this change could easily be confused with a vertebral compression fracture in dry bone.

The etiology of the lesions is still unclear but they appear to result from mechanical loading when in an upright posture. The occurrence of the condition in the 11- to 17-year-age group is thought to be related to the compression overloading on the spine, which is particularly vulnerable during the adolescent growth spurt (Fisk et al., 1984). Damborg et al. (2011) found a stronger familial link to the condition than environmental factors in their Danish population, with twice as many males affected than females, but this predilection for males has since been rejected (Palazzo et al., 2014). Between 0.4% and 8.3% of the population can be affected (Wenger and Frick, 1999), although a radiographic survey of 500 asymptomatic juveniles showed a much higher incidence of 56.3% for males and 20.3% for females (Fisk et al., 1984). Most will heal without symptoms, but they may develop early degenerative disease. Kyphosis is most common in the thoracic region of T9 to T10 (75%), while 20%–25% of cases have thoracolumbar involvement, and 5% have lumbar involvement (Resnick and Kransdorf, 2005). Type-II kyphosis, where the apex is at the thoracic–lumbar junction, is more likely to be associated with lower back pain and is known as "apprentices spine" due to its relationship to strenuous muscular activity and heavy lifting in particular (Bakshi et al., 2015; Wenger and Frick, 1999). Involvement of the lumbar spine can result in anterior lordosis and a "saddleback" deformity (Ortner, 2003), which has been linked to a higher incidence of spondylolysis in modern cases (Ogilvie and Sherman, 1987). Around 15%–10% of cases result in scoliosis, although this condition may also develop independently in the same spine (Palazzo et al., 2014). Scheuermann's disease may be related to a short sternum, which was identified in 1.7% of males with the condition. It is thought this may be caused by undue pressure on the sternum from the anterior thoracic spine (Palazzo et al., 2014).

This condition is difficult to identify in a disarticulated skeleton and relies on the identification of wedge-shaped vertebrae and round or oblong defects near the center of the endplate (Ortner, 2003). Current clinical diagnosis requires continuous involvement of at least three vertebrae with kyphosis of a 45 degree angle or more. A similar condition, spinal osteochondrosis, referring to more subtle changes in the spine, excludes wedging but includes flattening of the vertebral endplate, Schmorl's nodes, and detachment of the annular ring. This less severe condition can affect up to 30% of the population (Baker, 1988). Spinal osteochondrosis may develop into true Scheuermann's disease (Resnick and Kransdorf, 2005) and should be observable in the archeological record; although given its subtle nature it is unlikely we can confidently diagnose it.

Wells (1961) was the first to identify Scheuermann's disease in an archeological context, in a 16-year-old female from a Bronze Age round barrow in Dorset. This well-preserved spine showed anteriorly deficient bone from L3–L4 resulting in a wedge-shaped profile. The radiograph revealed an area of sclerosis directly below the lesions (Fig. 10.11). The female also had squatting facets that suggested strenuous activity. Anderson and Carter (1994) identified Scheuermann's disease in a 17- to 19-year-old from medieval Deal in Kent, with shortening of the anterior body of L1, wedging of T11 and T12, Schmorl's nodes, and a resulting kyphotic spine. A further possible case was identified in a 16-year-old from St Mary Spital, London, and anterior collapse of 2 or 3 lumbar or thoracic vertebrae was discovered in five other medieval adolescents (10–25 years) from the same site. It is thought that the London adolescents were carrying out strenuous activity from a young age, and there is a great potential for investigating the link between early trauma and Scheuermann's disease in adolescent skeletal samples (Lewis, 2016). Differential diagnosis of juvenile kyphosis should include acute trauma, tuberculosis when vertebral collapse occurs prior to ankylosis or clear cloaca formation, and tetanus and as the result of severe spasms (Roberg, 1937).

ENDOCRINE DISTURBANCES

The endocrine system comprises a series of ductless glands that secrete hormones into the blood. Over (hyper-) or under (hypo-) secretion of these hormones causes

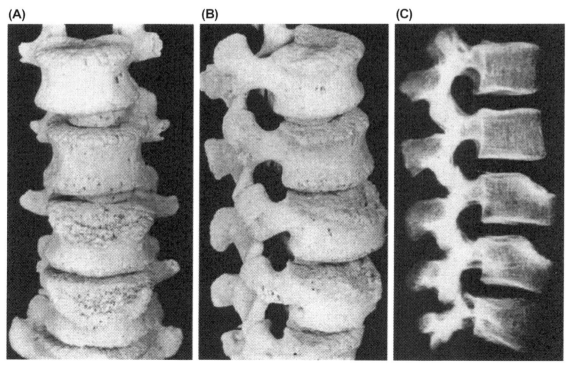

FIGURE 10.11 Scheuermann's disease in a 16-year-old female from Long Crichel in Dorset, England (1600 BC, skeleton 5). Anterior collapse with wedging of L3 and L4 is shown from the (A) anterior aspect and (B) lateral view and shows a porous surface to the affected area. (C) The radiograph shows an area of dense bone below the collapse. *From Wells, C., 1961. A case of lumbar osteochondritis from the Bronze Age. Journal of Bone and Joint Surgery 43 (3), 575.*

endocrine disease. The main endocrine glands associated with skeletal pathology are the pituitary, thyroid, parathyroids, adrenals (adrenal cortex), ovaries, and testes, but it is the hypothalamus and the pituitary gland that are the principle organizers of the endocrine system (Hinson et al., 2010). The hypothalamus is located beneath the thalamus at the base of the brain and is directly connected to the anterior pituitary lobe via blood vessels. Together the pituitary and hypothalamus control several endocrine systems including the hypothalamic–pituitary–thyroid axis, the hypothalamic–pituitary–gonadal axis, and the hypothalamic–pituitary–adrenal axis (Hinson et al., 2010). Excessive or inadequate secretions from these glands have serious consequences as deficiencies in the secretions of one gland affect the secretions of another, with skeletal changes dictated by the severity of the hormone deficiency and age of onset (Ortner, 2003).

Normal growth and development of the skeleton is reliant on an intricate relationship between the thyroid and pituitary glands, with the pituitary controlling linear growth and the thyroid stimulating maturation (Urist, 2012). The anterior lobe of the pituitary produces the somatotrophic (growth) hormone that stimulates the production of the insulin-like growth factor (IGF-1) by the liver. These then induce the thyroid to release thyroxin. The thyroid gland in turn feeds back to the pituitary gland which stimulates the continued release of the somatotrophic hormone. Parathyroid hormones (PTHs) activate osteoclasts to release calcium and phosphate into the bloodstream, while excessive amounts of adrenocortical glucocorticoid steroids released by the adrenal glands cause depression of the osteoblasts and subsequent osteoporosis (Canalis et al., 2007).

The first indication that an individual may suffer from an endocrine disorder would be a deficiency of linear growth and/or maturation, accelerated growth and/or maturation, or excessive growth in comparison to dental development. In bioarcheology, these changes would likely result in an over- or underestimation of child's dental or skeletal age, and so it is not surprising that identification of these conditions is extremely rare in nonadult remains. However, there are key morphological, radiological, and microscopic changes that may allow for a diagnosis of an endocrine disorder (Table 10.2).

Hypopituitarism (Pituitary Dwarfism)

The pituitary gland is situated in the pituitary fossa or sella turcica, a hollow in the sphenoid bone at the base of the brain. A normal pituitary gland is around 14mm across, but it increases in size during pregnancy and decreases with age (Hinson et al., 2010). Identification of a disorder of the pituitary gland may be evidenced by alterations in the size and appearance of the sella turcica. For example, abnormal secretion of the growth hormone as the result of a tumor may be identified by thinning and enlargement of the sella turcica or perforation of the floor (Ortner, 2003).

A deficiency in the somatotrophic hormone leads to proportionate dwarfism. This is usually due to tumors such as a craniopharyngioma in or above the pituitary fossa, but is genetic in 10% of cases. Dysfunction of the pituitary gland may also be caused by cerebral trauma or infection (Resnick and Kransdorf, 2005). The skeleton is short and gracile with delayed dental maturation. While the growth plates will remain open for longer than is normal, they will eventually fuse (Resnick and Kransdorf, 2005). In children with hypopituitarism, growth failure is normally recognized around 3 years of age when growth is 50% below normal and eruption of the permanent teeth is delayed. Although rare, there may also be slipping of the femoral head (Resnick and Kransdorf, 2005). The only cases of pituitary dwarfism identified in the archeological record have been of adults (Aristova et al., 2006; Hernandez, 2013; Ortner, 2003; Roberts, 1988) and careful observation of both the skull and postcranial skeleton is needed to enable a distinction between microcephaly and pituitary dwarfism (Ortner, 2003). Diagnosing the condition in a child skeleton would be extremely problematic as sufferers are likely to be underaged and hence missed. However, there may be osteoporosis and, as Waldron (2009) suggests, it may be possible to compare the skeletal proportions of an individual suspected of having the condition with children of the same dental age from the sample.

Hyperpituitarism (Pituitary Gigantism, Acromegaly)

Hyperpituitarism is a rare condition caused by an excessive production of the growth hormone, most often due to a secretory tumor (adenoma) resulting in extreme height and larger bones than normal. Pituitary gigantism refers to changes seen in an individual with open growth plates, causing excessive stature, bone density, bone length and diameter. Acromegaly results when there is excessive production of somatotrophic hormone and IGF-1 once the growth plates have closed. Nevertheless, characteristic features of acromegaly (e.g., thickening and exaggeration of facial bones, chin and sinuses, supraorbital ridges, thickened cranial vault, tufting, and arrowhead appearance of the terminal phalanges) have been identified in children with gigantism due to overactivation of intramembranous growth (Resnick and Kransdorf, 2005, p. 589).

As in pituitary dwarfism, growth is proportional (i.e., the bone increase in length and density relative to one another), and the severity relies on the age of onset, with early development causing greater growth than later onset. Thus far, no nonadult cases of this condition have been reported, although Gladykowska-Rzeczycka et al. (1998) suggested childhood onset for hyperpituitarism in a 25- to 30-year-old female from medieval Poland. Another case of gigantism and acromegaly was presented by Mulhern (2005) in a 20- to 30-year-old male with associated wedging of the lumbar spine and a fractured femoral head. Thinned parietals were considered

TABLE 10.2 Differentiation of Endocrine Disorders in Children

Condition	Effects	Skeletal Changes
Hormonal Deficiency		
Hypopituitarism		Proportional reduction in size of all bones; thinning, enlargement, or perforation of the sella turcica; delayed skeletal and dental maturation; slipped femoral epiphysis; and widespread osteoporosis
Hypothyroidism		Poorly mineralized or absent epiphyses on the distal femur and proximal tibia, brachycephaly, wormian bones, prognathism, stippled appearance of the proximal humeral and femoral epiphyses on X-ray, bilateral or unilateral slipped epiphyses (cretin's hip), bullet-shaped T12 and L1, wedged-shaped lumbar vertebrae, radiolucent metaphyseal bands
Hypoparathyroidism		Osteosclerosis, thickened cranium, enamel hypoplasia
Hypogonadism		Long gracile bones, especially of the lower limb, widespread osteoporosis
Cushing's Syndrome		Widespread osteoporosis, retarded growth, precocious puberty, premature suture closure, and stunting
Hormonal Excess		
Hyperpituitarism		Thinning, enlargement, or perforation of the sella turcica; extreme diaphyseal lengths compared to normal population, proportional enlargement of all bones
Hyperthyroidism		Enlargement of the sella turcica if site of tumor, cystic lesion of the frontal bone, osteoporosis, especially of the cervical vertebrae, hands, feet, and pelvis, craniostenosis
Hyperparathyroidism		Thinned cortex, absorption of the endosteal surface (tibia, humerus, femur), acroosteolysis of distal phalanges, bone cysts, fibrous cortical bone (brown tumors), radiolucent bands at metaphysis
Hypergonadism		Short stocky bones as the result of premature epiphyseal fusion and precocious puberty

Compiled from Resnick, D., Kransdorf, M., 2005. Bone and Joint Imaging. Elsevier Saunders, Philadelphia; Ortner, D., 2003. Identification of Pathological Conditions in Human Skeletal Remains. Academic Press, New York; Ortner, D., Hotz, G., 2005. Skeletal manifestations of hypothyroidism from Switzerland. American Journal of Physical Anthropology 127 (1), 1–6; Patidar, P., Philip, R., Toms, A., Gupta, K., 2016. Radiological manifestations of juvenile hypothyroidism. Thyroid Research and Practice 9 (3), 102–104; Levine, M.A., 2001. Hypoparathyroidism and pseudohypoparathyroidism. In: DeGroot, L., Jameson, J. (Eds.), Endocrinology. WB Saunders Company, Philadelphia, pp. 1133–1153; and Jaffe, H.L., 1940. Hyperparathyroidism. Bulletin of the New York Academy of Medicine 16 (5), 291.

suggestive of additional hypogonadism, and it was thought the individual may have been a eunuch. The "Tegernsee Giant" (Thomas Hasler), whose skeleton is housed in the Institute of Pathology at Munich University, is thought to have developed gigantism as the result of a pituitary tumor at 9 years of age, becoming 162 cm tall by the time he was 12. It is thought that the presence of the growth hormone also accelerated the formation of fibrous dysplasia in his skull (Nerlich et al., 1991). Similarly, polyostotic fibrous dysplasia in a modern child with gigantism from Taiwan seems to confirm that excessive levels of the growth hormone influence the rapid development of this cancer (Szwajkun et al., 1998).

Other conditions that may cause extreme growth such as Marfan's syndrome, should also be considered in a differential diagnosis of juvenile gigantism. Neurofibromatosis (Recklinghausen's disease) may occur in a single growing bone due to the secondary effects of neural tumors, causing regional gigantism of bone and soft tissue. Neurofibromatosis of a bone in the lower extremities may result in compensatory tilting of the pelvis and scoliosis (Caffey, 1945).

Hypothyroidism (Myxedema)

Thyroxin and triiodothyronine are the two main hormones secreted by the thyroid under the instruction of the pituitary gland (Resnick and Kransdorf, 2005, p. 597). Thyroxin stimulates skeletal maturation while also feeding back to the pituitary to secrete more somatotrophic hormone. Hence in hypothyroidism, both growth and maturation will be delayed. A normally functioning thyroid depends on the amount of iodine in the diet because the hormones it produces contain three or four iodine atoms (Hinson et al., 2010).

There are two main forms of hypothyroidism: endemic and sporadic. Endemic hypothyroidism occurs in areas where iodine is absent from the water supply, such as the high mountains of Switzerland (Ortner and Hotz, 2005). Sporadic hypothyroidism is caused by dysfunction of the thyroid gland itself through a genetic defect, or destruction of the thyroid or pituitary glands by a tumor or infection (Resnick and Kransdorf, 2005). In infancy, thyroid deficiency results in cretinism with mental retardation and developmental abnormalities (Resnick and Kransdorf, 2005). Thyroxin deficiency causes a delay in the development of the skull and pneumatization of the sinuses and mastoid processes, a delay in closure of the fontanels, delayed dental development, brachycephaly due to delay in growth of the base of the skull, wormian bones, a prognathic jaw, a larger nasal index due to a shorter face, an enlarged sella turcica, and an unusually shaped foramen magnum. Many of these cranial features may simply result in the child being placed into a younger age category. While normal maternal thyroid production limits changes in the affected fetus and newborn, absence of the distal femoral and proximal tibial epiphyses is an important clinical diagnostic feature (Resnick and Kransdorf, 2005). There are also alterations in the development of the segments of the sternum and sacrum, but these are unlikely to be useful in a poorly preserved nonadult skeleton where absence may be due to a lack of excavation or ossification of these tiny bones. However, there are a series of postcranial features that may help the recognition of the disease (Ortner and Hotz, 2005).

In congenital hypothyroidism short, bullet-shaped vertebral bodies, especially affecting the 12th thoracic and first lumbar vertebrae, can lead to kyphosis, and accessory ossification centers at the base of the metacarpals may be evident (Fig. 10.12; Caffey, 1945; Resnick and Kransdorf, 2005). Poor mineralization of the epiphyses (epiphyseal dysgenesis) gives a fragmented or stippled radiographic appearance, most commonly of the proximal humerus, femur, and navicular, and may cause collapse of the associated joint (Patidar et al., 2016). Collapse of the femoral head is the more frequent deformity, known as "cretin's hip." Hence, hypothyroidism should be considered in cases of bilateral or unilateral slipped femoral epiphysis and suspected Perthes' disease, where a flattened and mushroom-shaped femoral head without aseptic necrosis would more likely indicate cretin's hip (Resnick and Kransdorf, 2005). In later onset hypothyroidism, the lumbar vertebrae may develop wedge-shaped anterior margins of the superior aspect leading to spondylolisthesis, and delayed maturation of the vertebral end plates can cause the formation of a sclerotic band (Patidar et al., 2016).

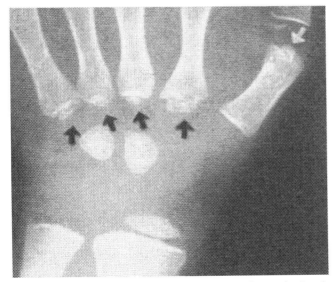

FIGURE 10.12 Accessory ossification centers at the proximal ends of the second to fifth metacarpals and distal end of the first metacarpal (arrows) in a child with hypothyroidism. *From Caffey, J., 1945. Pediatric X-Ray Diagnosis, Year Book Medical Publishers, Inc., Chicago, p. 747.*

Hyperthyroidism (Thyrotoxicosis)

Hyperthyroidism is a fairly common diagnosis today, but is rarely a primary condition and is unlikely to produce noticeable skeletal alterations (Ortner, 2003). It is nonexistent in infancy, uncommon or mild in older childhood, but may occur in adolescence (Resnick and Kransdorf, 2005). The release of excessive amounts of thyroxin may be secondary to excessive iodine in the diet causing toxic nodular goiter, or Grave's disease, an autoimmune condition (Hinson et al., 2010). There are some radiographic features that may help in identification, including cystic changes in the frontal bone that mimic multiple myeloma, and the more unusual expression of osteoporosis in the cervical vertebrae, hands, feet, and pelvis. In children it may lead to premature cranial suture closure (Resnick and Kransdorf, 2005).

Cushing's Disease

The adrenal glands are two separate glands situated on the kidney. The outer adrenal cortex produces steroid hormones including the stress hormone cortisol (glucocorticoid). Glucocorticoid excess, or Cushing's disease, is caused by oversecretion of the steroid by the adrenal gland, usually as the result of a tumor or due to congenital adrenal hyperplasia (Hinson et al., 2010). Adrenocortical tumors arise in children before the age of 5 years, and are more common in girls than boys. The condition is characterized by precocious puberty (before the age of 8 years in girls and 9 years in boys) resulting in premature growth arrest and short stature (Resnick and Kransdorf, 2005). Suppressed production of collagen will result in osteoblastic depression and severe osteoporosis. The skeletal changes are the same as observed in senile osteoporosis with the greatest effects seen in areas with high amounts of trabecular bone (Ortner, 2003).

Hypogonadism

Hypogonadism arises from a failure of testicular or ovary function (primary hypogonadism), pituitary failure (secondary hypogonadism), or hypothalamic failure (tertiary hypogonadism). Estrogen and testosterone are responsible for endochondral growth, the appearance of the secondary ossification centers, and the onset of puberty. A loss or reduction of one or both sex hormones with subsequent delay in maturation will result in a tall, long-legged gracile skeleton with thinned cortices.

There has been an emerging interest in the skeletal features associated with castration in the paleopathological literature (Eng et al., 2010). The creation of eunuchs through testicular removal shortly before puberty is seen to result in delayed maturation and subsequently longer bones. The earlier the procedure occurred, the more epiphyses will be affected, and the greater the stature of the individual. Documentary evidence suggests males would have undergone this procedure between the ages of 10 and 15 years (Eng et al., 2010). Examining the pattern of epiphyseal delay should enable the age at which the procedure took place to be estimated in adult skeletons, but the signatures are unlikely to be evident in nonadults. Dental development, which remains unaffected, will belie the older age of an individual who skeletally appears to be prepubescent.

Hypergonadism

This results in precocious puberty and a short and stocky skeleton due to premature closure of the epiphyses (Ortner, 2003). Identification in an adolescent skeleton will rest on a stocky individual with a younger age for dental development than the skeletal maturation suggests, although all populations will have individuals who enter puberty earlier than the average age (Lewis et al., 2016).

Hypoparathyroidism

The four parathyroid glands are located on the posterior surface of the thyroid. The PTH controls the levels of calcium, phosphorus, and vitamin D in the bloodstream and bone matrix. Hypoparathyroidism refers to a group of metabolic disorders in which hypocalcemia and hyperphosphatemia occur, usually due to the inability of the parathyroid glands to secrete sufficient amounts of PTH (Levine, 2001). Dysfunctional parathyroid glands may result from infection (i.e., miliary tuberculosis), magnesium deficiency, autoimmune disease (i.e., Addison's disease), or agenesis of the parathyroid glands as part of an inherited genetic disorder (DiGeorge syndrome). The latter causes, among other things, a hypoplastic mandible and death before the age of 6 years (Levine, 2001). Low levels of PTH stimulate osteoblasts and bone formation resulting in localized or generalized osteosclerosis (Hinson et al., 2010). Hypoplastic deciduous or permanent teeth may also be present depending on the age of onset (Levine and Keen, 1974; Resnick and Kransdorf, 2005). Severe hypocalcemia can lead to convulsions and slow mental development (Levine, 2001).

Hyperparathyroidism

Prolonged high levels of PTH increase osteoclastic activity causing increased bone resorption. This condition is usually the result of renal impairment, resulting in osteoporosis and eventually, low blood calcium levels. Although initially only identified microscopically, subperiosteal bone formation may be observed in the phalanges of the hand on the ulnar aspect (Resnick and Kransdorf, 2005) with resorption similar to that seen in acroosteolysis of leprosy. Moreover skeletal changes occur in up to 25% of cases with the formation of fine trabeculae and poorly mineralized cancellous bone resulting in secondary fractures. These minor traumas cause hemorrhage and microfractures leading to cyst formation and proliferation of the fibrous marrow, known as brown tumors (Jaffe, 1940).

These changes can occur anywhere but are most commonly seen in the mandible, long and short tubular bones, and the pelvis. Erosions in other joints may be confused with JIA but occur further away from the joint with resorption at the proximal end of the tibia, humerus, and femur (Resnick and Kransdorf, 2005). Radiolucent bands may be evident between the metaphysis and diaphysis, and the cranial bones can develop a speckled appearance as the result of trabecular resorption known as a "salt and pepper skull" (Resnick and Kransdorf, 2005). Rickets, Albright's disease (hereditary osteodystrophy), and fibrous dysplasia are differential diagnoses.

Secondary hyperparathyroidism can occur as the result of rickets due to reduced serum calcium levels (Jaffe, 1940). Such a case has been suggested for the changes seen in a 2- to 3-year-old from postmedieval St Martin's Church, in Birmingham, UK (Mays et al., 2007). Mays et al. (2007) highlighted the importance of microscopic evaluation (using a scanning electron microscope) in the identification of the disease, noting the presence of linear radiolucencies of the trabecular bone (tunneling resorption or dissecting osteitis), giving the cortical bone a longitudinal striated appearance seen on radiograph, osteoclastic resorption causing thinning of the trabeculae (osteopenia), enlarged vascular spaces, multiple reversal lines, poorly mineralized newly formed bone on normal bone, and "bitelike" defects (Fig. 10.13; Mays et al., 2007). Following this study, Mays and Turner-Walker (2008) presented a second case of possible secondary hyperparathyroidism as a result of kidney insufficiency (renal osteodystrophy) in a 13- to 15-year-old from medieval Wharram Percy, Yorkshire. The child was poorly preserved limiting the extent of the observations, but the presence of widespread subperiosteal lamellar and fiber

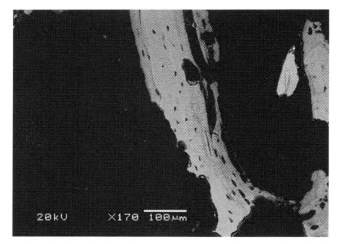

FIGURE 10.13 "Bitelike" resorption defects on the trabeculae visible under a scanning electron microscope are typical patterns seen in hyperparathyroidism. The slide is of a 2- to 3-year-old from St Martin's Church in Birmingham, England, with rickets and secondary hyperparathyroidism (19th century AD, skeleton HB772). *From Mays, S., Brickley, M., Ives, R., 2007. Skeletal evidence for hyperparathyroidism in a 19th century child with rickets. International Journal of Osteoarchaeology 17 (1), 79.*

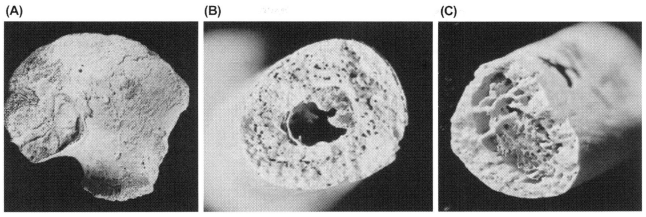

FIGURE 10.14 Possible secondary hyperparathyroidism as the result of renal osteodystrophy in a 13- to 15-year-old from Wharram Percy in West Yorkshire, England (AD 960–1700, skeleton WCO058). (A) There is a profuse layer of active periosteal new bone evident on both ilia; (B) a cross section of the left humerus and a rib fragment (C) shows a deposit of abnormal trabecular within the medullary cavity and porosity of the cortex. *From Mays, S., Turner-Walker, G., 2008. A possible case of renal osteodystrophy in a skeleton from medieval Wharram Percy, England. International Journal of Osteoarchaeology 18 (3), 309, 310, 312.*

bone, cortical porosity, and in-filling of the medullary cavity with a mass of randomly organized spicules are suggestive of hyperparathyroidism (Fig. 10.14). The presence of subperiosteal new bone was indicative of a secondary cause of the disease, and in the absence of rickets, renal insufficiency was suggested (Mays and Turner-Walker, 2008).

REFERENCES

Al-Matar, M., Petty, R., Tucker, L., Malleson, P., Schroeder, M., Cabral, D., 2002. The early pattern of joint involvement predicts disease progression in children with oligoarticular (pauciarticular) juvenile rheumatoid arthritis. Arthritis and Rheumatism 46 (10), 2708–2715.

Anderson, S., Wells, C., Birkett, D., 2006. The human skeletal remains. In: Cramp, R. (Ed.), Wearmouth and Jarrow Monastic Sites. English Heritage, London, pp. 481–545.

Anderson, T., Carter, A., 1994. A possible example of Scheuermann's disease from Iron Age Deal, Kent. Journal of Paleopathology 6 (2), 57–62.

Ansell, B., 1978. Chronic arthritis in childhood. Annals of the Rheumatic Diseases 37, 107–120.

Aristova, E., Chikisheva, T., Seidman, A., Mashak, A., Khoroshevskaya, Y., 2006. Pituitary dwarfism in an early bronze age individual from Tuva. Archaeology, Ethnology and Anthropology of Eurasia 27 (1), 139–147.

Aufdermaur, M., Spycher, M., 1986. Pathogenesis of osteochondritis juvenilis Scheuermann. Journal of Orthopaedic Research 4, 452–457.

Baker, K., 1988. Scheuermann's disease: a review. Australian Journal of Physiotherapy 34 (3), 165–169.

Bakshi, V.K., Chowdhary, J., Verma, A.P., Baberwal, M.C., 2015. A rare cause of kyphosis with low backache-"Scheuermann's disease":"Osteochondritis deformans juvenilis dorsi". International Journal of Research in Medical Sciences 3 (5), 1293–1298.

Bernstein, B., Stobie, D., Singsen, B., Koster-King, K., Kornreich, H., Hanson, V., 1977. Growth retardation in juvenile rheumatoid arthritis (JRA). Arthritis and Rheumatism 20 (2), 212–216.

Berntson, L., Gäre, B.A., Fasth, A., Herlin, T., Kristinsson, J., Lahdenne, P., Marhaug, G., Nielsen, S., Pelkonen, P., Rygg, M., 2003. Incidence of juvenile idiopathic arthritis in the Nordic countries. A population based study with special reference to the validity of the ILAR and EULAR criteria. The Journal of Rheumatology 30 (10), 2275–2282.

Buikstra, J., Poznanski, A., Cerna, M., Goldstein, P., Hioshower, L., 1990. A case of juvenile rheumatoid arthritis from pre-Colombian Peru. In: Buikstra, J. (Ed.), A Life Science Papers in Honour of J Lawrence Angel. Central American Archaeology, United States, pp. 99–137.

Burwell, R., 1988. Perthes' disease: growth and aetiology. Archives of Disease in Childhood 63 (11), 1408.

Burwell, R., Dangerfield, P., Hall, D., Vernon, C., Harrison, M., 1978. Perthes' disease. An anthropometric study revealing impaired and disproportionate growth. Journal of Bone & Joint Surgery, British Volume 60 (4), 461–477.

Bywaters, E., Ansell, B., 1965. Monoarticular arthritis in children. Annals of Rheumatoid Disease 24, 116–122.

Caffey, J., 1945. Pediatric X-Ray Diagnosis. Year Book Medical Publishers, Inc., Chicago.

Campillo, D., 1990. Etude des restes squelettiques d'un individu de l'époque tardi-romaine, atteint de polyarthrite rhumatoïde. Anthropologie et Préhistoire 101, 71–83.

Canalis, E., Mazziotti, G., Giustina, A., Bilezikian, J., 2007. Glucocorticoid-induced osteoporosis: pathophysiology and therapy. Osteoporosis International 18 (10), 1319–1328.

Cobb, J.E., Hinks, A., Thomson, W., 2014. The genetics of juvenile idiopathic arthritis: current understanding and future prospects. Rheumatology 53 (4), 592–599.

Damborg, F., Engell, V., Nielsen, J., Kyvik, K.O., MØ, A., Thomsen, K., 2011. Genetic epidemiology of Scheuermann's disease: heritability and prevalence over a 50-year period. Acta Orthopaedica 82 (5), 602–605.

DiGangi, E.A., Bethard, J.D., Sullivan, L.P., 2010. Differential diagnosis of cartilaginous dysplasia and probable Osgood–Schlatter's disease in a Mississippian individual from East Tennessee. International Journal of Osteoarchaeology 20 (4), 424–442.

Eng, J.T., Zhang, Q., Zhu, H., 2010. Skeletal effects of castration on two eunuchs of Ming China. Anthropological Science 118 (2), 107–116.

Fisk, J., Baigent, M., Hill, P., 1984. Scheuermann's disease: clinical and radiological survey of 17 and 18 year olds. American Journal of Physical Medicine & Rehabilitation 63 (1), 18–30.

Garralda, M., Herrerín, J., 2003. Juvenile rheumatoid arthritis in a woman from the necropolis (XVII-XVIII C. A.D.) of El Burgo de Osma Cathedral (Soria, Spain). Journal of Paleopathology 15 (3), 133–152.

Gholve, P., Scher, D., Khakaria, S., Widmann, R., Green, D., 2007. Osgood schlatter syndrome. Current Opinions in Pediatrics 19 (1), 44–50.

Gladykowska-Rzeczycka, J., Smiszkiewicz-Skwarska, A., Sokol, A., 1998. A giant from Ostrow Lednicki (XII-XIII c), dist. Lednogora, Poland. Mankind Quarterly 39 (2), 147–172.

Guyuron, B., 1988. Facial deformity of juvenile rheumatoid arthritis. Plastic and Reconstructive Surgery 81 (6), 948–951.

Hall, D., Harrison, M., Burwell, R., 1979. Congenital abnormalities and Perthes' disease. Clinical evidence that children with Perthes' disease may have a major congenital defect. Journal of Bone & Joint Surgery, British Volume 61 (1), 18–25.

Hawkey, D., 1998. Disability, compassion and the skeletal record: using musculo-skeletal stress markers (MSM) to construct an osteobiography from Early New Mexico. International Journal of Osteoarchaeology 8, 326–340.

Hernandez, M., 2013. A possible case of hypopituitarism in Neolithic China. International Journal of Osteoarchaeology 23 (4), 432–446.

Hinkes, M., 1983. Skeletal Evidence of Stress in Subadults: Trying to Come of Age at Grasshopper Pueblo (Ph.D. thesis). University of Arizona, USA.

Hinson, J., Raven, P., Chew, S., 2010. The Endocrine System. Basic Science and Clinical Conditions. Churchill Livingstone Elsevier, Edinburgh.

Jaffe, H.L., 1940. Hyperparathyroidism. Bulletin of the New York Academy of Medicine 16 (5), 291.

Jaganathan, S., Gamanagatti, S., Goyal, A., 2011. Musculoskeletal manifestations of hemophilia: imaging features. Current Problems in Diagnostic Radiology 40 (5), 191–197.

Kyere, K., Than, K., Wang, A., Rahman, S., Valdivia–Valdivia, J., La Marca, F., Park, P., 2012. Schmorl's nodes. European Spine Journal 21 (11), 2115–2121.

Lagier, R., Baud, C.-A., Kramar, C., 1991. A case of tibia vara (Blount's Disease) from the early middle ages. Journal of Paleopathology 4 (1), 25–28.

Landré-Beauvais, A., 1800. La Goutte Asthénique Primitive (Ph.D. thesis), Paris.

Leden, I., Persson, E., Persson, O., 1988. Aspects of the history of rheumatoid arthritis in the light of recent osteo-archaeological finds. Scandinavian Journal of Rheumatology 17, 341–352.

Levine, M.A., 2001. Hypoparathyroidism and pseudohypoparathyroidism. In: DeGroot, L., Jameson, J. (Eds.), Endocrinology. WB Saunders Company, Philadelphia, pp. 1133–1153.

Levine, R., Keen, J., 1974. Neonatal enamel hypoplasia in association with symptomatic neonatal hypocalcaemia. British Dental Journal 137, 429–433.

Lewis, B., 1998. Prehistoric juvenile rheumatoid arthritis in a Precontact Louisiana Native population reconsidered. Amerian Journal of Physical Anthropology 106, 229–248.

Lewis, M., 2016. Work and the adolescent in medieval England (AD 900-1550). The osteological evidence. Medieval Archaeology 60 (1), 138–171.

Lewis, M., Shapland, F., Watts, R., 2016. On the threshold of adulthood: A new approach for the use of maturation indicators to assess puberty in adolescents from medieval England. American Journal of Human Biology 28 (1), 48–56.

Lien, G., Flatø, B., Haugen, M., Vinje, O., Sørskaar, D., Dale, K., Johnston, V., Egeland, T., Førre, Ø., 2003. Frequency of osteopenia in adolescents with early onset juvenile idiopathic arthritis. Arthritis and Rheumatism 48 (8), 2214–2223.

Loveland, C.J., Gregg, J.B., Bass, W.M., 1985. Ancient osteopathology from the Caddoan burials at the Kaufman-Williams site, Texas. The Plains Anthropologist 29–43.

Maher, P.J., Ilgen, J.S., 2013. Osgood–Schlatter disease. BMJ Case Reports. pii:bcr2012007614.

Mattei, T., Rehman, A., 2014. Schmorl's nodes: current pathophysiological, diagnostic and theraputic paradigms. Neurosurgical Review 37 (1), 39–46.

Mays, S., Brickley, M., Ives, R., 2007. Skeletal evidence for hyperparathyroidism in a 19th century child with rickets. International Journal of Osteoarchaeology 17 (1), 73–81.

Mays, S., Turner-Walker, G., 2008. A possible case of renal osteodystrophy in a skeleton from medieval Wharram Percy, England. International Journal of Osteoarchaeology 18 (3), 307–316.

Mulhern, D., 2005. A probable case of gigantism in a fifth dynasty skeleton from the western cemetery at Giza, Egypt. International Journal of Osteoarchaeology 15 (4), 261–275.

Nerlich, A., Peschel, O., Löhrs, U., Parsche, F., Betz, P., 1991. Juvenile gigantism plus polyostotic fibrous dysplasia in the Tegernsee giant. Lancet 338 (8771), 886–887.

Ogden, J.A., 2006. Skeletal Injury in the Child. Springer Science, Philadelphia.

Ogilvie, J., Sherman, J., 1987. Spondylolysis in Scheuermann's disease. Spine 12 (3), 251–253.

Ortner, D., 2003. Identification of Pathological Conditions in Human Skeletal Remains. Academic Press, New York.

Ortner, D., Hotz, G., 2005. Skeletal manifestations of hypothyroidism from Switzerland. American Journal of Physical Anthropology 127 (1), 1–6.

Ortner, D., Utermohle, C., 1981. Polyarticular inflammatory arthritis in a pre-Columbian skeleton from Kodiak Island, Alaska, USA. Amerian Journal of Physical Anthropology 56 (1), 23–31.

Osgood, R.B., 1903. Lesions of the tibial tubercle occurring during adolescence. The Boston Medical and Surgical Journal 148 (5), 114–117.

Paget, J., Goodhart, J.F., 1885. Descriptive Catalogue of the Pathological Specimens Contained in the Museum of the Royal College of Surgeons of England. Vol. IV. Royal College of Surgeons, London.

Palazzo, C., Sailhan, F., Revel, M., 2014. Scheuermann's disease: an update. Joint Bone Spine 81 (3), 209–214.

Patidar, P., Philip, R., Toms, A., Gupta, K., 2016. Radiological manifestations of juvenile hypothyroidism. Thyroid Research and Practice 9 (3), 102–104.

Pearson, M., Rönning, O., 1996. Lesions of the mandibular condyle in juvenile chronic arthritis. British Journal of Orthodontics 23, 49–56.

Phaer, T., 1545. (reprinted 1955). Boke of Chyldren. E and S Livingstone, Edinburgh.

Plomp, K., Roberts, C., Strand Vioarsdottir, U., 2012. Vertebral morphology influences the develpment of Schmorl's nodes in the lower thoracic vertebrae. American Journal of Physical Anthropology 149 (4), 572–582.

Ponce, P., Novellino, P., 2014. A palaeopathological example of Legg-Calvé-Perthes disease from Argentina. International Journal of Palaeopathology 6, 30–33.

Ravelli, A., Martini, A., 2007. Juvenile idiopathic arthritis. Lancet 369 (9563), 767–778.

Resnick, D. (Ed.), 1995. Diagnosis of Bone and Joint Disorders. W.B. Saunders Company, Philadelphia.

Resnick, D., Kransdorf, M., 2005. Bone and Joint Imaging. Elsevier Saunders, Philadelphia.

Richardson, M., Helms, C., Vogler, J., Genant, H., 1984. Skeletal changes in neuromuscular disorders mimicking juvenile rheumatoid arthritis and hemophilia. American Journal of Radiology 143, 893–897.

Roberg, O., 1937. Spinal deformity following tetanus and its relation to juvenile kyphosis. Journal of Bone & Joint Surgery 19 (3), 603–629.

Roberts, C., 1988. A rare case of dwarfism from the Roman Period. Journal of Palaeopathology 2 (1), 9–21.

Rodriguez-Merchan, E., 1996. Effects of hemophilia on articulations of children and adults. Clinical Orthopaedics and Related Research 328, 7–13.

Rohnbogner, A., 2015. Dying Young: A Palaeopathological Analysis of Child Health in Roman Britain (Ph.D. thesis). University of Reading, England.

Rothschild, B., Hershkovitz, I., Bedford, L., Latimer, B., Dutour, O., Rothschild, C., Jellema, L., 1997. Identification of childhood arthritis in archaeological material: juvenile rheumatoid arthritis versus juvenile spondyloarthropathy. Amerian Journal of Physical Anthropology 102, 249–264.

Schaller, J., 2005. The history of pediatric rheumatology. Pediatric Research 58 (5), 997–1007.

Scheuer, L., Black, S., 2000. Developmental Juvenile Osteology. Academic Press, London.

Schlatter, C., 1903. Verletzungen des schnabel-formigen fortsatzes der aberen tibiaepiphyse. Beitrage zur Klinischen Chirurgie 38, 874.

Sidiropoulou-Chatzigianni, S., Papadopoulos, M.A., Kolokithas, G., 2014. Dentoskeletal morphology in children with juvenile idiopathic arthritis compared with healthy children. Journal of Orthodontics 28, 53–58.

Snorrason, E., 1952. Landré-Beauvais and his "goutte asthénique primitive". Acta Medica Scandinavica 142 (26), 115–118.

Sponseller, P., Stanitski, C., 2001. Fractures and dislocations about the knee. In: Beaty, J., Kasser, J. (Eds.), Rockwood and Wilkins' Fractures in Children. Lipencott Williams and Wilkins, Philadelphia, pp. 981–1076.

Still, G., 1896. On a form of chronic joint disease in children. Medico-chirurgical Transactions 80, 47–59.

Sweet, D., Madewell, J., 1995. Osteonecrosis: pathogenesis. In: Resnick, D. (Ed.), Diagnosis of Bone and Joint Disorders. W.B. Saunders Company, Philadelphia, pp. 3445–3494.

Szwajkun, P., Chen, Y.-R., Yeow, V.K.L., Breidahl, A.F., 1998. The "Taiwanese Giant": hormonal and genetic influences in fibrous dysplasia. Annals of Plastic Surgery 41 (1), 75–80.

Tsatsoulis, A., Siamopoulou, A., Petsoukis, C., Challa, A., Bairaktari, E., Seferiadis, K., 1999. Study of growth hormone secretion and action in growth-retarded children with juvenile chronic arthritis (JCA). Growth Hormone & IGF Research 9 (2), 143–149.

Umlawska, W., Prusek-Dudkiewicz, A., 2010. Growth retardation and delayed puberty in children and adolescents with juvenile idiopathic arthritis. Archives of Medical Science 1, 19–23.

Urist, M., 2012. Growth hormone and skeletal tissue metabolism. The Biochemistry and Physiology of Bone 2, 155–194.

Waldron, T., 2009. Palaeopathology. Cambridge University Press, Cambridge.

Walker, D., 2012. Disease in London, 1st-19th Centuries. Museum of London Archaeology, London.

Wells, C., 1961. A case of lumbar osteochondritis from the Bronze Age. Journal of Bone and Joint Surgery 43 (3), 575.

Wells, C., 1968. Osgood–Schlatter's disease in the ninth century. British Medical Journal 2 (5605), 623–624.

Wenger, D.R., Frick, S.L., 1999. Scheuermann kyphosis. Spine 24 (24), 2630.

Woo, P., 1998. Cytokines in juvenile chronic arthritis. Bailliere's Clinical Rheumatology 12 (2), 219–228.

Yeap, S., 2009. Rheumatoid arthritis in paintings: a tale of two origins. International Journal of Rheumatic Diseases 12 (4), 343–347.

Chapter 11

Miscellaneous Conditions

Chapter Outline

Infantile Cranial Lacunae	267
Cranial Modification	267
Anteroposterior Deformation	268
Circumferential or Circular Deformation	268
Juvenile Paget's Disease (Infantile Hereditary Hyperphosphasia, Hyperostosis Corticalis Deformans)	269
Phossy Jaw	269
Bladder Stone Disease	270
Lead Poisoning	271
Transverse Lines in Bone	271
Harris Lines	271
Lead Lines	272
Bismuth Lines	273
Metaphyseal Bands of Leukemia	273
Scurvy Line	273
Healing and Healed Rickets	273
Osteopathia Striata	274
Bone Length Discrepancy	274
Fluctuating and Directional Asymmetry	274
Pathological Asymmetry	275
Cerebral Palsy	277
Cerebrovascular Incident (Stroke)	277
Rasmussen's Encephalitis	277
Chicken Pox (Congenital Varicella)	277
Arthrogryposis Multiplex Congenita (Congenital Contractures)	278
Erb's and Klumpke's Palsy (Congenital Brachial Palsy)	278
Muscular Dystrophy	278
References	278

INFANTILE CRANIAL LACUNAE

Lytic lesions or lacunae in the thin skulls of perinates have been the subject of some attention in the paleopathological literature. Caffey (1945, p. 32) first noted these lesions in clinical cases calling them "lacunar skull" and describing them as most marked on the parietal and frontal bones (Fig. 11.1). While he discusses a link between the appearance of lacunae and spina bifida, hydrocephalus, meningocele, and meningoencephalocele, he also saw them on the radiographs of apparently healthy newborns. As the lytic lesions tended to disappear spontaneously, Caffey (1945) considered them the result of delayed development of the membranous cranial capsule. Kausmally and Ives (2007) identified similar lytic lesions in 7.4% (n = 7/94) of perinates from postmedieval London. The low prevalence of lesions led the authors to reject postmortem damage who identified several possible pathological conditions that may have caused them. These included infantile chordoma, infantile myofibromatosis, Langerhans cell histiocytosis (Letterer–Siwe form), and tuberculosis. They argued that lytic lesions on the pars basilaris of one perinate may have indicated infantile myofibromatosis (Kausmally and Ives, 2007). Mendonça de Souza et al. (2008) noted similar lesions on the skull of a 6-month-old Peruvian mummy. The child also had endocranial lesions, active new bone formation on the frontal and parietal bones, and a flattened occipital bone. In this case, cranial modification through head binding, followed by ischemic necrosis and secondary infection was considered the cause.

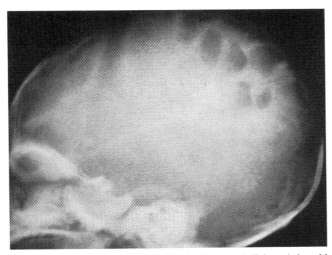

FIGURE 11.1 Clinical radiography of a lacunar skull in a 1-day-old child with spina bifida. *From Caffey, J., 1945. Pediatric X-Ray Diagnosis. Year Book Medical Publishers, Inc, Chicago, p. 32.*

CRANIAL MODIFICATION

Artificial cranial modification describes the alteration of the shape of the cranial vault using cradleboards or bands from infancy, when the bones are still soft and malleable (Pomeroy et al., 2010). Restricted growth in one area of the vault results in compensatory growth elsewhere, thus altering the cranial shape. As a sign of cultural identity, the term cranial modification or head shaping is preferred over artificial cranial deformation. It is unlikely that individuals considered they were deforming their bodies, but rather, that they were forming them into a more aesthetically pleasing shape. Cradle-boarding or head-binding allows the skull to be formed into a desirable adult shape and would have taken place over a prolonged period of time in the first few years of life. Originally, research into cranial modification was carried out as secondary to the primary desire to understand the effects of restricted and compensatory growth on the development of the skull base and face. These cases allowed such adaptations to be studied without the added complication of basicranial dysostosis commonly associated with congenital cranial deformation (Anton, 1989; White, 1996). The earliest cases of this practice are from the Upper Paleolithic, but it appears at various times in nearly every continent and in a variety of cultures, including the North and South America Indians, Pacific Islanders, and some Germanic tribes in Europe (Meiklejohn et al., 1992). Duncan and Hofling (2011) have suggested that for the Maya, newborns were at particular risk of soul loss or injury from evil winds, and that head binding formed part of a protection ritual. There are no standards for describing cranial modification, and some argue that they should be avoided to allow differences between groups to be identified and described (Pomeroy et al., 2010). However, they can broadly be defined into two types.

Anteroposterior Deformation

This type is characterized as anteroposterior (AP) flattening of the frontal and occipital bones, or the occipital bone alone, with lateral bulging of the parietal bones. The temporal and parietal bones are foreshortened giving the skull a triangular appearance when viewed from above. This shape is achieved by placing one or two boards, stones, or pads over the occipital and frontal regions in children under 2 years of age. Cranial base angle changes are mild and the orbits are broadened (Anton, 1989). White (1996) has suggested that this type of modification causes greater occurrence of premature sagittal suture closure and wormian bone formation as the result of extreme tensile forces on the parietal and occipital bones during their peak development. In a later study, O'Loughlin (2004) agreed that wormian bones in posteriorly placed sutures were significantly more common in modified skulls than those without any modification, although she did not observe them more frequently in any one type of modification (Fig. 11.2A).

Circumferential or Circular Deformation

Circumferential (C) modification describes a conical vault that extends posterosuperiorly with elongation of the frontal, temporal squama, and parts of the parietal and occipital bones. Parietal bulging is absent, and there is a "loaflike" appearance on superior view. The changes are usually achieved by wrapping the developing skull circumferentially with textiles. An anteroinferior displacement of the cranial base, resulting in a greater cranial base angle, is influenced primarily by posterosuperior migration of the vault. Orbits are lengthened (Anton,

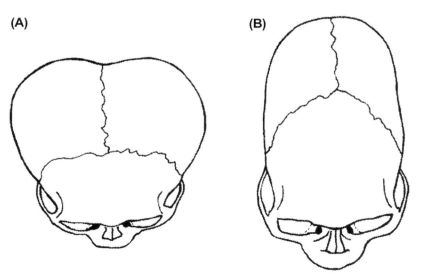

FIGURE 11.2 Cranial shapes typical of (A) anteroposterior and (B) circumferential modification. *From Anton, S., 1989. Intentional cranial vault deformation and induced changes of the cranial base and face. American Journal of Physical Anthropology 79, 256.*

1989). Both AP and C cranial modification types have "erect" and "oblique" subtypes that described the orientation of the deforming pressure and subsequent position of the occipital bone relative to the face (Fig. 11.2B; Anton, 1989).

Holliday's (1993) study of 47 nonadults from southwest New Mexico (AD 700–1150) identified active lytic lesions on flattened occipital bones in six infants as the result of secondary infections from cradleboards (Fig. 11.3). Practiced most commonly by southwestern Pueblo populations, infants were strapped to a board for 20 or more hours a day between birth and 10 months of age, with the weight of the infant's head on the board resulting in marked flattening of the occipital bone (Hrdlička, 1935). Holliday (1993) suggested that this continued compression may have caused ulceration of the scalp. Healed lesions were identified in the older children described as roughly circular areas of depressed remodeled bone. Similar but more widespread lesions were identified in a young infant from Lima in Peru, who also displayed active porous new bone as a layer on the endocranial surface of the parietal bones. The lesions were considered to be the result of ulcerations that led to the child's death (Mendonça de Souza et al., 2008). Tiesler (2011) has hypothesized that these lesions may also be caused by some form of manual intervention by the mother, to relieve pressure on the back of the child's head during boarding.

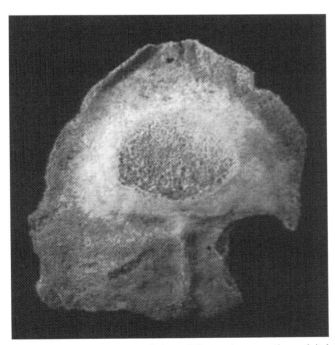

FIGURE 11.3 Large porous, lytic, and flattened area on the occipital bone of a 6-month-old from NAN Ranch Ruin village in southwest New Mexico (AD 700–1150). Endocranial lesions were also evident underlying the area. The lesions are thought to be the result of cradle boarding in infancy. *From Holliday, D., 1993. Occipital lesions: a possible cost of cradleboards. American Journal of Physical Anthropology 90, 286.*

In their analysis of children from the Chen Chen cemetery in Peru (c. AD 500–1150), Blom and Knudson (2014) found 80% (n = 242/286) of individuals under the age of 18 exhibited cranial modification, suggesting it was an almost universal practice and signifying a local identity. Three infants were identified as undergoing cranial modification. Beňuš et al. (1999) reported a rare AP cranial deformation in a 9- to 10-year-old from early medieval Slovakia, perhaps resulting from wrapping the head with bandages. The child was found buried within Devín castle suggesting they were of high status. Özbek (2001) examined artificial cranial modification in 42% (n = 13/31) nonadults from Chalcolithic Turkey. The infants displayed modifications that suggested the use of a single band from birth that ran from the frontal bone to the lower portion of the parietals, and that after a year the child's head was considered large enough to support a second bandage which was placed transversally and supported by the mandible resulting in a flattened occipital bone and superior frontal bone (Fig. 11.4). Variations in the extent of flattening probably resulted from different widths of band used and the varied tightness of the bandages (Özbek, 2001).

JUVENILE PAGET'S DISEASE (INFANTILE HEREDITARY HYPERPHOSPHASIA, HYPEROSTOSIS CORTICALIS DEFORMANS)

Although yet to be reported in the paleopathological record, this rare genetic disorder causes rapidly remodeling woven bone, osteopenia, and pathological fractures similar to those seen in Paget's disease of the elderly. It is thought to result from osteoprotegerin deficiency caused by deletion of the TNFRSF11B gene (Whyte et al., 2002). Only 40 cases have been reported in the modern clinical literature, and without treatment the condition is fatal, as babies fail to thrive and may develop pneumonia. Therefore, juvenile Paget's disease is a condition that paleopathologists would only expect to see in infant skeletons. Interestingly, patients with the condition have short humeri, laterally bowed femora, thickened crania, and coarse trabecular bone (Whyte et al., 2002).

PHOSSY JAW

Osteomyelitis of the jaw increased in the 19th century as the result of match manufacturing that exposed the makers of "strike-anywhere" matches to white phosphorus. When the fumes are breathed in, phosphorus particles reach the bony jaw through diseased gums and teeth. Exposure also results in weakening of the midshaft of the femur and secondary fractures known as "fragile femur" and "dark lines" at the ends of the long bones in children (Hinshaw and Quin, 2015). Studies demonstrated that biphosphonates caused bone weakening by displacing phosphate on the surface of the hydroxyapatite and binding to the mineral (Mukherjee et al., 2008). The condition died out when

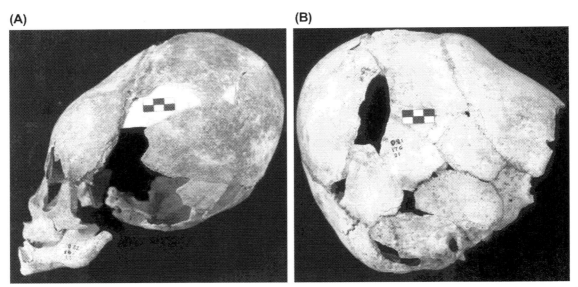

FIGURE 11.4 Cranial modification in two infants from Değirmentepe, Turkey. (A) The first child, aged 6–7 months has modifications that suggest the use of a single band, with flattening of the frontal bone and occipital bone (skeleton D′82.16J.22). (B) The second older child aged 1.5 years has modifications suggestive of the use of a second band that runs from bregma and would have been supported by the mandible (skeleton D′8217G.21). *From Özbek, M., 2001. Cranial deformation in a subadult sample from Değirmentepe (Chalcolithic, Turkey). American Journal of Physical Anthropology 115, 242, 243.*

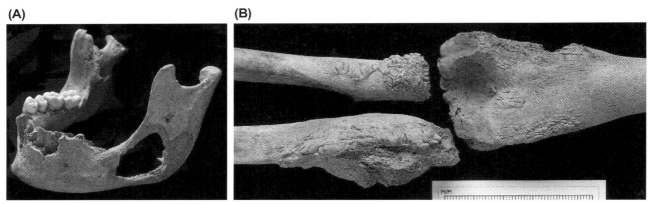

FIGURE 11.5 Possible "phossy jaw" in a 12- to 14-year-old from Coach Lane in Newcastle, England (AD 1711–1857, skeleton 69). (A) The left mandibular ramus displays a large cloaca with reactive new bone around the margins of the lesion. (B) Profuse reactive subperiosteal new bone on the bones of the left elbow. *From Roberts, C.A., Caffell, A., Filipek-Ogden, K.L., Gowland, R., Jakob, T., 2016. 'Til Poison Phosphorous Brought them Death': a potentially occupationally-related disease in a post-medieval skeleton from north-east England. International Journal of Paleopathology 13, 41, 42.*

white phosphorus was replaced by the more economical red phosphorus (Waldron, 2009). Phossy jaw was suggested as a possible differential diagnosis in an adolescent from 19th-century Coach Lane in Newcastle, England (Roberts et al., 2016). The child had osteomyelitis of the mandible and widespread new bone formation on the postcranial skeleton (Fig. 11.5). While chemical analysis of the dental calculus did not reveal unusually high levels of phosphorus, this unique case highlighted the need to include phossy jaw as a differential diagnosis for mandibular osteomyelitis, particularly in postmedieval English samples (Waldron, 2009).

BLADDER STONE DISEASE

This form of urolithiasis is most common in boys under the age of 10 from impoverished rural areas. The formation of the stones is related to nutritional deficiencies in vitamin A, vitamin B6, and magnesium. It is most strongly associated with consumption of high levels of carbohydrates derived from grain, hence its apparent relationship to rural areas. Bladder stones share an inverse relationship with renal stones that form in individuals with a diet high in animal protein (Steinbock, 2003). That the stones are more common in boys may reflect the different morphology of the bladder in males and females. The female bladder is shorter, wider, and straighter allowing any initial calcifications to be passed in the urine before forming into larger stones (Steinbock, 2003). Documentary evidence shows that bladder stones were a concern in impoverished areas of Europe, Asia, and America from 1550 to 1880s. Bladder stones can grow to the size of 8–10 cm and are made up of calcium oxalate or uric acid (Aufderheide and Rodriguez-Martín, 1998). They are generally ellipsoid in shape with a well-defined nucleus and laminated layers, but they may also be asymmetrical, triangular, or even in the shape of a "jack" with several projections. The external surface is usually nodular (Steinbock, 1989). To recover these stones we need to routinely sieve the abdominal areas of burials and be aware that they are just as likely to be associated with nonadult burials, as adult ones.

In 1989, Steinbock provided an excellent review of stones located from archeological sites, two of which were children from ancient Egypt. A 6.5 cm bladder stone was recovered from the grave of a 16-year-old boy from Abydos (3500 BC) and an "adolescent male" from Nagael-Deir (2800 BC) with four renal stones was reported by Shattock (1905). A child with a 1.2 cm bladder stone was also identified in late Roman to early medieval Cannington, Somerset (Brothwell and Powers, 2000), although not described in any detail. More recently, a 3.5 cm oval bladder stone was found in a 13- to 15-year-old from early medieval Sedgeford, Norfolk (Beckett et al., 2008). The stone was slightly pink in color and had a rough surface and laminated internal structure. Analysis of the stone showed the layers were made up of hydroxyapatite and calcium phosphate. The stone is of particular interest because Norfolk was well known for its high level of bladder stones, so much so that it was considered endemic in young males of the region (Beckett et al., 2008), and the Norwich School of Lithotomy was famous throughout Europe for its impressive collection of stones (Shaw, 1970).

LEAD POISONING

Lead accumulates in the hydroxyapatite crystals of the bone matrix resulting in or exacerbating iron deficiency anemia. Lead toxicity has been reported to cause mental retardation, convulsions, nerve damage, encephalopathy, and kidney failure (Kwong et al., 2004; Woolf et al., 1990). Exposure to lead in the past would have occurred due to ingestion of water from lead pipes, the use of lead utensils, air pollution, or through the direct application of lead to the skin through therapeutics and cosmetics (Aufderheide and Rodriguez-Martín, 1998). The Romans were known to boil fruit juices for their children in lead-coated or pewter (tin, lead, copper) vessels, and lead was used as a common sweetening agent ("sugar of lead") (Steinbock, 1979). The use of pewter vessels continued into the medieval period, with pewter bowls and spoons used to feed children containing higher levels of lead than the wine flagons used by adults (Beagrie, 1989). In the Southern United States, lead vessels were also used in the manufacture of rum in the 19th century (Curran, 1984). Children may also have been exposed to lead in utero or through breastfeeding. An increased demand for calcium during pregnancy releases greater amounts of lead from the bone into the maternal bloodstream, which is transmitted to the fetus and newborn (Manton et al., 2003). In a Mexican study, high umbilical cord lead levels were associated with premature births (Torres-Sánchez et al., 1999).

Environmental pollution had been noted in medieval urban environments since the 1250s (Brimblecombe, 2011). By the postmedieval period anthropomorphic lead levels are reported to have reached as high as 90 ppm (Millard et al., 2014), meaning lead exposure would have been a factor in many urbanizing societies in the past. While assessing lead content is problematic due to postmortem accumulation of lead in bone (Bower et al., 2005; Waldron, 1981), the analysis of anthropomorphic lead concentrations in human dental enamel from archeological sites is becoming well established (Budd et al., 2000), as is the identification of the source of lead through stable isotope analysis (Montgomery, 2010). In contrast, there are few features of lead toxicity directly evident on the skeleton, although the formation of a "lead line" in growing bones may be identified (see below). As the body's erythropoietic activity is suppressed in lead toxicity (see Chapter 8), an individual with lead poisoning is unlikely to show skeletal signs of anemia.

TRANSVERSE LINES IN BONE

Harris Lines

Harris lines, or radioopaque lines in the metaphyses, remain a popular but problematic indicator of physiological stress (Fig. 11.6). Park (1954, 1964) and Park and Richter (1953) described the precise mechanism behind the formation of the lines in the 1950s:

1. An episode of acute or chronic stress results in a deceleration of the growth plate as chondroblasts cease to lay down cartilage.
2. Osteoblasts continue to deposit osteoid along the static growth plate, producing a thin layer of bone along the transverse cartilage layer. This line is not visible on radiograph.
3. When normal growth resumes, the osteoblasts recover quickly adding to the pool of osteoid, which is now ossified to produce a layer of dense bone, substantial enough to be visualized on a radiograph.

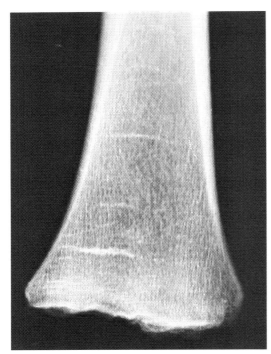

FIGURE 11.6 A series of radioopaque Harris lines in the distal tibia of a nonadult from later medieval St-Helen-on-the-Walls in York, England.

Hence, a Harris line is only evident if normal growth is resumed and the individual recovers from the stress episode. Once the epiphyses have fused, these lines can no longer develop. The exact etiology of Harris lines is unknown, but starvation (Park and Richter, 1953), septicemia, and pneumonia (Acheson and Macintyre, 1958) are among the many conditions associated with a slowing of growth and development of the lines. Sontag and Comstock (1938) highlighted the importance of emotional stress as a factor, and Harris (1933) identified neonatal and fetal lines, which he associated with birth trauma and poor maternal health. Young children were thought to be more predisposed to the development of Harris lines due to rapid growth and frequent illnesses (Dreizen et al., 1964). Good nutrition is directly related to the child's ability to recover rapidly from the stress episode and to begin catch-up growth, and this process is implicated in the greater number of fragmentary (resorbed) lines seen in better-nourished children (Dreizen et al., 1959). In fact, Papageorgopoulou et al. (2011) reported that around half of the Harris lines formed in adolescence would be removed from the tibia by adulthood, highlighting the importance of recording these features in nonadult material.

In bioarchaeology, Harris lines are often used to establish the frequency of stress episodes in a population by counting the mean number of lines, the percentage of individuals affected, and/or the age at which these lines occur most frequently (Ameen et al., 2005; Gronkiewicz et al., 2001; Hughes et al., 1996; Maat, 1984; Mays, 1995; McHenry, 1968; McHenry and Schulz, 1976). Suter et al. (2008) attempted to address some of the issues of Harris line recording, by providing an automated method for detecting lines and calculating the age of line formation in the tibia using digital radiographs. But the use of Harris lines to estimate the frequency of stress is fraught with problems due to intra- and interobserver error, and the fact that many clinical studies have failed to associate the development of lines with any discernible stress episode (Lewis, 2000, 2007). Magennis (1990) argued that Harris lines were associated with accelerated rates of linear growth and are part of the normal growth process, but was unable to establish whether the periods of rapid growth velocity were due to catch-up growth after an insult, or a causative factor. The fact that these lines may be "normal" has been substantiated by Lampl et al. (Lampl and Jeanty, 2003; Lampl et al., 1992) who have shown that periods of growth stasis occur as part of the normal growth process, and this may explain the appearance of Harris lines when no period of illness has been recorded. In their study of 241 Swiss tibiae of adults and children, Papageorgopoulou et al. (2011) also concluded that the majority of Harris lines were likely to be the result of the normal growth process and growth spurts, rather than an indicator of a physiological stress. Boucherie et al. (2016) argue that the etiology of a Harris line should be considered in relation to the age at which it was formed. Lines that are formed between the age of 5–9 years are less likely to be the result of a growth spurt and more likely to indicate a pathological event, while lines formed between 10 and 14 years are more likely to be the result of the pubertal growth spurt.

Lead Lines

Lead lines are thick radioopaque metaphyseal bands that develop under the growth cartilage in children with prolonged exposure to the metal (Fig. 11.7). Lead within the hydroxyapatite interferes with osteoblastic activity causing a lattice of uncalcified cartilage under the growth plate that leaves a thick and tight band of trabeculae when it is eventually calcified. Unlike Harris lines, lead lines are thick, dense, and brightly opaque on radiograph. In Caffey's (1931) original study of these features, lines were reported to be between 0.5 and 9 mm thick depending on the rate of growth of the bone examined. Caffey (1931) noted that these thick bands were actually made up of a series of narrow transverse lines of increased density rather than a single thick band, and that the lines fade as they reach the outer margins, and toward the midshaft. They are best visualized in the iliac bones and vertebral bodies, and have been identified in infants as young as 23 days old (Woolf et al., 1990). Due to a lack of remodeling in the affected area, lead lines may persist longer than Harris lines. Caffey (1938) also noted that in cases of active rickets both calcification and leadification of the cartilage

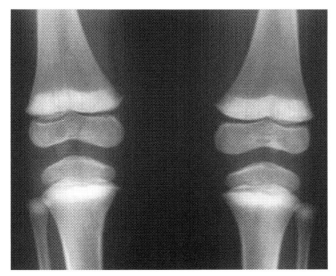

FIGURE 11.7 Thick transverse radioopaque lines at the metaphyses of the femur, tibia, and fibula in a child with lead poisoning. *From Herring, W., 2015. Learning Radiology: recognizing the basics. Elsevier Health Sciences, http://learningradiology.com/images/boneimages1/lead%20 Poisoning-knees.JPG.*

growth plate will produce a radiolucent band of uncalcified cartilage and osteoid without the formation of a lead line. The potential development of low phosphate rickets in reaction to plumbism may limit the use of lead lines to explore the condition in skeletal remains, at least until rickets begins to heal. To date, no systematic study of lead lines in the bones of children from archeological contexts has been carried out.

Bismuth Lines

In 1884 bismuth salts were first used as a treatment for syphilis in infants and children both in utero and after birth. Caffey (1937) identified sharp "metallic" metaphyseal lines in treated dogs that only formed at the time bismuth was administered and not in response to additional arsenic or mercury treatment. A series of lines was noted coinciding with each course of treatment. This episodic appearance of lines ruled out healing syphilitic osteochondritis as the cause. While Caffey (1937) argues that the radiological appearance of bismuth lines is indistinguishable from lead lines, histologically bismuth does not produce a large number of osteoclasts and subsequent lytic lesions seen in lead.

Metaphyseal Bands of Leukemia

These are single thick lines of radiolucency, measuring between 2 and 15mm that form immediately below the metaphyseal surface, which itself appears as a thinner radioopaque band (for more details see Chapter 8). These transverse bands have been shown to be present in

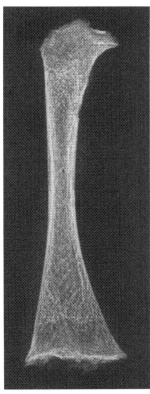

FIGURE 11.8 Wide radiolucent band or Trümmerfeld zone of scurvy at the metaphysis of the right femur of an infant from Bow Baptist Church in London, England (AD 1816–1853, skeleton 346). *From Walker, D., 2012. Disease in London, 1st–19th Centuries. Museum of London Archaeology, London, p. 207.*

10%–89% of leukemia patients, in areas of the skeleton undergoing rapid growth (Bolton-Maggs and Thomas, 2008; Willson, 1959).

Scurvy Line

Abnormal deposition of osteoid in scurvy results in a heavily calcified layer (the "white line of Frankel") at the metaphyses. Directly preceding this white line is an area of thinned trabeculae, appearing as a radiolucent band or "scurvy line" on radiograph (Caffey, 1945), also known as the Trümmerfeld zone (Fig. 11.8). A white line encompassing the epiphyses may also be evident (Wimberger's ring). Once healing begins, this radiolucent scurvy line will disappear rapidly leaving a band of dense calcification, recognized only as a Harris line.

Healing and Healed Rickets

Harris (1933) describes the difference between healing and healed lines of rickets compared to growth arrest lines in detail. Rickets healing lines will only be recognized in cases where the child died within a few months of recovery.

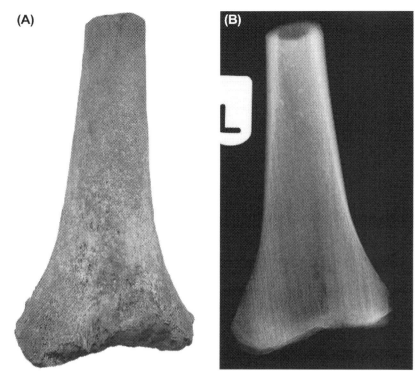

FIGURE 11.9 Osteopathia striata in the amputated distal left femur of a nonadult from Worcester Royal Infirmary (skeleton 801). (A) Macroscopically the bone appears normal although slightly porous, while the radiograph (B) reveals vertical radiolucent bands running along the shaft with fine horizontal radioopaque striae. Reproduced with the kind permission of Gaynor Western.

In healing rickets, a cartilage band of normal width lies below a layer of redundant cartilage that is still undergoing calcification. This new band, together with the osteoid layer will be invisible on radiograph. After healing, this new band appears as a fine line below a band of coarse trabecular bone. This is in contrast to a Harris line where the trabecular bone above and below the line appears normal (Harris, 1933).

OSTEOPATHIA STRIATA

Osteopathia striata with cranial sclerosis is a very rare genetic disease of X-linked inheritance, first described by Voorhoeve (1924) and Fairbank (1925, 1950). It is characterized by radioopaque vertical striations at the metaphyses of the long bones and the ilium. The striations are fine and often clearest at the metaphysis. The condition has been associated with several other anomalies including osteopetrosis, cleft palate, and mental retardation, but the link is not consistent (Bloor, 1954). In their radiographic survey of 134 amputated limb bones from Worcester Royal Infirmary in England, Western and Bekvalac (2015) were the first to identify a case of osteopathia striata in the distal femur of a 14-year-old. The femur showed fine horizontal striae with vertical radiolucent bands running up the shaft (Fig. 11.9; Western pers. comm.).

BONE LENGTH DISCREPANCY

Fluctuating and Directional Asymmetry

In ideal environmental conditions bilateral structures such as limbs develop symmetrically, as mirror images of each other. In reality it is normal for bilateral structures to display small differences of between 1% and 5% (Palmer, 1994). In archeological contexts, this degree of asymmetry is assessed by measuring each paired bone, with the measurement for the right side subtracted from the left. If the sides are symmetrical, there will be a 0 mm difference or there will be a positive (left larger than right) or negative (right larger than left) result (Ruff and Jones, 1981). Bilateral symmetry is categorized into three forms: directional asymmetry (DA) where at a population level, one side is consistently larger than the other (Palmer and Strobeck, 1986); anti- or random asymmetry where the larger side varies within the population; and fluctuating asymmetry (FA) where deviations from symmetry are normally distributed around a mean of zero (Van Valen, 1962). FA is an indicator of environmental stress causing small disturbances in the pattern of development by external factors (Albert and Greene, 1999) and is associated with high morbidity (Livshits and Kobyliansky, 1991). By contrast, DA results from cultural factors such as handedness.

FA has been linked to congenital disorders such as Down syndrome, cleft lip and palate, and mental retardation (Van Dongen et al., 2009; Wilson and Manning, 1996). In 1988, Livshits and collegues noted higher FA in preterm infants compared to their full-term counterparts. This led Steele (2000) to warn against the use of preterm infants when exploring asymmetry in archeological samples as the nature of their death suggests severe stress, which would naturally result in FA. In a later study, Van Dongen et al. (2009) did not find any association between FA and the most severely deformed stillborn children. They suggested that either the development of symmetrical limbs is buffered in utero, or that individuals with FA were eliminated much earlier in the developmental process, or alternatively that asymmetries associated with congenital abnormalities occurred much later in development. In their study of 680 children aged 2–18 years from Liverpool, Wilson and Manning (1996) demonstrated that FA decreased until 10 years of age, after which it increased up to 15 years of age, with a peak at 13 years for males and 14 years for females. After 15 years of age, FA began to decrease. Wilson and Manning (1996) argue that children under 10 years have a higher FA due to rapid growth making asymmetry harder to maintain, while a high metabolic rate linked to increased asymmetry occurred with the onset of puberty between 10 and 15 years, resulting in the differences seen between males and females (Wilson and Manning, 1996). It is possible that the peak identified at 13 years is related to the period of peak height velocity during puberty, and that the decline in FA after 15 years indicates a slowing of growth in postpubertal individuals.

Studies into DA have demonstrated that right side dominance of the upper limb is most common. This is not surprising given a review of manual tasks over a 5000-year period showed that 93% of activities required the preferential use of the right arm (Coren and Porac, 1977). Lower limb dominance by contrast is more common on the left (Cuk and Leben-Seljak), perhaps due to bracing of the left leg when the right arm is in use. In her study of DA in 435 nonadult skeletons (under 18 years) from 11 different English samples, Blackburn (2011) reported that infants showed the greatest symmetry, with asymmetry becoming increasing right side dominant with age. This is consistent with clinical studies showing children developing right-sided handedness after 12 months (Ramsay, 1980; Ramsay et al., 1979). Blackburn (2011) noted the greatest difference occurred at the humeral midshaft, perhaps due to continued remodeling here once remodeling at the articular surface and length had ceased. Franks and Cabo (2014) criticize the use of ratios to control for size in skeletal asymmetry studies and suggest the use of raw right and left differences to assess asymmetry before transforming these scores into ratios. As an alternative to ratios they suggest the use of regression analysis of conversion and principal components analysis.

The percent variation in DA can be calculated using the equation (Auerbach and Raxter, 2008; Auerbach and Ruff, 2006): $(right-left) \times 100/\{(right+left)/2\}$.

Albert and Greene (1999) explored the use of bilateral asymmetry of epiphyseal fusion in paired bones as an indicator of environmental stress. While dental asymmetry is the most commonly employed method, skeletal maturation has been shown to be more sensitive to environmental stress. They studied 90 individuals aged 11–30 years from early and late medieval Kulubnarti in Sudan, with the early medieval population considered to be the more stressed. They found statistically significant differences in the occurrence of asymmetrical fusion in the early medieval population compared to those from a later period, with the right side fusing earlier than the left. This difference between two genetically linked groups argued against handedness being the predominant factor.

Pathological Asymmetry

There is no agreement on how much variability between opposing limbs constitutes a clinical significant feature, as opposed to reflecting FA or DA as part of a general stress process. At which point do side differences in length and width of the bones becomes pathological? How can this be assessed in a child's remains where the length of the bones fluctuates with growth and within the nonadult sample? Expected differences due to FA or DA will be difficult to assess unless each age cohort is controlled for, resulting in very small sample sizes from which a mean "expected" difference can be calculated. In clinical studies it has been suggested that the normal amount of difference between limb lengths in 95% of the population is less than 4 mm at 1 year of age, increasing to 11 mm in adults (Brady et al., 2003). Potentially then, smaller discrepancies in the bone lengths of children may signal pathology compared to greater differences in adults. In Blackburn's (2011) study of nonadult skeletons, normal variations between each side were reported to be at 1.27%, 2.01%, and 0.88% of adult humeral length, diameter, and epicondylar breadth differences, respectively, similar to the values reported by Auerbach and Ruff (2006). Infant values (under 1 year) were much lower at 0.67%, 3.59%, and 2.45%, respectively; in children aged 1–8 years asymmetry increased slightly to 0.77%, 3.06%, and 1.57% reaching adult values by 9 years. To identify asymmetry not caused by natural handedness, an infant humerus that is over 0.7% shorter and 3.6% thinner than the infant mean, or a child humerus that is over 0.8% shorter and 3.6% shorter than the child mean, might indicate pathological change (i.e., disuse atrophy). More especially if the smaller arm is the right and it is accompanied by a thinner cortex and shaft.

Cases of child limb asymmetry are not uncommon in paleopathology, and understanding the exact cause of the discrepancy can be difficult. To date there are around 20 cases of unilateral atrophy in nonadults identified in surveys, skeletal reports, and in the published literature, some associated with more severe skeletal anomalies (e.g., Brothwell and Brown, 1994; Connell et al., 2012; Dickel and Doran, 1989; Holst, 2004; Lewis, 1999; Morse, 1978; Valette et al., 2000) but many with no indication as to the cause. A review carried out by the author, of limb discrepancy in a collection of medieval skeletons from St. Oswald's Priory in Gloucester, England, identified six examples of limb asymmetry in either the humerus or femur in children aged between 5 and 15 years of age. While some changes appeared mild, discrepancies in cortical thickness, shaft circumference, and long bone length of up to 8 mm were observed (Fig. 11.10). Brothwell and Browne (2002) expressed concern about the choice of polio as a common diagnosis in cases of single limb atrophy as their review of clinical cases indicated that bilateral leg involvement was more common in child cases of polio paralysis. Instead, they considered the left arm atrophy evident in a 12-year-old from Jewbury, York, to be the result of birth trauma, although they considered muscular dystrophy (MD) as a potential cause. Child onset limb atrophy can be challenging to identify in nonadults where, unlike adult cases, the condition may not have been in existence for long enough for discrepancies with the unaffected side to become apparent.

Allison and Brooks (1922) outlined ways to diagnose disuse atrophy and its resolution. During the period of disuse, the diameter of the medullary cavity will increase as the shaft diameter decreases, with trabeculae becoming thin and sparse. After prolonged disuse the thinned cortical bone becomes porous. In children, bones are shortened, there is an alteration of shape with cross sections becoming more rounded (as opposed to triangular in the case of the tibia), in comparison with the shaft, and a decrease in thickness of the shaft is more pronounced making the epiphyses appear enlarged by comparison. During recovery, bones remain shortened and the surviving trabeculae become thickened but do not increase in number. Eventually cortical thickness and the size of the medullary cavity will return to normal. There are numerous conditions, other than polio, which may result in paralysis and disuse atrophy of limbs in children (Table 11.1) and these are outlined below. Poliomyelitis is discussed in Chapter 7.

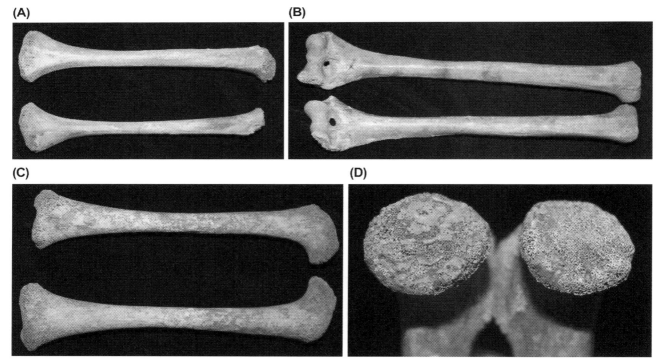

FIGURE 11.10 Various degrees of atrophy in the limb bones of nonadults from St Oswald's Priory in Gloucester, England. (A) A severely atrophied left humerus (bottom) with the unaffected right humerus of a 5- to 6-year-old child with basilar compression on the occipital bone (AD 1540–1857, skeleton 368); (B) less severe but evident atrophy and shortening of the left humerus in comparison to the right in a 13- to 14-year-old (AD 1120–1230, skeleton 95); and (C) atrophy and shortening of the right femur (top) in comparison to the normal left femur of a 5- to 6-year-old with (D) close-up view of the femoral proximal metaphyses (AD 1540–1857, skeleton 364).

TABLE 11.1 Conditions Contributing to Disuse Atrophy

	Condition	Characteristics
Congenital	Cerebral palsy	Multiple limbs, hip joints
	Amyoplasia congenita	Multiple limbs, club foot, bilateral
	Anterior horn lesions	Multiple limbs
	Hereditary brachial plexus neuropathy	Whole upper limb
	Astasia abasia	Inability to stand or walk, hydrocephalus, bilateral
	Cervical rib syndrome	Upper limb
Infection	Congenital varicella (chicken pox)	Passed to child in 2–3 trimester; hypotrophy of upper or lower limb, deformed digits, skin lesions
	Poliomyelitis	Postpolio syndrome, arms and/or legs (can recover)
	Osteomyelitis	Nonuse of affected or related bone
Trauma	Joint or shaft fracture	Nonuse of affected or related bone
	Peripheral nerve or muscle damage	Any limb
	Erb's palsy	Upper arm (breech birth)
	Klumpke's palsy	Lower arm (breech birth)

Cerebral Palsy

Cerebral palsy is an umbrella term for several permanent nonprogressive disorders that occur with damage to the fetal brain (for more details see Chapter 3). It results from infection during pregnancy, insufficient oxygen to the fetus, premature birth, and birth trauma causing skeletal anomalies, paralysis, and delayed maturation (Badawi et al., 1998). In 40% of cases cerebral palsy affects a single limb with 60% of individuals suffering from paralysis of multiple limbs. Hemiplegia is the most common pattern (50%) followed by quadriplegia (25%) and paraplegia (21%). Cerebral palsy is slightly more common in males than females with a modern ratio of 1.3:1. Scoliosis may occur but its severity depends on the extent of neurologic involvement, and there may also be hip dysplasia, femoral neck anteversion (abnormal anterior placement), and foot deformities (Fawcitt, 1964).

Cerebrovascular Incident (Stroke)

Stokes are caused by occlusion of a major artery in the brain and death of tissue cells. The cause may be ischemic or hemorrhagic, and although stokes are considered a risk of old age, they occur in 3.3 per 100,000 children and are associated with congenital heart disease, leukemia, and sickle cell anemia. Neurological disorders include muscle atrophy and hemiplegia (DeVeber et al., 2000).

Rasmussen's Encephalitis

This rare inflammatory neurological disorder is related to progressive epilepsy and cognitive decline. Damage to one brain hemisphere is common, resulting in unilateral or more rarely bilateral hemiparesis and hemiplegia. The age of onset for Rasmussen's encephalitis is normally between 6 and 8 years, with 10% of cases appearing around 12 years of age (Bien et al., 2002).

Chicken Pox (Congenital Varicella)

Congenital Varicella Syndrome was initially described by Hubbard in 1878 and results from the in utero transmission of the *varicella zoster* virus that causes chicken pox in children, and shingles in adults (Gershon, 2005). Many people suffer chicken pox in childhood resulting in a general level of immunity in the population, for this reason congenital varicella is not a common disease, especially in the postvaccine era. However, unimmunized pregnant women are at risk, particularly if they have other children who may be exposed to the infection by their peers. The transplacental transmission rate is estimated to be between 25% and 50% (Gershon, 2005), but only 1%–2% of infants will develop the congenital syndrome. The virus principally invades the nerves (Mandelbrot, 2012), and if varicella is transmitted to the fetus in the first trimester it can be severe, affecting the brain and potentially resulting in microcephaly (Mandelbrot, 2012). Transmission during the second and third trimester causes less severe symptoms, with necrotic tissue on the upper limbs potentially damaging the underlying nerves and muscles. A child may be born normal although 20%–30% develop a fatal chicken pox infection after 10–15 days, resulting from skin hemorrhaging, pneumonia, and damage to their central nervous system (Al-Qattan and Thomson, 1995; Gershon, 2005). In all cases children are at risk of being born with severe skin lesions in the form of ulcerations, muscular atrophy, and unilateral shortening of the limb and associated digits, absence of digits, joint flexure, and secondary disuse atrophy (Al-Qattan and Thomson, 1995; McKendry and Bailey, 1973). The limbs are estimated to be affected in between 46% and 72% of cases (Lamont et al., 2011). Children may be born with a spectrum of changes or only develop a single sign (Mandelbrot, 2012). Hypoplasia of the lower limb is more common than the upper limb, with the degree of limb involvement dependent on the time at which the disease was contracted in utero. Contractions of the fingers may be evident in skeletal remains as palmer grooves, similar to those seen in leprosy. In the foot, unilateral equinovarus and scoliosis may be evident (McKendry and Bailey, 1973).

Arthrogryposis Multiplex Congenita (Congenital Contractures)

This rare congenital condition has a 32% mortality rate and is caused by mutations in the zinc-finger gene (ZC4H2). Arthrogryposis multiplex congenita is characterized by multiple deformities of the joints present at birth (Hirata et al., 2013). Muscles fail to differentiate or are absent and replaced with fibrous or scar tissue. Limbs become contracted, with knee hyperflexion and hip dislocation, and fingers and toes may become permanently flexed. Equinovarus is a common complication (Lloyd-Roberts and Lettin, 1970). Long bones become tubular in shape, slender and porotic due to disuse, and may be subject to secondary fracture. The condition is nonprogressive and may affect a single lower limb, or both upper and lower limbs, and the spine may develop secondary scoliosis. Osteogenesis imperfecta, poliomyelitis or rheumatoid arthritis should be included in the differential diagnoses (Lloyd-Roberts and Lettin, 1970).

Erb's and Klumpke's Palsy (Congenital Brachial Palsy)

Breech delivery may cause trauma to the muscles and other soft tissues of the back and lower limbs and causes secondary paralysis if the child survives. Paralysis may be present as Erb's plasy (affecting the upper arm), Klumpke's palsy (affecting the forearm and hand), or complete limb palsy as the result of trauma to the third and fourth cervical nerves (Yates, 1959). Around 13% of infants will make a spontaneous recovery of muscle strength, but contracture deformity of the hand or elbow can persist limiting full movement of the limb (Adler and Patterson, 1967). In addition to disuse atrophy, dislocation of the radial head and bowing of the ulna with elbow contracture may be identified through flattening of the trochlear and anterior angulations of the radial epiphysis (Adler and Patterson, 1967).

Muscular Dystrophy

Similar to cerebral palsy, MD is a term that covers several conditions usually with a genetic inheritance. Duchenne's MD is the most common type with an incidence of 20–30 males per 100,000 births (Emery et al., 2015). Symptoms appear before the age of 6 years comprising progressive muscle weakness, wasting and contractures of the lower extremities. Today the prognosis is for children to be confined to a wheelchair by 12 years with mortality from respiratory disorders common before they reach adulthood. A less severe form of MD, Becker's MD, usually occurs after 16 years of age with death expected much later when the individual is in their 40s. Facioscapulohumeral MD is less common and affects upper body (face, shoulder, upper arm), causing "winging" of the scapula (Emery et al., 2015).

REFERENCES

Acheson, R.M., Macintyre, M.N., 1958. The effects of acute infection and acute starvation on skeletal development. British Journal of Experimental Pathology 39, 37–45.

Adler, J., Patterson, R., 1967. Erb's palsy. Long-term results of treatment in eighty-eight cases. Journal of Bone and Joint Surgery 49-A (6), 1052–1064.

Al-Qattan, M., Thomson, H., 1995. Congenital varicella of the upper limb. Journal of Hand Surgery (British and European Volume) 20B (1), 115–117.

Albert, A., Greene, D., 1999. Bilateral asymmetry in skeletal growth and maturation as an indicator of environmental stress. American Journal of Physical Anthropology 110 (3), 341–349.

Allison, N., Brooks, B., 1922. Bone atrophy: a clinical study of the changes in bone which result from non-use. Archives of Surgery 5 (3), 499–526.

Ameen, S., Staub, L., Ulrich, S., Viock, P., Ballmer, F., Anderson, S., 2005. Harris lines of the tibia across centuries: a comparison of two populations, medieval and contemporary in Central Europe. Skeletal Radiology 34, 279–284.

Anton, S., 1989. Intentional cranial vault deformation and induced changes of the cranial base and face. American Journal of Physical Anthropology 79, 253–267.

Auerbach, B., Raxter, M., 2008. Patterns of clavicular bilateral asymmetry in relation to the humerus: variation among humans. Journal of Human Evolution 54, 663–674.

Auerbach, B., Ruff, C., 2006. Limb bone bilateral asymmetry: variability and commonality among modern humans. Journal of Human Evolution 50 (2), 203–218.

Aufderheide, A.C., Rodriguez-Martín, C., 1998. The Cambridge Encyclopedia of Human Paleopathology. Cambridge University Press, Cambridge.

Badawi, N., Watson, L., Petterson, B., Blair, E., Slee, J., Haan, E., Stanley, F., 1998. What constitutes cerebral palsy? Developmental Medicine and Child Neurology 40, 520–527.

Beagrie, N., 1989. The Romano-British pewter industry. Britannia 20, 169–191.

Beckett, S., Hatton, M., Rogers, K., 2008. The discovery and analysis of a urinary calculus from an Anglo-Saxon burial in Sedgeford, Norfolk. Norfolk Archaeology 45, 397–409.

Beňuš, R., Masnicová, S., Lietava, J., 1999. Intentional cranial vault deformation in a Slavonic population from the medieval cemetery in Devin (Slovakia). International Journal of Osteoarchaeology 9, 267–270.

Bien, C.G., Widman, G., Urbach, H., Sassen, R., Kuczaty, S., Wiestler, O.D., Schramm, J., Elger, C.E., 2002. The natural history of Rasmussen's encephalitis. Brain 125 (8), 1751–1759.

Blackburn, A., 2011. Bilateral asymmetry of the humerus during growth and development. American Journal of Physical Anthropology 145 (4), 639–646.

Blom, D., Knudson, K., 2014. Tracing Tiwanaku childhoods: a bioarchaeological study of age and social identities in Tiwanaku society. In: Thompson, J., Alfonso-Durruty, M., Crandall, J. (Eds.), Tracing Childhood Bioarchaeological Investigations of Early Lives in Antiquity. University of Florida Press, Gainesville, pp. 228–245.

Bloor, D., 1954. A case of osteopathia striata. Journal of Bone and Joint Surgery British Series 36 (2), 261–265.

Bolton-Maggs, P., Thomas, A., 2008. Disorders of the blood and bone marrow. In: McIntosh, N., Helms, P., Smyth, R., Logan, S. (Eds.), Forfar and Arneil's Textbook of Pediatrics. Churchill Livingstone, London, pp. 959–990.

Boucherie, A., Castex, D., Polet, C., Kacki, S., 2016. Normal growth, altered growth? Study of the relationship between harris lines and bone form within a post-medieval plague cemetery (Dendermonde, Belgium, 16th Century). American Journal of Human Biology. http://dx.doi.org/10.1002/ajhb.22885.

Bower, N., Getty, S., Smith, C., Simpson, Z., Hoffman, J., 2005. Lead isotope analysis of intra-skeletal variation in a 19th century mental asylum cemetery: diagenesis versus migration. International Journal of Osteoarchaeology 15, 360–370.

Brady, R., Dean, J., Skinner, T., Gross, M., 2003. Limb length inequality: clinical implications for assessment and intervention. Journal of Orthopaedic and Sports Physical Therapy 33 (5), 221–234.

Brimblecombe, P., 2011. The Big Smoke: A History of Air Pollution in London since Medieval Times. Routledge, London.

Brothwell, D., Brown, S., 1994. Pathology. In: Lilley, S., Stroud, G., Brothwell, D., Williamson, M. (Eds.), The Jewish Burial Ground at Jewbury. Current British Archaeology, York, pp. 465–466.

Brothwell, D., Browne, S., 2002. Skeletal atrophy and the problem of the differential diagnosis of conditions causing paralysis. Antroplogia Portuguesa 19, 5–17.

Brothwell, D., Powers, R., 2000. The human biology. In: Rathtz, P., Hirst, S., Wright, S. (Eds.), Cannington Cemetery. English Heritage, London.

Budd, P., Montgomery, J., Evans, J., Barreiro, B., 2000. Human tooth enamel as a record of the comparative lead exposure of prehistoric and modern people. Science of the Total Environment 263 (1), 1–10.

Caffey, J., 1931. Clinical and experimental lead poisoning: some roentgenologic and anatomical changes in growing bones. Radiology 17 (5), 957–983.

Caffey, J., 1937. Changes in the growing skeleton after the administration of Bismuth. American Journal of Diseases in Children 53 (1), 798–806.

Caffey, J., 1938. Lead poisoning associated with active rickets. American Journal of Diseases in Children 55 (4), 798–806.

Caffey, J., 1945. Pediatric X-Ray Diagnosis. Year Book Medical Publishers, Inc., Chicago.

Connell, B., Gray Jones, A., Redfern, R., Walker, D., 2012. A Bioarchaeological Study of Medieval Burials on the Site of St Mary Spital. Museum of London Archaeology, London.

Coren, S., Porac, C., 1977. Fifty centuries of right-handedness: the historical record. Science 198 (4317), 631–632.

Cuk, T., Leben-Seljak, P., Stefanovic, M., 2001. Lateral asymmetry of human long bones. Variability and Evolution 9, 19–32.

Curran, A.S., 1984. Lead poisoning: an historical overview. New York State Journal of Medicine 437–438.

DeVeber, G., Roach, E.S., Riela, A., Wiznitzer, M., 2000. Stroke in children: recognition, treatment, and future directions. Seminars in Pediatric Neurology 309–317.

Dickel, D., Doran, G., 1989. Severe neural tube defect syndrome from the early archaic of Florida. American Journal of Physical Anthropology 80, 325–334.

Dreizen, S., Currie, C., Gilley, E.J., Spies, T.D., 1959. Observations on the association between nutritive failure, skeletal maturation rate and radiopaque transverse lines in the radius in children. American Journal of Roentogeneology 76 (3), 482–487.

Dreizen, S., Spirakis, N., Stone, R., 1964. The influence of age and nutritional status on 'bone scar' formation in the distal end of the growing radius. American Journal of Physical Anthropology 22, 295–306.

Duncan, W., Hofling, C., 2011. Why the head? Cranial modification as protection and ensoulment among the Maya. Ancient Mesoamerica 22, 199–210.

Emery, A.E., Muntoni, F., Quinlivan, R.C., 2015. Duchenne Muscular Dystrophy. Oxford University Press, Oxford.

Fairbank, H., 1925. A case of unilateral affection of the skeleton of unknown origin. The British Journal of Surgery 12, 594–599.

Fairbank, H., 1950. Osteopathia striata. The Journal of Bone and Joint Surgery 32-B (1), 117–125.

Fawcitt, J., 1964. Skeletal changes in cerebral palsy children. Annals of Radiology 7 (5–6), 466–471.

Franks, E., Cabo, L., 2014. Quantifying asymmetry: ratios and alternatives. American Journal of Physical Anthropology 154 (4), 498–511.

Gershon, A., 2005. Varicella-Zoster virus. In: Hutto, C. (Ed.), Infectious Diseases: Congenital and Perinatal Infections: A Concise Guide to Diagnosis. Humana Press Inc., Totowa, pp. 91–100.

Gronkiewicz, S., Kornafel, D., Kwiatkowska, B., Nowakowski, D., 2001. Harris's lines versus children's living conditions in medieval Wroclaw, Poland. Variability and Evolution 9, 45–50.

Harris, H.A., 1933. Bone Growth in Health and Disease. Oxford University Press, London.

Herring, W., 2015. Learning Radiology: recognizing the basics. Elsevier Health Sciences.

Hinshaw, W.B., Quin, L.D., 2015. Recognition of the causative agent of "Phossy Jaw" and "Fragile Femur" in fumes arising from white phosphorus. Phosphorus, Sulfur, and Silicon and the Related Elements 190 (12), 2082–2093.

Hirata, H., Nanda, I., van Riesen, A., McMichael, G., Hu, H., Hambrock, M., Papon, M.-A., Fischer, U., Marouillat, S., Ding, C., 2013. ZC4H2 mutations are associated with arthrogryposis multiplex congenita and intellectual disability through impairment of central and peripheral synaptic plasticity. The American Journal of Human Genetics 92 (5), 681–695.

Holliday, D., 1993. Occipital lesions: a possible cost of cradleboards. American Journal of Physical Anthropology 90, 283–290.

Holst, M., 2004. Osteological Analysis. Bempton Lane, Bridlington (Unpublished Report): York Osteoarchaeology Ltd.

Hrdlička, A., 1935. The Pueblos. With comparative data on the bulk of the tribes of the Southwest and northern Mexico. American Journal of Physical Anthropology 20 (3), 235–460.

Hubbard, T., 1878. Varicella occurring in an infant twenty-four hours after birth. British Medical Journal 1, 822.

Hughes, C., Heylings, D.J.A., Power, C., 1996. Transverse (Harris) lines in Irish archaeological remains. American Journal of Physical Anthropology 101 (1), 115–131.

Kausmally, T., Ives, R., 2007. Lytic Lesions in the Skull. Problems of Diagnosis in Infantile Human Remains. Paper Presented at the British Association of Biological Anthropology and Osteoarchaeology. University of Reading.

Kwong, W., Friello, P., Semba, R., 2004. Interactions between iron deficiency and lead poisoning: epidemiology and pathogenesis. Science of the Total Environment 330, 21–37.

Lamont, R.F., Sobel, J.D., Carrington, D., Mazaki-Tovi, S., Kusanovic, J.P., Vaisbuch, E., Romero, R., 2011. Varicella-zoster virus (chickenpox) infection in pregnancy. An International Journal of Obstetrics & Gynaecology 118 (10), 1155–1162.

Lampl, M., Jeanty, P., 2003. Timing is everything: a reconsideration of fetal growth velocity patterns identifies the importance of individual and sex differences. American Journal of Human Biology 15, 667–680.

Lampl, M., Veldhuis, J.D., Johnson, M.L., 1992. Salutation and stasis: a model of human growth. Science 258, 801–803.

Lewis, M., 1999. The Impact of Urbanisation and Industrialisation in Medieval and Post-medieval Britain. An Assessment of the Morbidity and Mortality of Non-adult Skeletons from the Cemeteries of Two Urban and Two Rural Sites in England (AD 850–1859) (Ph.D. thesis). University of Bradford.

Lewis, M., 2000. Non-adult palaeopathology: current status and future potential. In: Cox, M., Mays, S. (Eds.), Human Osteology in Archaeology and Forensic Science. Greenwich Medical Media Ltd, London, pp. 39–57.

Lewis, M., 2007. The Bioarchaeology of Children. Cambridge University Press, Cambridge.

Livshits, G., Davidi, L., Kobyliansky, E., Ben-Amitai, D., Levi, Y., Merlob, P., Optiz, J.M., Reynolds, J.F., 1988. Decreased developmental stability as assessed by fluctuating asymmetry of morphometric traits in preterm infants. American Journal of Medical Genetics 29 (4), 793–805.

Livshits, G., Kobyliansky, E., 1991. Fluctuating asymmetry as a possible measure of developmental homeostasis in humans: a review. Human Biology 441–466.

Lloyd-Roberts, G., Lettin, A., 1970. Arthrogryposis multiplex congenita. The Journal of Bone and Joint Surgery 52B (3), 494–508.

Maat, G.J.R., 1984. Dating and rating of Harris's lines. American Journal of Physical Anthropology 63, 291–299.

Magennis, A.L., 1990. Growth velocity as a factor influencing the formation of transverse lines. American Journal of Physical Anthropology 81 (2), 262.

Mandelbrot, L., 2012. Fetal varicella–diagnosis, management, and outcome. Prenatal Diagnosis 32 (6), 511–518.

Manton, W., Angle, C., Stanek, K., Kuntzelman, D., Reese, Y., Kuehnemann, T., 2003. Release of lead from bone in pregnancy and lactation. Environmental Research 92 (2), 139–151.

Mays, S., 1995. The relationship between Harris lines and other aspects of skeletal development in adults and juveniles. Journal of Archaeological Sciences 22, 511–520.

McHenry, H., 1968. Transverse lines in long bones of prehistoric California Indians. American Journal of Physical Anthropology 29, 1–18.

McHenry, H.M., Schulz, P.D., 1976. The association between Harris lines and enamel hypoplasia in prehistoric California Indians. American Journal of Physical Anthropology 44, 507–512.

McKendry, J., Bailey, J., 1973. Congenital varicella associated with multiple defects. Canadian Medical Association Journal 108 (1), 66.

Meiklejohn, C., Agelarakis, A., Akkermans, P.A., Smith, P.E., Solecki, R., 1992. Artificial cranial deformation in the Proto-Neolithic and Neolithic Near East and its possible origin: evidence from four sites. Paléorient 18 (2), 83–97.

Mendonça de Souza, S., Reinhard, K.J., Lessa, A., 2008. Cranial deformation as the cause of death for a child from the Chillion River valley, Peru. Chungara. Revista de Anthropologia Chilian 40 (1), 41–53.

Millard, A., Montgomery, J., Trickett, M., Beaumont, J., Evans, J., Chenery, S., 2014. Childhood lead exposure in the British Isles during the industrial revolution. In: Zuckerman, M. (Ed.), Modern Environmental and Human Health. Wiley Blackwell, New York, pp. 279–300.

Montgomery, J., 2010. Passports from the past: investigating human dispersals using strontium isotope analysis of tooth enamel. Annals of Human Biology 37 (3), 325–346.

Morse, D., 1978. Ancient Disease in the Midwest. Ilinois State Museum, Springfield.

Mukherjee, S., Song, Y., Oldfield, E., 2008. NMR investigations of the static and dynamic structures of bisphosphonates on human bone: a molecular model. Journal of the American Chemical Society 130 (4), 1264–1273.

O'Loughlin, V.D., 2004. Effects of different kinds of cranial deformation on the incidence of wormian bones. American Journal of Physical Anthropology 123 (2), 146–155.

Özbek, M., 2001. Cranial deformation in a subadult sample from Değirmentepe (Chalcolithic, Turkey). American Journal of Physical Anthropology 115, 238–244.

Palmer, A., Strobeck, C., 1986. Fluctuating asymmetry: measurement, analysis, patterns. Annual Review of Ecology and Systematics 17, 391–421.

Palmer, A.R., 1994. Fluctuating Asymmetry Analyses: A Primer. Developmental Instability: its Origins and Evolutionary Implications. Springer, New York, pp. 335–364.

Papageorgopoulou, C., Suter, S.K., Rühli, F.J., Siegmund, F., 2011. Harris lines revisited: prevalence, comorbidities, and possible etiologies. American Journal of Human Biology 23 (3), 381–391.

Park, E.A., 1954. Bone growth in health and disease. Archives of Diseases in Childhood 29, 269–281.

Park, E.A., 1964. The imprinting of nutritional disturbances on the growing bone. Pediatrics 33 (6), 815–862.

Park, E.A., Richter, C.P., 1953. Transverse lines in bone: the mechanism of their development. Bulletin of the Johns Hopkins Hospital 93, 234–248.

Pomeroy, E., Stock, J.T., Zakrzewski, S.R., Lahr, M.M., 2010. A metric study of three types of artificial cranial modification from north-central Peru. International Journal of Osteoarchaeology 20 (3), 317–334.

Ramsay, D., 1980. Onset of unimanual handedness in infants. Infant Behavior and Development 3, 377–385.

Ramsay, D., Campos, J., Fenson, L., 1979. Onset of bimanual handedness in infants. Infant Behavior and Development 2, 69–79.

Roberts, C.A., Caffell, A., Filipek-Ogden, K.L., Gowland, R., Jakob, T., 2016. 'Til Poison Phosphorous Brought them Death': a potentially occupationally-related disease in a post-medieval skeleton from north-east England. International Journal of Paleopathology 13, 39–48.

Ruff, C.B., Jones, H.H., 1981. Bilateral asymmetry in cortical bone of the humerus and tibia—sex and age factors. Human Biology 69–86.

Shattock, S., 1905. A prehistoric or predynastic Egyptian calculus. In: Transactions of the Pathological Society, vol. 56. London, pp. 275–291.

Shaw, A.B., 1970. The Norwich School of Lithotomy. Medical History 14 (3), 221–259.

Sontag, L.W., Comstock, G., 1938. Striae in the bones of a set of monozygotic triplets. American Journal of Diseases in Children 56, 301–308.

Steele, J., 2000. Skeletal indicators of handedness. In: Cox, M., Mays, S. (Eds.), Human Osteology in Archaeology and Forensic Science. Greenwich Medical Media Ltd, London, pp. 307–323.

Steinbock, R., 1989. Studies in ancient calcified soft tissues and organic concretions. II. Urolithiasis (renal and urinary bladder stone disease). Journal of Paleopathology 3, 41–69.

Steinbock, R.T., 1979. Lead ingestion in history. The New England Journal of Medicine 301 (5), 277.

Steinbock, T., 2003. Bladder-stone disease. In: Kiple, K. (Ed.), The Cambridge Historical Dictionary of Disease. Cambridge University Press, Cambridge, pp. 357–358.

Suter, S., Harders, M., Papageorgopoulou, C., Kuhn, G., Székely, G., Rühli, F., 2008. Technical note: standardized and semiautomated Harris lines detection. American Journal of Physical Anthropology 137 (3), 362–366.

Tiesler, V., 2011. Becoming Mayan: infancy and upbringing through the lens of pre-Hispanic head shaping. Childhood in the Past 4, 117–132.

Torres-Sánchez, L.E., Berkowitz, G., López-Carrillo, L., Torres-Arreola, L., Ríos, C., López-Cervantes, M., 1999. Intrauterine lead exposure and preterm birth. Environmental Research Section A 81, 297–301.

Valette, A., Capasso, L., Scarsini, B., 2000. A hydrocephalus from the necropolis of Pontecagnano (IX-III Centuries B.C.). In: Thirteenth Biannual European Members Meeting of the Paleopathology Association. Chieti, Italy.

Van Dongen, S., Wijnaendts, L., Ten Broek, C., Galis, F., 2009. Fluctuating asymmetry does not consistently reflect severe developmental disorders in human fetuses. Evolution 63 (7), 1832–1844.

Van Valen, L., 1962. A study of fluctuating asymmetry. Evolution 16 (2), 125–142.

Voorhoeve, N., 1924. L'image radiologique non encore decrite d'une anomalie du squelette: Ses rapports avec la dyschondroplasie et l'osteopathia condensans disseminata. Acta Radiologica 36 (3), 407–427.

Waldron, H., 1981. Postmortem absorption of lead by the skeleton. American Journal of Physical Anthropology 55, 395–398.

Waldron, T., 2009. Palaeopathology. Cambridge University Press, Cambridge.

Western, A., Bekvalac, J., 2015. Digital radiography and historical contextualisation of the 19th century modified human skeletal remains from the Worcester Royal Infirmary, England. International Journal of Paleopathology 10, 58–73.

White, C., 1996. Sutural effects of fronto-occipital cranial modification. American Journal of Physical Anthropology 100 (3), 397–410.

Whyte, M.P., Obrecht, S.E., Finnegan, P.M., Jones, J.L., Podgornik, M.N., McAlister, W.H., Mumm, S., 2002. Osteoprotegerin deficiency and juvenile Paget's disease. New England Journal of Medicine 347 (3), 175–184.

Willson, J.K., 1959. The bone lesions of leukemia: a survey of 140 cases. Radiology 72 (5), 672–681.

Wilson, J.M., Manning, J.T., 1996. Fluctuating asymmetry and age in children: evolutionary implications for the control of developmental stability. Journal of Human Evolution 30, 529–537.

Woolf, D., Riach, I., Derweesh, A., Vyras, H., 1990. Lead lines in young infants with acute lead encephalopathy: a reliable diagnostic technique. Journal of Tropical Pediatrics 36, 90–93.

Yates, P., 1959. Birth trauma to the vertebral arteries. Archives of Disease in Childhood 34, 436–441.

Index

'*Note*: Page numbers followed by "f" indicate figures, "t" indicate tables.'

A

Achondroplasia, 46–48
  bullet-shaped, 46–47
  case study, 47–48
  cist grave, 47
  cone-shaped, 46–47
  minor dental developmental delay, 47–48
  nonadult material, 47
  physical appearance of, 46–47
  skeletal features, 47
Acromesomelic dysplasia, 48
Actinobacillus actinomycetemcomitans, 77–78
Active immunity, 5–6
Alveolar bone, 77
Anemia, 193
Anencephaly, 35–37
Aneurismal bone cyst, 236, 237f
Anomalies
  birth defects, 17–18
  cranium
    congenital deafness, 28–29
    Crouzon's syndrome, 25–26
    development of, 19
    fontanels, 19
    hydrocephaly, 26–28
    microcephaly, 26
    premature cranial suture closure, 20–26
  defects, 17
  dental anomalies
    dental fusion, 81–83
    hyperdontia (supernumerary teeth), 80
    hypodontia, 79–80
    macrodontia and microdontia, 83
    natal and neonatal teeth, 80
    talon cusps, 83
  embryonic period, 18
  endosteal, 19
  extremities
    polydactyly and syndactyly, 34
    radioulnar synostosis, 33–34
    talipes equinovarus (clubfoot), 33
  homeobox/Hox genes, 18
  malformations, 17–18
  neural tube defects
    congenital herniation (dystrophism), 34–35
    anencephaly, 35–37
    cleft palate, 37–39
    spina bifida, 39–40
  prenatal development, critical periods in, 18, 19f
  skeletal development, 19
  spine
    cervical spine, 29
    cleft neural arches, 31–32, 32f
    congenital kyphosis, 29
    congenital lordosis, 29
    congenital scoliosis, 29
    lumbarization and sacralization, 30, 31f
    occipitalization (atlantooccipital fusion), 29–30, 30f
    sagittal clefting, 30–31, 32f
    spondylolysis, 30
  teratogens, 17
  terminology, 18
  thorax
    bifid ribs, 33
    costal fusion, 33
    supernumerary ribs, 32
Antemortem tooth loss, 78, 79f
Anterior–posterior (AP), 7, 268
Apert's syndrome, 23–25
Aural atresia, 28–29, 29f
Aural stenosis, 28–29, 28f

B

Benign primary tumors
  chrondroblastoma, 234, 234f
  chrondromas and Ollier's disease, 232–233
  chrondromyxoid fibroma, 234
  desmoid fibroma (desmoplastic fibroma), 234
  fibrous cortical defects, 234–235, 235f
  giant-cell tumor (osteoclastoma), 231, 231f
  HMO, 232, 233f
  nonossifying fibroma, 235, 236f
  osteoblastoma (codman's tumor), 230, 230f
  osteochondroma, 231–232, 232f–233f
  osteofibrous dysplasia, 235–236
  osteoid osteoma, 230, 230f
Bifid ribs, 33
Binder syndrome (maxillonasal dysplasia), 53–54
Bladder stone disease, 270–271
Blood-borne disorders. *See* Hemopoietic disorders
Blount's disease (tibia vara), 255, 255f
Boldsen's model, 10
Bone cysts, 226
  aneurismal bone cyst, 236, 237f
  unicameral (solitary) bone cyst, 236, 237f
Bone length discrepancy
  fluctuating and directional asymmetry, 274–275
  pathological asymmetry
    arthrogryposis multiplex congenita (congenital contractures), 278
    cerebral palsy, 277
    cerebrovascular incident (stroke), 277
    chicken pox (congenital varicella), 277–278
    Erb's and Klumpke's palsy (congenital brachial palsy), 278
    limb asymmetry, 276
    MD, 278
    Rasmussen's encephalitis, 277
Bone remodeling, 5
Bone, 3
  bone formation and remodeling, 4–5
  bone length discrepancy
    fluctuating and directional asymmetry, 274–275
    pathological asymmetry, 275–278
  long bone fractures, 96
  rapid bone remodeling, implications of, 8
  transverse lines in
    bismuth lines, 273
    Harris lines, 271–272
    healing and healed rickets, 273–274
    lead lines, 272–273
    leukemia, metaphyseal bands of, 273
    scurvy line, 273
  woven and lamellar bone, 4–5
Brachycephaly, 22–23
Brittle bone disease, 60
Brodie's abscess, 136–137
Buckle fractures, 94

C

Caffey's disease, 145
Calculus, 76–77
Cancer, 225
Carpenter's syndrome, 22
Cerebral palsy, 63–64, 277
Cerebrospinal fluid, 26–27
Cerebrovascular incident (stroke), 277
Chicken pox (congenital varicella), 277–278
Child paleopathology
  comorbidity and cooccurrence, 11–12
  differential diagnosis, 10–11
  frailty and selective mortality, hidden heterogeneity of, 8–9
  frailty and susceptibility, child's level of, 1
  growing bone, nature of, 2–3

283

Child paleopathology (*Continued*)
  immune system development
    adaptive immunity, 5
    adolescent, 6–7
    bioarchaeology, exploring immunodeficiency in, 7
    childhood immunity, 6
    humoral immunity, 5
    innate immunity, 5
    newborn, 5–6
  measuring specificity, 9–10
  paleopathological practice, 10
  pathological lesions, 1–2
  pediatric paleopathology, factors in, 8
  Scheuermann's disease, 1–2
  scurvy, 1–2
  skeletal development and ossification
    bone formation and remodeling, 4–5
    endochondral ossification, 3–4
    intramembranous ossification, 3
    ossification, pattern and timing of, 5
    primary germ layers, 3
  soft tissue, 10
Chordoma, 241
Chrondroblastoma, 234, 234f
Chrondrogenic tumors, 226
Chrondromas, 232–233
Chrondromyxoid fibroma, 234
Chronic sinusitis
  acute bacterial sinusitis, 139
  allergies, 139
  cobweb-like lesion, 139, 139f
  frontal sinus, 137–138, 138f
  maxillary sinuses, 137–139, 138f
  nonadult studies, 139
  odontogenic sinusitis, 139–140
  pathogens, 139
  trapped bacteria, 137–138
  upper respiratory tract infections, 138–139
Circulatory disorders
  osteochondroses, 252–254
    Blount's disease (tibia vara), 255, 255f
    Legg–Calvé–Perthes disease, 255–256, 257f
    Scheuermann's disease (juvenile kyphosis, spinal osteochondrosis), 256–258, 257f–258f
Claw–hand deformity, 169
Cleft palate
  bilateral cleft palate, 37–38
  cleft mandible, 39, 39f
  differential diagnosis, 38
  environmental factors, 37–38
  lateral incisor, 37–38
  U-shaped deformity, 37–38
Congenital herniation (dystrophism), 34–35
Congenital syndromes
  Binder syndrome (maxillonasal dysplasia), 53–54
  cerebral palsy, 63–64
  Down syndrome (trisomy 21) and aneuploid conditions
    archaeological record, 59
    chromosomes, 57–58
    cranial features, 59
    dental changes, 57–58
    heart defects, 58
    nasal bones, 58–59
    sonographs, 58–59
  Klippel–Feil syndrome
    clinical changes, 55
    midthoracic vertebrae, 55–57
    skeletal features, 57, 58t
    types, 55
  osteogenesis imperfecta, 60–61, 63f
  osteopetrosis (osteosclerosis fragilis), 61
  physical impairment, 45–46
Copper/silver beaten skull, 27
Corrected caries rate (CCR), 75
Costal fusion, 33
Crania, 115
Cranial fractures
  archaeological contexts, 103
  mandible, fractures of, 103–104
  ping-pong injury, 102–103
Cranial modification
  anteroposterior deformation, 268
  circumferential/circular deformation, 268–269
Craniofacial dysotosis type 1, 25–26
Cranium
  congenital deafness, 28–29
  Crouzon's syndrome, 25–26
  development of, 19
  fontanels, 19
  hydrocephaly, 26–28
    archeological record, 27–28
    cerebrospinal fluid, 26–27
    diagnosis, 27
    enlarged head, 27
    features of, 27
  microcephaly, 26
  premature cranial suture closure
    artificial cranial modification, symptom of, 21–22
    brachycephaly, 22–23
    cloverleaf deformity, 25, 25f
    craniostenosis, 21, 21t
    craniosynostosis, 20–21
    function, 20–21
    oxycephaly, 23–25, 25f
    plagiocephaly, 23, 24f
    sagittal suture, 21–22
    scaphocephaly, 22
    sutural agenesis, 20–21
    trigonocephaly, 23, 24f
  TB, 156–157
Cushing's disease,
Cuspal enamel hypoplasia, 84–85

D

Decayed, missing, or filled (DMF), 75
Deformation, 18
Dental disease
  antemortem tooth loss, 78, 79f
  calculus, 76–77
  chronic dental conditions, 67
  dental anomalies
    dental fusion, 81–83
    hyperdontia (supernumerary teeth), 80
    hypodontia, 79–80
    macrodontia and microdontia, 83
    natal and neonatal teeth, 80
    talon cusps, 83
  dental caries
    deciduous caries, 68–70
    low molecular weight, 68
    risk factor, 68
    Streptococcus mutans, 68
  dental development, disruption in
    dental enamel hypoplasia, 84–85, 84t
    Turner's and Skinner's teeth, 85–86
  nonadult caries
    antemortem tooth loss, 70
    anterior deciduous teeth, 71–72, 74f
    bottle caries, 71–72
    children, recording and reporting caries in, 75–76
    clinical pattern, 70–71
    dental enamel hypoplasia and caries, 70
    medieval groups, 70
    refined foods, 70
    true prevalence rates, 70–71, 71t–74t
  oral infections, 67
  periapical cavitation, 77
  teething, 67–68
  trauma
    dental modification, 84
    maxillary incisors, 83–84
    solitary bone cysts, 83–84
Desmoid fibroma (desmoplastic fibroma), 234
Developmental dysplasia of the hip (DDH), 49–52
Developmental Origins of Health and Disease (DOHaD), 7
Dietary iron-deficiency anemia
  clinical symptoms of, 197
  common cause of, 197–198
  cranial lesions, 198
Directional asymmetry, 274–275
Dislocations
  glenohumeral junction/upper limb, 112
  hip dislocations/lower limb, 112–114
  pelvic fractures, 112–114
  shoulder dislocations, 112
Disruption, 18
Down syndrome, 1–2
Dry bone, 3
Dysplasia, 18

E

Early childhood caries (ECC), 68–69
Ectoderm (outer layer), 3
Ekman-Westborg–Julin syndrome, 83
Enamel matrix secretion, 84
Endochondral ossification
  cartilage template, 3–4
  growth plate, 4
  vitamin D deficiency, 4
Endocranial lesions
  acute leptomeningitis, 144
  cerebrospinal fluid, 142
  dura mater, 142
  epidural hematomas, 144

extradural hematomas, 144
meningitis, 144
middle arachnoid layer, 142
nature and distribution of, 144–145
pediatric bone, 144
periosteal reactions, 142–144
pia mater, 142
subdural hematomas, 144
TB, 144
types, 141–142, 143f
Endocrine disturbances
anterior lobe, 259
Cushing's disease, 261
differentiation of, 259, 260t
hypergonadism, 262
hyperparathyroidism, 262–263
hyperpituitarism (pituitary gigantism, acromegaly), 259–260
hyperthyroidism (thyrotoxicosis), 261
hypogonadism, 261–262
hypoparathyroidism, 262
hypopituitarism (pituitary dwarfism), 259
hypothyroidism (myxedema), 260–261
PTHs, 259
skeletal pathology, 258–259
Endoderm (inner layer), 3
Epiphysis, 5
Erb's plasy, 278
Erlenmeyer-flask deformity, 52–53, 53f
Ewing's sarcoma, 241

F
Fiber bone. *See* Woven/immature bone
Fibrous cortical defects, 234–235, 235f
Fibrous dysplasia, 53
Fluctuating asymmetry (FA), 274–275

G
Generalized aggressive periodontal disease, 78
Genetic disorders, 61
Giant-cell tumor (osteoclastoma), 231, 231f
Greenstick fractures, 92–93

H
Healing
features and time since, 98, 99t
fracture healing, 98, 99t
humerus tuberosity, 98
terminal phalanges, 98
tibial malleolus, 98
Hematoma, 92–93
Hemophilia, 207–209
Hemophilic arthritis, 252
Hemopoietic disorders
anemia, 193
cribra orbitalia, 194, 195f, 196–197
cribrous syndrome, 194–196
dietary iron-deficiency anemia
clinical symptoms of, 197
common cause of, 197–198
cranial lesions, 198
fetus blood cell formation, 193
folic acid and vitamin B12, 197
hair-on-end trabeculae, 194

hemophilia A and B, 207–209
leukemia
acute lymphoblastic leukemia, 206
archeological case of, 207
critical feature of, 206–207
endosteal and intracortical bone resorption, 207
fibula, 207
metaphysic, 206
osteolytic lesions, 207
types of, 206
folate deficiency, 199
lead poisoning, 199–200
malaria, 198–199
orbital lesions, 196–197
parasitic infections, 199
porotic hyperostosis, 194, 196–197
porous lesions, 194–196
postnatal skeletal development, 193
protein molecule hemoglobin, 193
red bone marrow, 193, 195f
sickle cell anemia
genetic abnormality, 204
hair-on-end skull changes, 204–205
hemoglobin S, gene for, 203–204
low hemoglobin levels, 204
marrow infarction, 204–205
punched-out lesions, 204–205
thalassemia
cranial changes, 200
facial changes, 200
gene mutations, 200
genetic transmission, types of, 200
hemoglobin, 200
osseous changes, 200–201
pathological fractures, 200–201
postcranial bones, 201–203
premature epiphyseal fusion, 201
red blood cells, 200
skeletal expression, 200–201
symptoms, 200
vitamin B12 deficiency, 199
yellow bone marrow, 193, 194f
Hereditary multiple osteochondroma (HMO), 232, 233f
Hodgkin's lymphoma, 242
Hutchinson's incisors, 179–180, 181f
Hydrocephaly
archeological record, 27–28
cerebrospinal fluid, 26–27
diagnosis, 27
enlarged head, 27
features of, 27
Hyperdontia (supernumerary teeth), 80
Hyperphalangism, 34
Hyperthyroidism (thyrotoxicosis), 261
Hypertrophic osteoarthropathy (HOA), 161–162
Hypodontia, 79–80
Hypopituitarism (pituitary dwarfism), 259
Hypothyroidism (myxedema), 260–261

I
Immunoglobulin A (IgA), 68–69
Infantile cortical hyperostosis (ICH), 145–147
Infantile cranial lacunae, 267
Infantile osteomyelitis, 136
Infantile scurvy (vitamin C deficiency)
breast milk, 213–214
cereals, 213–214
comorbidity and cooccurrence, 218
differential diagnoses, 216–217
early radiographic signs, 214
healing microfractures, 216
histological techniques, 214–215
macroscopic and radiological features, 216, 217t
Möller–Barlow disease, 214–215
postcranial lesions, 215–216
prevalence rates, 217–218
radiographs, 216, 216f
ribs, 215–216
scorbutic infants, 214
subperiosteal hemorrhage, 214
Trümmerfeld zone, 216
type 1 collagen forms, 213–214
Infective osteitis, 133–134
Insulin-like growth factor (IGF-1), 259
Iron-deficiency anemia, 197

J
Joint mouse, 110–111
Juvenile ankylosing spondylitis (JAS), 250
Juvenile idiopathic arthritis (JIA)
prevalence of, 245
skeletal lesions, 245–246
scoliosis, 245–246
bird-face deformity, 246
swollen fingers, 246, 246f
skeletal lesions, 246, 247t
femoral heads, 246–247
systemic arthritis, 247
seronegative idiopathic arthritis, 248–249
Juvenile-onset adult-type rheumatoid arthritis (JORA), 249–250, 250f–251f
juvenile psoriatic arthritis, 250
hemophilic arthritis, 252
Schmorl's nodes, 252, 254f
Juvenile osteochondritis dissecans (JOCD), 110–111
Juvenile psoriatic arthritis, 250
Juvenile rheumatoid arthritis (JRA), 245

K
Klippel–Feil syndrome, 245–246
clinical changes, 55
midthoracic vertebrae, 55–57
skeletal features, 57, 58t
types, 55
Klumpke's palsy, 278

L

Lacunar skull, 267, 268f
Lamellar/mature bone, 4–5
Langerhans cell histiocytosis (LCH), 225
    eosinophilic granuloma
        Hand–Schüller–Christian disease, 238–239
        Letterer–Siwe disease, 239
    histiocytosis X, 236–237
    mastoiditis and otitis media, 237–238
    nonadult archeological material, 236–237
Lead poisoning, 271
Legg–Calvé–Perthes disease, 252–256
Leprogenic odontodysplasia (LOD), 167–168
Leprosy
    bacilli, 164
    children, pathogenesis in, 166
    chronic granulomatous infectious disease, 164
    hyperendemic areas, 164
    infantile leprosy, 164–166
    leprous spots, 165–166
    nerve damage, 167
    paleopathology, 171–172
    primary and secondary lesions, 164, 165t
    respiratory tract, 164
    skeletal lesions of, 164
    skeletal manifestation
        dentition, 167–169
        hands and feet, 169–170
        periostitis and osteomyelitis, 170
        rhinomaxillary syndrome, 167, 168f
Léri–Weill dyschondrosteosis (LWD), 48
Lethal forms, 48, 60–61
Leukemia
    acute lymphoblastic leukemia, 206
    archeological case of, 207
    critical feature of, 206–207
    endosteal and intracortical bone resorption, 207
    fibula, 207
    metaphyseal bands of, 273
    metaphysic, 206
    osteolytic lesions, 207
    types of, 206
Localized periodontal disease, 78

M

Malaria, 198–199
Malformation, 18
Malignant primary tumors
    chordoma, 241
    Ewing's sarcoma, 241
    non-Hodgkin's lymphoma, 242
    osteosarcoma (osteogenic sarcoma), 240, 241f
Malnutrition, 7
Mastoiditis, 141, 141f
Mental retardation, 61
Mesoderm, 3
Mesomelic dysplasias, 48
Metabolic disorders
    infantile scurvy (vitamin C deficiency)
        breast milk, 213–214
        cereals, 213–214
        comorbidity and cooccurrence, 218
        differential diagnoses, 216–217
        histological techniques, 214–215
        macroscopic and radiological features, 216, 217t
        Möller–Barlow disease, 214–215
        postcranial lesions, 215–216
        prevalence rates, 217–218
        radiographs, 216, 216f
        ribs, 215–216
        scorbutic infants, 214
        subperiosteal hemorrhage, 214
        Trümmerfeld zone, 216
        type 1 collagen forms, 213–214
    nutrition and infection, 209
    rickets and osteomalacia (vitamin D deficiency), 209–213
        anterior-lateral concavity, 212
        bowing deformities, 212, 212f
        clinical changes, 212–213
        cupping deformities, 212
        dental enamel defects, 211–212
        environmental pollution, 212–213
        kidney malformation, 209–210
        normal physeal development, 211
        nutritional rickets, 211
        plump bones, 212
        premature babies, 209
        skeletal abnormalities, 210–211
        swaddling, impact of, 212–213
Metaphyseal (physeal) fractures, 92, 94–96
Metaphyseal dysplasia, 52–53
Microcephaly, 26
Moon's molars, 179–180
Mulberry molars, 179–180, 181f
Muscular dystrophy (MD), 276, 278

N

Neoplastic disease, 225
Neural tube defects
    anencephaly, 35–37
    cleft palate, 37–39
    congenital herniation (dystrophism), 34–35
    spina bifida, 39–40
Neurofibromatosis, 260
Neuro-osseous growth, 7
Non-Hodgkin's lymphoma, 242
Nonossifying fibroma, 235, 236f
Nursing bottle caries, 69–70

O

Occipital bone, 61
Oligoarticular arthritis, 249
Ollier's disease, 232–233
Osteitis, 133–134
Osteoblastoma (codman's tumor), 230, 230f
Osteochondroma, 231–232, 232f–233f
Osteochondroses, 252–254
Osteofibrous dysplasia, 235–236
Osteogenesis imperfecta, 60–61, 63f
Osteoid osteoma, 230, 230f
Osteomyelitis
    acute and chronic, 134–135
    animal bites, 134
    Brodie's abscess, 136–137
    epiphysis and metaphysic, 135
    infantile osteomyelitis, 136
    lytic lesions, 136
    nonpyogenic, 134–135
    overgrowth, 134–135
    pathogens, 134
    phyogenic osteomyelitis, 134–135
    profuse involucrum formation, 134–135
    spinal osteomyelitis, 137
Osteopathia striata, 274
Osteopetrosis (osteosclerosis fragilis), 61
Osteosarcoma (osteogenic sarcoma), 240, 241f
Otitis media and mastoiditis, 140–141

P

Paget's disease, 269
Parathyroid hormones (PTHs), 259
Pediatric bone, 2–3, 12
    influences, 92
Periapical cavitation, 77
Periodontal disease (periodontitis), 77–78
Phossy jaw, 269–270, 270f
Physeal fractures
    chondral fractures, 95–96
    cupping, 95–96
    necrosis, 95–96
    salter–harris fractures, 94–95
Physiological stress, 8–9
Pituitary gigantism, 259
Plasmodium falciparum, 198–199
Plastic deformation
    interosseous membrane, 93
    mediolateral/anteroposterior, 93
    radius, 102
    ulna, 102
Poliomyelitis
    bulbar–spinal polio, 153–154
    limb shortening, 155
    polio paralysis, extent and severity of, 153–154
    scoliosis, 154
    spinal paralysis, 154
    Talipes cavus, 154
Polydactyly, 34
Porotic hyperostosis, 194
Pott's disease, 137
Primordial cysts, 77
Pyle's disease, 52–53

R

Radioulnar synostosis, 33–34
Rasmussen's encephalitis, 277
Recklinghausen's disease, 260
Reiter's syndrome, 249
Rhinomaxillary syndrome (RMS), 167, 168f
Rib fractures, 108
Rubella, 152–153, 154f

S

Scaphocephaly, 22
Scheuermann's disease (juvenile kyphosis, spinal osteochondrosis), 1–2, 256–258, 257f–258f
Schmorl's nodes, 252, 254f
Scurvy (vitamin C deficiency), 1–2, 92–93
Septic arthritis, 136
Seronegative idiopathic arthritis, 248–249
Sickle cell anemia
   genetic abnormality, 204
   hair-on-end skull changes, 204–205
   hemoglobin S, gene for, 203–204
   low hemoglobin levels, 204
   marrow infarction, 204–205
   punched-out lesions, 204–205
Skeletal dysplasias
   achondroplasia, 46–48
      dental developmental delay, 47–48
      physical appearance of, 46–47
      skeletal features, 47
   acromesomelia, 48
   DDH and congenital hip dislocation, 49–52
   dwarfism, 46
   fibrous dysplasia, 53
   mesomelia, 48
   metaphyseal dysplasia, 52–53
   thanatophoric dwarfism
      pelvis, 48–49
      shortened iliac bones, 48
      type 1 or 2, 48
      upper limb bones, 48–49
Skinner's teeth, 85–86
Smallpox (osteomyelitis variolosa)
   ankylosis, 151
   osteomyelitis variolosa, elbow in, 152f
   symptoms of, 151
   variola major, 151
   variola minor, 151
   virulent strain, 152
Spina bifida
   spina bifida cystic, 39–40
   spina bifida occulta, 39–40
Spinal injuries
   adult injuries, 105
   cervical fractures, 105
   Clay-Shoveler's fractures, 107
   multiple fractures, 104–105
   spondylolysis and spondylolisthesis, 106–107
   tetanus, 106
Spinal osteomyelitis, 137
Spine
   cervical spine, 29
   cleft neural arches, 31–32, 32f
   congenital kyphosis, 29
   congenital lordosis, 29
   congenital scoliosis, 29
   lumbarization and sacralization, 30, 31f
   occipitalization (atlantooccipital fusion), 29–30, 30f
   sagittal clefting, 30–31, 32f
   spondylolysis, 30
Staphylococcus albus, 133–134
Staphylococcus aureus, 133–134
Streptococcus mutans, 68–69
Subperiosteal new bone formation
   blood vessels, repair of, 131–132
   diagnosis of, 132
   lamellar bone, 131–132
   microscopic features, 132
   physiological periostitis, 132, 132f
Symphalangism, 34
Syndactyly, 34

T

Talipes equinovarus (clubfoot), 33
Talon cusps, 83
Tartar. *See* Calculus
Thalassemia
   cranial changes, 200
   facial changes, 200
   gene mutations, 200
   genetic transmission, types of, 200
   pathological fractures, 200–201
   postcranial bones, 201–203
   premature epiphyseal fusion, 201
   red blood cells, 200
   skeletal expression, 200–201
   symptoms, 200
β-Thalassemia major (T-major), 200
Thanatophoric dwarfism
   pelvis, 48–49
   shortened iliac bones, 48
   type 1 or 2, 48
   upper limb bones, 48–49
Thorax, 115
   bifid ribs, 33
   costal fusion, 33
   supernumerary ribs, 32
Thyroxin, 260
Torticollis, 23
Torus fractures. *See* Buckle fractures
Trauma
   age-related injuries
      birth trauma, 108–109
      Erb's and Klumph's palsy (congenital brachial palsy), 109–110
      JOCD, 110–111
      slipped femoral epiphysis, 111–112
      toddler's fractures, 110
   angulation, 102
   autopsies and surgical intervention, 115–117
   biological and social development, 92
   burns, 114
   callus, 91–92, 101
   caveats, 91–92
   child trauma, study of
      activity-induced injuries, 121–122
      caregiver-induced violence and neglect, 119–121
      culturally sanctioned ritual violence, 118–119
      extreme cultural conflict, violence associated with, 117–118
      structural violence, 122–123
   cortical striations, 102
   cranial fractures
      archeological contexts, 103
      mandible, fractures of, 103–104
      ping-pong injury, 102–103
   dental trauma
      dental modification, 84
      maxillary incisors, 83–84
   dislocations
      glenohumeral junction/upper limb, 112
      hip dislocations/lower limb, 112–114
      pelvic fractures, 112–114
      shoulder dislocations, 112
   fragment overlap, 97
   healing
      features and time since death, 98, 99t
      fracture healing, 98, 99t
      humerus tuberosity, 98
      terminal phalanges, 98
      tibial malleolus, 98
   long bone fractures, 96
   myositis ossificans traumatica (heterotrophic ossification), 114
   overgrowth, 97–98
   pediatrics trauma, principles of
      greenstick fractures, 92–93
      metaphyseal (physeal) fractures, 92, 94–96
      pediatric bone influences, 92
      plastic deformation, 92–93
      torus/buckle fractures, 92, 94
   postcranial injuries, 100–102, 100t
   premature fusion, 96–97
   rib fractures, 108
   spinal injuries
      adult injuries, 105
      cervical fractures, 105
      Clay-Shoveler's fractures, 107
      multiple fractures, 104–105
Trauma (*Continued*)
      spondylolysis and spondylolisthesis, 106–107
      tetanus, 106
      thoracic and lumbar vertebra, 105
      vertebral fractures, 104–105
   trauma patterns, 92
Trephination, 115–117
Treponema pallidum, 172
Treponemal diseases
   clinically different conditions, 172
   congenital syphilis
      clinical manifestations of, 177, 177t
      dentition, 179–182
      early onset, 178–179
      late onset, 179
      sexual maturity and pregnancy, 176–177
   endemic syphilis (bejel, treponarid), 176
   etiology, 172
   paleopathology, 182–185
   pre-Columbian hypothesis, 172
   transmission, mode of, 172
   yaws, 175
Triiodothyronine, 260
Tuberculosis (TB)
   cranium, 156–157
   gastrointestinal TB, 156
   hands and feet, 162

Tuberculosis (TB) (*Continued*)
  joints, 160–161
  long bones, 161–162
  mandible, 158
  miliary, 155
  paleopathology
    biomolecular analysis, 163–164
    cow's milk, 162
    endocranial lesions, 163–164
    Pott's disease, 162
  pregnant women, 155–156
  primary, 155
  ribs, 160
  scapula, 158
  secondary, 155
  spine
    coccidioidomycosis, 159–160
    lytic lesions, 159–160, 159f
    Pott's disease, 158
    recovery, 159
    Scheuermann's kyphosis, 159–160
    secondary neural arch, 159
    segmentary arteries, 158
Tumors
  benign primary tumors
    chrondroblastoma, 234, 234f
    chrondromas and Ollier's disease, 232–233
    chrondromyxoid fibroma, 234
    desmoid fibroma (desmoplastic fibroma), 234
    fibrous cortical defects, 234–235, 235f
    giant-cell tumor (osteoclastoma), 231, 231f
    hereditary multiple osteochondromas (HMO), 232, 233f
    nonossifying fibroma, 235, 236f
    osteoblastoma (codman's tumor), 230, 230f
    osteochondroma, 231–232, 232f–233f
    osteofibrous dysplasia, 235–236
    osteoid osteoma, 230, 230f
  bone cysts
    aneurismal bone cyst, 236, 237f
    unicameral (solitary) bone cyst, 236, 237f
  bone tumors, 228–229, 228f
  clinical practice, 228–229
  dense sclerotic margin, 229
  geographical distribution, 226
  histology, 228–229
  Langerhans cell histiocytosis (LCH)
    eosinophilic granuloma, 238
    histiocytosis X, 236–237
    mastoiditis and otitis media, 237–238
    nonadult archaeological material, 236–237
  lesions and terminology, classification of, 226, 227t
  malignant primary tumors
    chordoma, 241
    Ewing's sarcoma, 241
    non-Hodgkin's lymphoma, 242
    osteosarcoma (osteogenic sarcoma), 240, 241f
  new bone formation, 228–229
Turner's teeth, 85–86

U
Unicameral (solitary) bone cyst, 236, 237f

V
Vertebral neural canal (VNC), 7
Vitamin B_{12} deficiency, 199
Vitamin C (ascorbic acid), 213–214

W
Wimberger's sign, 178, 178f
Woven/immature bone, 4–5

Printed in the United States
By Bookmasters